Nursing Case Management

From Essentials to Advanced Practice Applications

Nursing
Case
Management
From Essentials to Advanced
Practice Applications

ELAINE L. COHEN, EdD, RN, FAAN
Director of Case Management
Utilization Management, Department of Quality & Outcomes
Associate Professor, School of Nursing
University of Colorado Hospital
University of Colorado
Health Sciences Center
Denver, Colorado

TONI G. CESTA, PhD, RN, FAAN
Vice President
Patient Flow Optimization
North Shore—Long Island Jewish Health System
Great Neck, New York

FOURTH EDITION

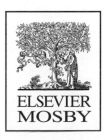

ELSEVIER
MOSBY

ELSEVIER
MOSBY

11830 Westline Industrial Drive
St. Louis, Missouri 63146

First Edition 1993. Second Edition 1997. Third Edition 2001.

ISBN-13: 978-0-323-02765-6
ISBN-10: 0-323-02765-2

Executive Vice President, Nursing & Health Professions: *Sally Schrefer*
Senior Editor: *Yvonne Alexopoulos*
Developmental Editor: *Danielle M. Frazier*
Publishing Services Manager: *Catherine Albright Jackson*
Senior Project Manager: *Mary Stueck*
Book Design Manager: *Gail Morey Hudson*

Printed in the United States of America

Last digit is the print number: 9   8   7

To all the pioneers and their efforts
in the development, research, and evaluation of
nursing case management

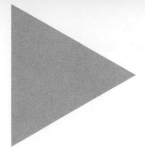

Contributors

SHERRY L. ALIOTTA, RN, BSN, CCM
President
S.A. Squared, Inc.
Farmington Hills, Michigan

AMY J. BARTON, PhD, RN
Associate Dean for Clinical Affairs
Assistant Professor, School of Nursing
University of Colorado Health Sciences Center
Denver, Colorado

ARTHUR E. BLANK, PhD
Assistant Professor, Director
Center for the Evaluation of
    Health Programs
Department of Family and Social Medicine
Albert Einstein College of Medicine
Bronx, New York

JEANNE BOLING, MSN, CRRN, CDMS, CCM
Executive Director
Case Management Society of America
Little Rock, Arkansas

KATHLEEN A. BOWER, DNSc, RN, FAAN
Principal and Co-Owner
The Center for Case Management
South Natick, Massachusetts

MICHAL BOYD, RN, ND, NP, FCNA (NZ)
Senior Lecturer, School of Nursing
Auckland University of Technology
Nurse Practitioner, Aged Care
Waitemata District Health Board
Auckland, New Zealand

VICKI J. BROWNRIGG, RN, FNP, PhDc
Director of Nursing Programs
Department of Nursing
Trinidad State Junior College
Trinidad, Colorado

REBECCA F. CADY, RNC, BSN, JD
Editor in Chief
JONA's Healthcare Law, Ethics and Regulation
Middletown, Rhode Island

MARY ALLEN CAREY, PhD, RN, CS
Professor, Assistant Dean for Curriculum &
    Instruction
College of Nursing, University of Oklahoma
Oklahoma City, Oklahoma

ELIZABETH FALTER, RN, MS, CNAA, BC
President, Falter & Associates, Inc.
Adjunct Clinical Associate Professor
University of Arizona
Adjunct Professor
Georgetown University Center for Professional
    Development
Tucson, Arizona

TINA GERARDI, MS, RN, CAE
Deputy Executive Director
New York State Nurses Association
Latham, New York

MARY LU GERKE, BSN, MSN, MA
Vice President, Operations
Gundersen Lutheran Medical Center
LaCrosse, Wisconsin

COLLEEN J. GOODE, RN, PhD, FAAN
Vice President, Patient Services and CNO
University of Colorado Hospital
Denver, Colorado

EVELYN KOENIG, MSW, ACSW
Manager, Oncology Case Management
Grady Health System
Atlanta, Georgia

GERRI S. LAMB, PhD, RN, FAAN
Associate Dean, Clinical and Community Services
Associate Professor, College of Nursing
University of Arizona
Tucson, Arizona

CARRIE B. LENBURG, RN, EdD, FAAN
President and Consultant
Creative Learning and Assessment Systems
    (CLAS, Inc.)
Roan Mountain, Tennessee

PATRICIA HRYZAK LIND, RN, MS
Associate Director, Patient/Nursing Services
Department of Veterans Affairs
VA Healthcare Center Upstate New York:
Canandaigua, New York

MARGO MacROBERT, RN, MS, CNAA
Director, Case Management
College of Nursing, University of Oklahoma
Oklahoma City, Oklahoma

MARY B. McCARTHY, BSN, RN
Student, Master of Science Program
Women's Health Nurse Practitioner Program
School of Nursing
University of Colorado Health Sciences Center
Denver, Colorado

CATHY MICHAELS, PhD, RN, FAAN
Assistant Professor, College of Nursing
University of Arizona
Tucson, Arizona

PATRICIA MORITZ, PhD, RN, FAAN
Dean and Professor, School of Nursing
University of Colorado Health Sciences Center
Denver, Colorado

KATHRYN NOLD, MSHA, BSN, RN
Manager, Quality and Outcomes
University of Colorado Hospital
Denver, Colorado

RUTH A. O'BRIEN, PhD, RN
Associate Professor, School of Nursing
University of Colorado Health Sciences Center
Denver, Colorado

THERESA J. ORTIZ, MSW, ACSW, LCSW
Manager, Social Services
University of Colorado Hospital
Denver, Colorado

BARI K. PLATTER, RN, MS, CNS
Clinical Nurse Specialist/Educator
Psychiatric Services
University of Colorado Hospital
Denver, Colorado

GAYLE PREHEIM, EdD, RN, CNAA, BC
Associate Professor, School of Nursing
University of Colorado Health Sciences Center
Denver, Colorado

RICHARD W. REDMAN, PhD, RN
Associate Dean, Academic Affairs
Professor, School of Nursing
The University of North Carolina at Chapel Hill
Chapel Hill, North Carolina

LYNN RIIPPI, BSN, RN
Health Plan Case Manager
University of Colorado Hospital
Denver, Colorado

JILL SCOTT, PhD, RN
Associate Director for Nursing, AHEC
Assistant Professor, School of Nursing
University of Colorado Health Sciences Center
Denver, Colorado

MARLYS SEVERSON, RN, BSN, CCM
President, SCM Associates, Inc.
Bellflower, California

DIANE J. SKIBA, PhD, FAAN, FACMI
Associate Professor, School of Nursing
University of Colorado Health Sciences Center
Denver, Colorado

ROY L. SIMPSON, RN, C, CMAC, FNAP, FAAN
Vice President, Nursing Informatics
Cerner Corporation
Kansas City, Missouri

KATHLEEN SMITH, RN, MS
Informatics Nurse Specialist
University of Colorado Hospital
Denver, Colorado

VIVIENNE SMITH, RN, BSN
Informatics Nurse Specialist
University of Colorado Hospital
Denver, Colorado

LENA SORENSEN, PhD, RN
Associate Professor, School of Nursing
University of Colorado Health Sciences Center
Denver, Colorado

HUSSEIN A. TAHAN, DNSc, RN, CNA
Director of Nursing
Cardiovascular Services
Columbia University Medical Center
New York Presbyterian Hospital
New York, New York

SISTER CAROL TAYLOR, CSFN, PhD, MSN, RN
Director, Center for Clinical Bioethics
Assistant Professor
School of Nursing and Health Studies
Georgetown University, Washington, D.C.

MARY CRABTREE TONGES, RN, PhD, FAAN
Senior Vice President, Chief Nursing Officer
University of North Carolina Hospitals
Chapel Hill, North Carolina

KAY VAUGHN, RN, MS, CS
Adjunct Professor, Regis University
Adjunct Professor
University of Colorado Health Sciences Center
School of Medicine
Denver, Colorado

CAROLEE SHERER WHITEHILL, RN, MS
Clinical Case Manager, Case Management
University of Colorado Hospital
Denver, Colorado

JOANNE WOODALL, MSN, ANP, RN, CM
Director, Case Management
TMC Healthcare
Tucson, Arizona

BONNIE COX YOUNG, RN, MS
Senior Director, Psychiatric Services
University of Colorado Hospital
Denver, Colorado

DONNA ZAZWORSKY, MS, RN, CCM, FAAN
Director, Community Nursing and Outreach
St. Elizabeth of Hungary Clinic
Managing Partner, Case Manager Solutions, LLC
Tucson, Arizona

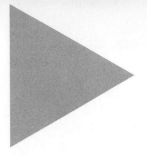

Foreword

Since the late 1980s, nursing case management has been found in the professional literature. The concept has been described in detail, outcomes have been researched, and environments where nurse case managers are successfully serving families and communities have been described. Books and articles on nursing case management have noted how this structure and methodology for delivering care has expanded from its origins to every conceivable area where individuals are in need of health care. Clearly, nursing case management has withstood the test of time and is here to stay. This is not to say that either the concept or the practice is entrenched, static, or unchangeable. Where human beings are involved, change is inevitable. New ideas, new information, new providers, new partners—all have an impact on the application of nursing case management principles.

Given the expectation of change and evolution, it follows that books on the subject of nursing case management need updating, expanding, and clarification of previous work. Thus, there is a need for a fourth edition of *Nursing Case Management: From Essentials to Advanced Practice Applications*, by Elaine Cohen and Toni Cesta.

One of the expansion areas found here is in the area of technology. The rapid change in the technological tools available and an increase in the use of technology drives the need to discuss how such changes affect the way nurses work as well as the impact on client outcomes. The application of distance technology places an additional burden on the nurse case manager to use all means available to obtain a true health picture of the clients being served. Although there are cautions that nurses must learn to successfully implement the concept of telehealth, Chapter 35 describes the benefits to both families and health care providers. Ease of contact with a nurse case manager and potential reduction of costs for minor or easily resolved health care issues are two of the benefits of such technology. Of course in the updating process, technology is found interwoven throughout the book and emerges as one of this edition's major themes. Chapters that have been enhanced in the area of technology have added the latest use as well as problems encountered and successes achieved.

This edition brings new information to nurses who are interested in keeping up with changes in practice, changes in expected outcomes, and technological advances.

As it has in the past, the new edition of this book will continue to be a valuable resource to many audiences. Nurse practitioners will find it useful to read about the issues confronting the profession and a validation of their own experiences. It is also a source of information that can revitalize the reader who is practicing in the cost-conscious environments described here.

Nurse case managers, in particular, will value the comments and stories of their colleagues as they develop care systems that respond to today's client needs and the pressures of a constantly changing health care system.

Educators will find this book helpful for senior level students and/or in the graduate level curriculum. The structure of the book is designed to stimulate thinking, discussion, and analysis of health care issues.

Elaine Cohen and Toni Cesta have again sought out thinkers, researchers, and practice experts so that they can present, in one resource, the most up-to-date information on the subject of nursing case management. With each edition, they advance the work of nurses, the concept of nursing case management, and as a result, assured positive outcomes for the people served. This is, after all, the central purpose of nursing.

Vivien De Back, RN, PhD, FAAN
Professor (Retired)

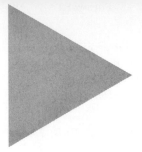

Preface

Our first edition was a comprehensive text to explore nursing case management and promote the development of a critical mass of information around this model of care delivery. It spoke to the diversity and challenges we faced in professional practice settings.

This book has since grown into a "classic" resource, establishing a foundation and springboard for other work in nursing case management to evolve. Building upon this heritage, the intention of the fourth edition is to enhance and advance the knowledge base and stay ahead of the continuing evolution of case management.

Since our book is used as a basic text on the subject of nursing case management and managed care, it requires a framework that includes both a historical perspective and new concepts common to health care today. With over 10 years of publication behind us, we have attempted to present what occurred with nursing case management and how it continues to change professional practice.

Faced with the realities of a dynamic health care market, we recognized the value of other disciplines and collaboration in the process and management of integrated care. In nursing case management we discovered that it was more effective when all the people involved in providing care were part of the case management approach. That is the beauty of an integrated and collaborative team—responsibility is shared.

We have honored that past by holding on to the historic pieces—however, they are set in the context of the twenty-first century. We have moved beyond the critical mass and continue to take a fresh look at case management approaches to the delivery of care. To tap the depth of the full understanding of this model and provide information regarding best practices in case management, one needs to be the vehicle for the expression of others' views, perspectives, and ideas: thus the many contributors to this book.

Since nursing case management continues to prove itself as a successful and practical model and is played out in multiple ways and in different contexts, its usefulness and effectiveness has been strongly validated in multiple arenas. Case management is practiced nation-wide. Its global impact is also impressive, with numerous examples evident in international health care settings. This edition engages the diverse and dynamic facets of contemporary practice in nursing case management. It reflects a less dated and more system focused approach which makes this text a "lived" document.

With the globalization of every element of our lives, professionals and consumers alike benefit from the cooperation received from partnering. General concepts of partnerships are explored as we describe how case managers partner with other disciplines and groups. As we witness the emergence of collaborative models in health care, we see how new generations of nursing case management exemplify care of individuals and communities, begin to address population-based services, and respond to increased consumerism in health care. In a health care environment where all social, political, economic, and cultural issues intersect, we realize how an understanding of public policy enhances the practice of the case manager.

With numerous changes in health care taking center stage in practice settings, this edition affords the opportunity to view the impact of public policy on health care delivery. It encourages nurse case managers to act on behalf of their clients, families, and communities. The implementation of new case management models addresses the importance of educational requirements, promotion of practice competencies, and role definition for the full development of future nurse case managers.

We now reside in a data-driven health care environment and methods for gathering, evaluating, and presenting relevant data about care systems is paramount. The evaluation component of case management that focuses on clinical, financial, utilization, and quality elements and its applicability to the day-to-day practice of the case manager is covered in this edition. This book expands on the importance of evaluating the outcomes of care and how collecting data can provide an infrastructure on which to base future decisions. Issues such as outcomes effectiveness data and the influence of evidenced-based practice are presented. Understanding the effects of health care reimbursement and its application at the patient level, telehealth, throughput and capacity management, the impact of the revenue cycle, compliance and regulatory issues, and principles needed to effect successful change and increase the sophistication of case manager client interaction, are covered extensively.

In looking back at our rich past, we realized that our books on nursing case management incorporate a broader scope of coverage and are written to complement other texts on this subject. We have been able to set the underpinning and foundation of case management practice by offering practical application to the theory presented as well as how case management is changing to meet the dynamic challenges of our health care settings. Our book is for leaders of nursing case management.

There is a purposeful ebb and flow in the fourth edition as we attempt to capture the depth and breadth of contemporary practice and strike a balance between former approaches to nursing case management and their newer examples. Some foundational models are no longer in their original form. They have transitioned and by doing so offer lessons in the evolution of practice. Several pioneers of these models continue to share their expertise and by doing so seed further knowledge and innovation toward advancing nursing case management and create greater value for our health care systems. Most importantly, the innovators of these models gave us a wonderful future to behold. It is in this spirit that we offer our current edition.

ACKNOWLEDGEMENTS

In this fourth edition we wish to formally acknowledge our many readers for making this book a success. We are thankful and humbled by the many insights you impart. To our numerous contributors, sincere thanks for sharing your expertise and wisdom. Your diversity of opinion and powerful reflection speaks to the future of health care. To our reviewers, your perspectives helped frame the context of this edition. We are deeply grateful to Dr. Vivien DeBack for her perceptive foreword and her staying in touch with professional practice. Your generosity of time and sage advice is extremely appreciated. We are indebted to Yvonne Alexopoulos, Julie Nebel, Danielle Frazier, and the entire staff of Nursing Editorial for their expert assistance. Their caring manner, commitment to quality publications, and professionalism is outstanding. Heartfelt thanks to our families and friends for your graciousness, indomitable spirits, and loving support.

Elaine L. Cohen and **Toni G. Cesta**

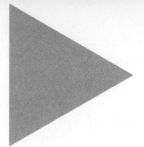

Contents

UNIT VII
IMPLEMENTATION: TAKING A SYSTEMS PROCESS APPROACH

UNIT VIII
**EVALUATION, OUTCOMES MEASUREMENT, AND RESEARCH: IMPORTANT
COMPONENTS OF DECISION MAKING**

I

EVOLUTION OF CASE MANAGEMENT

Health care delivery in the twenty-first century holds great promise and formidable challenges for nursing case management. The complex variations in the practice of nursing case management and its integration into the business of health care are the focus of this unit. Understanding the development of case management is critical to evaluating how it is evolving to meet the needs of the future. Although many of its historical manifestations hold true to present-day practice, nursing case management remains challenged by the multitude of issues posed by a transforming health care system, nurses' individual health care settings, and professional practice. Its strength, however, resides in the ability to mature in concert with the changing health care marketplace.

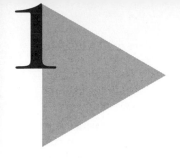

Evolution of Nursing Case Management in a Changing Health Care System

CHAPTER OVERVIEW

Many dramatic changes in the practice and delivery of health services have contributed to the new realities and complexities of the current health care system. This chapter discusses how the changing health care system and emerging issues have shaped current nursing case management practices, as well as identifying opportunities for innovation and providing an overview of the trends that have led to the development of the nursing case management approach in the delivery of patient care.

This section also discusses the reasons for the success of the nursing case management model in increasing cost-effectiveness, quality of care, and job satisfaction. Included in this discussion are nurse-physician collaborative practice, management of the patient's environment by coordinating and monitoring the appropriate use of patient care resources, monitoring of the patient's length of stay and patient-outcome standards to produce measurements for evaluating cost-effectiveness, and enhanced autonomy and increased decision-making by direct health care providers.

Nursing case management offers the nursing profession an opportunity to define its role in the health care industry and challenges the profession to identify the work that nurses do in terms of its autonomous value to the patient.

DYNAMICS OF THE CARE CLIMATE

The 1990s marked a decade of major transition in health care as the system shifted from traditional fragmented approaches of health service delivery to greater integration and control brought on by managed care. However, as the 1990s receded and gave way to the 21st century, many of the same issues of access, cost containment, and quality persist. Why these challenges continue is evident by the following:

- Diminished access to health care services for the uninsured population
- Rationed and multitiered distribution of health services
- Mixing of government pricing regulation and market-based competition, resulting in fragmented and cumbersome cost-control initiatives
- Increased control mechanisms for continuous quality improvement and compliance
- Greater demand for concrete, documented information on measurable outcomes at the individual and community levels
- Rising ethical concerns and legal liability resulting in the practice of defensive medicine

- Shifting in the delivery of services from acute care settings to more inclusive services across the health/illness continuum
- Lack of consensus and definition of what constitutes health and the impact of socioeconomic, environment, and public health etiologies on the delivery of cost-effective, quality health care (Cohen & De Back, 1999; De Back & Cohen, 1996; Kindig, 1999; Shi & Singh, 1998)

As noted, health care in the 20th century was marked as disease-focused, fragmented, inaccessible, and costly. The first decade of the 21st century is expected to exhibit similar characteristics; however, the need to respond efficiently to varying levels of change in the present health delivery system hallmarks the need for (1) increased emphasis on disease prevention and health promotion, both for cost savings to the system and for quality-of-life benefits to consumers; (2) active engagement of consumers in health care decision-making; (3) development of health care partnerships between medical centers and corporate and business entities to deliver the most economical health care for enrolled and prepaid populations—including the development of treatment protocols, standardizing care, and promoting health care reform; (4) utilization of health-outcome data as justification for spending health care dollars; (5) significant expansion of primary care in ambulatory and community-based settings; and (6) sweeping changes in the education and practice of health professionals to staff these emerging primary care systems (Grayson, 2002; Sheehy & McCarthy 1998).

Archetypal Changes

Major paradigm shifts that have unfolded in the decade of the 1990s underpin the current practice of health care professionals. These changes represent the focus and direction that the leadership in nursing case management will be taking for delivery of health care services well into this century.

REVISITING PRIMARY HEALTH CARE

These new paradigms converge to offer health, wellness, and care rather than exclusively focusing on illness and cure. To reduce costs and ensure access, the new environment for health care supports primary care–based health care interventions on the community level, the hallmark of which emphasizes an integrated approach to continuous and seamless health care delivery across an individual's lifetime (De Back & Cohen, 1996). Primary care is population based and wellness care focused and demands a shift in the commitment of health care professionals to safeguard the population's and society's health and well-being (Campbell, 1997; Issel & Anderson, 1996; Taylor & Barnet, 1999). As the emphasis of care shifts toward wellness and prevention, nonmedical determinants such as socioeconomic status, lack of housing, inadequate nutrition, family violence, and public health will play a greater role in contributing to population health outcomes (Issel & Anderson, 1996; Kindig, 1999).

Reimbursement in a primary care–based wellness-focused system will embrace new criteria for payment as health promotion strategies, surveillance, health maintenance, and care activities take the forefront. Present fee-for-service arrangements will be outpaced by population-based capitation, contractual arrangements for group services, and other innovative financial models (De Back & Cohen, 1996). Kindig (1999) proposes a realignment of financial incentives that is based on an aggregate measure of health for large populations or health plans that could be used for the maintenance and improvement of the health of populations. The measurement of health status proposed by Kindig (1997) must incorporate both quantity (i.e., mortality) and quality of life.

The technological challenges in providing population-based care are numerous; as outlined by Adkins and Morgan (1995), they include defining "*community*" within a statistical and epidemiological perspective, establishing data collection methods and aggregation of information, developing information in the most meaningful and accessible format, and determining the efficacy of treatment and care outcomes. These authors refer to the integration of communication, computing, and content processes as an "infocosm" similar to what is commonly defined as the information superhighway. This technology medium will enhance the management of data for population-focused care by linking knowledge management (communication capability), ensuring public data access (transcending from individual care record to community plans), accessing virtual information to determine population-based care protocols, and processing a large volume of data to meet the needs of an expanded customer infrastructure (Adkins & Morgan, 1995).

One key to a well-developed, coordinated system of health care involves partnership. The importance and power of partnering are evident in the outcomes generated by these relationships. Affiliations that facilitate the improvement of health and plan wellness and illness care to meet the needs of individuals, communities, and populations are emerging through the efforts of health care professionals involved on numerous local, regional, national, and international levels. These endeavors are not limited by geographic or system boundaries and demand involvement and integration across educational, legislative, economic, and public arenas (Cohen & De Back, 1999). Case management will have a significant role in the development of population-based health management as exemplified by the case manager's ability to provide health services for individuals, communities, special populations, institutions, and health plans, while addressing health status, quality of life, and effectiveness of health care utilization issues (Chapman, 1999).

CONSUMER STRENGTH

Additional forces are moving the traditional models of fragmented and dehumanized care to those that are comprehensive, coordinated health care networks. Basic premises that relied on exclusionary provider-based decision-making have shifted to principles that place emphasis on increased responsiveness to the health care needs of consumers and the development of collaborative partnerships with the recipients of health care.

As customers who purchase health care, consumers are much more sophisticated and savvy about their options for health care services and are demanding better communication with health care professionals (Campbell, 1998; Golodner, 1999). Several strategies, such as The Centers for Medicare & Medicaid Services' Conditions of Participation (federal regulations that ensure a hospital's compliance with certain practice criteria) and the patients' bill of rights proposed by the House and Senate, are aimed at ensuring that consumers are included in health care/treatment decision-making processes. A report titled "Eye on Patients," conducted by the American Hospital Association (1996) and the Picker Institute, demonstrated that regardless of the setting in which patients received health care (ambulatory or acute care), they claimed that they were not involved in decisions about their care to the extent that they wanted to be (21% of patients in clinics or physician offices and 36% of patients in hospitals).

Smith and Brooks (1999) advocate structure, process, and outcome targets to improve customer relations. Some of these elements include promoting the use of the Internet as a source of health care information; widespread customization of health services; minimizing cultural, environmental, and attitudinal barriers to care; cultivating ways to partner with the consumer in promoting cost-effective services; and improving consumer knowledge and personal health care abilities.

Changes in the geographical locations where health care can be and is provided have given rise to multiple service settings distinguished by the movement from acute to primary care, from inpatient to ambulatory settings, and from institution-based to integrated delivery systems. These changes have resulted in the prevailing mindset to realign and adjust itself to what Taylor and Barnet (1999) identify as the "nonnegotiables of moral health care" (Box 1-1), which one of these principles that speaks to the collaborative efforts of accepting the consumer as a partner in care. These practice elements strike at the very core of nurses' professional and moral obligations to society and demand fundamental changes in their approaches to health care delivery.

BOX 1-1   NONNEGOTIABLES OF MORAL HEALTH CARE

JUST SYSTEM OF HEALTH CARE
- Views health care as an obligation of a moral society rather than a mere business commodity
- Ensures a basic, decent minimum of care for all
- Responsive to the needs of the most vulnerable members of society
- Distributes the benefits and burdens of caregiving in a just manner

"PATIENT-FIRST" ORIENTATION
- Commits system resources and professional competencies and will to an orientation that consistently puts patients first
- Demands the subordination of self-interest to the promotion of patient well-being when patient interests are at stake

BROAD NOTION OF HEALTH THAT ENCOMPASSES MORE THAN PHYSIOLOGICAL FUNCTIONING
- Commitment to wholeness of being versus wholeness of body; to cure as *one* of the manifestations of care
- Commitment to quality of life that is multidimensional (i.e., physiological, emotional, social, and spiritual functioning) and subjective
- Range of therapeutic interventions to include more than the "technological fix," that is, compassionate presence, development of coping strategies that address problems related to life's meaning and purpose, and so on

TRUSTING PROFESSIONAL RELATIONSHIPS
Includes relationships among the health care system and the public at large; patients, families, and employees; and health care professionals and patients, families, and other health care professionals
- Grounded in the system's and the health care professional's commitment to secure the patient's and/or society's health and well-being (i.e., fidelity to fiduciary responsibilities)
- Based on a respect for human dignity, which affirms the worth of everyone with whom one interacts
- Provide the individualized knowledge that guides collaborative efforts to achieve valued health outcomes

CLINICAL COMPETENCE
- Encompassing interpersonal, intellectual, technical, and ethical competencies
- Demonstrated ability to "work the system" to achieve valued health outcomes

From Cohen, E.L., & De Back, V. (1999). *The outcomes mandate: Case management in health care today,* St. Louis: Mosby.

DIMENSIONS OF CARE SYSTEMS

Within this context, the infrastructure of nursing case management has evolved to provide care and manage services in the new care system. The intricacies of delivering health care have greatly influenced the relationships between managed care and the case management model, thereby reconfiguring the approach from managing costs to managing care. An example of this trend is illustrated in the Institute of Medicine (1996) treatise "2020 Vision: Health in the 21st Century," whereby the influx of high-risk individuals (i.e., chronically ill elderly with complex medical problems and the indigent, whose risk factors are related to socioeconomic origins) will potentially shift managed care from an episode-driven system to a risk-driven one. To increase the quality of health care and reduce costs, identifying and intervening with individuals who are at risk for high service utilization will require providers to predict and manage health risk across a full continuum (Clough, 1996). The Healthy People 2010 Program takes national health initiatives even further by attempting to improve the quality of life for all Americans. Through implementation of national benchmarking standards, Healthy People 2010 will, it is hoped, eliminate the health disparities that exist among racial, ethnic, and economic groups (Healthy People 2010, Department of Health and Human Services, January 2000). These possibilities reflect the complex variations in the practice of case management and its integration into the business of health care.

To establish accountability and guarantee value, nursing case management must embrace the panorama of health care processes and retain a broader, more global political, public, and social systems perspective. Rethinking the future processes and outcomes of nursing case management places this model in sync with evolving population-based care delivery systems. The concomitant effects of such an approach lie not just in one system in which the case manager works but rather in the variety of systems that affect the work of providers and enhance the understanding, role, and practice of the nurse case manager. Subsequent chapters focus on the interdisciplinary integration and coordination elements that are so vital to the successful evolution of case management.

As we thrive in the new millennium, some of the primary system challenges that will continue to influence the provision of health care in general and nursing case management specifically are the growth and consequences of managed care; caring for the population with long-term and chronic illnesses; attending to the uninsured; increased technology, practice, quality, and outcome issues; and consumer service and empowerment—subjects that are covered in later chapters.

PRESERVING THE PAST AND VISIONING THE FUTURE

What Is Nursing Case Management?

Understanding the development of nursing case management as a model is critical to evaluating how it is evolving to meet the needs of the future. Nursing case management, which began as a community-based model in the early 1900s and was adapted for acute care in the mid-1980s, is considered an outgrowth of primary nursing and allows for quality outcomes-focused care while containing costs. This approach to managing the delivery of health care has emerged as a professional practice model that increases nurse involvement in decisions regarding standards of practice and integrates the cost and quality components of nursing services (Zander, 1985). The historical manifestations of nursing case management hold true to present-day practice in that this model provides outcome-oriented patient care within an appropriate length of stay, uses appropriate resources based on specific case types, promotes the integration and coordination of clinical services, monitors the use of patient care resources, supports collaborative practice and continuity of care, and enhances patient and provider satisfaction (Ethridge & Lamb, 1989; Henderson & Wallack, 1987; Stetler, 1987; Zander, 1987, 1988a).

The practice of case management itself can vary from one practice setting to another, with its identifying characteristics dependent on the discipline that uses it, the personnel and staff mix that is used, and the setting in which the model is implemented. Nursing case management, however, is a collaborative approach that focuses on the coordination, integration, and direct delivery of patient services and places internal controls on the resources used for care. Such management emphasizes early assessment and intervention, comprehensive care planning, and inclusive service system referrals.

Several health care settings have adopted unique methods of monitoring patient care activity and resource distribution, such as *critical paths* (a description of patient care requirements in outline form), *case management care plans* (similar to the standard nursing care plan but adapted to nursing case management outcome standards), and *multidisciplinary action plans* (MAPs).

Nursing case management has been described as *within the walls* (WTW), which emphasizes case management activities in the acute care hospital setting, and as *beyond the walls* (BTW), which refers to case management in outpatient and community-based environments as well as health maintenance organization (HMO) arrangements (Ethridge, 1991; Ethridge & Lamb, 1989; Rogers, Riordan, & Swindle, 1991). In addition, collaborative models of case management that embrace the elements of joint decision-making responsibility and shared accountability have emerged to ensure comprehensive patient care and overall system improvement. Mergers of organizations, which have become commonplace in health care, have led to the development of integrated case management models. Case management practices have been successfully incorporated into population-based disease management models as well.

However one views it, because nursing case management balances the cost and quality components of nursing service and patient care outcomes, it has successfully evolved into a professional model that is both sensitive and responsive to current practice demands. A more detailed and differential analysis of case management models is provided in the following chapters.

Why Nursing Case Management?

Although the traditional models of nursing care delivery are appropriate for their time, their efficacy is challenged by the multitude of issues posed by the evolving health care system, nurses' individual health care settings, and professional practice. Prospective payment, which is now considered the economic driver across acute, community, and long-term care settings; continuous cutbacks in Medicare reimbursements, along with numerous shifts in the configurations of managed care; and demographic changes in work force composition have compelled providers of health care services to engage in the restructuring and innovative rethinking of priorities related to the delivery and management of patient care. The focus on different approaches to care delivery has prompted those in health service settings to look at alternative delivery systems as a means of improving patient outcomes and controlling costs.

Restructured Reimbursement

In an era of managed care and government cutbacks, current health care financing and reimbursement methodologies present a dizzying array of options and alternatives. In its most simplistic form, the concept of managed care within the acute care setting has evolved as an approach by which the directives on patient care are determined by predicted patterns of resource use. The managed care system places emphasis on managing the patient's environment by coordinating and monitoring the appropriate use of resources and is an integral component of the nursing case management model (Cohen, 1991). This model seeks to increase accountability for nursing practice and to reduce costs and fragmentation associated with patient care by establishing a mechanism for the regulation and integration of services over the course of an individual's illness (Henderson & Wallack, 1987; Zander, 1988a). Through the coordination of such processes as utilization review/utilization management (the evaluation of medical necessity, appropriateness of level of care, efficiency, and quality of health care services) and discharge planning (evaluation of the patient's care needs early in the admission process that ensures appropriate support services and/or placement along the continuum), optimum patient outcomes can be achieved.

Chapter 20, *The Managed Care Market: Nurse Case Management as a Strategy for Success,* examines case management in the context of the current health care market, expresses the nurse case manager's role within the managed care environment, and discusses new opportunities that managed care has generated for nurses.

Assessment criteria related to hospital-based nursing case management must be able to assess quality while monitoring and evaluating the outcomes of professional practice. The method used demands the following from the provider:

- Independent assessment and adjustment to variations in patients' needs as defined in terms of patient diagnosis, severity level, and spiritual, emotional, and family concerns
- Identification and utilization of appropriate health care resources
- Comprehensive monitoring of patient discharge programs to ensure continuous access to care (Ethridge & Lamb, 1989; Zander, 1988b).

The basic principles used in case management have universal application and are widely used by insurers to control escalating health care costs. These principles are also used by providers in acute care settings who continue to contain inpatient expenditures and provide quality patient care (McIntosh, 1987; Ricklefs, 1987; Health Care Advisory Board, 2002).

The findings of research studies indicate that the changes in inpatient nursing practice patterns associated with nursing case management have helped reduce costs related to the hospitalization of defined groups of patients within certain diagnosis-related group (DRG) categories (Cohen, 1991; Ethridge & Lamb, 1989; Zander, 1988b). These changes have promoted cost-effectiveness, expedited care delivery, maintained nurses' professional autonomy, enhanced collaborative nurse–physician relationships, improved care provider satisfaction, and are instrumental in enhanced hospital capacity management and patient throughput. In addition, the professional standards and quality indicators promoted by the American Nurses Credentialing Center (ANCC) Magnet Recognition Program have forwarded the benefits of nursing case management in facilitating continuity of care across a continuum and achieving interdisciplinary team success when addressing clinical and business decisions within health care organizations (ANCC, 2000; Cohen, 1991; Ethridge & Lamb, 1989; Health Care Advisory Board, 2002; Olivas et al., 1989a; 1989b; Zander, 1988c). See Chapter 46 for additional evidence of the utility of nursing case management.

CURRENT ISSUES IN NURSING CASE MANAGEMENT

Nursing case management continues to evolve in concert with the changing health care marketplace. Among the trends and issues shaping case management today are the continual need for concrete, documented information on the measurable outcomes of nursing case management interventions and the importance of future nursing case management research in shaping the structure and process of care. Other important influences are the expanding role and implications of information technology and data reporting processes, telehealth, the increasing use of standardized language and documentation systems that allow for systematic tracking and management of patients across a health care continuum; outcomes effectiveness and evidence-based practice; education and competencies of future nurse case managers; understanding compliance, regulatory and reimbursement issues; emphasis on ethical competence in nursing case management; and the impact of revenue cycle involvement, coding, and documentation responsibilities that are adjunct to the role and success of case management. Later chapters address each of these issues in turn.

Traditional nursing care delivery systems are ill equipped to deal with the many constraints, economic limitations, and continual changes in today's health care settings. Cost containment and concerns about quality of care are pushing health care institutions to consider case management as a way to improve patient care and control costs. Assigning a case manager to oversee the provision of patients' care is an increasingly used and widely recognized strategy to help ensure that patients receive needed care and services and that those services are delivered in an efficient, quality, cost-effective manner.

References

Adkins, K., & Morgan, G. (1995, Jan.). Focusing care: Away from the patient and toward the population. *Healthcare Informatics, 12*(1), 76-78.

American Nurses Credentialing Center (2000). *Magnet nursing services recognition program for excellence in nursing services health care organization instructions and application process manual 2000-2001.* Washington, D.C.: American Nurses Credentialing Center.

American Hospital Association (1996). *The Picker Institute: Eye on patients: A report from the American Hospital Association and the Picker Institute.* Chicago: American Hospital Association.

Campbell, S. (1997). A population-based approach to managing risk, access and care in a managed care market. *Healthcare Strategic Management, 15*(7), 14-15.

Campbell, S. (1998). Healthcare organizations are listening to the newly found voice of the consumer. *Healthcare Strategic Management, 16*(3), 14-15.

Chapman, L. (1999, Nov./Dec.). Population health management and the role of the case manager. *The Case Manager, 10*(6), 60-63.

Clough, J. (1996). Risk identification: Management versus avoidance. In E. Cohen (Ed.), *Nurse case management in the 21st century* (pp. 168-180). St. Louis: Mosby, Inc.

Cohen, E. (1991). Nursing case management: Does it pay? *Journal of Nursing Administration, 21*(4), 20-25.

Cohen, E., & De Back, V. (1999). *The outcomes mandate: Case management in health care today.* St. Louis: Mosby, Inc.

De Back, V., & Cohen, E. (1996). The new practice environment. In E. Cohen (Ed.), *Nurse case management in the 21st century* (pp. 3-9). St. Louis: Mosby, Inc.

Department of Health and Human Services (2000, January). *Healthy People 2010.* (Author.)

Ethridge, P. (1991). A nursing HMO: Carondelet St. Mary's experience. *Nursing Management, 22*(7), 22-27.

Ethridge, P., & Lamb, G. (1989). Professional nursing case management improves quality, access, and costs. *Nursing Management, 20*(3), 30-35.

Golodner, L. (1999). Consumer voice: From whimper to roar. In E. Cohen & V. De Back (Eds.), *The outcomes mandate: Case management in health care today* (pp. 20-26). St. Louis: Mosby, Inc.

Grayson, M. (2002, Oct.). Forward motion. *Hospitals & Health Networks, 76*(10), 34-38.

Health Care Advisory Board. (2002). *Maximizing hospital capacity: Expediting patient throughput in an era of shortage.* Washington, D.C.: The Advisory Board Company.

Henderson, M.G., & Wallack, S.S. (1987). Evaluating case management for catastrophic illness. *Business and Health, 4*(3), 7-11.

Institute of Medicine (1996). *2020 Vision: Health in the 21st century.* Washington, D.C.: National Academy Press.

Issel, L.M., & Anderson, R. (1996). Take charge: Managing six transformations in health care delivery. *Nursing Economics, 14*(2), 78-85.

Kindig, D. (1997). *Purchasing population health: Paying for results.* Ann Arbor, Mich.: University of Michigan Press.

Kindig, D. (1999). Purchasing population health: Aligning financial incentives to improve health outcomes. *Nursing Outlook, 47*(1), 15-22.

McIntosh, L. (1987). Hospital based case management. *Nursing Economics, 5*(5), 232-236.

Olivas, G., Del Togno-Armanasco, V., Erickson, J.R., & Harter, S. (1989a). Case management: A bottom-line care delivery model. Part I: The concept. *Journal of Nursing Administration, 19*(11), 16-20.

Olivas, G., Del Togno-Armanasco, V., Erickson, J.R., & Harter, S. (1989b). Case management: A bottom-line care delivery model. II: Adaptation of the model. *Journal of Nursing Administration, 19*(12), 12-17.

Ricklefs, R. (1987, Dec. 30). Firms turn to case management to bring down health care costs. *Wall Street Journal.*

Rogers, M., Riordan, J., & Swindle, D. (1991). Community-based nursing case management pays off. *Nursing Management, 22*(3), 30-34.

Sheehy, C.M., & McCarthy, M.C. (1998). *Advanced practice nursing: Emphasizing common roles.* Philadelphia: F.A. Davis Co.

Shi, L., & Singh, D. (1998). *Delivering health care in America: A systems approach.* Gaithersburg, Md.: Aspen Publication.

Smith, T., & Brooks, A.M. (1999). Redefining quality: Designing new partnerships for consumer and provider. In E. Cohen & V. De Back (Eds.), *The outcomes mandate: Case management in health care today* (pp. 198-206). St. Louis: Mosby, Inc.

Stetler, C.B. (1987). The case manager's role: A preliminary evaluation. *Definition, 2*(3), 1-4.

Taylor, C., & Barnet, R. (1999). The ethics of case management: The quality/cost conundrum. In E. Cohen & V. De Back (Eds.), *The outcomes mandate: Case management in health care today* (p. 30). St. Louis: Mosby, Inc.

Zander, K. (1985). Second generation primary nursing: A new agenda. *Journal of Nursing Administration, 15*(3), 18-24.

Zander, K. (1987). Nursing case management: A classic. *Definition, 2*(2), 1-3.

Zander, K. (1988a). Managed care within acute care settings: Design and implementation via nursing case management. *Health Care Supervisor, 6*(2), 24-43.

Zander, K. (1988b). Nursing case management: Strategic management of cost and quality outcomes. *Journal of Nursing Administration, 18*(5), 23-30.

Historical Perspective of Nursing Care Delivery Models Within the Hospital Setting

CHAPTER OVERVIEW

This chapter reviews the history and theory of various models of professional practice and institutional patient care systems. The restructuring of health care delivery systems has become a promising and successful solution in dealing with cost containment, patient care, and quality improvement issues. Benefits include managing the appropriate use of health care and personnel resources; providing effective and efficient patient care through comprehensive assessment, planning, and coordination efforts; promoting opportunities for professional development and growth across all health care disciplines through participatory and collaborative practice models; and meeting the needs of both the provider and the recipients of care through integrated networks of health services.

EVOLUTION OF NURSING CARE

A historical perspective will help readers see how professional practice and nursing care delivery models evolved and how some of the methods used by previous approaches have contributed to the development of nursing case management today.

Various configurations for the delivery of nursing care have matured within the rapidly changing health care industry. These changes have paralleled major economic, societal, and demographic trends. Changes in patient requirements have occurred as a result of imposed economic constraints brought on by managed care. Currently, patients are being discharged with increased severity of illness levels, and alternative access to care is not always available or affordable. The rise of consumerism, with its emphasis on patient involvement, the advances in scientific technology, and the change in societal values and expectations all contribute to the multifaceted nature of nursing care delivery systems. Several approaches have emerged to meet specific market demands.

Models of Nursing Care

The traditional modes of delivery were defined by patient selection and allocation and assignment systems of personnel (Arndt & Huckabay, 1980; Stevens, 1985).

The *case method* was one of the earliest staffing assignments developed. It involved assigning the nurse to either one patient or a caseload of patients to provide complete care. Sometimes referred to as private duty, the case method used a patient-centered approach by giving the professional nurse full responsibility for the care of the patients on an 8-hour basis (Poulin, 1985; Stevens, 1985). This method, considered the precursor of primary nursing (Poulin, 1985), was inefficient because only one nurse provided all direct care for the patient.

The *functional method* required a division of labor according to specific tasks and was a popular improvement of the case method (Stevens, 1985). The functional model, a task-oriented approach, involved the use of a variety of personnel. It was regarded as a highly efficient, regimented system and was designed to take advantage of different levels of caregiver skill (Stevens, 1985). In functional care, the nurse was required to organize and manage a number of given tasks within a certain time.

The issue associated with the functional approach in nursing care delivery was the fragmentation that occurred in the effort to meet the needs of both patient and staff. Components of patient care that were not addressed raised the frustration levels of both the provider and the patient (Poulin, 1985; Stevens, 1985). The sole reliance on regimented tasks was one of the functional model's major drawbacks and resulted in dissatisfaction for both the patient and the nurse. The functional method also did not offer the opportunity to provide comprehensive, continuous care. Nursing's use of the functional method was the adaptation of an industrial mode of practice to a service system (Poulin, 1985; Stevens, 1985).

Team nursing changed the assignment orientation from tasks to patients and addressed the problems of the functional system (Shukla, 1982; Van Servellen & Joiner, 1984). For instance, patient care needs that might have been missed in a functional nursing model could be picked up by the team approach. The *team method* was developed in the early 1950s by Dr. Eleanor Lambertsen as a way to use all nursing personnel with various skill levels (professional nurses, practical nurses, and nurses' aides). This approach developed in response to the improved technology and shortage of professional nurses (Lambertsen, 1958). The system began to evolve, with greater efforts being made to improve the quality of patient care by focusing on patient outcomes. The professional nurse was responsible for the delivery of patient care services and the supervision, coordination, and evaluation of the outcomes of nursing care provided by the team members.

The advantage of team nursing over functional nursing included increased availability of professional nursing skill for a larger number of patients, greater continuity of care, increased interaction between nurses and patients, and less time spent by professional staff on nonprofessional tasks. The anticipated outcome of such a system was cost-effective nursing care (Chavigny & Lewis, 1984; Hinshaw, Chance, & Atwood, 1981; Lambertsen, 1958; Shukla & Turner, 1984).

The team approach was more than a system for the assignment of personnel. The approach relied heavily on the education, experience, clinical skill, and values of all staff involved in the care of patients. The specifics of nursing care were delineated in the nursing care plan, which included therapeutic, preventive, and rehabilitative steps. Because the care plan was initiated on admission and developed throughout the course of the patient's hospitalization, it was considered cumulative. The plan served as an evaluative measure of patient care and later was adapted as a standard for nursing practice by the Joint Commission on Accreditation of Healthcare Organizations (JCAHO). Although team nursing increased the professional nurse's responsibility for patient outcomes, the limitation in the team approach was related to a greater complexity of role functions and an inability to fit into existing practice systems.

Primary nursing is a configuration of care that promotes greater professional accountability and autonomy and improves continuity of care. This model picks up where team nursing leaves off by making the individual nurse responsible for the assessment, planning, coordination, and evaluation of the effectiveness of care for a certain number of patients. Primary nursing encourages collaborative practice and promotes patient advocacy (Dieman, Noble, & Russel, 1984; Halloran, 1983; Poulin, 1985; Zander, 1985).

Primary nursing is viewed as a care-planning system rather than a caregiving one. The focus in this model is on the planning process for comprehensive and individualized delivery of care. The process uses the nursing care plan, which outlines preferred patient outcomes (Dieman et al., 1984; Stevens, 1985). Nurses are held responsible and accountable for the outcome of patient care during hospitalization. The nurse is also expected to use the nursing process as a framework for administering professional and direct care responsibilities (Halloran, 1983).

Studies have compared the economic and cost-effective variables of primary nursing (Daeffler, 1975; Felton, 1975; Hancock et al., 1984; Hinshaw et al., 1981). These studies report that primary nursing contributes to greater patient and staff satisfaction and is less expensive than team nursing (Daeffler, 1975; Felton, 1975). However, the validity of these studies has been questioned. It appears that the reported cost savings and improvement in the quality of care are a result of the competency levels of the professional staff rather than of the structure of primary nursing (Shukla, 1981).

For primary nursing to be effective, compatible support systems, such as unit secretaries, need to be in place to provide for the routine and nonprofessional activities of the care setting. However, because of current budget constraints, increased severity of patient conditions, and shortened length of stay, hospitals have difficulty maintaining this system of care. Initially, the concept of primary nursing required an all-professional nursing staff. However, a mix of nursing service staff skills and competencies is currently being used successfully in many hospitals (Poulin, 1985; Stevens, 1985). As a result, this patient care delivery system is assuming characteristics of other patient care models and is evolving into a prototype that can be adapted to alternate delivery models of nursing care.

PROFESSIONAL PRACTICE AND ALTERNATIVE PATIENT CARE DELIVERY MODELS

The unstable nature of health care economics and managed care has made it necessary to focus attention on developing and implementing alternative systems for the delivery of patient care. Almost two decades ago, the need to deliver health care effectively and efficiently stimulated the promotion of national initiatives directed by the Department of Health and Human Services and supported by the National Commission on Nursing. The purpose of these efforts was to decrease length of stay, reduce costs, and improve the quality of patient care (National Commission on Nursing Implementation Project [NCNIP], 1986; Secretary's Commission on Nursing, 1988).

The same principles hold true today that to achieve these goals while maintaining viability, patient care delivery systems must be sensitive to limited fiscal and resource appropriation. The systems must also incorporate cost-effective standards, establish quality assurance outcomes of professional practice, and broaden accountability for the outcomes of care. Several professional practice and alternative care delivery models have been successfully developed and implemented. These models have prompted major adjustments in the practice environments of their settings.

Some of the fundamental characteristics of these professional practice and care delivery approaches are the adaptability and receptiveness of the approaches to differentiated and professional competency levels of practice; the reconfiguration of patient care and maximum use of nursing personnel resources; the use of collaborative practice arrangements among nurses, physicians, and other health care workers; the redesigning of the relationship between the providers and recipients of health care to improve patient care outcomes; and the enhancement of the relationship between the providers of patient care and the organizational culture that supports them. A description of some of the models used in practice follows.

Integrated Competencies of Nurses Model (ICON)

ICON models I and II are examples of the earliest alternate care delivery approaches that blend the professional and educational competency levels of staff with the health care needs and requirements of patients (Rotkovich, 1986). The nursing care responsibilities in these models, which were set up as demonstration projects, are differentiated on the basis of the nurse's educational preparation. Head nurses are required to have a master's degree and are responsible for the management and distribution of personnel and resources and overall quality of care delivered on the unit. Nurses with baccalaureate degrees are accountable for the assessment, planning, and evaluation activities of the nursing process. Nurses with associate degrees complement the professional nurse in patient care and carry out nursing decisions. In the ICON I model, licensed practical nurses (LPNs), nurses with diplomas, and nursing assistants are excluded from the staffing complement.

Although ICON I was considered the nursing care delivery system for the future, another model, ICON II, had been implemented and ran concurrently to help LPNs and nurses with diplomas or associate degrees make the transition into their respective practice roles (Rotkovich & Smith, 1987). The goal of this model was to assist through in-service programs, continual education, and clinical preceptors the grandfathering of the associate degree and diploma nurses into the professional nurse's role and the LPNs into the associate nurse's role. This objective is in line with the profession's broader goal of achieving two entry levels of nursing practice.

Cost-effectiveness, quality, and job satisfaction variables were measured and evaluated on an ongoing basis. No data have been published relating the effects of staff mix and competency levels of nursing staff on the productivity and quality of patient care using the ICON I and II models. Information on nursing personnel satisfaction and retention is also missing.

Partners in Practice

The *partners-in-practice system*, defined by Manthey (1989) as a progression from primary nursing, is a partnership established between an experienced senior registered nurse and an individual who supports the nurse as a technical assistant. The technical assistant is assigned to the nurse, not to a caseload of patients. Consequently, by delegating tasks to the technical assistant, the registered nurse can concentrate on providing professional patient care.

The registered nurse is responsible for defining the role, standards, and nursing care activities. By providing direction and supervision, the registered nurse is also accountable for the overall care delivered in the partnership. An official contract is used to confirm the relationship, and both members are paired on the same time schedule.

This system of care delivery is highly sensitive to unit-based human resource distribution requirements, skill mix, competency levels, and patient care needs. Because of the emphasis placed on the delivery of productive and efficient health care services, the partners-in-practice system can yield substantial benefits. These benefits include savings in overall budget and personnel salary expenditures as a result of reduced turnover rates, decreased use of staffing agencies, and improved management of supplemental nursing resources. The system enhances nursing staff retention by offering opportunities for advanced clinical training and education.

Contract and Group Practice Models

Contract and group practice models have been implemented at Johns Hopkins Hospital. They focus on building up the relationship among nursing care providers, the organization, and the environments in which they work. The *contract model* concentrates on promoting job satisfaction and retention by engaging nursing staff in autonomous decision-making related to unit-based staffing levels and coverage, scheduling activities, standards of practice, quality assurance, and peer review (York & Fecteau, 1987). Another characteristic of this model is that it uses primary nursing. The staff benefits from the associated practice arrangements, which include salaried (versus hourly wage) compensation programs.

The *group practice model* is another innovative system developed for nurse practitioners who work in the emergency department and provide services to a group of patients who require primary health care (York & Fecteau, 1987). This model, which is built on the same objectives and goals as the contract model, initiates a productivity incentive that compensates nurse practitioners for the amount of care they provide per patient visit. This model calls for the creation of an incentive fund that is allocated as patient target volumes are met.

Both of these models prove their economic viability and organizational effectiveness by decreasing costs related to staff turnover and sick time, increasing patient visits and admissions, and decreasing length of stay. Reallocation of staff mix, skill, and competence levels leads to greater productivity and better use of the professional nursing staff. Additional gains include increased job satisfaction because of greater continuity of patient care, increased professional responsibility and autonomy, and reciprocal compensation packages.

NURSING CASE MANAGEMENT

A review of the literature indicates that aspects of some of the past and current nursing practice approaches and delivery models of care were incorporated into the development of nursing case management. The strength of nursing case management comes from the philosophy and collaborative practice strategies of both primary and team nursing. In fact, some of the care planning and coordination processes used in these models are reflected in the critical paths and care plans of nursing case management. These plans are used to monitor patient care requirements and activity as well as the resources for meeting those needs.

With former models, nursing care revolved around the nursing care plan, which provided a broad-based outline for the delivery of nursing services for the patient. These plans gave little direction in establishing a structure for achieving expected outcomes of nursing care for each day of hospitalization. The *nursing case management model*, however, provides a framework for nurses to manage the patient's hospital stay. Directing the delivery of patient care services allows the nurse to anticipate needs, thereby providing the opportunity for overall coordination and integration of outcomes and cost (Cohen & Cesta, 1994; Zander, 1990).

Nursing case management also integrates many of the professional practice demands and initiatives characteristic of alternative patient care delivery models. By emphasizing care that is patient centered, the nursing case management approach embraces techniques of business in which the patient is seen as a valuable consumer who has the right to demand the best in health care. Placing the patient at the core of nursing's power base authorizes the profession to reconfirm its commitment to society. Nursing case management incorporates a new way of looking at the relationships among cost, quality, and nursing care. It places an emphasis on the autonomy, authority, and accountability of professional nursing practice by promoting an open system of care in which information is shared among all disciplines. A team whose members work collaboratively replaces the individual method of providing patient care. Because of its universal applicability, an in-depth discussion and treatment of the nursing case management model are provided in Unit II.

References

Arndt, C., & Huckabay, L. (1980). *Nursing administration theory for practice with a system approach.* Chicago: American Hospital Association, pp. 65-111.

Chavigny, K., & Lewis, A. (1984). Team or primary nursing care? *Nursing Outlook, 32*(6), 322-327.

Cohen, E., & Cesta, T. (1994, Fall). The economics of health care and the realities of nursing in the 1990s. Case management in the acute care setting: a model for health care reform. *Journal of Case Management, 3*(3), 110-116, 128.

Daeffler, R.J. (1975). Patient's perception of care under team or primary nursing. *Journal of Nursing Administration, 6*(3), 20-26.

Dieman, P.A., Noble, E., & Russel, M.E. (1984). Achieving a professional practice model: How primary nursing can help. *Journal of Nursing Administration, 14*(7), 16-21.

Felton, G. (1975). Increasing the quality of nursing care by introducing the concept of primary nursing: A model project. *Nursing Research, 24*(1), 27-32.

Halloran, E. (1983). Staffing assignment: By task or by patient. *Nursing Management, 14*(8), 16-18.

Hancock, W.N. et al. (1984). A cost and staffing comparison of an all-RN staff and team nursing. *Nursing Administration Quarterly, 8*(2), 45-55.

Hinshaw, A.S., Chance, H.C., & Atwood, J. (1981). Staff, patient and cost outcomes of all-RN registered nurse staffing. *Journal of Nursing Administration, 11*(11), 30-36.

Lambertsen, E. (1958). *Education for nursing leadership.* Philadelphia: J.B. Lippincott Co.

Manthey, M. (1989). Practice partnerships: The newest concept in care delivery. *Journal of Nursing Administration, 19*(2), 33-35.

National Commission on Nursing Implementation Project (1986, Nov. 7). *Invitational Conference.* Milwaukee: W.K. Kellogg Foundation.

Poulin, M. (1985). Configuration of nursing practice. In American Nurse's Association (Ed.), *Issues in professional nursing practice* (pp. 1-14). Kansas City, Mo.: The Association.

Rotkovich, R. (1986). ICON: A model of nursing practice for the future. *Nursing Management, 17*(6), 54-56.

Rotkovich, R., & Smith, C. (1987). ICON I—The future model, ICON II—The transition model. *Nursing Management, 18*(11), 91-96.

Secretary's Commission on Nursing (1988, Dec.). *Final report (Volume I).* Washington, D.C.: Department of Health and Human Services.

Shukla, R.K. (1981). Structure vs. people in primary nursing: An inquiry. *Nursing Research, 30*(7), 236-241.

Shukla, R.K. (1982). Primary or team nursing? Two conditions determine the choice. *Journal of Nursing Administration, 12*(11), 12-15.

Shukla, R.K., & Turner, W.E. (1984). Patient's perception of care under primary and team nursing. *Research in Nursing and Health, 7*(2), 93-99.

Stevens, B.J. (1985). *The nurse as executive* (pp. 105-137). Rockville, Md.: Aspen Publication.

Van Servellen, G.M., & Joiner, C. (1984). Convergence among primary nurses in their perception of their nursing functions. *Nursing and Health Care, 5*(4), 213-217.

York, C., & Fecteau, D. (1987). Innovative models of professional nursing practice. *Nursing Economics, 5*(4), 162-166.

Zander, K. (1985). Second generation primary nursing: A new agenda. *Journal of Nursing Administration, 15*(3), 18-24.

Zander, K. (1990). Managed care and nursing case management. In G.G. Mayer, M.J. Madden, & E. Lawrenz (Eds.), *Patient care delivery model* (pp. 37-61). Rockville, Md.: Aspen Publishers, Inc.

Historical Development of Case Management

CHAPTER OVERVIEW

The case management approach represents an innovative response to the demands of providing care in the least expensive setting and coordinating and planning for needed community resources. For more than 30 years, there has been a growth in the variety of case management delivery systems of care.

This chapter reviews the historical development of the case management concept. Descriptions of different non-nursing case management models are given to make the reader aware of the vastness and complexity of this approach. This is not intended to suggest limited use of the case management model. On the contrary, its great potential and applicability should be promoted. Studies show that this model can be an effective and efficient system by focusing on and caring for the health and social needs of the individual.

INTRODUCTION OF CASE MANAGEMENT

Most of the literature on nursing case management practiced in the acute care setting is evolving. However, case management has been used by mental health and social services for years. For more than three decades, the case management approach has been used as an alternate design for the delivery of health care. The first federally funded demonstration project began in 1971 and has been associated with a number of methods to coordinate and provide comprehensive services of care for the individual (Merrill, 1985). Regardless of the different approaches, the main principle underlying case management is ensuring the quality as well as the efficiency and cost-effectiveness of the services provided (Weil & Karls, 1985). Emphasis is placed on the recipient of case managed care and the coordination and networking of services (Weil & Karls, 1985; White, 1986).

Research related to the outpatient and community-based population has studied the effects of health care case management in areas other than nursing. The specific target groups included the frail elderly, the chronically ill who are functionally or emotionally challenged, and clients who require long-term care services. These case management projects were designed to use less-expensive, community-based services to prevent unnecessary institutionalization (Steinberg & Carter, 1983; Zawadski, 1983). Various services, from companionship to homemaking, were provided to assist individuals in their daily activities.

Findings of these studies show that case-managed, in-home support services, such as mental health, respite care, and homemaker or personal care services, have been effective in improving access (evidenced by shorter service waiting lists), assessment, and care-planning needs of elderly clients (Expanded In-home Service for the Elderly Program [EISEP], 1988; Raschko, 1985). Additional studies illustrate the efficacy of case management in coordinating and integrating health and social services for long-term care, assessing quality-of-life outcomes (quality-of-living conditions), and reducing time spent in long-term care facilities (Carcagno & Kemper, 1988; Eggert, Bowlyow, & Nichols, 1980; Sherwood & Morris, 1983).

Because the nursing profession recognizes the need for changes in the system of health care delivery, nurses are increasingly being designated as case managers. This change results from the expertise and knowledge of nurses in managing patient care. Case managers are involved in the assessment, coordination, referral, and individualized planning, monitoring, and follow-up activities associated with case management (Grau, 1984; Johnson & Grant, 1985; Mudinger, 1984).

Primarily used with long-term care populations, case management arrangements have been developed by private insurance carriers as cost-containment strategies and have been integrated into the acute care setting (Henderson & Collard, 1988; McIntosh, 1987). Consequently, different models of case management have evolved. Merrill (1985) identified three categories of case management: social, primary care, and medical-social.

Social Case Management

Social case management models emphasize comprehensive long-term community care services used to delay and/or prevent hospitalization. Both health and social needs are addressed in this setting. Primarily successful with the elderly population, this model focuses on ensuring the independence of the individual through family and community involvement. It is based on a multidisciplinary approach to coordinate the care of the patient.

Various services, from companionship to homemaking, are offered to assist individuals in their daily activities. One example of the social case management approach is the U.S. Department of Housing and Urban Development's Congregate Housing Services Program, in which non–health services are provided to the elderly living in a housing project.

Primary Care Case Management

Primary care case management takes on the role of gatekeeper based on the medical model of care. This approach focuses on the treatment of a particular health problem and tries to prevent institutionalization. In this model the physician functions as the case manager and is responsible for coordinating services and managing the patient (Johnson & Grant, 1985).

Primary care case management emphasizes the need to regulate resource use to ensure cost-effectiveness. Examples mentioned include health management organizations (HMOs), which originally served Medicaid beneficiaries and have become increasingly popular among insurance companies as a means of controlling the disproportionate use of medical care.

Because the patient population accommodated by primary care case management is defined by health status, the type of case management services required varies according to the health needs of the patient. The financial imperatives to curtail high-cost medical technology are strong under the primary care case management system. However, a major liability of this approach is the exclusion of necessary medical services and hospitalization. Johnson and Grant (1985) recommend that quality assurance standards be incorporated into this mode of health care delivery.

Medical-Social Case Management

The medical-social case management model focuses on the long-term-care patient population at risk for hospitalization. This model combines available resource utilization with additional services, which are not traditionally covered by health insurance, to maintain the individual in the home or community. The case manager(s) in this system may be drawn from nurses, physicians, social workers, and family members who have input into the assessment, coordination, care planning, and care monitoring.

An example of the medical-social case management model is the social-HMO demonstration project, which integrates both medical and social services on a prepaid capitated basis to meet the multiple needs of the chronically ill patient. This model emphasizes providing the least restrictive and least costly long-term care by identifying the appropriate services and coordinating its delivery.

Additional definitions of the case management model are offered by White (1986), who bases the case management approach on a continual process of responsibility and authority for the provision of care and resource appropriation and use. Along this spectrum, situations arise that either preclude the use of case management or facilitate case management arrangements with direct health service delivery.

Five case management models were also characterized. These models are differentiated on the basis of authority level of the client, support and financial systems, and payment allocation (White, 1986).

1. Restricted market: In this arrangement the clients become their own case managers and negotiate for services among independent providers.
2. Multiservice agency: This system allows an agency to provide its own health care.
3. Advocacy agency: With this model, some case management is provided along with direct patient care services.
4. Brokerage agency: The agency in this system acts as a broker in coordinating, controlling, and monitoring services and resources.
5. Prepaid long-term care organization: With this arrangement, a company contracts for case management services and coordinates resources on a prepaid, capitated basis.

Weil and Karls (1985) further characterized case management into three practice models: the generalist case manager or broker model, the primary-therapist-as-case-manager model, and the interdisciplinary team model.

The generalist case manager model is structured to provide direct service, access, planning, and monitoring activities to clients. The case manager in this system acts as a broker and is involved in the intake, coordination, and evaluation processes.

A broad range of professional disciplines may be represented; therefore the case managers in this model may include social workers, nurses, and mental health or rehabilitation specialists. Continuous and efficient service is ensured because of the close working relationship between the case manager and client. The case manager also benefits from autonomous decision-making and other independent management responsibilities.

The primary therapist model emphasizes a therapeutic relationship between the case manager and client. The case manager in this system is required to have a master's degree and training in psychology, social work, psychiatry, or psychiatric clinical nursing specialties.

As in the generalist model, the case manager–patient relationship is a close one, with the case manager responsible for coordination and evaluation services. Because of this one-on-one relationship, the primary therapist model works well with small, community-based programs and has been successful in coordinating and planning efforts and resources with larger networking systems.

Initiatives to ensure the delivery of case management are strong under the primary therapist model. However, therapeutic services have been known to take precedence at the expense of case management functions. Weil and Karls (1985) recommend the supplementation of case management responsibilities with therapeutic care.

The interdisciplinary team model focuses on providing case management services through a collaborative team approach. The responsibilities and designated case management functions are divided among the team members according to their area of specialization and expertise.

In this system, the case managers may include nurses, social workers, or therapists who have accountability and provide services within their own area of concentration. One team member, however, is appointed to maintain overall service coordination and evaluation.

The benefits of the interdisciplinary team approach include improved continuity of care and enhanced coordination of services and staff support systems to promote mutual program planning, problem solving, and client advocacy.

INDEPENDENT/PRIVATE CASE MANAGEMENT

The independent/private case management model offers the provision of case management services by case managers who are either self-employed or are salaried employees in a privately owned case management firm. The terms *independent* and *private* refer to the absence of oversight by a managed care organization or a health care organization such as a home care agency or an acute care hospital.

Although similar services are provided, independent and private case management are differentiated as follows. *Independent case management* consists of firms that are not a formal part of an insurance company or a health care facility. They exist solely for the provision of case management services based on a contractual agreement between the independent case management firm and the health care organization. *Private case management* refers to the services provided by an independent case manager privately contracted or hired by a patient or a family member (Cesta & Tahan, 2003).

Private case management systems have evolved to meet the needs of clients outside publicly funded programs or those who prefer more personalized services (Parker & Secord, 1988). Parker and Secord cite the findings of a major survey conducted by Inter-Study's Center for Aging and Long-Term Care and funded by the Retirement Research Foundation.

This study investigated the characteristics, services, referral, and funding sources of private geriatric case management firms across the United States. According to Parker and Secord (1988), this model evolved as a result of an increase in the elderly population, escalating health care costs, growing need for integrated social and health services for the elderly, and increasing emphasis placed on long-term care issues. Survey findings are discussed in the following five paragraphs.

- Private case management firms were in business an average of 3 years, and most (98.9%) were independently owned, run for profit, and self-managed. Some affiliations existed with hospitals, public and private social service agencies, and nursing homes. Clientele consisted of elderly individuals with mean annual incomes ranging from $5000 to $15,000. Case managers in this system were college graduates who were prepared in social work or nursing and who carried a small caseload of clients.
- In most instances, private case management functions included coordination of services, social, functional, and financial; mental health assessment and counseling; and referral, monitoring, and evaluation services. Medical assessments were made by physicians in 44% of the private case management businesses. Some of the other services consisted of nursing home and housing placement, retirement planning, companion and homemaker services, and transportation and respite care. These direct services were provided more frequently by for-profit and unaffiliated private case management businesses than by the nonprofit and affiliated companies. The firms that employed registered nurses as case managers tended to provide more direct care services as well.

- Services most often referred by private case managers included home health care, homemaker, and personal care services; family and legal counseling; and physical therapy. Referral sources were composed of physicians, social workers, family members, and self-referrals.
- Private case managers were able to provide more individualized services and were also accessible on off hours, weekends, and holidays.
- Reimbursement for services provided by private case managers ranged from hourly and set rates per session to service and package rates. Unaffiliated and for-profit businesses used more hourly and set rate methods and also segregated their services to charge for case management functions involving more time and attention. Sliding fee scales were more common in affiliated and nonprofit organizations. Funding sources to private case management businesses included out-of-pocket payments by client or family members, private insurance, Medicare, Medicaid, and other sources that consisted of public funds, trusts, and grants.

Benefits of private case management approaches for staff members include increased flexibility and autonomy in decision-making, independent planning and coordinating of services, greater income, and professional satisfaction. Clients and their families also reported improved accessibility to case managers, less duplication and redundancy of services, individualized care, and long-term association with one case manager. However, further evaluation is needed regarding access to other health care services, overall quality of private case management care, cost, and reimbursement issues.

As noted by Cesta & Tahan (2003), independent/private case managers function in a dual advocacy role that at times can generate conflict. These individuals are expected to deliver care that is efficient and cost-effective in a manner that is satisfactory for both the patient and the hiring insurance company or health care facility.

COMPONENTS OF CASE MANAGEMENT

Weil and Karls (1985) extensively outlined the main service components common in all case management models.

Client Identification and Outreach

Individuals who are eligible or require case management services are identified. Admission to a case management program is determined by interview process, referral, and networking systems or by the case manager actively promoting eligibility for individuals who might not inquire about case management services for themselves (for example, individuals who are indigent or have mental illness).

Individual Assessment and Diagnosis

Case managers use their comprehensive knowledge and skill to assess the physical, emotional, and psychological needs as well as the social and support requirements of their clients. This process aids in the coordination, facilitation, monitoring, and access of case management services.

Service Planning and Resource Identification

With the collaboration of the client, the case manager assumes the responsibility for coordinating and planning care services. This includes the development of care plans and determining resource and networking systems.

Linking Clients to Needed Services

Case managers act as brokers to expedite and follow through with the coordination and planning needs of the client. Both community and agency resources may be used. In some systems, this responsibility involves actually transporting the client to a recommended service.

Service Implementation and Coordination

The case manager ensures that the identified needs are satisfied and follows the formal agreements made with the networking agencies. This is done by extensive documentation and record keeping of the efficiency, effectiveness, and quality of case management care services. A participative relationship of client and case manager and autonomous decision-making on the part of the case manager are crucial to both groups' engagement in the system.

Monitoring Service Delivery

The case manager is responsible for directing and overseeing the distribution of services to the client. A multidisciplinary and multiservice relationship is promoted to ensure appropriate and effective delivery of case-managed services.

Advocacy

Case managers act on behalf of the client in ensuring that needed interventions are obtained and that the client is making progress in the program. As explained by Weil, the advocacy strategy is used not only for the individual client but also for the benefit of all individuals in common predicaments.

Evaluation

The case manager is responsible and accountable for appraising the specific as well as the overall usefulness and effectiveness of case managed services. The evaluation process involves continuous monitoring and analysis of the needs of the individuals and services provided to the clients. Early identification of changes or problems with the client or the provider of services is made, ensuring timely intervention and replanning by the case manager.

References

Carcagno, G.J., & Kemper, P. (1988). The evolution of the National Long Term Care Demonstration: An overview of the Channeling Demonstration and its evaluation. *Health Services Research, 23,* 1-22.

Cesta, T.G., & Tahan, H.A. (2003). *The case manager's survival guide: Winning strategies for clinical practice.* 2nd Edition. St. Louis: Mosby, Inc.

Eggert, G.M., Bowlyow, J.E., & Nichols, C.W. (1980). Gaining control of the long term care system: First returns from Access Experiment. *The Gerontologist, 20,* 356-363.

Expanded In-home Service for the Elderly Program (1988, November 30). *An evaluation of New York City's home care services supported under the Expanded In-home Service for the Elderly Program.* New York: Health Research, New York University. Funded by New York City's Department for the Aging (contract #11000100).

Grau, L. (1984). Case management and the nurse. *Geriatric Nurse, 5,* 372-375.

Henderson, M.G., & Collard, A. (1988). Measuring quality in medical case management programs. *Quality Review Bulletin, 14*(2), 33-39.

Johnson, C., & Grant, L. (1985). *The nursing home in American society.* Baltimore: Johns Hopkins University Press, pp. 140-200.

McIntosh, L. (1987). Hospital based case management. *Nursing Economics, 5*(5), 232-236.

Merrill, J.C. (1985). Defining case management. *Business and Health, 3,* 5-9.

Mudinger, M.O. (1984). Community based case: Who will be the case managers? *Nursing Outlook, 32*(6), 294-295.

Parker, M., & Secord, L. (1988). Private geriatric case management: Providers, services and fees. *Nursing Economics, 6*(4), 165-172, 195.

Raschko, R. (1985). Systems integration at the program level: Aging and mental health. *The Gerontologist, 25,* 460-463.

Sherwood, S., & Morris, J.N. (1983). The Pennsylvania Domiciliary Care Experiment: Impact on quality of life. *American Journal of Public Health, 73,* 646-653.

Steinberg, R.M., & Carter, G.W. (1983). *Case management and the elderly: A handbook for planning and administering programs.* Lexington, Mass.: Lexington Books.

Weil, M., & Karls, J. (1985). Historical origins and recent developments. In M. Weil & J. Karls (Eds.), *Case management in human service practice* (pp. 1-28). San Francisco: Jossey-Bass Publishers.

White, M. (1986). Case management. In G.L. Maddox (Ed.), *The encyclopedia of aging* (pp. 92-96). New York: Springer Publishing.

Zawadski, R.T. (1983). The long-term care demonstration projects: What are they and why they came into being? *Home Health Care Services Quarterly, 4*(3-4), 5-26.

II

CONTEMPORARY MODELS OF CASE MANAGEMENT

Unit II highlights the emergence of collaborative models of nursing case management that embrace elements of joint decision-making and shared accountability. This approach ensures comprehensive patient care delivery and overall system improvement. In the twenty-first century, case management models will include the integration of care across the continuum. Both care management and disease management approaches build on interdisciplinary systems of care and are evolving as complementary strategies to nursing case management.

Dimensions of Nursing Case Management

CHAPTER OVERVIEW

As the demand for cost-effective high-quality health care continues to grow, innovative approaches to improving patient care delivery must be explored. The goals of cost-effectiveness combined with high-quality care can only be achieved within a framework of total organizational commitment to restructuring care to meet the needs of today's health care provider and the present patient population.

Case management is an effective approach that can be used in the reorganization process. As discussed, this model helps define the role and scope of the nurse's responsibilities in the delivery setting. Case management models can enhance the productivity and competency levels of staff by organizing personnel to use their varying skills and expertise in better ways. This could increase professionalism and the satisfaction of all providers.

By ensuring that appropriate outcomes are achieved, case management provides a framework for continuous and refined planning of nursing and interdisciplinary care and ensures appropriate and cost-effective use of patient resources. Finally, case management models can contribute to the foundation of total quality improvement and ensure the continued delivery of high-quality patient care.

PRECURSOR OF CONTEMPORARY APPROACHES TO NURSING CASE MANAGEMENT

Cost management issues and quality care, which at one point were on opposite sides of the health care delivery spectrum, are now being integrated into one system. The economic power once reserved for physicians and hospitals has been transferred to the purchasers of health services, which include business corporations, insurance companies, and individuals. The buyers' objectives are coordinating and managing the use of health services and allocating resources for future distribution.

Managed care emerged as control shifted from the provider to the purchaser of health services. The managed care system links the provider with the patient to manage cost, access, and quality components of health care delivery. Major health policies like the federal Health Maintenance Organization Act, adopted in the early 1970s, established a trend for the growth of managed care programs. The health maintenance organizations (HMOs) and preferred provider organizations (PPOs), two popular examples, offered an alternative to costly inpatient care through the provision of cost-effective treatments and multiple preventive and outpatient services.

Case management is used in these managed care plans as a cost-containment initiative. It further grounds the managed care approach by focusing on the individual health care needs of the patient.

Case management is effective because it targets the coordination, integration, and outcome evaluation processes of care. The inherent strengths in case management systems have led to a renewed interest in the utility and effectiveness of such systems.

TREND-SETTING IN NURSING CASE MANAGEMENT

Managed care is a system that provides the generalized structure and focus for managing the use, cost, quality, and effectiveness of health care services. Managed care then becomes an umbrella for several cost-containment initiatives that may involve case management. On the other hand, nursing case management can be conceptualized as a process model, the underpinnings of which are essential in attending to the many components and services used in the delivery aspects of patient care.

With case management, the accountability and responsibility for the delivery of care are based on an entire occurrence of hospitalization for a targeted diagnosis-related group (DRG) of patients and is not geographically confined to that patient's unit (Etheredge, 1989; Zander, 1990). This widens the circumscribed area of patient services to include patient care planning and coordination across health care settings. Case management, then, implies consistency of provider: even though different, formal, informal, and even very esoteric resources are used, the coordinator or provider (usually an individual) remains the same (Zander, 1991).

Collaborative practice arrangements in the form of group practice are supported, and interdisciplinary decision-making is facilitated to ensure appropriate use of patient resources and achievement of expected clinical outcomes. Collaboration usually includes members of the health care team and the patient or family to help accomplish anticipated care outcomes. Participants of the health care team use critical paths, clinical pathways, and case management plans. Variance analysis and evaluation of patient care are expanded beyond the confines of the patient unit and encompass all patients in the specific caseload (Etheredge, 1989; Zander, 1990).

An example of a case management model—the Beth Israel Multidisciplinary Patient Care Model (Cesta, 1991)—was developed for use within an acute care setting. Using the practice concepts of both primary and team nursing, this model supported the coordination and management of patient care from admission to discharge. The objectives of the model were as follows:

- Improve quality of care
- Control resource utilization
- Decrease length of stay
- Increase patient satisfaction
- Increase staff satisfaction

This case management model, which was implemented through a reorganization of the nursing department structure, provided the opportunity for advancement of selected registered nurses working at the bedside. When a case management career ladder is used, nurses who have a baccalaureate degree and who have demonstrated advanced clinical and leadership skills can remain in the direct patient care environment and expand their professional careers by working as case managers.

The case manager was removed from direct care delivery to coordinate overall patient services. This individual is also part of a multidisciplinary team that continually assesses, evaluates, and plans patient care. The assessment is based on expectations regarding outcomes of care of the physician, nurse, and all other individuals involved in the patient's care.

Case managers assumed responsibility for a caseload of patients who met high-risk criteria developed for each clinical area. Patients were referred to utilization management or social work as needed.

Care was managed through prospective protocols called multidisciplinary action plans (MAPs). Outcome data, including variances, were collected and used to improve clinical and system processes.

An MAP projected patient care outcomes for each day of hospitalization. Because care plans were a group effort, they promoted greater satisfaction for the patient, family, and health team members. These plans involved all patient care areas and specialties and covered a wide range of diagnoses or surgical procedures, such as neurosurgery, orthopedics, acquired immunodeficiency syndrome (AIDS), general medicine, pediatrics, maternal and child health, oncology, detoxification, and rehabilitation. Ultimately, the model increased professional development and improved recruitment, motivation, and retention of staff (Ake et al., 1991).

Case managers, who were unit based, coordinated the care being delivered by the registered nurses and nursing assistants working on the team. The manager also served as a role model to the novice nurse or orientee. By consulting with less-experienced registered nurses, the manager helped to improve the professionalism and clinical skills of the unit's personnel and promoted collegial relationships with all health care providers. Other responsibilities of the case manager included patient and family teaching and support and discharge planning with the social worker.

This model enhanced the use of personnel by expanding support or ancillary staff role responsibilities. Because the nursing attendants were included as part of the care team, they better understood the medical and nursing needs of their patients.

The multidisciplinary patient care model was an integral component of the organizational restructuring of patient care delivery. Because it was research based and part of the planned change process, several clinical and quality care indicators were evaluated to determine the model's effectiveness. This model required ongoing assessment of quality improvement data, job and patient satisfaction ratings, and length-of-stay data.

Another example of a comprehensive case management model was developed at The Long Island College Hospital, Brooklyn, New York. This model incorporated the same goals as the Beth Israel model, with emphasis on the use of product and personnel resources. Process and structure redesign for this model began with a review of the role functions of nurses, social workers, utilization managers, and discharge planners. The existing care process for each discipline was entered in a flow chart, and process barriers were identified. Each discipline identified ways in which personnel might be redeployed to ensure the best use of available personnel as well as to reduce duplication. Interventions were moved to preadmission whenever possible. For example, discharge planning and home care referrals were moved to the preadmission arena. Social workers began to divide their time between the inpatient and outpatient care settings.

Another significant component of this model was the redeployment of the existing clinical nurse specialists as case managers. Long Island College Hospital identified the case manager role as an advanced practice role, and the clinical nurse specialists were best prepared to assume the additional responsibilities associated with case management. Generic staff development functions that they were performing were returned to the Department of Nursing Education and Research.

A triad model of case management, which builds on the expertise of all members of the case management team, is another example of addressing clinical and business decisions within health care organizations. This model was adopted and implemented at the University of Colorado Hospital (UCH), Denver, Colorado, in response to the increased penetration of managed care in Denver and shorter length of stay for UCH patients.

Based on a strategy from Vanderbilt University Medical Center, the triad model promotes interdisciplinary team involvement and includes three main disciplines: nurse case manager, social work, and utilization management (see Chapters 8 and 9 for a more detailed description).

Taking a population-based approach, this model facilitates the identification and resolution of system issues that may hinder the movement of patients across the continuum of care.

A Team Data Collection Tool was developed and has evolved to demonstrate cost management with a focus on the quality and outcomes of care. Financial impact of the triad model resulted in $5 million returned to the bottom line in recovered and overturned appeals/denials/provider liable accounts. In addition, data collection of surveyed admissions showed that as of year to date, 98.6% of admissions met InterQual criteria and 97% of patients were discharged when they no longer met the criteria. This model also demonstrated a significant impact on meeting regulatory and compliance needs and promoted staff and physician education. In all, the concomitant effects of this initiative on nursing practice have resulted in patient assignments to appropriate levels of care, shortened length of stay, and improved discharge planning through the identification of risk factors that affect discharge.

The Professionally Advanced Care Team (ProACT) Model

The ProACT model was developed at the Robert Wood Johnson University Hospital (RWJUH) in New Brunswick, New Jersey to meet the demand-induced nursing shortage, differentiated practice, and prospective payment initiatives (Tonges, 1989a, 1989b). This model expanded the role and professional practice of the registered nurse by establishing two roles for the nurse. The first role is that of the clinical care manager (CCM), and the second is that of primary nurse.

The CCM role required a nurse with a baccalaureate degree who managed the care for a caseload of patients throughout their hospitalization. This position involved managerial, personnel, clinical, and fiscal accountability. Primary nurses, who had graduated from accredited registered nurse programs, were given responsibility for 24-hour management of patients on the unit and all direct and indirect caregiving activities. They were also accountable for the assessment, planning, and evaluation components of patient care as well as the delegation of tasks to licensed practical nurses (LPNs) and nursing assistants providing direct patient care.

This system maximized primary nursing through the redistribution of support staff and a restructuring of ancillary services at the unit level. Patient care services that could be supported by non-nursing departments, such as housekeeping, dietary, supplies, and pharmacy, were assigned to the appropriate unit personnel. For example, support-service hosts were responsible for hotel-type functions such as bed making, and pharmacy technicians were responsible for ordering, obtaining, and preparing medications, among other duties. By placing accountability for nonclinical services on personnel from respective support departments, nurses were free to provide comprehensive and coordinated patient care.

The traditional reporting structures and organizational processes were altered to adapt to the ProACT model's premise of restructuring care with the patient as the central focus. Luckenbill and Tonges (1990) reported in a preliminary evaluation that job satisfaction increased through collaborative care efforts among nurses, physicians, and other health care workers and through a well-coordinated support-service system for staff and patients. Additional findings included a 10% decrease in length of stay with specific DRG patients and a concomitant increase in patient revenues that were attributable to nursing interventions.

As part of an iterative process of work redesign at RWJUH, the CCM role was reexamined and substantially changed in the mid-1990s. The first change broadened the CCM's scope from a unit-based to a service-based approach. This review subsequently identified an opportunity to decrease duplication of effort and redundancy in the nursing case management, utilization management, and discharge planning functions (Brett, Bueno, Royal, & Sengin, 1997). It was thought that all three roles centered on expediting patient throughput, primarily by reviewing and using data from the medical record, resulting in overlap among responsibilities. To streamline processes and improve efficiency, the case management, utilization management, and discharge planning functions were integrated into a new outcomes manager role. Several key processes were automated to support this transition, including home care referrals.

A number of variables were evaluated to assess the outcomes of this change, and the most striking results appear to be a 41.5% increase in home care referrals and a reduction of 17 full-time equivalents (Brett et al., 1997).

South Dakota Demonstration Project—Differentiating Outside the Walls

A nursing delivery model expanding on the theme of differentiated practice has been developed and implemented at Sioux Valley Hospital in Sioux Falls, South Dakota. This hospital was one of several institutions participating in a statewide demonstration project. The project demonstration sites consisted of a consortium of institutions, with representation from the acute care setting, long-term care (nursing home), and home health agencies (Koerner, Bunkers, Nelson, & Santenna, 1989).

Differentiating Outside the Walls*

Nursing case management has been in existence in this 400-bed hospital since the practice differentiated in 1989 (Koerner & Karpiuk, 1994). That model was founded on principles of the original primary nursing concepts of the 1970s and 1980s: consistent caregivers; holistic, patient-centered planning; and coordinated acre and services within a hospital setting. The primary nurse, or case manager, had the authority and autonomy for care decisions and was accountable to guide care delivery toward financially sound goals. Early outcomes of primary nursing models included reduced hospital length of stay and cost of care, reduced recidivism, and increased patient satisfaction. However, this early single-case or unit-based approach to care delivery in the hospital setting lacked aggregate analysis of populations and did not extend across the continuum. It also lacked measures related to physiological outcomes, quality of life, functional status, and identification of high-risk subgroups within populations.

In the first generation of an Advanced Practice RN (APRN) case management model, focus was on the one-to-one relationship of an APRN and single high-resource-user cases, or HULAS (heavy users, losers, and abusers). This model was usually initiated after an inpatient acute care stay and extended into the patient's home setting after discharge. Case finding was based on case complexity, recidivism, or other pattern of unusual utilization or high cost. This method of case finding during or after crisis and in the midst of intensive resource use is a high-cost method for subscriber systems. As the concept of outcomes management developed in the literature, the one-to-one nursing case management model within its differentiated practice context began to shift. Episodic care gave way to longitudinal management of whole populations of patients. Risk assessment of managed subscribers increased. Evidence-based care practices and evolving national guidelines mandated continuous scrutiny of local practice patterns, care methodologies, and outcomes of care. Interdisciplinary collaborative management of increasingly complex patients replaced the old paradigm of care planning and task completion, while broadening the accountability of outcomes of care. The advent of integrated clinical pathways (ICPs), reflective of "re-modeling" in the next generation, provided a collaborative, multidisciplinary foundation for care delivery coordination, and, later, for outcomes management. Clinical pathways are evolving to facilitate coordination of complex, longitudinal care driven by evidence-based care methodologies. They assist in targeting, documenting, and tracking abstractable outcomes reflecting physiological, functional, utilization, and cost outcomes. As hospital-based care moves into the community, longitudinal clinical pathways, with greater emphasis on health maintenance and self-care of chronic disease, help to focus

---

*Reprinted from Cohen, E., & De Back, V. (1999). *The outcomes mandate: Case management in health care today.* St Louis: Mosby.

attention on longitudinal outcomes. In the future, visual trajectories from these outcomes may be consumer-friendly tools to help client-provider partnerships to understand and manage self-care and health maintenance (Jensen & Koerner, 1999).

References

Ake, J.M., Bower-Ferris, S., Cesta, T., Gould, D., Greenfield, J., Hayes, P., Maislin, G., & Mezey, M. (1991). The nursing initiatives program: Practice based models for care in hospitals. In *Differentiating nursing practice: Into the twenty-first century.* Kansas City, Mo.: American Academy of Nursing.

Brett, J.L., Bueno, M., Royal, N., & Sengin, K. (1997). PRO-ACT II™, integrating utilization management, discharge planning, and nursing case management into the outcomes manager role. *JONA 27*(2), 37-45, 1997.

Cesta, T. (1991, Nov.). *Managed care,* personal correspondence and paper presented at the Annual Symposium on Health Services Research, New York.

Etheredge, M.L. (1989). *Collaborative care nursing case management.* Chicago: American Hospital Publishing, Inc. (American Hospital Association).

Jensen, G.C., & Koerner, J. (1999). Longitudinal profiling: A differential community nursing model. In E. Cohen & V. De Back (Eds.), *The outcomes mandate: Case management in health care today* (pp. 153-155). St. Louis, Mosby Inc.

Koerner, J.G., & Karpiuk, K.L. (1994). *Implementing differentiated nursing practice: Transformation by design.* Gaithersburg, Md.: Aspen Publishers, Inc.

Koerner, J.E., Bunkers, L., Nelson, B., & Santenna, K. (1989). Implementing differentiated practice: The Sioux Valley Hospital experience. *Journal of Nursing Administration, 19*(2), 13-20.

Luckenbill, J., & Tonges, M. (1990). Restructured patient care delivery: Evaluation of the ProACT ™ model. *Nursing Economics, 8*(1), 36-44.

Tonges, M. (1989a). Redesigning hospital nursing practice: The professionally advanced care team (ProACT™) model, part I. *Journal of Nursing Administration, 19*(7), 31-38.

Tonges, M. (1989b). Redesigning hospital nursing practice: The professionally advanced care team (ProACT™) model, part II. *Journal of Nursing Administration, 19*(9), 19-22.

Zander, K. (1990). Managed care and nursing case management. In G.G. Mayer, M.J. Madden, & E. Lawrenz (Eds.), *Patient care delivery models* (pp. 37-61). Rockville, Md.: Aspen Publishers.

Zander, K. (1991, April). Presentation at *Nursing care management: Transcending walls opening gates.* Wichita, Kan.: Saint Joseph Medical Center.

Two Strategies for Managing Care

Care Management and Case Management*

Cathy Michaels
Elaine L. Cohen

CHAPTER OVERVIEW

In the twenty-first century, case management models will include the management of care across the continuum. Various complementary strategies have evolved that build on an interdisciplinary system of care. Care management is one such approach that is designed to provide health planning for groups of individuals with like situations across the continuum of care.

CARE MANAGEMENT: A COMPLEMENT TO CASE MANAGEMENT

Case management is a way of managing unique and high-risk situations often associated with costly hospital use. Typically situations requiring case management involve patients whose self-care capacity and/or caregiving is diminished when their disease process and its treatment is the most intense, even life threatening. The outcome of these situations is frequent hospital and physician visits. Patients at high risk, however, represent a small percentage of the patient population.

Most patients do not face high-risk situations. The majority of health care experiences encompass situations that are usual; that is, there are resources to manage the situation or there is resolution of illness. In these instances, patients have the capacity for self-care, the support of caregivers, or an illness that can be successfully treated, like pneumonia, hip surgery, or wound care. Patients in less than high-risk situations like this do not require the one-to-one relationship of case management but do require continuity of care. Well-known examples of care management are the multidisciplinary teams for organ transplantation and rehabilitation.

Care management can provide needed continuity, establishing a system of care for a particular condition, across the continuum of care to ensure seamless transition to the right services and right providers at the right time. Patients and their caregivers who can be supported by care management can manage their own health concerns. From the risk of self-care capacity, patients at moderate or low risk merit care management, whereas case management is for patients at high risk. Who matches which risk status is a care management decision, as is who requires case management.

Care management is embedded in the work of all clinicians. Health care professionals who develop therapeutic relationships with patients know what works for people and what does not, within their own disciplinary context. Nurses have much to contribute given their emphasis on body, mind, and spirit, as well as the ability to serve people across the continuum of care.

Individuals from many disciplines serve as case managers for patients in unique and high-risk situations. Social workers, for instance, provide case management for the frail elderly and the behaviorally challenged. Nurses may best be the case managers for people with life-threatening chronic illnesses, because physical evaluation along with psychosocial assessment is critical for avoiding and minimizing the need for hospitalization. In general, our most recent experience with managing care has overrelied on approaches used in case management. Issues that relate to the clinical population are the domain of care management. Care management practices, however, are not as prevalent, because clinicians often have not knit together their collective expertise across the continuum of care and across time for groups of people in similar moderate- and low-risk situations.

Care management is a matter of clinical judgment, but decisions cannot be made in isolation of the other disciplines. Clinicians must connect and coordinate their efforts. What drives the system that is created and which discipline does what mainly depend on the available clinical resources. Boxes 5-1 and 5-2 present examples of care management teams.

BOX 5-1   **A Care Management Example for a Hospital in a Remote Area**

An interdisciplinary team established a care management system for people with chronic obstructive pulmonary disease (COPD). The hospital nursing staff assumed assessment of the patient's self-care capacity, and the respiratory therapists, the knowledge, skill, and ability related to the use of inhalers and nebulizers. If the patient is at high risk, the respiratory therapist will continue to follow the patient through home care. If, however, the person with COPD is in the end stage, the nurse case manager will follow because of the disease's complexity and end-of-life issues. This care management strategy was developed by an interdisciplinary team in a small community hospital. Clinically and financially, it was important to create a system of care for people with COPD, a fairly large population in this area without many clinical resources. Outside unit staff nurses and respiratory therapists, it was important to focus the work of the nurse case manager on COPD at the end of life, the highest of high risk. But this care management strategy can be revisited and redesigned every year by evaluating annual outcomes for this population.

BOX 5-2   **A Second Example from a Hospital in an Urban Area**

The multidisciplinary team comes together to strengthen a hospital program for congestive heart failure (CHF) and ends up considering posthospital follow-up by telephone and, if needed, home visit and prehospital emergency department CHF clinic. This bolsters the work of nurse case managers who are already in place for patients whose hospital experience exceeds more than two hospital visits in 6 months. The team reached the consensus that a system of care was needed to bolster the work of the nurse case managers.

LAUNCHING CARE MANAGEMENT

Launching a care management effort needs to build on an interdisciplinary system of care that complements case management. This can be achieved by maximizing success in improving health and well-being for people in both high-risk and less than high-risk situations at the same time, decreasing cost to the health system. *Care management* is defined as a way for clinicians to link their disciplinary efforts, programs, and services across the continuum of care for the clinical benefit of patients in like situations who are at moderate- or low-risk status with a similar health care situation and to identify when case management is called for and which discipline is in the best position to provide it. To be effective, care management must be cycled across the continuum—at a minimum from the hospital to home and across primary or specialty care settings.

The necessary clinical mindset for care management is to consider one's patient care unit at the entire continuum of care, not just a single point on that continuum, like a medical-surgical unit or home health. As such, no patient is ever discharged but rather moves along the continuum of care matched to self-care or whatever services are needed to support health and well-being. Then by developing clinical guidelines and linkages to weave together disciplinary efforts between the multiple points across the continuum of care, the therapeutic relationship between interdisciplinary providers and patients is supported rather than "taken over," as is the case with many clinical protocols and mandates (Box 5-3).

Organizing care management with a seamless and effective interdisciplinary, not just multidisciplinary, effort that best serves patients and their caregivers reflects three principles:

Principle 1: Care management is a community effort.

Principle 2: Patients are grouped by similar health and functional efforts.

Principle 3: A system of care is built to support the therapeutic relationship between providers and patients.

PRINCIPLE 1: A COMMUNITY EFFORT

In many health settings today, we are learning how to streamline clinical connections. For example, to avoid hospitalizations, we need to be able to simplify initiating home health care in the community for patients with life-threatening chronic illnesses. Initiating home health care usually requires a physician to receive clinical information about the patient and respond by ordering home health services. Often

---

| **BOX 5-3** | **EXAMPLE OF CARE MANAGEMENT OVER THE CONTINUUM OF CARE** |

Clinical diabetes educators could be the case managers for high-risk diabetic groups who experience uncontrolled blood sugar levels and make frequent visits to the emergency department. Support groups at physician offices and/or at neighborhood centers could be developed for people with diabetes who are at moderate risk for managing their health concerns (these groups are diagnosed with diabetes, but their blood sugar level is controlled most of the time with diet, exercise, and medication). Quarterly education programs could be developed for people who are at low risk or predisposed to developing diabetes and those with diabetes who are at moderate risk.

this occurs when the physician is doing other things, like seeing patients in the office or making rounds in the hospital. Delays can only increase the likelihood that hospitalization will be extended—an unwelcome disruption of life for most patients and a cost to the health system.

Clinical connections comprise programs and services across the continuum of care and the disciplines that provide care. Streamlined, these connections represent a stage of integration where we have the disciplinary interdependence to provide accessible, quality, and cost-effective care across the continuum and across time.

Interdependence is the key to building a system of clinical connections, or a system of care. We can start shifting to interdependence by inviting all the appropriate clinicians to knit together their collective efforts to assist a group of patients, or a clinical population, presenting a challenge to the health system. This interdependence is similar to a community approach that is inclusive, not exclusive. We look to who will be the right provider to do what for whom, when, where, and why. The interdisciplinary community then becomes a vehicle for mutual exchange, dialogue, and active listening. The clinicians can then organize their efforts across the continuum of care and across time, honing in on the best approach for patients given the resources of the health system.

PRINCIPLE 2: GROUPING PATIENTS

One of the first tasks in care management is to identify groups of people in like situations who feel vulnerable and present a clinical and financial challenge to the health system. These clinically relevant groups or populations are then risk stratified into high-, moderate-, and low-risk situations. Individuals in the high-risk (unique) group may require case management interventions. The interdisciplinary team can then decide which discipline is best suited to become the case manager and develop a system of consultation with the other disciplines to support the designated primary case manager in their care responsibilities. The key in this situation is not to duplicate effort, because it can be confusing to the patient and expensive to the system, not just in dollars but also in needless resource use. The interdisciplinary team can also develop care management approaches for improving the health and well-being of moderate- and low-risk groups of patients within that population.

PRINCIPLE 3: HONORING THE THERAPEUTIC RELATIONSHIP

A key to care management is building a system of care that supports the therapeutic relationship. Care management is not intended to provide a recipe or protocol for treating everyone the same. Rather, the intent is to build a system of care that streamlines the mechanics of health services so providers have more therapeutic time to spend with their patients.

In a letter to the editor, published in the *Arizona Daily Star* (1998), Isla Jacobs, a southern Arizona resident, writes about the importance of relationship: "I lament the direction the medical profession has taken. It's a big business now and seems to be preoccupied with cold efficiency. Listening to a patient's problems, whether real or imagined, has gone by the wayside. Two of the most important areas of medicine are trust and patience. In days past the doctor was truly a member of the family." Although her remarks are addressed to physicians, her words have meaning for every health care provider. Essential to a therapeutic relationship is the capacity to be heard by and be known to the professionals to whom you entrust your health. With meaningful relationships between patients and providers, successful outcomes can be maximized for patients, providers, and the entire health care system.

SUMMARY

Care management is important for every health system, regardless of whether the system is contracted to provide health care. An example of the Medicare reimbursement process helps to illustrate this point. If a patient's hospitalization costs more than what Medicare pays (either by an extended length of stay or costly care within that stay), then the health system pays the difference. Managing care within the hospitalization period can increase efficiency and lower expenses. However, managing care across the continuum can avoid and minimize the need for hospitalization in the first place and/or increase the likelihood that the patient's length of stay will be within predetermined limits. Care management is simply indispensable to a health system in that it serves as insurance for decreasing the need for costly hospital stays. The future bodes well for care management as a springboard for successful contracting.

Our current care challenges revolve around chronic conditions and aging and therefore require multiple strategies to manage care across the continuum. Case management and care management are two strategies for helping people with chronic conditions and aging issues to learn to optimize health, well-being, and self-care capacity. Case management is designed for unique and high-risk situations. Care management is the approach associated with a common diagnosis or life situation—that is, for people in moderate- and lower-risk situations. By honoring the therapeutic relationship, both case and care management can improve health and well-being while generating cost savings.

Case management is better known. Care management has yet to unfold; but not unlike care planning for hospital patients, care management is simply health planning for groups of people with like situations across the continuum of care. Based on a foundation of clinical judgment and interdisciplinary effort, care management can be a winning proposition.

Reference

Jacobs, I. (1998, Jun. 2). Lost family member (Letter to the editor). *Arizona Daily Star*, p. 8.

Bibliography

Bower, K., & Falk, C. (1996). Case management as a response to quality, cost and access imperatives. In E. Cohen (Ed.), *Nurse case management in the 21st century*. St. Louis: Mosby–Year Book, Inc.

Cohen, E., & Cesta, T. (2001). *Nursing case management: From essentials to advanced practice applications*, 3rd Edition. St. Louis: Mosby, Inc.

National Chronic Care Consortium (1995). *Risk identification*. Bloomington, Minn.: Author.

Newman, M., Lamb, G., & Michaels, C. (1992). Nurse case management: The coming together of theory and practice. *Nursing & Health Care, 12*(8), 404-408.

Stempel, J., Carlson, A., & Michaels, C. Walking in partnership. In E. Cohen (Ed.), *Nurse case management in the 21st century*. St. Louis: Mosby–Year Book, Inc.

6

Disease Management

Applying Systems Thinking to Quality Patient Care Delivery

Patricia Hryzak Lind

CHAPTER OVERVIEW

The concept of disease management is not new. It has taken on heightened interest and awareness with the evolution of managed care, cost containment, and consumerism. The Institute of Medicine's (IOM) report "Crossing the Quality Chasm" has identified areas in health care where gaps in care occur, raising concerns about patient safety and quality. Disease management processes for an at-risk population include use of evidence-based clinical guidelines to improve patient outcomes and are in concert with the IOM premises: "Disease management is a system of coordinated healthcare interventions and communications for populations with conditions in which patient self-care efforts are significant. Disease management includes:
- Supporting the practitioner/patient relationship and plan of care,
- Emphasizing prevention of exacerbations and complications using evidence-based practice guidelines and patient empowerment strategies, and
- Evaluating clinical, humanistic and economic outcomes on an ongoing basis with the goal of improving overall health" (Disease Management Association of America, 2003).

To implement a successful disease management program, a clinician must understand the natural course of the condition and treatment alternatives with attention to cost and quality of these options. The practitioner should understand how one educates an individual or a population about their condition and evidence-based treatment options. In addition, the developer must have knowledge and data about health care utilization and costs across all care settings, including elements of prevention and health promotion to maintain clients at their optimal level of wellness for as long as possible.

EVOLUTION OF DISEASE MANAGEMENT

Population-based disease management has been used by individual clinical practices in examples such as identifying and inviting all patients with diabetes for diabetic education classes or mailing educational materials to all women of childbearing age in need of Pap screening tests. Although these interventions target groups at risk, a more comprehensive approach to disease management should include the following components: assessment of patient needs, stratification of risk, identification of the problem, planning of a comprehensive group of interventions, evaluating the effectiveness of the approaches, and measurement of the clinical, cost, satisfaction, and functional outcomes.

Disease management is progressing from simply targeting those members most at risk for the disease to encompass educating populations at large about prevention and health promotion. Disease management continues to evolve from that of a chronic disease focus to a program designed to improve the health of populations served by organizations, provider groups, or the community at large. This evolution cannot occur without the integration of nursing knowledge and practice into all aspects of the program, beginning from the planning phase and throughout evaluation.

Disease management may be reaching the point of being unstoppable as an innovation. Everett Rogers (1995) chronicled the diffusion of innovations as a progression from innovators, or the first 2.5% of a field to adopt the change, to early adopters, who constitute the next 15%, and progressively to full acceptance. After an innovation has been adopted by the first 15% to 20%, it becomes mainstream and unstoppable. As more HMOs, employers, and communities implement disease management programs, the proliferation of these efforts will be more the norm than the outlier.

EVALUATING DISEASE MANAGEMENT PROGRAM

Success factors for a disease management program include several key components (Box 6-1) (Todd and Nash, 1997). The integration of information and data begins with the optimal selection of patients throughout program implementation and concludes with outcome evaluation to ensure program success. Linking program participation to cost and utilization data has become increasingly more critical as managed care organizations and employers evaluate the effectiveness of either targeted or prevention programs on their bottom lines. Targeted programs are aimed at specific patients with chronic conditions such as diabetes. Further specificity occurs in these programs by choosing patients at increased risk such as those with nonadherence to treatment plans or a lack of preventive care such as annual eye examinations. This aspect of disease management has become easier with the development of health care information systems that track and trend these data. However, the future holds additional opportunities with the integration of encounter-level data, increased accuracy at targeting at-risk patients, linkages to utilization data that can be trended for longitudinal studies, and additional research in guideline implementation and the refinement of valid and reliable instruments to assess progress toward outcome measures.

A sound method for calculating return on investment is also critical to program implementation and evaluation. Disease management programs must prove their worth in today's cost-conscious and competitive

---

BOX 6-1 ▶ KEY SUCCESS FACTORS FOR DISEASE MANAGEMENT

- Understanding the course of the disease
- Targeting patients likely to benefit from the intervention
- Focusing on prevention and resolution
- Increasing patient compliance through education
- Providing full-care continuity across health care settings
- Establishing integrated data management systems
- Aligning incentives

From Todd, W.E., & Nash, D. (1997). *Disease management—A systems approach to improving patient outcomes.* Chicago: American Hospital Publishing Co.

health care environment. Purchasers and developers of disease management programs are becoming more sophisticated in understanding how programs affect their health care costs, participant quality of life or functional status, consumer satisfaction, clinical outcomes, and, for businesses, productivity of their employees. Statements about "return on investment" must be substantiated with actual health care costs and accurate calculations of cost avoidance. Estimates and approximations are increasingly being replaced with calculations based on actual health care expenditures. Innovative programs will continue to develop and flourish if these programs use data to demonstrate actual health care savings, increased worker productivity, and improved quality of life.

Determining the "teachable moment" for patients or providers, or the point in a treatment algorithm when the greatest health impact can be achieved, continues to provide opportunities for research; a "teachable moment" is that point when the patient is ready and able to change behavior to achieve a healthier state. For providers of health care, it means recognizing where the patient is along the change continuum and providing information and support in concert with the patient's current status. The *transtheoretical model of change* (Prochaska & DiClemente, 1983; Prochaska, DiClemente, & Norcross, 1992; Prochaska & Velicer, 1997) is a model of intentional behavior change that describes how people modify a problem behavior or acquire a positive behavior. The model focuses on the decision-making of the individual and his or her readiness to change at each stage. Used in smoking cessation and other addictions, in weight loss, and with people who have chronic conditions, the model is useful in determining when a patient is ready to make a life change and is helpful in determining an approach that yields positive results.

Using a quality improvement framework, determining what interventions have the most impact, is necessary to continuously advance patient care. The timing and type of intervention and how it is delivered via clinician, media, or technology continue to change as new health and patient education innovations enter the market. Research as to the most appropriate and cost-effective type of intervention refines approaches to patient care as well as contain costs. The optimal timing and method of reinforcement of education to sustain a behavior change are critical to learning more about patient education and motivation. All of these areas continue to be fruitful opportunities for research and program evaluation studies.

Disease management continues to change as new and different partnerships emerge. Partnerships among managed care organizations, employers, and disease management programs continue to develop. Employers are using data such as the Health Plan Employer Data Information Set (HEDIS) or the National Committee for Quality Assurance (NCQA) Quality Compass to identify health plans that improve the health and satisfaction of the work force. Contractual relationships between employers and disease management companies have emerged as employers search for ways to have healthy employees who are productively at work (Lumsdon, 1995). Employers may evaluate each health plan's preventive and disease management interventions to select the insurer who offers well-developed programs with proved and sustained outcomes to help employees maintain and improve their health and ultimately their work productivity.

Accreditation bodies, including the Joint Commission on the Accreditation of Healthcare Organizations (JCAHO), National Committee for Quality Assurance, and the American Accreditation Healthcare Commission (URAC), have implemented certification processes for disease management programs. Through accreditation, aggregate outcome analysis may form a standard set of performance measures and ensure program consistency with evidence-based guidelines (Edlin, 2003).

Consumers are being charged by their employers, as well as their care providers, with taking responsibility for their own health status. Lifestyle concerns such as obesity, nutrition, and substance use contribute to overall health state. Although a health care provider can counsel and educate patients about these issues, the ultimate change rests with each patient. Employers in turn are shifting health care costs to their employees through higher premiums and copayments. Some employers have charged a higher premium contribution for those employees who smoke, thus adjusting for increased health costs.

Consumers are actively seeking health information. Deering (1996) found that 80% of consumers with mental and physical health problems sought information about their condition and 67% to 79% read advertisements or watched television, respectively, about health or medicine concerns. Clearly, consumers are seeking knowledge and are looking to partner with their practitioner, employer, or managed care company to support their health behaviors.

The alignment of incentives supports the success of any disease management program. Risk contracting within managed care organizations or capitation as a reimbursement mechanism encourages the determination of the most cost-effective treatment in the most cost-effective setting (Ichter, 1998). The use of incentives or rewards with education of patients to seek optimal levels of health as well as necessary preventive care, must be in concert with the financial aspects of physician reimbursement. If physicians are penalized for preventive service utilization or are not at risk for costly hospital services, the incentives for prevention are incorrectly aligned with disease management programs.

Employers have instituted wellness incentives through self-insured products. These programs consist of monetary incentives or rebates when specified health behaviors are achieved. Targeted changes may include smoking cessation, weight loss, or sustained exercise program attendance. Programs have been well accepted by employees with increased employee health and satisfaction.

Managed care plans supply provider profiling reports that include data on individual patients within selected populations. A sample annual profile might contain a list of all patients with asthma, the number of office and emergency department visits within the past year, the number of filled prescriptions for inhaled corticosteroids, and whether the patient had an influenza vaccination the previous fall. These reports may be given to assist the physician or nurse practitioner in care provision or quality improvement opportunities identified by the managed care plans. Monetary incentives may be linked to the data if the managed care plan tried to increase prescribed inhaled corticosteroids after an acute asthma exacerbation or attempted to raise the percentage of at-risk members who receive an influenza vaccination.

For disease management programs to be successful, the alignment of the incentive to the sought-after behavior is critical. To achieve this goal, data must be accurate and contain an actionable plan for the patient or provider. Barriers to care must be assessed and understood. Modes of receiving information may be varied and based on patient preference. Reinforcement of the desired behavior should be rewarded and sustained. Patient behavior includes adherence to treatment regimens, including drug therapy, diet, exercise, and lifestyle changes; therefore, understanding aspects of self-care, including how and when to self-medicate, is important in managing a chronic condition.

Program evaluation should be multidimensional, allowing the developer to thoroughly analyze the interventions and program impact. These should include patient satisfaction, health care utilization and cost, functional status and quality of life, and clinical outcomes. A program that increases health care utilization but causes a decrease in functional status and unsatisfied consumers needs critical review and revision. Additional information about evaluation is included later in this chapter.

Disease management programs continue to grow and evolve, as does the role of the nurse in the development, implementation, and evaluation of these programs. Consumerism and the patient's quest for health care information, the proliferation of the information through technology such as the Internet, and changing provider–patient relationships into partnerships also provide opportunities for nurses to influence the health and knowledge of populations. Nursing can do much to promote the concept of health management through the development and implementation of programs that support primary prevention while implementing disease management programs that target individuals who are in need of interventions at the secondary or tertiary levels of prevention.

DISEASE MANAGEMENT PROGRAM DEVELOPMENT

Defining the Population

In a great mystery, knowing "who done it" ahead of time ruins the book. For disease management, knowing "who needs it" ahead of time ensures program success and potentially guarantees customer satisfaction. Defining the population and knowing that you have selected the patients who truly have the condition and could benefit the most from your intervention would be disease management "utopia." "Targeted populations might include high-volume clinical services, high-cost health care expenditures, services that have great variation in clinical practice, services that may pose a significant risk to patients, clinical opportunities for improvement, or patient care situations where long-term complications are linked to provider risk" (Doxtator & Rodriguez, 1998, p. 186).

Disease management programs must be in concert with the needs of the organization. Using a framework for planning is helpful (Figure 6-1). Understanding the program goals is essential. If the vision of the program is to decrease inpatient readmissions after hospitalization for depression, the design of the program is different than that of a program designed to increase worker productivity related to unscheduled absences for migraines. Knowing what the organization wants to achieve with the disease management program and why this change is needed are the first steps in program design.

Some conditions are more suitable for disease state management than others. Although chronic conditions account for 75% to 80% of health care costs and treatment, these conditions may show a more

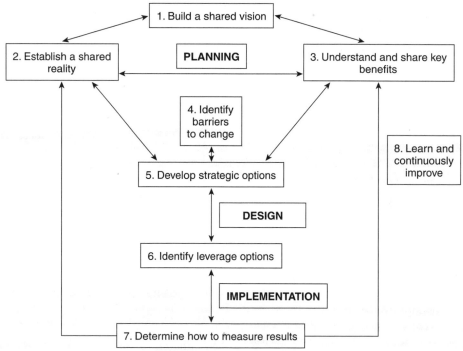

FIGURE **6-1**   Systems-thinking model: The disease management process.
Redrawn from *Todd, W.E., and Nash, D. (1996). Disease management—A systems approach to improving patient outcomes. Chicago: American Hospitals Publishing Co.*

rapid return on investment than preventive health program. Specific elements are necessary before a condition can be selected for disease management; these include patient education for self-care, sharing of real-time patient care data and best practices with clinicians, and the ability to influence the continuum of care to improve outcomes and lower costs.

The next step is to abstract data to substantiate the need for the program. Employers might obtain the data from their Workers' Compensation files or from absentee records. Managed care organizations may analyze annual health care utilization data to determine clinical conditions that are the drivers for inpatient, emergency, outpatient, primary care, or pharmaceutical health care costs. Providers, through their office database, may determine those clinical conditions seen frequently in their office. Each of these examples may identify one or more clinical conditions that, through a disease management program, could improve patient care, decrease health care costs, or shift utilization to a more appropriate level of care. Analyzing data over several years allows for a clear identification of the program rather than aberrant data due to patient outliers or unusual clinical conditions. Trending data and comparing the findings with regional or national benchmarks validates incidence and prevalence to further ensure the methodology for correct patient identification.

A number of companies have entered the market with a variety of data abstraction systems to identify patients for interventions. Based on organizational needs and goals, a careful analysis of the data extraction systems, company and provider community acceptance of these types of systems, and robustness of the educational interventions assists in decision-making. There are information systems that identify patients with the health condition as well as systems that attempt to detect patients at risk or those who are undiagnosed. Selection of a system based on goals with attention to confidentiality and state and federal legal considerations varies based on practice location. For practices that span state lines, knowledge of legislation is essential. Privacy statutes such as the Health Insurance Portability and Accountability Act (HIPAA) require strict patient confidentiality and restrict utilization of individually identifiable health information.

Another organizational data need is a system to manage and evaluate individual case management clients. Separate systems may be necessary, one as a patient identification system and another as a data tracking system, for case management. The case management system should contain demographic information such as patient identification; data input capabilities for health outcome, satisfaction and functional status surveys, and a link to cost and utilization data. The ability to analyze this progress of individuals and populations is essential. The interface with current information systems and analysis software is part of the evaluation process in selecting software. In addition, patient confidentiality and security safeguards require careful scrutiny. Short-term tactical solutions such as database development projects, stand-alone PC-based software, or stand-alone reporting initiatives can provide helpful lessons for the selection of long-term strategic initiatives such as data warehouse systems (Matthews, 1999).

Disease management programs are built from a quality improvement perspective. The identification of strategic opportunities that achieve program planners' goals as well as participants' purpose is paramount to success. Early generations of disease management targeted "low-hanging fruit" or those patient care opportunities that, with simple interventions, could realize cost savings and changes in health behavior. Examples of such first-generation programs included mailed influenza vaccination reminders to at-risk patients and outbound telephone calls to schedule retinal eye examinations for diabetic patients or to remind chronically ill patients about medication refills. Following these types of interventions, targeted case management programs emerged for high-risk patients.

Disease management programs attempt to educate everyone within a selected population. Individual case management interventions are aimed at high-risk patients and provide customized interventions to address their specific patient care needs. An example of this approach would be mailing educational interventions to all managed health care plan members with diabetes to remind them of preventive care and to provide information on diabetic education. Individualized case management would occur with newly diagnosed members, those recently prescribed insulin pumps, or those recently hospitalized for complications related to their diabetes. Individual case management reinforces the continuing relationship between the patient and the primary care provider, through the use of an individual plan of care.

Understanding who bears the financial risk for health care costs is also an important part of the planning process. Providers may share financial risk with managed care organizations. As the managed care organization communicates data related to quality improvement activities, the practitioner may be rewarded or penalized for compliance with these initiatives. Examples of data sharing would include profiles of patients with diabetes in need of retinal eye examination or lists of patients with congestive heart failure without evidence of prescribed angiotensin-converting enzyme inhibitor medications. Monetary rewards or penalties may be tied to the level of patient compliance and/or physician education about preventive care and chronic conditions.

Todd and Nash (1997) predict that the next generations of disease management will include "truly integrated care" leading to "health management." They define *integrated care* as a program that aligns care and reimbursement, and they include risk stratification for patients with interventions that are matched to patient risk. Health management encompasses prevention as well as disease management through the "collection of health status, health risk and severity data, and the linkage of this information to clinical and economic outcomes data for the purpose of determining the predictors of health, disability, illness, disease, complications and probability of eventual outcome" (Peterson & Kane, 1997, p. 307).

PLANNING THE INTERVENTION

Planning the intervention includes researching the literature and interviewing colleagues who have implemented similar programs. Published research may contain the outcomes, instruments, and tools suggested to achieve goals. Actual implementation strategies may not be included. Unpublished program information may be presented at professional seminars that assists with other avenues for planning interventions. Direct contact with authors may yield helpful information.

Understanding available human, information, communication, educational, and financial resources is essential. Determining who are the organizational champions, to assist in gaining more of these resources, is also paramount to program success. A clinical team approach to disease management would involve primary care and specialist practitioners, including physicians, nurses, and social workers, as well as pharmacists. Additional assistance from data and financial analysts, quality improvement specialists, and outcome measurement experts would augment the team process and product. Integration of these champions into the planning process assists greatly in achieving program goals.

The proliferation of pharmaceutical companies within this aspect of health care is unprecedented. Often in partnership with data management companies or universities, pharmaceutical companies are attempting to strengthen their programs with the data to support their interventions and costs. The organization must decide if the disease management program will be purchased from a vendor or developed within the company or clinical practice. Each approach has its benefits and drawbacks. A careful analysis of resources also assists the planner and the decision-makers in selecting the "buy or build" route.

Development of a business plan to determine whether to partner with a vendor or develop one's own program is required. A careful analysis of the partner's history, scope of services, implementation work plan, measurable outcome results, program costs, and data integrity is conducted. A review of the company's business alliances may also prove enlightening. If the vendor is linked to a pharmaceutical company, one might explore expectations about drug promotion or formulary placement. Review of sample data extractions against one's own data warehouse validates whether the correct patients have been selected for the intervention. A thoughtful review of each partner's objectives, skills, and patient care contributions assists with the decision as to whether a disease management vendor adds value to the clinical initiative.

Contractual arrangements between the employer, physician, or managed care organization and the disease management vendor are necessary. Key elements in the contract should include "the type of agreement, identification of the intervention group, establishment of analysis for cost baselines, profiling of disease data elements, requirement for resource costing, seasonal adjustment procedures and definition of terms, contract dynamics and management" (Langley, Langley-Hawthorne, Martin & Armstrong, 1996, p. 1099). Legal review of the contract in concert with a clinician's scrutiny determines how patients, providers, and employers accept and embrace the program interventions.

New patient educational media and technology continue to enter the health management market. Patient reminders through interactive voice response systems, list serves and interactive websites on the Internet, and patient registration for educational program through cable television networks are just the start of new modes of providing patient education. Several of these approaches also include prelearning and postlearning assessments and integration of standardized instruments to assess functional status or quality of life to measure the effect of the intervention on an individual. Individual and population data are then available for analysis about the effectiveness of the education and/or the technology. These types of program also allow consumers to access education whenever they desire and often in their home rather than through structured classroom sessions.

Determining the data source for identification of at-risk patients and measurement of intended outcomes early in the planning process is critical. When one understands the source of the data and data limitations, one can address these issues proactively or account for them in the intervention or analysis. Many managed care organizations use administrative claims data coupled with their own demographic database. These data are derived from paid health care claims and may vary based on provider coding or be delayed by billing procedures. Patients who should obtain care but do not are not identified for intervention because they have no paid health care claims. Patients without prescription coverage cannot be targeted for pharmaceutical interventions. Supporting administrative claims data with survey data or chart audits enriches patient identification but adds cost to the program.

Conduction of a barrier analysis also assists in program development. A barrier analysis involves the identification of obstructions to program development or resources. This information allows the planner to understand these obstacles and develop a proactive plan to address them. Comprehending the barriers to program implementation at this point is also crucial. Disease management programs with misaligned incentives or those that lack physician, patient, or employer cooperation are difficult to implement successfully. Identification of alternatives within the program for discussion with key constituents may assist greatly with overcoming these barriers.

Once the population is defined, a pilot approach allows a "test run" of the intervention, including perceptions of the program participants and health care providers. For example, during the planning of a program to encourage pregnant women on Medicaid to obtain early and consistent prenatal care, focus groups might be held with women in their second pregnancies to determine the educational materials, appointment adherence rewards, and program barriers to patient implementation. Their realistic and constructive feedback would allow for changes in proposed printed materials and program processes before community implementation. A similar approach might be used to gain insights from high-volume obstetrical offices to assess proposed implementation processes in the physician or midwife's practice.

Determining the type and format of patient education materials to be used is also essential. Most purchased or self-developed disease management programs offer mailed or web-based educational materials to assist consumers in learning more about a particular aspect of their condition. Some programs have developed websites with educational materials, self-assessments, or hyperlinks to national organizations to assist patients. Telemedicine, interactive voice response programs, software programs, interactive laser disks, DVDs, CD-ROM materials, and other types of media continue to enter this market. Demand management companies offer outbound telephone calls to at-risk members providing reminders, education, and support. Whatever the method chosen, the material must be understandable to the patient, be in concert with published national standards or guidelines, offer resources for additional information, and, if necessary, be approved by governmental agencies if provided to Medicare or Medicaid patients.

Some programs offer educational group sessions. Group educational sessions should use tested curricula that have been reviewed by health care providers and patients. Many national organizations, such as the American Diabetes Association and the American Lung Association, offer educational programs for patients and their families. Information about program availability, cost, location, and frequency of program offerings should be validated before distribution. A discussion with the agency is also helpful to review common goals, operational issues such as program promotion and attendance increases, the possibility of discounts, and a plan for data collection to assist with outcome evaluation. Some managed care plans have negotiated discounts or reduced rates for their members. Others offer rebates when a patient has completed a self-help course.

Consumer testing and validation of program incentives are helpful. Individuals and groups differ as to what is valued. What is acceptable to a pregnant woman on Medicaid may be different from what is appreciated by a Medicare patient with a chronic condition. In addition, the acceptability of incentives or prizes to the population, the providers, and any government regulations affects the use of rewards.

If the planned disease management intervention also includes individual case management of high-risk members, planning for these resources in advance is also required. As more patients and health care providers become aware of the program, referrals for individual case management increase. Some of these referrals will be for patients who are truly at risk for complications or increased health care utilization. Other referrals will be for patients who desire additional information or resources to better self-manage their condition. Knowing the program goals and available resources and developing a plan to assist consumers who want to enhance their self-management allow the case manager to blend the roles of disease management implementation with individual case management.

IMPLEMENTATION OF THE PROGRAM

If planning is everything, implementation is the icing on the cake. Well-planned programs with pilots allow developers to test interventions and their acceptability to the consumer and health care provider or employer before full population implementation. Pre-testing instruments, determining readability of the consumer materials, developing processes for distributing materials or gathering data, and assessing practitioner acceptability of the program should all be completed. Implementation serves as a time of continuous quality improvement, making program adjustments as needed with a clear vision of the outcomes expected and desired.

One practitioner intervention may be the distribution of clinical practice guidelines. As has been widely published, national guidelines often need modifications for acceptability to local practitioners. At the implementation stage, these guidelines are distributed to care providers beyond the program champions, developers, or provider test groups. Program champions serve a vital role in the community "personalization," dissemination, and implementation of clinical practice guidelines.

The Department of Veterans Affairs has implemented a complete electronic medical record (EMR) which includes a program of clinical reminders. Based on nationally recognized clinical practice guidelines, clinicians are electronically reminded to assess, educate and provide care to at-risk patients. The defined interventions may include preventive health education, screening assessments or examinations, immunizations or specialty referrals. Monthly reports provide the clinicians with individualized and comparable data on their practice patterns and use of clinical reminders. A contracted independent assessment of reminder completion demonstrates a significant improvement in process and outcomes measures of evidence-based care.

There are many benefits to using clinical practice guidelines, including the distillation of relevant scientific literature and national standards into a document that supports evidence-based practice and the identification of specific patients for interventions and practical recommendations for care management. Practice guidelines also allow the establishment of key intervention points and outcome measures to reduce variability in care.

Guidelines include challenges and controversy. Practitioners may be unreceptive to "cookbook" medicine, be concerned about the legal implications, or debate the content or literature used to substantiate their development. Practical aids such as profiling systems, reminder letters, or patient education materials that support guideline parameters, removal of barriers to care access, and office supports such as reminder stickers or check sheets are valuable supports to the disease management program goals.

Guidelines like those used in disease management programs are never stagnant. A scheduled annual or semiannual review of their recommendations and usefulness is essential to their implementation and ongoing credibility with practitioners. Guideline success is built on access to ongoing evidence-based practice information, patient management tools, reliable data and evaluation parameters, continuing reminders about the guidelines, and their intended patient care outcomes and clinician involvement in the development, dissemination, and evolution of this practice tool.

EVALUATION OF THE DISEASE MANAGEMENT PROGRAM

Process and outcome measures for the disease management program should be determined at the development and planning phase and be based on program goals. A multidimensional approach to evaluating the disease management program is integral to assessing program efficacy and effectiveness. The development and use of standardized outcomes methodology for disease management initiatives are anticipated.

In 1997 the National Committee on Quality Assurance (NCQA) released its first data using the Quality Compass 1997, a database containing performance, accreditation, and patient satisfaction information from more than 300 managed health plans throughout the United States. The concept of the Quality Compass 1997 is based on the use of standard measures and tools to assess specific aspects of care and service throughout managed care plans. This model provides the opportunity to assess care globally across many managed care plans and has relevance to other care delivery sites. NCQA continues to use this methodology to educate consumers and employers on plan-specific managed care organizational performance.

The Clinical Value Compass (Figure 6-2) was developed to assess quality evaluation in clinical settings. Using Donabedian's constructs of structure, process, and outcome, "the logic underpinning the compass is that providers will measure the value of care for similar patient populations, analyze the internal delivery processes that contribute significantly to the current levels of measured outcomes and costs, run tests of changed delivery processes and determine if these changes lead to better outcomes" (Nelson, Mohr, Batalden, & Plume, 1996, p. 246). The four poles of the compass represent member satisfaction, functional status, cost associated with care, and clinical status.

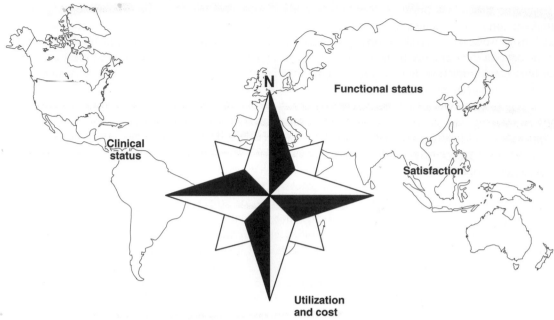

FIGURE **6-2**   Clinical Value Compass.

The applicability of the compass directions to measure program outcomes can be used within managed care plans, physician offices, integrated delivery systems, or employer-developed disease management programs. The Clinical Value Compass approach has four cardinal points: functional status, costs, satisfaction with care, and clinical outcomes. Based on outcomes management, this framework allows determination of specific results in each quadrant. These quadrants are representative of not only outcomes management but also the focus of health maintenance organizations, disease, or case management systems.

The directional points of the compass were developed through various research studies (Batalden & Stoltz, 1993; Batalden, Nelson, & Roberts, 1994; Nelson & Batalden, 1993; Nelson & Wasson, 1994). Functional status measures may include standardized instruments such as the Medical Outcomes Study Short-Form 12 or 36 (Ware, Snow, Kosinski, & Gandek, 1993) or a quality-of-life measure specific to the program condition or disease process such as arthritis. Use of these types of tools allows comparison with other populations or published research. Instruments should be valid and reliable rather than "homegrown" to ensure accurate measurement of the outcome. Permission to use the instrument must be obtained before use, to comply with copyright regulations.

Patient satisfaction with the intervention is another measure that is part of the compass framework. Satisfaction surveys may measure participant satisfaction with the type of intervention they perceived they received, the amount of assistance offered by the intervention, and their satisfaction with their personal health outcome following the disease management intervention. Again, a standardized satisfaction survey that is found to be valid and reliable serves as a measure of participant satisfaction.

Health care utilization can be measured through pretest and posttest measures of service delivery. The number and cost of emergency department visits for a defined population of patients with asthma would constitute a utilization measure. Because of the seasonal or episodic variation of this illness as well as enrollment patterns within a managed care plan, continuous enrollment logic may be applied. To ensure accuracy and program evaluation over time, the selection of patients who have been constantly enrolled within the agency or health plan for 2 years provides longitudinal data. The measurement would then include use of the emergency department for this population for 2 years before the intervention and for 2 years after the intervention. If a more timely measure is needed, the comparison of emergency department use within one spring allergy season to the following season may be used. When designing health care utilization measures, factor in any issues related to access that might affect this measure such as changes in copayments, increased number of urgent care centers, or expanded primary care office hours.

Clinical outcome measures should also be thoughtfully chosen before intervention. For example, increased retinal eye examinations may be a process measure to the outcome measures of diabetic retinopathy as a complication of blindness. The timelines of the measure, as well as the access to data that may not be available for several years, must be considered as clinical outcome measures are chosen.

Another clinical measure may include a standardized HEDIS measure. HEDIS allows consumers and employers to compare performance across the managed care industry; to publish national, regional, and state averages; and to establish benchmarks for care and service measures. The incorporation of an HEDIS measure would allow evaluators to compare findings across their own data and to benchmarks.

Two aspects of financial measures must be considered for the final pole of the compass framework. One measure is the health care costs affected through the disease management program intervention. For example, one might measure the costs associated with the emergency department visits in the previous example about the asthma disease management program. To determine this, elements such as copayments, negotiated rates for emergency department care, cost of medications, and treatments or professional services given in the emergency department would all be calculated into the preintervention and postintervention calculations.

When calculating the total program return on investment, all aspects of expenditures to support the program must be included. A *basic return on investment model* assists with the program analysis. Understanding the definitions of various types of costs and benefits such as direct versus indirect, fixed versus variable, and hard versus soft assists with program calculations. "The use of an actual cost model is the most accurate and sophisticated accounting method; many health systems lack this advanced accounting capabilities" (Doxtator & Rodriguez, 1998, p. 189).

From the cost of the initial data extraction to target the population to the final measures based on the compass framework, accounting for costs is essential to a true analysis of return on investment. The collection of data to capture decreases and increases in utilization and revenue, ongoing program support costs, "soft" estimates, and initial program investment over periods of time, including the baseline and annually throughout the life of the program, are necessary. Determining the payback period is recommended. Because of the seasonal nature of some conditions, garnering physician buy-in to the program as well as patient enrollment, a 3-year payback period is often recommended. Assistance from the financial and quality analysts is important to extract the financial costs and contrast them to the savings related to health care utilization and costs.

HEALTH MANAGEMENT FOR THE FUTURE

Disease management programs tend to be developed and proliferate where an oversupply of physicians or hospitals exist. Because of increased competition and demand from employers, the health care systems that focus on outcomes and can deliver these quality improvement changes initiated programs to meet these requirements. Often when the reimbursement structure changes to capitation or a set fee per patient, disease management programs are instituted to promote education and self-help and shift costly care to the most appropriate, cost-effective site of care. Some or all of these elements exist wherever health care is administered. Disease management program development is based on knowledge of the condition, finding the right population for information and self-management, aligning provider and patient incentives for care, developing information systems to allow sharing data and care across the continuum, and focusing on prevention.

Predictive modeling, a mathematical approach to patient identification in need of additional health resources, is a new addition to the disease management repertoire. Previously used in financial services to predict credit risk, in meteorology for weather events, and by colleges for academic performances, predictive modeling attempts to find consumers who are at risk for chronic conditions and those with chronic conditions at risk for co-morbidities (McCain, 2001). Using medical and/or pharmacy claims in conjunction with demographics and self-reported information, the analysis predicts risk or health care costs for the future. Approaches to predictive modeling vary from identification of at-risk or undiagnosed patients to detection of patients lacking a clinical guideline recommendation, to those who could benefit from findings in newly published research. The focus of predictive modeling is the improvement of clinical outcomes by supporting clinicians and consumers in decision-making.

The next generations of disease management may expand to a "total population management" approach through customized resources for risk identification and stratification, wellness programs, disease and case management and end-of life care (Edlin, 2002, p. 46). Although disease management continues to be present as long as there are chronic conditions, health management will focus on chronically ill populations as well as healthy groups. Health promotion programs have long been the cornerstone of nursing. No matter the name, program components or sponsor nurses are vital to the process of improving care for populations. Optimal care for populations can be achieved through nursing leadership in the development, implementation, evaluation, and reimbursement for population-based health management.

References

Batalden, P.B., Nelson, E.C., & Roberts, J.S. (1994). Linking outcome measurement to continual improvement: The serial "V" way of thinking about improving clinical care. *The Joint Commission Journal of Quality Improvement, 20*(4), 167-180.

Batalden, P.B., & Stoltz, P.K. (1993). A framework for the continual improvement of health care: Building and applying professional and improvement knowledge to test changes in daily work. *The Joint Commission Journal of Quality Improvement, 19*(10), 424-447.

Committee on Quality Health Care in America, Institute of Medicine (2001). *Crossing the Quality Chasm: A new health care system for the 21st century.* Washington, D.C.: National Academy Press.

Deering, M.J. (1996). Consumer health information demand and delivery: Implications for libraries. *Bulletin of the Medical Library Association, 84*(2), 209-216.

Disease Management Association of America (2003). A definition of disease management. Available at www.dmaa.org.

Doxtator, R.F., & Rodriguez, D.J. (1998). Evaluating costs, benefits, and return on investment for disease management programs. *Disease Management, 1*(4), 185-192.

Edlin, M. (2003). Disease management accreditation helps plans focus even more on quality care. *Managed Healthcare Executive, 13*(1), 38-40.

Edlin, M. (2002). Total population management reduces future treatment costs. *Managed Healthcare Executive, 12*(11), 46-47.

Ichter, J.T. (1998). The link between disease management and capitation contracting: Financing population health. *Disease Management, 1*(1), 27-30.

Langley, P.C., Langley-Hawthorne, C.E., Martin, R.E., & Armstrong, E.P. (1996). Establishing the basis for successful disease management. *The American Journal of Managed Care, 2*(8), 1099-1108.

Lumsdon, K. (1995). Hard labor. *Hospitals & Health Networks, 69*(13), 34-42.

Matthews, P. (1999). Case management information systems: How to piece together now and beyond year 2000. *Nursing Case Management, 4*(2), 80-89.

McCain, J. (2001). Predictive modeling holds promise of earlier identification, treatment. *Managed Care, 10*(9), 12-15.

National Committee for Quality Assurance (1997, Jan.). *HEDIS 3.0—Health Plan Employer Data Information Set.* Washington, D.C.: National Committee for Quality Assurance.

National Committee for Quality Assurance (1997, Oct.). *The state of managed care quality*, Press release: Washington, D.C.: American Association of Health Plans.

Nelson, E.C., & Batalden, P.B. (1993). Patient based quality improvement measurement systems. *Quality Management in Health Care, 21*(1), 18-30.

Nelson, E.C., Mohr, J.J., Batalden, P.B., & Plume, S.K. (1996). Improving health care, Part 1: The clinical value compass. *The Joint Commission Journal on Quality Improvement, 99*(4), 243-256.

Nelson, E.C., & Wasson, J.H. (1994). Using patient-based information to rapidly redesign care. *Healthcare Forum, 37*(4):25-29.

Peterson, K.W., & Kane, D.P. (1997). Beyond disease management: Population based health management. In W.E. Todd & D. Nash (Eds.), *Disease management—A systems approach to improving patient care* (pp. 305-346). Chicago: American Hospital Publishing Co.

Prochaska, J.O., & Velicer, W.F. (1997). The transtheoretical model of health behavior change. *American Journal of Health Promotion, 12*, 38-48.

Prochaska, J.O., & DiClemente, C.C. (1983). Stages and processes of self-change of smoking: Toward an integrative model of change. *Journal of Consulting and Clinical Psychology, 51*, 390-395.

Prochaska, J.O., DiClemente, C.C., & Norcross, J.C. (1992). In search of how people change: Applications to addictive behavior. *American Psychologist, 47*, 1102-1114.

Rogers, E.M. (1995). Lessons for guidelines from the diffusion of innovations. *Journal of Quality Improvement, 21*(7), 324-328.

Todd, W.F., & Nash, D. (1997). *Disease management—A systems approach to improving patient outcomes.* Chicago: American Hospital Publishing Co.

Ware, J.E., Snow, K.K., Kosinski, M., & Gandek, B. (1993). *SF-36 Health survey manual and interpretation guide.* Boston: The Health Institute, New England Medical Center.

III

CONTEMPORARY MODELS OF CASE MANAGEMENT

Within-the-Walls Case Management

To sustain responsiveness to the mandates of managed care environments and a rapidly changing health care system, new generations of acute care–based case management models have unfolded. Unit III offers a portrait of the many innovative strategies, rich and successful models that have evolved across the country. These models have at their core the principles of interdisciplinary cooperation, relationship building, active communication, comprehensive support for continued health care needs, and client and family advocacy. These approaches speak to the contributions of all providers to maintaining the health of the public.

Within-the-Walls Case Management

An Acute Care–Based Nursing Case Management Model

with Joanne Woodall

CHAPTER OVERVIEW

This chapter reviews various models of within-the-walls case management. This approach became popular when hospitals began restructuring to improve productivity, manage effective use of resources, lower costs, and maintain quality.

Strong evidence indicates that this patient care delivery model has a great effect on resource use and quality patient care. Daily assessment and evaluation of the patient's clinical care, reduced length of stay, enhanced capacity management, increased patient throughput and other financial benefits, general applicability of this model, and improved nurse, physician, and patient satisfaction demonstrate the merit and relevancy of this approach to patient care delivery and professional practice.

COST-EFFECTIVE CARE

The changing nature of health care economics has forced hospitals to view case management as an alternative to the delivery of direct care services. Hospital-based case management is founded on traditional approaches. It ensures the most appropriate use of services by patients. A case management system in the hospital setting avoids duplication and misuse of medical services, controls costs by reducing inefficient services, and improves the effectiveness of care delivery (Lavizzo-Mourey, 1987). Lavizzo-Mourey (1987), McIntosh (1987), and Henderson and Collard (1988) reported several advantages of hospital-based case management. First, the hospital setting offers a wide range of specialized skills that can be made available to both the provider and recipient of case management services. Second, because most of the resources needed for patient care are centralized within the acute care setting, early assessment of patient needs, planning and coordination of care delivery, and evaluation of alternative systems are enhanced. Third, because space and overhead costs are factored into hospital-based care, the management of expenditures associated with high-cost patients is minimized. Fourth, systems for monitoring and measuring the cost-effectiveness of case management arrangements are present within the hospital setting.

Many hospital-based case management systems have engaged registered nurses (RNs) as case managers (Henderson & Collard, 1988; Henderson & Wallack, 1987; McIntosh, 1987). Nurse involvement in case management allows nurses to influence and direct the delivery and quality of patient care. Such involvement allows for more control, visibility, and recognition for nursing services delivered. The involvement also offers more consistent outcome attainment and demonstrates nursing personnel contributions to patient care (Zander, 1988a).

Because it would be virtually impossible to cover all patient models of nursing case management that may currently exist, this chapter focuses on some of the systems that have served as the foundation for the development of within-the-walls case management. The chapter also highlights the approaches to patient care delivery and professional practice that have received national attention.

PRIMARY NURSE CASE MANAGEMENT MODEL

Nurse case management has emerged in the acute care setting as a professional model of practice. One model, characterized as a *primary nurse case management model*, has been used at the New England Medical Center in Boston, Massachusetts. Stetler (1987), Woldum (1987), and Zander (1988a, 1988b, 1990) identified the following factors that distinguish this case management system of care.

Primary nurse case management is based on the concept of managed care. *Managed care* is defined as care that is unit based, outcome oriented, dependent on a designated time frame, and focused on the appropriate use of resources for both the inpatient and outpatient populations.

Primary nurse case management services and caseloads are designated for specific patient case types or case mixes. Examples of case types coordinated by primary nurse case management are cardiac, leukemia, pediatric, gastrointestinal, stroke, craniotomy, and some gynecological.

Nurse case managers are the primary caregivers for patients. The managers provide direct care to patients in their caseloads while the patients are housed in their units, and they continue to coordinate the care of these patients throughout hospitalization, regardless of the patient's physical location.

The process of care is monitored by the use of case management plans, which include diagnosis-related group (DRG) length of stay; critical pathway reports, which outline the components of appropriate care; and variance analysis, which ensures the continuous evaluation of patient care activities.

Care is coordinated through collaborative group practice arrangements across geographic units, case consultation, and health care team meetings. Patient discharge planning is outlined before admission and updated throughout hospitalization until the time of discharge.

The New England Medical Center's nursing case management model presents an innovative alternative to the delivery of nursing care within the acute care setting. The model has evolved since its introduction and has been widely adapted.* The development of care multidisciplinary action plans (MAPs) increases the potential for evaluating the cost-effectiveness and quality of care standards proposed by this model. Care MAPS have expanded on case management plans and critical paths by focusing on standards of care and practice for a specific case type, responding to variances in the delivery of care, linking continuous quality improvement (CQI) to practices, and integrating resource allocation, patient care outcomes, and cost reimbursement systems (Zander, 1991, 1992a, 1992b).

The competence and experience of the case manager are critical to the effective delivery of patient care services (Henderson & Wallack, 1987). The case management model at the New England Medical Center, along with most nurse case management programs, primarily uses RNs as case managers. A case manager must have at least 1 year of nursing experience and charge responsibilities and must demonstrate leadership ability. Henderson and Wallack (1987) and Henderson and Collard (1988) recommend that to ensure cost-effective care and quality assurance standards, the nurse case manager should have expertise

---

*Conceptually, case management is now considered a strategy for the coordination of care and is evolving into a sophisticated resource for managing access, quality, and cost (Bower & Falk, 1996).

related to the care of designated types of patients and specific diagnostic categories. Because of the model's reliance on a primary nursing care delivery system, staffing mix allocation was not differentiated in the New England Medical Center's model. Some case management programs have successfully used a variety of personnel other than professional nursing staff. Studies are needed to determine the best staffing mix for nursing case management programs.

Contrary to what Zander (1990) reported about the nursing case management model at the New England Medical Center, a study in another institution has shown a preliminary increase in direct nursing care hours and greater use of resources during the initial phase of hospitalization. These changes resulted in an overall decrease in length of stay, an increase in patient turnover, and a potential increase in patient revenues generated for the hospital (Cohen, 1991).

LEVELED PRACTICE MODEL

Another nursing case management model, identified as the *leveled practice model*, has focused on the management and coordination of patient care needs. This system differs from the primary nurse case management model in that the case manager's functions are focused on the management activities of patient care and not on the responsibility for patient care delivery (Loveridge, Cummings, & O'Malley, 1988; O'Malley & Cummings, 1988). A work group consisting of RNs, licensed practical nurses, and nurses' aides provides direct care on a specific patient unit. The professional nurse is designated as the case manager and is responsible for coordinating and monitoring patient care of an assigned caseload through collaboration with the work group, patient, family, and interdisciplinary health team members. In addition, the case manager relies on information related to case mix, hospital costs, patient resource use, insurance, and reimbursement data (O'Malley & Cummings, 1988).

The leveled case management model has promoted differentiated practice arrangements by delineating functional role responsibility and accountability between those nurses with baccalaureate degrees and those with associate degrees (Loveridge et al., 1988). Differentiated competence levels in nursing practice were classified extensively by Primm (1986). Because of the principles inherent in leveled practice case management, the role of the professional staff nurse becomes an autonomous one. Consequently, this change in practice places different obligations on the nurse manager. The nurse manager's role becomes what MacGregor-Burns (1978) described as *transformational leadership*, which focuses on teaching, mentoring, and coaching activities. In the leveled practice nursing case management model, management responsibility emphasized overall administrative and fiscal support, as well as patient outcome assessment and quality care improvement (Loveridge et al., 1988; O'Malley & Cummings, 1988).

PRIMARY CASE MANAGEMENT

The primary case management model, which was developed and implemented at Hermann Hospital in Houston, Texas, embraced the primary nursing philosophy of care and used a clinical career ladder for RNs (Cavouras et al., 1990). The clinical ladder consisted of six levels of clinical expertise, which progressed from a patient-focused orientation at the beginning levels to interdisciplinary and general service practice responsibility and accountability as nurse case managers at the top level.

The primary case management model used unit-based case managers who were responsible for coordinating, developing, and evaluating the delivery and the quality of patient care. Staff nurses and nurse extenders provided the care, which was based on standard protocols. The care plans outlined the daily care requirements and activities and served as a mechanism for monitoring and evaluating issues related to quality and as a patient care resource for nursing and hospital-wide support services such as laboratory, pharmacy, and respiratory therapy. Quality improvement was also monitored through unit-based quality assurance programs.

Cost-effectiveness, quality of care, and nurses' job satisfaction were also evaluated through retrospective variance analysis of patient charges and length of hospital stay, quality-assurance monitoring, and nurse satisfaction surveys. To date, no data have been published.

SAINT VINCENT'S CATHOLIC MEDICAL CENTERS INTEGRATED CASE MANAGEMENT MODEL

Case management models in the late 1990s were beginning to reflect the need to integrate previously disconnected services. Saint Vincent's Catholic Medical Centers in New York City designed and implemented an integrated design model in 1997. The model integrates three functions of the case manager under one umbrella; these include the clinical coordination/facilitation role of the case manager, utilization management (UM), and discharge planning. Each acute care case manager is unit based and performs these interrelated functions for all patients on the unit to which they are assigned. In the past, each of these functions was performed by a separate care provider. This fragmentation resulted in higher cost, longer length of stay, and an inefficient system.

To make the system more efficient and more responsive to a managed care environment, a number of structural changes were made. These included a redefinition of the functions listed earlier with a realignment of the functions under the role of the case manager. This more streamlined approach to care delivery resulted in a more efficient, integrated care delivery process and reduced the need to "pass the baton" from one team member to the next.

Case managers use guidelines and multidisciplinary action plans as tools in the clinical coordination/facilitation aspect of their role (Appendix 7-1). The guidelines delineate the appropriate resources and length of stay for various case types. The case managers are responsible for collecting variations from the guidelines as part of their daily variance collection process. Other variances collected identify system delays and clinical issues, quality issues, and unmet clinical outcomes.

The data are reviewed daily and individual issues are addressed. The data are also aggregated and reviewed for potential quality improvement efforts. For example, magnetic resonance imaging (MRI) delays are collected in the following four categories that identify the cause of the delay:

Delays related to scheduling

Delays related to lack of weekend availability

Delays related to unavailable reports

Delays related to equipment failure

Repetitive, substantive delays are addressed in terms of the cause of the problem and potential solutions. An interdisciplinary team is often assembled to address the problem and develop an action plan for correcting the problem.

In the role of clinical coordinator and facilitator, a number of functions may be performed; among these are development of the interdisciplinary plan of care and expediting diagnostic testing and treatments as identified by the plan of care. This clinical focus fosters a partnership with the physicians and other members of the health care team. It allows the case manager to identify and suggest opportunities to deliver care more efficiently and/or at lower cost.

The case managers are also responsible for performing UM functions. This includes using established review criteria such as the Milliman and Robertson Guidelines (Doyle & Schibanoff, 1997) to perform insurance reviews. They are in daily communication with the third-party payer and work to ensure that the hospital is reimbursed for every day that the patient is in the acute care setting. Services are reviewed to ensure that they are medically necessary and reasonable, provided in the most appropriate setting, and at or above quality standards.

Discharge planning functions were moved from under the responsibility of social work to the responsibility of the registered nurse case manager. This required a redefinition of the role of the social worker from one of discharge planning *coordinator* to discharge planning *collaborator*. Social workers were redeployed to perform other, more comprehensive social work functions such as the following:

Counseling and psychosocial support
Coping with end-of-life issues
Substance abuse
Financial issues
Family support issues

Case managers perform the initial assessment and refer patients to the social worker based on high-risk screening criteria developed for specific clinical areas. For example, medical/surgical services have their specific list of criteria (Table 7-1), whereas the emergency department has a different list of criteria (Table 7-2). The coordination function of discharge planning is performed by the RN case manager.

In an effort to better manage the routes of entry to the hospital, case managers are also assigned to the emergency and admitting departments. The case managers in the emergency department review

TABLE 7-1	**GUIDELINES FOR REFERRALS**

Registered Nurse Case Managers/Social Workers in Medical/Surgical Inpatient Adult Services

Registered Nurse Case Manager	Social Worker
Performs admission and concurrent utilization management, including insurance calls	Patient/family has difficulty coping with new diagnosis (e.g., cancer, ventilator dependency), difficulty understanding/accepting decision-making re: the long-term discharge planning options)
Coordinates/facilitates plans of care	Psychiatric, cognitive, or behavioral factors that may impede delivery of care and discharge planning process
Facilitates daily rounds and team meetings	Inadequate supports that may have an impact on compliance with continuing care needs (NOTE: Social workers can provide case managers with information to give to patients and families, concerning entitlements.)
Assessments of all patients for psychosocial needs	Ethical or legal concerns (e.g., patient, family, team conflicts related to medical plan of care, guardianship cases or end-of-life issues around advance directives, DNR)
Discharge planning, including equipment, home care, rehabilitation, and long-term care facilities	Suspicion or evidence of domestic violence, elder abuse or neglect, child abuse or neglect, rape, or sexual assault; known to protective services for adults (PSA)
Orders transportation	Substance abuse counseling referrals where patient requests or is viewed as amenable to intervention

Courtesy of St. Vincent's Hospital and Medical Center, New York, New York; revised 5/99.

Continued

TABLE 7-1	GUIDELINES FOR REFERRALS—CONT'D

Registered Nurse Case Managers/Social Workers in Medical/Surgical Inpatient Adult Services

Registered Nurse Case Manager	Social Worker
Completes PRIs	Unidentified patient or patients are seriously ill and there is difficulty locating significant others
Oversight of clinical guidelines	Patients signing out against medical advice (AMA) (the hospital's AMA policy is currently under review)
Tracks data (e.g., variances in patient care and systems standards)	Homelessness (e.g., new onset, patient is unable to return to prior living situation)
Provides ALC notification	Long-term nursing facility placements for patients with complex family or financial situations
Issues HINN letters	

PRI, Patient review instrument; *ALC*, alternate level of care; *HINN*, hospital-issued notice of noncoverage.

TABLE 7-2	GUIDELINES FOR REFERRALS

Registered Nurse Case Managers/Social Workers in the Emergency Department

Registered Nurse Case Manager	Shared Responsibilities: Registered Nurse Case Manager/Social Worker	Social Worker
Admission utilization review: intake assessment of admitted patients	Coordinate/facilitate plans of care for discharged patients	Patient/family has difficulty understanding/accepting and/or following through on medical plans of care and continuing care options
Utilization/insurance calls	Transportation	Interventions regarding issues affecting access to continuum of care (e.g., immigration problem, primary caregiver, or disabled person)
Coordinate/facilitate plans of care for admitted patients	Patient education (e.g., reinforcement regarding follow-up with medical appointments, medical regimen)	Advocacy and counseling around entitlements or other essential services (e.g., Medicaid, Food Stamps, housing, medications)

TABLE 7-2	GUIDELINES FOR REFERRALS—CONT'D

Registered Nurse Case Managers/Social Workers in the Emergency Department

Registered Nurse Case Manager	Shared Responsibilities: Registered Nurse Case Manager/Social Worker	Social Worker
Screening/assessments of patients for psychosocial needs in conjunction with plan of care	Crisis intervention needed for patient/family having difficulty coping with illness, family dysfunction, trauma, death, accidents, injuries, substance abuse	Suspicion or evidence of domestic violence, elder abuse or neglect, child abuse or neglect, sexual assault
Discharge planning, including equipment, home care, infusion treatment	Referrals for nursing homes, adult homes, shelters	Ethical or legal concerns (e.g., patient, family, team conflicts related to medical plan of care, guardianship or protective services for adults [PSA] cases, end-of-life issues around advance directives)
Initiate inpatient discharge planning		Referrals for home supports for psychosocially complex patients
Participates in the development of emergency department guidelines for care		Referrals for marital, individual, or family treatment
Track data (e.g., variances in patient care standards, systems standards)		Assistance needed in locating families of unidentified, seriously ill patients
Clinical resource for staff		Tracking of difficult-to-locate patients for follow-up medical care
Facilitates patients' progress through the emergency department to disposition		
Oversees/facilitates transfers from institution to institution		

all potential admissions for appropriateness and make referrals to outside agencies when needed. Their initial case management assessment is made and included as part of the in-hospital patient documentation on all admitted patients. The care processes of treat-and-release patients are expedited by the case manager and through the use of emergency department clinical practice guidelines that differentiate the appropriate interventions and time frames for treating various emergency conditions.

The case manager in the admitting department performs parallel functions. She or he reviews all planned admissions and transfers for appropriateness and performs a case management assessment on surgical patients in preadmission testing. This documentation and a preliminary discharge plan are transferred electronically to the unit-based case manager. The collaborative effort performed by the admitting and emergency department case managers helps prevent inappropriate or unnecessary admissions and ensures that the patient is receiving the care needed in the most appropriate setting.

The design of the case management model at Saint Vincent's connects three role functions that had been disconnected in the previous care delivery system. This integrated approach reduces redundancy, duplication, and delays. Within the first year of implementation, the hospital achieved its target goal length of stay reduction of 1.1 days. Insurance denials were reduced by 30% in medical/surgical and by 80% in psychiatry. Patient complaints regarding discharge planning and communication of the plan of care were reduced by 20%.

TUCSON MEDICAL CENTER CASE MANAGEMENT MODEL

JoAnne Woodall

Past

A case management model developed at Tucson Medical Center (TMC) in the late 1980s addressed the cost and quality aspects of patient care delivery (Del Togno-Armanasco, Olivas, & Harter, 1989). This approach incorporated elements of the New England Medical Center's case management model and differentiated practice models in addition to basic philosophic practice components of primary nursing and shared governance.

Called *collaborative nursing case management*, this model primarily focused on standardizing the use of patient care resources and the delivery of services during the patient's hospitalization for selected DRG case types. Both patient mix and service volume management strategies were used to attain cost-effective, quality patient care (Olivas et al., 1989a).

A collaborative case management plan (CCMP) and a care plan MAP were used to identify the contributions of all health care providers and to support a unit-specific standard of patient care. Variations from practice standards were also monitored and evaluated. The care plan MAP was revised in 1991 to meet requirements of the Joint Commission on Accreditation of Healthcare Organizations (Gwozdz & Del Togno-Armanasco, 1992). It was also used as a basic documentation form.

Hospitalwide and unit-specific multidisciplinary practice committees were established to assist in clinical decision-making and overall evaluation processes of the patient care model. These groups consisted of physical therapists, dietitians, social workers, physicians, and home care professionals (Olivas et al., 1989b). Patients were encouraged to participate and were included in the planning of their care regimens, which are carried out on a continuous basis from the time of admission to after discharge.

Various evaluation mechanisms were developed to measure the potential impact of this case management model on outcomes of care. A patient satisfaction questionnaire and a retrospective chart review were implemented along with a physician-satisfaction-with-care questionnaire to ascertain variables related to patient care and job satisfaction. Information on cost of care, rate of absenteeism, and staff turnover also were collected. Findings showed increased satisfaction with both nursing and medical care (at the .05 alpha level) for case-managed, total hip replacement, coronary bypass, and valvular surgery patients. There was no turnover of nurse case managers, and a marked decrease in turnover rates was demonstrated for nursing staff on the oncology and orthopedic units.

Outcome data also showed a decreased length of stay among patients who underwent total hip and knee replacements. The decrease was 3.48 and 2.82 days, respectively, over a 3.5-year period. Length of stay for valvular replacement and coronary bypass patients also decreased. In addition, a positive cost variance of $9273 was realized for the valvular replacement and coronary bypass patient populations (Del Togno-Armanasco, 1992).

As noted, case management of TMC started as a unit-based nursing clinical model. Within a short time, notable success was demonstrated in the areas of satisfaction and cost savings. Lengths of stay decreased, costs diminished, and patient and physician satisfaction increased. When case management was initiated, TMC had a Department of Patient and Family Services made up of social workers, who performed discharge planning, crisis counseling, and medical-legal intervention on a consulting basis. In addition, the Department of Utilization Management, made up of nurses, performed the required utilization review/management functions. These departments coexisted and interfaced with case management. It became apparent that these departments were frequently involved with the same patients, the same charts, and the same issue. The resulting redundancy offered an opportunity for improvement.

Present

In 1996, in response to efforts to maximize efficiency and reduce redundancy, a number of significant changes were made. The unit-based case managers were centralized into a case management team (CMT) led by a steering committee of administrative leaders, director of budget and finance, and vice president for patient care. The Department of Patient and Family Services soon became part of this team, combining the social workers and nurse case managers into the same centralized department. UM was downsized to two nurses, and these nurses were also moved into the CMT. UM functions became part of the nurse case manager's role, with the designated UM nurses performing education and oversight for this function. The result of these moves was to create one department with a net savings of full-time equivalents (FTEs).

The decision to combine these specialties into one department was grounded in solid rationale. Both social workers and nurse case managers use the tools of expert assessment, planning, coordination, and communication to do effective and timely discharge planning. This facilitates timely discharge by eliminating delays for nonmedical reasons and ensuring a safe discharge with a plan in place to support the patient's continuing recovery or end-of-life needs. Recognizing that both medical and social complexity can contribute to extended lengths of stay and recidivism, the expertise of the nurse case manager and the social worker can each be used to greatest advantage, depending on the predominant risk factors presented by individual patients.

Similarly, both UM nurses and nurse case managers are involved in ensuring appropriate level of care, expediting the medical plan of care by eliminating system barriers, and ensuring accountability for utilization of expensive and finite resources. Both of these roles require review of the chart, communication with the physician, and coordination with payers to ensure reimbursement for services. Clearly, the roles of nurse case manager, social worker, and UM have significant areas of overlap (Del Togno-Armanesco et al., 1995). It is also apparent that the goals of each specialty are the same—to meet the health needs of the patient in the most effective and resource-efficient way.

Combining departments that share the same goals and many of the same functions seems like an obvious path to increased efficiency. However, bringing people together into the same department does not ensure the successful creation of a functional team. The literature is full of examples of territory conflict between nurse and social worker case managers. The difficulty in combining the roles of UM nurse and nurse case manager is also well documented (McKenzie, 1989; Hospital Case Management, 1996). The merging of these groups requires a change in identity, clarity of purpose, flexibility, and a high level of trust and willingness to learn. As TMC moved forward to make these changes, the following barriers were identified:

1. No unified model for case management was in place throughout the system.
2. The case managers frequently operated in isolation from each other and developed many procedures and processes that differed from one area to another. This was frequently confusing

for physicians and other staff and impaired the smooth transition of patients from one unit to the next and from one case manager to the next. Case managers receiving patients from another area frequently thought that they were "reinventing the wheel" because elements of the case management plan were lost and patients were subjected to redundant assessments and intakes.

3. Social workers were redefined as case managers when they joined the case management team, but for the most part they continued to function as social work consultants, much as they had in the past. Nurse case managers and social workers triaged tasks rather than designating patients to their respective case loads based on either medical or social risk criteria.

4. Nurse case managers verbalized that they viewed UM as another task to be added to those that they already did. They were resistant to letting go of clinical functions, which they knew, liked, and valued, to make room for the utilization review/UM function. The UM nurses, on the other hand were uncomfortable letting go of their utilization review/UM responsibilities to the case managers, who did not value them in the same way, and verbalized their concern that the quality of UM was diminishing.

5. The members of the new CMT did not feel or function like a team. They felt like various pieces put together for organizational purposes. Their comfort level with their jobs as they knew them was threatened. They were expected to do new things in a different way but were unsure how to go about it or even if they wanted to.

The challenge at TMC was to overcome the barriers and to emerge with a unified and highly functional CMT, fully using the tremendous resources of knowledge, expertise, and experience brought to the group by members of each of the specialties. The expected outcomes were to enhance the effectiveness of all of the group members by sharing and expanding skill sets and to more successfully and efficiently promote the goals of case management and the organization.

The following strategies were used to overcome barriers and accomplish the outcomes:

1. *Clearly define a mission and purpose statement for the CMT that directly supports the overall vision and goals of the organization* (Appendix 7-2).

2. *Develop a model for case management that incorporates nursing, social work, and UM into one cohesive team* (Appendix 7-3).

3. *Define and differentiate core case management functions common to all of the team members and specialty case management functions that belong to the expertise of each specialty area* (Appendix 7-4).

4. *Write job descriptions for nurse case manager, social worker case manager, and UM case manager that clearly reflect the above functions and competencies.*

5. *Develop a model by which patients are triaged to either the nurse or social worker case manager, depending on medical or social high-risk criteria* (Appendix 7-5). This model was developed through a process of defining medical and social high-risk criteria for case management of inpatients. It is acknowledged that patients are at risk for high-cost/high-utilization care for reasons that relate to medical complexity as well as social complexity. High-risk patients are designated to the caseload of the nurse or social work case manager, whoever is most qualified to deal with the identified issues. For patients with both medical and social complexities, the social worker and nurse collaborate and consult.

6. *Offer continuing education opportunities on case management topics.* The case management team compiled a list of educational requests and needs. This list was used as a springboard to develop a staff development calendar, using internal and external experts to present information on designated topics at biweekly meetings. The TMC case management team also cooperated with the Southern Arizona Chapter of Case Management Society of America (CMSA) to offer a preparatory

course for the CCM exam. An on-site case management seminar was brought to TMC and attended by all of the CMT.

7. *Conduct biweekly team meetings to discuss issues, celebrate successes, process decisions, and share information.* CMT staff meetings are held on weeks alternating with the staff development presentations. These meetings provided opportunities for disseminating organizational information, discussing case management issues, communicating projects and successes of individuals and clinical clusters within the CMT, problem solving, and giving subteam reports.

8. *Develop case management processes that move with the patients across the lines of specialty units to create seamless flow and continuity and reduce redundancy.* One of the identified goals of case management is to facilitate seamless patient movement through the system. Because the case manager is a critical communication link, the case management processes must reduce redundancy and ensure continuity. The key touch points identified are admission, transfer, and discharge. Case management assessment and communication forms and processes were developed and standardized by the team to ensure that these touch points do not become gaps and that continuity and quality are protected.

9. *Implement individualized learning plans for case managers having difficulty in role definition.* Because of the inconsistencies in how case management originated in various clinical units at TMC, role definition was an obstacle for some of the case managers. In several instances, individualized reorientation plans were created and implemented to assist case managers to more clearly define their role and function. These learning plans included mentoring, rotations with other case management specialists, and observational experiences with community case managers. This approach was very successful and, in some cases, the recipients of this reorientation opportunity went on to become mentors and role models for others.

10. *Promote a case management identity, both for individual team members and for the team as a whole.* On occasion, the case management team meeting is replaced by a potluck meal, where food and fun are the agenda. Team-building programs and human dynamics seminars were developed and offered as a means of improving communication, appreciating differences, and working effectively as a group.

These strategies had measurable success—for example, (1) patients with 10 of the 15 top DRGs admitted to TMC showed decreased lengths of stay; (2) there was a decrease in social worker calls to the emergency department since it was staffed with nurse case managers; (3) medical/social high-risk criteria were used to screen every patient and to assign the appropriate nurse or social work case manager; (4) one third of the nurse case managers achieved national certification in case management; (5) case management team members assumed responsibility for planning and presenting staff development programs for the remainder of the team; and (6) numerous process improvement projects were initiated, including critical pathways and a readmissions project. These indicators of team success enhanced the goals of cost and quality improvement, which are the ongoing objectives of case management.

This is not the end of the story. TMC continues to have new issues that challenge its ability to provide quality state-of-the art care while managing cost and reimbursement. Case management must continually redefine itself to anticipate and respond to these changing needs. To fully appreciate where it has been, from where it has come, and where it is going, the case management department conducted a self-evaluation. The process was informal and interactive, and the conclusions left the participants with the renewed belief that this case management team is in some meaningful ways stronger and more relevant than ever, as a result of the challenges that brought about change.

Early in the 2000s, case management was faced with staff reductions, along with the entire organization. This resulted in a case management staff reduction of nearly 30%. The department was forced to scrutinize work processes, priorities, and flexibility to continue to meet the needs of the patients and the organization. The most notable outcome of this era of reorganization of case management was the emergence of a nursing and social work case management staff that has become highly cross-trained. With reduced numbers, the nurses and social workers no longer had the luxury of sharing cases, but they increasingly trained each other to handle issues and situations traditionally seen as "strictly social work" or as "strictly nursing." Although these specialties within the case management team still consult freely and frequently with each other, there is a much greater sense of "cross-competence" between the disciplines. The TMC model still recognizes the unique functions of each of its specialties (see Appendix 7-4), but the lines between the sets of specific specialty functions have blurred.

Case managers are also much more comfortable moving between clinical service lines in the hospital. With a strong case management identity, staff members see themselves less as "cardiac" or "neuro" case managers and more as case management specialists who have a body of skills and knowledge that can be generalized to many different environments. There also is a per diem staff, made up of nurse and social work case managers who float to provide the ability to staff up or down depending on census or need. These changes have improved the flexibility and efficiency of the department. With this flexibility, we have been able to provide weekend coverage for the hospital as well as on-call coverage for evening hours, with no increase in FTEs.

Our emergency department case management model has undergone major reengineering. During the staff reduction period, the emergency department case management position was eliminated. The original purpose for having a case manager in the emergency department was to have a "gatekeeper" to divert unnecessary admissions during the time when TMC had capitated contracts. With changes in contracting, the capitated risk went away, health plans became the gatekeepers, and the primary purpose for emergency department case management diminished. However, new challenges, as fed by the nursing shortage, reduced numbers of staffed beds, and emergency department bottlenecking, created a mandate to bring back the emergency department case management position. This time, the purpose is to help to decompress the emergency department by facilitating the speedy discharge of patients not requiring hospitalization and to contribute to the timely movement of patients through the system. This change, along with a host of other process changes taking place throughout the system, contributed to the reduction of emergency department divert time from approximately 60% to less than 10%. The emergency department case manager also handles issues that were previously thought to be "social work" issues, greatly reducing the need for social workers to leave their units to respond to needs in the emergency department.

The utilization case managers have also evolved significantly over the past 3 years. The staff has increased from two to four FTEs. It was recognized that even though all case managers have a responsibility for resource and UM, the formal review functions were not being given the attention that they required when placed on the already overfull plate of the case managers. So, with the exception of two highly specialized populations—pediatrics and high-risk antepartum—the reviews are being done by the utilization staff. The UM approach has become more proactive and interactive with the rest of the case management staff as well as the entire health care team in an effort to identify and reduce avoidable days and denials. In addition, the UM staff is actively involved in concurrent DRG assignment and physician education to ensure accurate documentation. This effort has improved coding accuracy, allowed for more accurate reimbursement, and supported a morbidity and mortality profile that more accurately reflects the acuity and complexity of the patients treated at TMC.

Case management at TMC has its roots in the need to become more efficient and cost-effective in providing quality services to patients and families. We are continually finding new and better ways to do this as the health care environment presents us with new challenges. Members of the TMC case management department believe that even though the change process has been painful at times, we have emerged a stronger, more flexible, and more effective team.

References

Bower, K.A., & Falk, C.D. (1996). Case management as a response to quality, cost, and access imperatives. In E. Cohen (Ed.), *Nurse case management in the 21st century* (pp. 161-167). St Louis: Mosby–Year Book, Inc.

Cavouras, C.A., Walts, L., Taylor, S., Garner, A., & Bordelon, P. (1990). Alternative delivery system: Primary case management. In G. Mayer, M. Madden, & E. Lawrenz (Eds.), *Patient care delivery models* (pp. 275-282), Rockville, Md.: Aspen Publishers, Inc.

Cohen, E. (1991). Nursing case management: Does it pay? *Journal of Nursing Administration, 21*(4), 20-25.

Del Togno-Armanasco, V. (1992). [Collaborative Case Management: Outcome data]. Unpublished raw data.

Del Togno-Armanasco, V., Olivas, G., & Harter, S. (1989). Developing an integrated nursing case management model. *Nursing Management, 20*(5), 26-29.

Del Togno-Armanasco, V., Hopkin, L., & Harter, S. (1995). How case management really works. *American Journal of Nursing* 24I-24L.

Doyle, R.L., & Schibanoff, J.M. (1997). *Healthcare management guidelines, Vol. 1,* Chicago: Milliman & Roberston.

Gwozdz, D.T., & Del Togno-Armanasco, V. (1992). Developing an integrated nursing case management model. *Nursing Management, 20*(5), 26-29.

Henderson, M.G., & Collard, A. (1988). Measuring quality in medical case management programs. *Quality Review Bulletin, 14*(2), 33-39.

Henderson, M.G., & Wallack, S.S. (1987). Evaluating case management for catastrophic illness. *Business and Health, 4*(3), 741.

Lavizzo-Mourey, R. (1987). Hospital based case management. *DRG Monitor, 5*(1), 1-8.

Loveridge, C., Cummings, S., & O'Malley, J. (1988). Developing case management in a primary nursing system. *Journal of Nursing Administration, 18*(10), 36-39.

MacGregor-Burns, J. (1978). *Leadership.* New York: Harper & Row.

McIntosh, L. (1987). Hospital based case management. *Nursing Economics, 5*(5), 232-236.

McKenzie, C.B., Torkelson, N.G., & Holt, M.A. (1989) Care and cost: Nursing case management improves both. *Nursing Management 90*(1), 30-34.

Olivas, G., Del Togno-Armanasco, V., Erickson, J.R., & Harter, S. (1989a). Case management: A bottom-line care delivery model. Part 1: The concept. *Journal of Nursing Administration, 19*(11), 16-20.

Olivas, G., Del Togno-Armanasco, V., Erickson, J.R., & Harter, S. (1989b). Case management: A bottom-line care delivery model. Part 2: Adaptation of the model. *Journal of Nursing Administration, 19*(12), 12-17.

O'Malley, J., & Cummings, S. (1988). Nursing case management. 3: Implementing case management. *Aspen's Advisor for Nurse Executives, 3*(7), 8-9.

Primm, P.L. (1986). Entry into practice: Competency statements for BSNs and ADNs. *Nursing Outlook, 34*(3), 135-137.

Should case managers absorb UR, discharge planning? (1996, Oct.), *Hospital Case Management*, 145-148.

Stetler, C.B. (1987). The case manager's role: A preliminary evaluation. *Definition, 2*(3), 1-4.

Woldum, K. (1987). Critical paths: Marking the course. *Definition, 2*(3), 1-4.

Zander, K. (1988a). Managed care within acute care settings: Design and implementation via nursing case management. *Health Care Supervisor, 6*(2), 24-43.

Zander, K. (1988b). Nursing care management: Strategic management of cost and quality outcomes. *Journal of Nursing Administration, 18*(5), 23-30.

Zander, K. (1990). Managed care and nursing case management (pp. 37-61). In G.G. Mayer, M.J. Madden, & E. Lawrenz (Eds.), *Patient care delivery models.* Rockville, Md.: Aspen Publishers, Inc.

Zander, K. (1991, Fall). Care Maps TM: The core of cost/quality care. *The New Definition, 6*(3), 1-3.

Zander, K. (1992a, Winter). Physicians, care maps and collaboration. *The New Definition, 7*(1), 1-4.

Zander, K. (1992b, Spring). Quantifying, managing, and improving quality. 1: How care maps link CQI to the patient. *The New Definition, 1*(2), 1-3.

APPENDIX 7-1

St. Vincent's
Hospital and Medical Center

MULTIDISCIPLINARY ACTION PLAN

Diagnosis: *Carotid Stenosis*

Procedure: *Carotid Endarterectomy*
          ☐ Left
          ☐ Right
          ☐ Bilateral

Date/Time of arrival on unit: _____

Anticipated length of stay (including day of surgery): 1 day

Case Manager: _____

Social Worker (if applicable): _____

Goals mutually set with patient and/or family:
Yes ☐
No ☐ Explain: _____

Initials	Signature/Title	Initials	Signature/Title

MAP009 7/98

ST. VINCENT'S HOSPITAL AND MEDICAL CENTER MULTIDISCIPLINARY ACTION PLAN
DAY OF SURGERY

Procedure: Carotid Endarterectomy

MD: _____

RN: _____

Date: _____

MAP Does not Replace MD Orders		Notes
TESTS/PROCEDURES/ TREATMENTS	Nursing assessment and A-line monitoring q1 hr × 4-6 hr Maintain systolic BP > 100 & < 180 Discontinue A-line after 4-6 hrs if systolic BP stable If stable and A-line D/C'd, nursing assessment q2 hr × 6 & if stable then q4 hr Complete nursing admission assessment Notify MD if T ≥101° Measure intake and output × 8 hr; D/C if urinary output sufficient HOB ↑ 30° Incentive spirometer 10 × q1 hr while awake	
MEDICATION	IV: 1 liter _____ @ _____ cc/hr. D/C when stable & tolerating PO fluids Demerol _____ mg & Vistaril _____ mg IM q3-4 hr PRN pain When tolerating PO, Percocet 1-2 tab PO q3-4 hr PRN pain ASA 325 mg PO qd	
ACTIVITY	OOB to chair within 4 hr, then progressive ambulation as tolerated	
NUTRITION	NPO until alert, then clear fluids Advance to cardiac prudent diet as tolerated	
CONSULTS		
PATIENT EDUCATION	Assess, instruct, and evaluate re: ■ Unit orientation ■ Pain modalities ■ Post-operative preventive care Give and review carotid endarterectomy patient MAP, if not previously received	
SOCIAL WORK	Psychosocial assessment and intervention, and D/C plan, as indicated	
CASE MANAGEMENT	Evaluate individual patient/family needs; initiate referrals and consults, as indicated	

MAP009 (10/98)

ST. VINCENT'S HOSPITAL AND MEDICAL CENTER MULTIDISCIPLINARY ACTION PLAN
DAY OF SURGERY

Procedure: Carotid Endarterectomy

MD: _____
RN: _____
Date: _____

Patient Problem and Nursing Interventions	Expected Patient Outcome and/or Discharge Outcome	Assessment/Evaluation		
Alteration in Body Systems	Complications will be Prevented/Minimized			
1. Nursing assessment		1.	1.	1.
A. *Vital signs & neurovascular check*	A. VS & neurovascular status WNL	A. (Flow sheet)	A. (Flow sheet)	A. (Flow sheet)
B. *A-line*	B. Hemodynamically stable	B. (Flow sheet)	B. (Flow sheet)	B. (Flow sheet)
C. *Assess orientation to person, place & time*	C. Oriented to person, place, & time	C. (Flow sheet)	C. (Flow sheet)	C. (Flow sheet)
D. *Assess lung sounds & RR*	D. Respirations unlabored & even; lungs clear. Using incentive spirometer, coughing and deep breathing	D. (Flow sheet)	D. (Flow sheet)	D. (Flow sheet)
E. *Assess if neck dressing is intact, and/or for the presence of drainage/bleeding. HOB ↑ 30°*	E. Neck dressing dry and intact	E. (Flow sheet)	E. (Flow sheet)	E. (Flow sheet)
F. *Palpate abdomen, nating distention or discomfort. Auscultate for bowel sounds. Assess presence or absence of nausea, vomiting and flatus Advance diet*	F. Abdomen soft, not distended Minimal/no nausea/vomiting Tolerating diet	F. (Flow sheet)	F. (Flow sheet)	F. (Flow sheet)
G. *Assess bladder for distention*	G. No signs/symptom of complications Voiding without difficulty	G. (Flow sheet)	G. (Flow sheet)	G. (Flow sheet)
H. *Assess circulation and mobility of extremities*	H. No signs/symptoms of complications	H. (Flow sheet)	H. (Flow sheet)	H. (Flow sheet)
I. *Assess IV site for redness, edema, & pain. Ascertain IV is patent & infusing*	I. No signs/symptoms of complications IV D/C'd when stable & tolerating fluids	I. (Flow sheet)	I. (Flow sheet)	I. (Flow sheet)
Alteration in Comfort	Pain R/T Postoperative Period will be Prevented/Minimized			
1. Incisional pain: A. *Assess level of pain (use 1-10 pain scale)* B. *Administer pain medications* C. *Assess effect of pain medication* D. *Use comfort measures and diversional measures*	1. Verbalize minimal discomfort after Intervention implemented 2. Attain identified goal of pain relief	1. (Flow sheet)/ (MAR)	1. (Flow sheet)/ (MAR)	1. (Flow sheet)/ (MAR)
Knowledge Deficit R/T Surgical Procedure and Discharge Planning	Increased Knowledge R/T Postoperative Care & Discharge Planning			
1. Assess knowledge/instruct/ evaluate re: ■ Pain relief ■ Preventive postoperative measures.	1. Verbalize understanding &/or Demonstrate: ■ Preventive postoperative measures & pain relief	1.	1.	1.
2. Review plan of care, including possible discharge date and follow-up plan	2. Verbalize understanding of plan of care, discharge date & time, & follow-up plan	2. (Discharge summary)	2. (Discharge summary)	2. (Discharge summary)

MAP009 (10/98)

ST. VINCENT'S HOSPITAL AND MEDICAL CENTER MULTIDISCIPLINARY ACTION PLAN
POSTOPERATIVE DAY 1

Procedure: Carotid Endarterectomy

MD: _____

RN: _____

Date: _____

MAP Does not Replace MD Orders		Notes
TESTS/PROCEDURES/ TREATMENTS	Nursing assessment q8 hr 6A-2P-10P Notify MD if T >101° HOB ↑ 30° Incentive spirometer 10 × q1 hr while awake	
MEDICATION	Percocet 1-2 tab PO q3-4 hr PRN pain ASA 325 mg PO qd Initiate usual prescription medications	
ACTIVITY	Ambulate ad lib	
NUTRITION	Cardiac prudent diet	
CONSULTS		
PATIENT EDUCATION	Assess, instruct, and evaluate re: ■ Carotid endarterectomy instructions ■ Discharge and follow-up plan of care	
SOCIAL WORK	Psychosocial assessment and intervention, and D/C plan, as indicated	
CASE MANAGEMENT	Probably for discharge today if outcomes attained Evaluate individual patient/family needs; initiate referrals and consults, as indicated	

MAP009 (10/98)

ST. VINCENT'S HOSPITAL AND MEDICAL CENTER MULTIDISCIPLINARY ACTION PLAN POSTOPERATIVE DAY 1

Procedure: Carotid Endarterectomy

MD: _____
RN: _____
Date: _____

Patient Problem and Nursing Interventions	Expected Patient Outcome &/or Discharge Outcome	Assessment/Evaluation		
Alteration in Body Systems	Complications will be Prevented/Minimized			
1. Nursing assessment		1.	1.	1.
A. *Vital signs & neurovascular check*	A. VS & neurovascular status WNL	A. (Flow sheet)	A. (Flow sheet)	A. (Flow sheet)
B. *Assess lung sounds & respirations*	B. Respirations unlabored & even; lungs clear. Using incentive spirometer; coughing and deep breathing	B. Flow sheet)	B. (Flow sheet)	B. (Flow sheet)
C. *Assess if neck dressing is intact, and/or for the presence of drainage/bleeding*	C. Neck dressing dry and intact or suture line exposed	C. (Flow sheet)	C. (Flow sheet)	C. (Flow sheet)
D. *Assess and mobility of extremities*	D. No signs/symptoms of complications	D. (Flow sheet)	D. (Flow sheet)	D. (Flow sheet)
Alteration in Comfort	Pain R/T Postoperative Period will be Prevented/Minimized			
1. Incisional pain: A. *Assess level of pain (use 1-10 pain scale)*	1. Verbalize minimal discomfort after intervention implemented	1. (Flow sheet)/ (MAR)	1. (Flow sheet)/ (MAR)	1. (Flow sheet)/ (MAR)
B. *Administer pain medications* C. *Assess effect of pain medication* D. *Utilize comfort measures and diversional measures*	2. Attain identified goal of pain relief			
Knowledge Deficit R/T Surgical Procedure and Discharge Planning	Increased Knowledge R/T Postoperative Care & Discharge Planning			
1. Assess knowledge/instruct/evaluate re: ■ Carotid endarterectomy instructions	1. Verbalize understanding of discharge instructions	1.	1.	1.
2. Review discharge follow-up plan	2. Verbalize understanding of follow-up plan	2. (Discharge summary)	2. (Discharge summary)	2. (Discharge summary)

MAP 009 (9/98)

St. Vincent's Hospital and Medical Center Multidisciplinary Action Plan

Procedure: Carotid Endarterectomy

PROGRESS NOTES:

_____

_____

_____

_____

_____

_____

_____

_____

_____

_____

_____

_____

_____

_____

_____

_____

_____

_____

MAP 009 (9/98)

Appendix 7-2

Tucson Medical Center Health Care Case Management

Mission Statement

In collaboration with patients, families, and the health care team, case management facilitates meeting the complex health needs of patients in the most effective and resource-efficient way.

Goals

- To protect quality of care while managing utilization and reimbursement
- To decrease health care costs for defined populations
- To increase satisfaction of multiple customers
- To explore the most appropriate care options for and with individual patients and families
- To increase compliance with treatment plans
- To reduce fragmentation of care
- To support recovery when recovery is possible
- To bridge gaps in the continuity of care
- To support patients and families through life transitions

Courtesy of Tucson Medical Center, Tucson, Arizona.

Appendix 7-3

Case Management Model

The Tucson Medical Center case management team is composed of nurse case managers, social work case managers, and utilization case managers. These three groups of specialists, assisted by clerical support, interact collaboratively to support the mission and goals of case management. There is a core set of case management functions that is shared by all of the members of the case management team, as well as specific functions that fall under the unique expertise of each group.

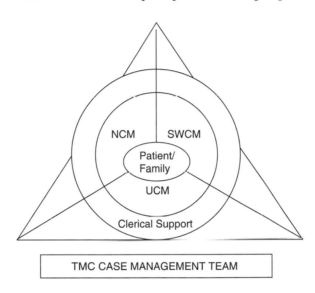

APPENDIX 7-4

Core Case Management Functions and Specific Specialty Functions

CORE CASE MANAGEMENT FUNCTIONS

The case manager will act to:

- Identify at-risk populations for high cost, extended lengths of stay, destabilization, and repeat hospitalization
- Coordinate resources to ensure that necessary services are provided at the most appropriate level of care and that there is a smooth progression of the patient throughout the system during hospitalization
- Initiate a discharge planning process, beginning at or before hospital admission, that ensures safe and comprehensive support for continued health care needs
- Anticipate potential delays in the health care process, and act proactively to avoid these delays
- Identify obstacles to efficiency and good outcomes, and intervene to overcome or eliminate these when possible
- Reduce redundancy and fragmentation of care by acting as a communication link between the patient, family, members of the health care team, and payers
- Gather, interpret, and use data to identify problems and trends and to demonstrate outcomes and cost-effectiveness
- Act as advocate for the patient and family
- Educate the patient, family, and interdisciplinary team regarding health care resources
- Share skills and expertise with case management team

SPECIFIC SPECIALTY FUNCTIONS

Utilization Case Manager	Nurse Case Manager	Social Worker Case Manager
1. Perform utilization review for appropriateness of admission, continued stay, and placement	1. Perform case management assessments	1. Perform case management assessments
2. Identify and refer high-risk complex patients for ongoing case management	2. Interact with patients, families, physicians, and other health team members to develop proactive plans for continued care	2. Interact with patients, families, physicians, and other health team members to develop proactive plans for continued care
3. Function as expert resource for rules/regulations regarding utilization management	3. Evaluate and modify plan according to changing patient needs and clinical data; document and communicate plan to all team members	3. Evaluate and modify plan according to changing patient needs; document and communicate plan to all team members

Utilization Case Manager	Nurse Case Manager	Social Worker Case Manager
4. Issue denials when necessary	4. Intervene when medical complexity results in fragmented care	4. Provide in-depth psychosocial assessment when appropriate
5. Assign working diagnosis-related group and prompt for accurate documentation	5. Identify and act to eliminate gaps in clinical care; make appropriate referrals	5. Provide support for crisis intervention, bereavement counseling and substance abuse counseling
		6 Function as social work resource for regulatory and legal issues
		7. Intervene when social/economic issues affect health care and disposition

Courtesy of Tucson Medical Center, Tucson, Arizona, with modification.

APPENDIX 7-5

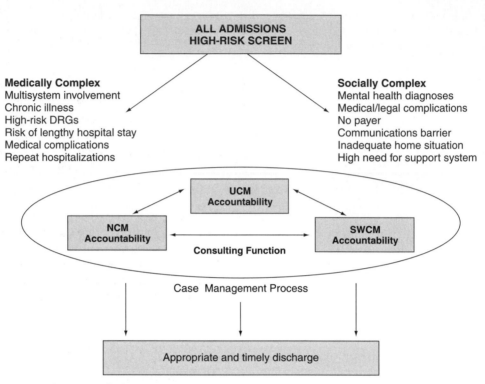

ALL ADMISSIONS HIGH-RISK SCREEN

Medically Complex
Multisystem involvement
Chronic illness
High-risk DRGs
Risk of lengthy hospital stay
Medical complications
Repeat hospitalizations

Socially Complex
Mental health diagnoses
Medical/legal complications
No payer
Communications barrier
Inadequate home situation
High need for support system

UCM Accountability

NCM Accountability

SWCM Accountability

Consulting Function

Case Management Process

Appropriate and timely discharge

Courtesy of Tucson Medical Center, Tucson, Arizona.

Collaborative Models of Case Management

Evelyn Koenig

CHAPTER OVERVIEW

Collaborative models of case management, with interdependence among team members, joint decision-making responsibility, and joint accountability, offer an alternative to one-discipline or multidisciplinary models. They ensure the ready availability of competencies, knowledge, and skills necessary for comprehensive patient care and for system improvement. They build on the unique strengths of all team members and, when aligned, create solutions better than any individual can develop in isolation.

EVOLUTION IN CASE MANAGEMENT

Case management is an old concept reborn. Aspects of case management were seen in attempts to care for the poor during the late 1800s. Community-based models of case management have been applied in mental health, social service, and public health settings since that time. Case management has also been used in the insurance industry and in the management of the care of deinstitutionalized mentally ill and developmentally disabled. In the mid-1980s, the introduction of the prospective payment system gave impetus to the application of case management concepts in health care settings (Cesta et al., 1998; Cohen & Cesta, 1997; Lyon, 1993).

Case management development in health care was largely a nursing-driven process initiated to support "cost effective, patient outcome oriented care" (Cohen & Cesta, 1997). As managed care spread, case management models proliferated. Many models stressed the need for a multidisciplinary approach, usually under the direction of the nurse case manager. However, as fiscal constraints increased and institutions adopted downsizing as a cost-containment method, some responded by collapsing roles. Nurse case managers often found themselves as sole provider, absorbing aspects of the utilization, social work, and discharge planning roles.

Developing in parallel to these more recent trends of single-discipline models, downsizing, and role collapse is a growing body of work on collaboration as the most viable method for meeting the pressures of today's environment (Harper & Harper, 1992; Huszczo, 1996; Liedtka & Whitten, 1997). It supports the growing awareness that case management cannot be the function of a single individual (Bach, 1996) and that the nurse case manager will need to develop a collaborative practice with others to better coordinate the delivery of health care (Blancett & Flarey, 1996).

COLLABORATION

Collaboration is a "process of joint decision-making among interdependent parties, involving joint ownership of decisions and collective responsibility for outcomes" (Liedtka & Whitten, 1997). As length of stay decreases, patient complexity increases, and reimbursement systems become increasingly complicated, collaborative models of case management ensure the availability of the competencies, knowledge, and skills necessary to the task at hand. With a clear sense of direction, collaborative case management teams can provide higher-quality solutions than any one individual working alone or in traditional multidisciplinary relationships.

THE EVOLUTION OF A COLLABORATIVE MODEL

In 1994, Tennessee was faced with the rapid conversion to a Medicaid managed care model. Vanderbilt University Medical Center (VUMC) recognized the need for change to ensure a competitive position in the new environment. At the VUMC, costs were significantly higher than those of local competitors and the length of stay was high. The development and initiation of a case management model were seen as important elements in developing a competitive edge and responding to the managed care challenge.

In recognizing the strength brought by a diverse skill mix and the role conflict created by collapsing jobs (Erickson, 1996), case management was seen, from its inception, as the responsibility of a triad of nurse case manager, social worker, and utilization manager (Figure 8-1). *Case management* was defined as

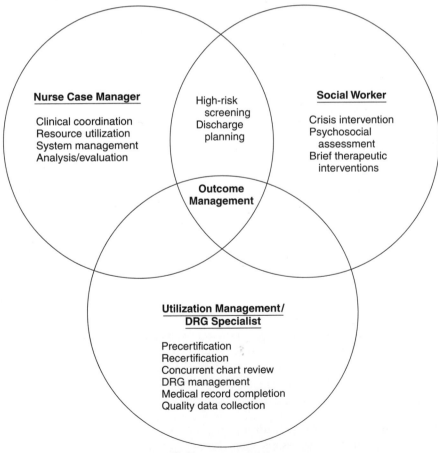

FIGURE **8-1** Case management triad.

the process of coordinating patient care across the continuum to ensure optimal quality outcomes, patient satisfaction, and appropriate use of resources. Nurses and social workers became partners within this model. Although the model recognized and respected the unique skills of each discipline, some sharing of responsibility was also required. The nurse case manager assumed responsibility for clinical coordination, resource utilization, pathway development, and outcome measurement. The social worker provided psychosocial assessment and intervention. High-risk screening and discharge planning were shared between nurse and social worker. Historically lacking in effectiveness, the utilization review function required redesign to make the utilization manager a partner in the triad. Staff was upgraded to licensed or credentialed personnel, and jobs were redesigned to include precertification, recertification, medical record completion, coding, and quality data collection (Erickson, 1996). Each triad was assigned a patient population and assumed responsibility for high-risk screening, assessment, planning/managing and evaluating care, and continuum of care planning. Triads would "run the list" of patients at least daily, dividing the work, reaching joint decisions about assigned responsibilities, and together designing plans of care.

Case management outcomes were impressive. Over 5 years, case management triad efforts helped reduce the gap in charges with local competitors from 39.7% to less than 1% and the average length of stay from 7.1 to 5.2 days. Case management triads were, in general, functioning well and providing higher-quality solutions than any individual member could develop working alone. The nursing members of the triads, however, began to question their sole responsibility for outcome management. If the triad was responsible for a patient population and outcome management/system improvement was a part of that responsibility, then all triad members should be equally accountable. The triads should become truly collaborative with "collective responsibility for outcomes" (Liedtka & Whitten, 1997). Case management leadership agreed. In a communication to all triad members, team accountability was outlined. "All triad members have responsibility for the work of case management which includes evaluation; evaluation is better with input from different team members; and evaluation is the interdisciplinary collaboration 'walk' " (Erickson, 1997).

Today, all members of the case management triad are held accountable as a team for all aspects of case management. They are responsible for ensuring their activities fit with the needs of the patient care center (service line) to which they are responsible, using the patient care center business plan as reference. Members continue to screen their patient population using triad-developed high-risk indicators. Patients at risk are assigned, and assessment, care planning/evaluation, and continuum of care planning are provided. The nurse assumes primary responsibility for the clinical coordination of care on the medically complex patients. Physician rounds provide a major forum for the identification of high-risk patients and for recommendations related to care and to resource utilization. Consultation with staff nurses on care plan development also assists in ensuring smooth progress across the continuum. The nurse facilitates evidence-based pathway development and revision to enhance consistency and appropriateness of care. By facilitating discharge of the medically complex patient, the nurse ensures that transitions in care are appropriate.

The social worker assumes primary responsibility for the psychosocially complex patients (e.g., those with psychiatric and/or substance abuse problems, family conflict, or lacking resources needed to address care needs). The social worker provides assistance in coordination of care, psychosocial assessment, crisis intervention, brief therapeutic intervention, linkage with resources, and discharge planning for these patients.

The utilization manager ensures precertification and recertification for the triad population and continues to provide triad members with information on payer-related issues. The utilization manager also ensures that medical record documentation appropriately supports the coding/billing functions.

"Running the list," or the daily discussion of all new and active triad patients, is key to triad function. It is this daily discussion that ensures that all triad members have an opportunity to contribute to the care of each patient from their own unique perspective.

In addition, each triad has established a case management dashboard, "a system of warning lights and gauges that will allow the case management team to monitor when practice for their assigned population is going well and when there are problems" (Erickson, 1998). Some indicators are common to all case management teams. In addition, each team identifies cost, quality, and patient satisfaction indicators unique to their population (Figure 8-2). All triad members contribute to the dashboard and, through trending of the data collected, the triad can identify areas for improvement and design improvement activities.

DRG XXX

	INDICATOR	FY Baseline	1st Quarter	2nd Quarter	3rd Quarter	4th Quarter
	Total admissions	624	75	61	52	
D	Admission type					
E	Elective	374	48	51	30	
M	Emergency	124	15	5	10	
O	Observation	0	0	0	2	
G	Same day surgery	62	12	2	5	
R	Trauma	64	0	3	5	
A	Payor mix					
P	TennCare	29%	27%	21%	18%	
H	Commercial	35%	38%	38%	44%	
I	Medicare	25%	27%	25%	25%	
C	Self	6%	3%	8%	7%	
S	Other	5%	5%	8%	6%	
	Case mix index	1.4	1.5	1.6	1.7	
C	Average LOS	5	5	4	3	
O	Charges/Admission	21,000	19,962	18,747	17,213	
S	Cost/Admission	11,977	11,660	11,335	11,300	
T	Profit/Loss	883	2575	3000	3035	
	Denied days	15	13	15	20	
	Readmits (within 30 days)	16	8	5	3	
	Unrelated	12	6	4	3	
	Related-unavoidable	2	0	1	0	
	Related-avoidable	2	2	0	0	
Q	Discharge delays	NA				
U	Funding		3	1	0	
A	Bed availability		1	4	5	
L	Patient condition		4	2	6	
I	Family issues		1	0	0	
T	Other		8	5	3	
Y	Estimated blood loss	NA				
	Complications (number/type)		4 CSF LEAK	1 CSF LEAK	0 CSF LEAK	
S	Patient survey	NA	85% complete	92% complete	95% complete	
A	Complaints	NA				
T	Patient		3	2	1	
I	Physician		5	2	2	
S	Other		0	1	0	
F						
A						
C						
T						
I						
O						
N						

FIGURE **8-2**   Dashboard sample.

In a recent assessment of the VUMC case management model, triad members strongly endorsed the collaborative approach. One team member summarized the feelings of many. "We are more powerful as a team than we would be working independently. With complex cases it is impossible for one person to handle all patient/family needs . . . case management enables me to work with someone who has a knowledge base different than mine and they contribute valuable information from their perspective" (VUMC, 1998).

BUILDING A COLLABORATIVE MODEL

Collaborative care models result in a number of positive outcomes, among them the potential to reduce cost while improving quality outcomes, to increase patient satisfaction, and to increase staff satisfaction and commitment (Liedtka & Whitten, 1997). However, health care–givers, often involved in multidisciplinary care, rarely work with the interdependence and accountability required by collaboration. A study of 39 Vanderbilt triad members demonstrated that, although experienced in health care, 79.9% of the respondents had never worked in a collaborative model (Kidd & White, 1998). Because collaborative care models are rare and require knowledge and skills seldom used or rewarded in traditional health care, preparation for collaborative practice is critical to the model's success.

CREATING THE VISION

"Vision is a picture of the future, laid out as a possibility" (Whiteside, 1993). It communicates a common purpose and gives coherence to activities. It assists individuals in putting aside differences and working together cooperatively (Senge, 1990). It also helps establish a sense of accountability for system, as well as individual, performance (Liedtka & Whitten, 1997).

A clearly stated vision is a necessary first step in creating a collaborative case management model. It creates a consistent reference point against which the team can measure their performance. The VUMC vision communicates the desired future—case management triads providing leadership to the patient care center in the development and implementation of patient care models that will assure effective coordination of care across the continuum. It defines the desired outcomes—enhanced quality, increased patient and provider satisfaction, and effective use of resources. And it defines the method—a collaborative care model that optimally uses the unique skills of each professional and holds team members "collectively responsible for outcomes" (Liedtka & Whitten, 1997). To keep the vision central, it is incorporated in the scope and standards of practice, is core in orientation, and is reiterated at every opportunity. In this way the vision is the touchstone, the consistent measure of team progress toward the desired future.

BUILDING THE TEAM

The success of the team depends on individual excellence and the ability of the individuals to work together to tap the potential of the whole. It requires alignment, "a commonality of purpose, a shared vision and understanding of how to compliment one another's efforts" (Senge, 1990).

> "Collaborative teams don't just happen when people come together for a meeting. They are created through clear communication and upfront agreements about roles and decision-making that build trust. The agreements that the team begins with will enable it to sustain its focus and achieve its outcomes" (VUMC, 1994).

Team chartering is an efficient, effective method of helping the team define how they will work together. The charter has several elements:

- The purpose of the team
- The scope of the team's work
- Givens or boundaries (those things that cannot be changed)
- Decision-making process and fallback (how decisions will be made and the fallback if agreement cannot be reached)
- Roles (individual and collective responsibilities of team members, including professional roles and roles within the team, such as leadership)
- Norms and ground rules (how members work together)
- Meetings (times and frequency)
- Supports for the team (the supports necessary to ensure success)

Our experience demonstrates that chartered teams function more effectively, as there is commonality of purpose and a defined structure. If the team has problems in functioning, the charter serves as a reference for corrective action. It is also a critical tool in the orientation of new team members.

Because collaborative practice requires interdependence, it has also been helpful to assist team members in understanding and valuing individual style. A helpful tool is the Myers-Briggs Type Indicator. Team members complete the inventory and receive an individual interpretation of style preferences. In a group session, all team member preferences are shared and the group learns how individual style impacts the team, the potential inherent in style diversity, and methods to use diverse styles in optimizing team function.

Managing conflict is a major challenge to teams. Each team needs help in "acknowledging and using conflict productively versus suppressing and ignoring it" (Liedtka & Whitten, 1997). The Myers-Briggs tool provides a method for understanding team members' reactions and provides direction in helping people adapt (Barger & Kirby, 1995). The concept of *planned renegotiation* is also useful. It is a way to provide controlled change by using "pinches" (indicators of personal discomfort), to anticipate team disruption, and to renegotiate expectations before serious disruption occurs (Sherwood & Glidewell, 1972). The Thomas-Kilmann Conflict Mode Instrument can be useful because it focuses on the individual style used most often in conflictual situations, the adaptiveness of that style, and ways to develop flexibility in matching style to circumstance (Thomas & Kilmann, 1974). Any or all of these tools can be introduced for use by the team.

PREPARING TEAM MEMBERS

Curricula necessary to the preparation of new case management staff have been well documented (Cohen & Cesta, 1997; Satinsky, 1995; Tahan, 1996). Core content includes the history of case management; case management models; health care trends; payer networks and contracts; systems of reimbursement; case management practice (risk screening, assessment, care planning and evaluation, and continuum of care planning); pathway creation; continuous improvement techniques; and outcomes measurement and management. However, a collaborative model requires that content be reframed to emphasize interdependence and joint accountability.

Orientation begins with the vision for case management and its relationship to the institutional mission and goals. The collaborative aspect of the vision, with its functional interdependence and joint accountability, is emphasized. Information on the characteristics of well-functioning teams is provided. Participants are asked to complete an inventory of their assumptions about teams, and those are contrasted to the reality of the collaborative model (Harper, 1992). If individuals are joining a functioning team, they review the team charter to understand its purpose and structure. Because the introduction of a new member changes team dynamics, renegotiation of roles may be necessary. Material on conflict management is provided to new staff, and they are given the opportunity to practice conflict management techniques. They are also given an understanding of personal style and its impact. Again, if they are joining an established team, they learn how their style complements the team. When core content is presented, it includes reference to the way tasks are carried out in a collaborative model and how joint accountability is measured. Mentors assigned are responsible for assisting in the mastery of case management process and collaborative practice.

EVALUATING THE TEAM

Members of the collaborative teams have both individual and joint accountability. There is individual accountability for the quality of professional practice and for behavior as a team member. There is joint accountability for team functioning and outcomes. Expected outcomes are specific to each team, and a communication loop exists that requires the team to regularly report on its progress and to self-adjust as necessary. Successful individual practice does not result in positive evaluation if the team is failing and this is clearly communicated. Positive evaluation requires individual and team success. This is a unique message to most professionals, necessitating repetition.

SUMMARY

Case management practice continues to evolve. The developing collaborative models provide an alternative to traditional case management models, and outcomes demonstrate the synergy that can develop among members of a well-functioning collaborative team.

References

Bach, D. et al. (1996). Developing a successful hospital case management system. In D. Flarey & S. Blancett (Eds.), *Handbook of nursing case management*. Gaithersburg, Md.: Aspen.

Barger, N., & Kirby, L. (1995). *The challenge of change in organizations, helping employees thrive in the new frontier.* Palo Alto: Davies-Black Publishing.

Blancett, S., & Flarey, D. (1996). Case management: The shape of things to come. In D. Flarey & S. Blancett (Eds.), *Handbook of nursing case management*. Gaithersburg, Md.: Aspen.

Cesta, T. et al. (1998). *The case manager's survival guide, winning strategies for clinical practice.* St. Louis: Mosby Inc.

Cohen, E., & Cesta, T. (1997). *Nursing case management, from concept to evaluation,* 2nd Edition. St. Louis: Mosby Inc.

Erickson, S. (1996, July/Aug.). Case management. *Issues and Outcomes,* 6-8.

Erickson, S. (1997). Unpublished presentation.

Erickson, S. (1998). The Vanderbilt model of outcomes management. *Critical Care Nursing Clinics of North America* *10*(1), 13-20.

Harper, A., & Harper, B. (1992). *Skill-building for self-directed team members.* New York: MW Corporation.

Huszczo, G. (1996). *Tools for team excellence.* Palo Alto: Davis-Black Publishing.

Kidd, K., & White, S. (1998). Unpublished manuscript.

Liedtka, J., & Whitten, E. (1997). Building better patient care services: A collaborative approach. *Health Care Management Review 22*(3), 16-24.

Lyon, J. (1993). Models of nursing care delivery and case management: Clarification of terms. *Nursing Economics* *11*(3), 163-169.

Satinsky, M. (1995). *An executive guide to case management strategies.* Chicago: American Hospital Publishing, Inc.

Senge, P. (1990). *The fifth discipline,* New York: Doubleday.

Sherwood, J., & Glidewell, J. (1972). Planned renegotiation: A norm setting OD intervention. In W. Burke, (Ed.), *Contemporary organization development, approaches and interventions.* Washington, D.C.: NTL Learning Resources Corporation.

Tahan, H. (1996). Training and education needs of case managers. In D. Flarey, & S. Blancett, (Eds.), *Handbook of nursing case management.* Gaithersburg, Md.: Aspen.

Thomas, K., & Kilmann, R. (1974). *Thomas-Kilmann conflict mode instrument.* Santa Clara, Calif.: Xicom, Inc.

Vanderbilt University Medical Center, Center for Patient Care Innovation. (1994). Unpublished material.

Vanderbilt University Medical Center, Office of Case Management. (1998). Unpublished results.

Whiteside, J. (1993). *The Phoenix agenda.* Essex Junction, Vt.: Oliver Wight Publications, Inc.

Case Management

A Process, Not a Person

Theresa J. Ortiz
Lynn Riippi

CHAPTER OVERVIEW

For a successful case management program, the patient, in partnership with many professionals, must engage in a process. Case management or care coordination is not a new concept. Think of a rural physician with limited resources who "manages" his or her patients across their life span. And in exchange for their education, on graduation, physicians in many European countries are assigned patients by region or district. In this setting, the physician may take on additional roles such as pharmacist, nurse, therapist, or social worker. Home visits are common. Regardless of the structure or where the patient enters the system, the case management process begins with identification of patient needs and risks, development of a plan to address those needs, and monitoring of the plan for success. Case management is really a process, not a person. The process has evolved from a simple plan, such as the rural physician who develops a life-long relationship with the patient, to a complex, fragmented arrangement as we try to balance demands from managed care, regulatory agencies, and the sophisticated consumer. Organizations develop and change, and thus case management models transition. Staff also goes through a process of change and growth. An unchanging factor is the demand for accountability in the case management process.

THE CASE MANAGEMENT PROGRAM

The case management model chosen by an institution is determined by many factors and does not remain static. The University of Colorado Hospital is a 450-bed tertiary care hospital located in Denver, Colorado. The initial case management program used dyads of social workers and nurse case managers. The program was successful and brought many positive changes to the organization. Program evaluation was an ongoing part of the process, resulting in modifications to meet patient, payer, and organizational needs. Having the case managers function in the dual role of case and utilization manager demonstrated value. The case managers began to understand the payer role in the process and increased their negotiation and brokering skills. However, over time, program evaluation demonstrated that the workload needed to be adjusted. Various models were evaluated, and a site visit was made to Vanderbilt University to observe their triad model (see Chapter 8). This model added a third component to the dyads, the utilization management nurse, creating a triad. The teams started out as hospital unit based and gradually transitioned to population-based teams, many of whom follow their patients across the continuum of care.

The evolution of University of Colorado Hospital's case management program began with the identification of multiple factors, including the hospital's mission and the competitive managed health care market. The hospital's mission includes education, research, and service to the indigent. When designing a case management model in an academic setting, additional factors may need to be considered, depending on the relationship between medical school, physician group practice, and hospital. Balancing the hospital's mission becomes difficult because the key players are often working toward different objectives. At times their motivating factors may even be in conflict with one another (Table 9-1).

Recognizing that aligning incentives between these three entities was a monumental task, the model was designed to start with what was controllable. Historically, no group other than the utilization review department had been accountable for the utilization of resources and patient length of stay. Staff in general had little understanding of managed care, reimbursement, covered and noncovered benefits, or internal and external resources. In addition, lacking was the concept that case management is a process that includes many disciplines, all of which have a part in coordinating care.

The optimal situation would be to design a model, hire staff with specific expertise, close the health care system for at least 1 week to ensure large blocks of training time, and then, when fully prepared, begin the program. In most institutions, limited budgets, systems constraints, and administrative expectations for quick results do not allow the staff time for adjustment and mastery of new skill sets. The model was piloted in just such an environment. Almost immediately the human barriers to implementation began to surface (Table 9-2).

Database Design

As the demand to demonstrate added value in the patient care process increases, case management programs must develop a mechanism to trend system issues (i.e., variances) that affect patient care, resource utilization, length of stay, etc. Data must be formatted so as to identify areas for performance improvement activities, track triad team-productivity, and serve as a decision-making tool for administration. The case management team database at University of Colorado Hospital, like the program model, has gone through multiple permutations. The original hand-tallied tool was designed to capture variations in patient care that prevented a smooth transition through the hospital stay (e.g., a discharge is postponed because a test could not be performed on a timely basis). The foundation for the database was a data entry sheet completed by the case management teams that identified and assigned

TABLE 9-1	What Are the Motivating Factors for Each Group?	
Medical School	**Physician Group**	**University Hospital**
How is the hospital reimbursed for the additional costs associated with training?	Physicians trying to balance academic medicine, research, clinical responsibilities, and the reality of managed care	Competing in a stage 4 managed care market on costs
Students must meet minimal requirements for graduation.	Physicians develop their own practice patterns. Residents "adopt" the personality of the attending physician.	Reimbursement declining
Need to perform required number of procedures, which may not always incorporate utilization management principles		Need to contain resource utilization

TABLE 9-2	HUMAN BARRIERS EXPERIENCED IN IMPLEMENTATION OF THE CASE MANAGEMENT MODEL			
Fear	**Staff Response**	**Rationale for Fears**	**Leadership Strategies**	**Outcomes**
Fear of losing my job	"If I do not go along with this model, I will lose my job."	Case management programs nationwide had eliminated or changed roles for social workers and clinical nurse specialists	Use of a consultant with strong managed care background	Consultant provided an objective view for program development and was able to solicit cooperation from multiple departments
Fear of change	"What do I do everyday in this new role?"	New role, new expectations, new job skills, new partner	Clear structure and accountabilities provided for framework for daily expectations	Took approximately 6 to 9 months for teams to demonstrate team behavior
		Feeling of being overwhelmed was real for health care professionals who were very skilled and comfortable in their "old" roles	Job descriptions with performance standards developed	
			Day-long training session for case management teams	
Fear of managed care	"I would have gone to business school if I had wanted to deal with finances. I am trained to care for patients."	Fear of managed care in a stage 4 managed care market is a reality. Hospitals in this market were downsizing, consolidating, and/or closing	"Managed Care 101" training	Teams have become less intimated by third-party payers
		Lack of understanding about managed care rules and how to incorporate these into a patient treatment plan were new skill sets that needed to be learned.	Training on developing a relationship with a third-party payer	Teams see that their role as "financial stewards" for the patient is just as important as their clinical care

These human barriers, although less tangible, were as much of a challenge to leadership as selecting the right model for the particular setting, developing the right report formats, or refining the data base.

Continued

TABLE 9-2	HUMAN BARRIERS EXPERIENCED IN IMPLEMENTATION OF THE CASE MANAGEMENT MODEL—CONT'D			
Fear	**Staff Response**	**Rationale for Fears**	**Leadership Strategies**	**Outcomes**
Fear of technology	"Why do we have to keep data? I'm a caregiver. People should know that I do a good job."	"What value do your services add to patient care?"	Education stressing "data is your friend" ■ Technical computer training	Teams began to understand their data, began to present it to various committees (i.e., clinical pathway team), and became involved with strategies for improvement
		This is a question being asked by health care companies as well as administration. Fear of data and technology may be real to health care professionals who have not been exposed to computers, data collection, or evaluation of care provided	■ Development of tools for data collection	
			■ Development of a database	
			■ Development of usable report formats	
			■ Education on data analysis	
			■ Leadership training in data presentation	
			■ Training in the quality improvement process	

variance days to the responsible party. The responsible party may have been a hospital department (e.g., no available operating rooms), a nursing unit (e.g., delay in getting a medication started), a physician (e.g., delay in moving a patient to a lower level of care), or discharge planning (e.g., patient refuses to leave the hospital once he or she is determined to be medically stable). Completing the data entry sheet was an educational experience for most of the case management team members, who were not used to tracking outcomes this way. Identifying and assigning variances forced the case management teams to become more proactive in searching for creative funding and placement options.

The case management database (on Microsoft Access) was designed with a software expert from the financial department and consisted of all University of Colorado Hospital inpatients after diagnosis-related

TABLE 9-2	HUMAN BARRIERS EXPERIENCED IN IMPLEMENTATION OF THE CASE MANAGEMENT MODEL—CONT'D			
Fear	**Staff Response**	**Rationale for Fears**	**Leadership Strategies**	**Outcomes**
Fear of being the "bad guy"	"I do not want to be seen as the utilization management police." or "It's not my place to question the physician."	Staff was used to functioning in a clinical role but not in a total patient care coordination role that included attention to financial issues. Understanding that there are limits in providing care and that patients do have responsibilities in their care were new skill sets to be learned	One-on-one supervision and case review with managers	Teams developed relationship with business contracting department
			Relationship building with all health care team members. Focus on the fact that patients are the center of what we do.	Staff became more sophisticated in negotiating for benefit exceptions based on cost analysis.
			Education about the "big system" perspective ■ Guest lecture from finance discussed how heath care dollars are spent in our institution.	

group (DRG) assignments had been made. Once the medical records were coded, they were downloaded into the database. Along with the DRG assignment, demographic data, length of stay, and hospital charges were also included. The program calculated the cost of a variance by multiplying the average variable direct cost per day of the assigned DRG by the number of days assigned. For example, if the patient's length of stay was decreased by 5 days and the variable cost of the DRG was $500 per day, the facility would potentially save $2500. This formula may not work for all institutions but was a way to begin showing how variances affect the financial part of providing care for patients. Not all variances were negative; if the case management team intervened (facilitated a test being done earlier or negotiated for benefits with a third-party payer) and it resulted in a decreased length of stay, the team received credit for the intervention.

Specialized reports were taken to medical quality improvement committees to analyze trends. General monthly summaries were reported to the triad teams, administration, physician, and nursing unit manager. The summaries helped each group develop interventions for system areas that needed improvement.

Eventually, the triads determined the data tool should be simplified. Because baseline data were established, it was no longer necessary to track all cases. The interdisciplinary Case Management Department partnered with the Quality and Outcomes Department to automate the tool by making it able to be scanned. Organizational strategic goals were used to determine which streamlined data should now be collected. For example, the hospital is currently focusing on improved quality and utilization management for Medicare patients. The organization wants to provide the best quality care at the lowest cost. Thus, the triad teams currently collect data on the Case Management Department outcomes and interventions related to the Medicare population. An example of data collected includes patients readmitted for the same diagnosis within 30 days. This allows the teams to examine whether the readmission could have been prevented by an alternative discharge planning intervention after the first admission. As organizational goals modify over time, it is likely the data collected and outcomes will again change. The process must remain fluid to continue to render the data useful and meaningful.

Outcomes

A newly formed case management department early in its organizational process might set goals different from those of a more mature program. The early dyad case management program resulted in a number of positive outcomes (Riippi & Jackson, 1997). To date, these outcomes have been maintained, including the following:

1. A decrease in the number of patients on the "$100,000" report. (This report lists patients whose hospital charges have reached a threshold.) This means there are significantly fewer dollars outstanding in accounts receivable. This outcome really got the attention of the hospital chief financial officer, who reviewed these reports weekly. When possible, case managers and social workers are placing these patients in more appropriate settings sooner and/or obtaining funding to help these patients access resources. Discharges directly from the intensive care unit increased instead of requiring the patient to stay another day in a less acute bed for the purpose of discharge planning.
2. The overall readmission rate has decreased. Teams are coordinating follow-up care and return appointments with primary care physicians, clinics, and home care.
3. Emergency department referrals to social workers and case managers have increased, allowing staff to intervene initially and look for appropriate solutions to patients' situations. They now often divert inappropriate admissions. Teams also identified patients who visited the emergency department frequently and developed alternative follow-up plans, thus reducing the frequency of return visits.
4. Improved customer satisfaction is reflected in telephone calls and letters, as well as satisfaction surveys. These customers include not only patients but also internal customers in other departments and external third-party payer case managers.
5. A significant decrease occurred in the monies spent on home care for the indigent. Case management teams were able to work out more cost-effective alternatives for these patients that did not compromise care.
6. Dollars paid to an outside vendor for home infusion services to the indigent decreased from $500,000 to $70,000 the first year the program was piloted. By the third year the spending had decreased to under $30,000. Currently the spending is under $10,000 per year. Teams were taught to use an algorithm for possible alternatives to home infusion services. Patients received the same level of service but at times in an alternative setting.

An unexpected bonus to the initial implementation of the case management program was the networking that developed. Collaboration has increased and patients are moving more smoothly between units and services.

With the transition to the triad model and the addition of the utilization management nurses, additional outcomes have been achieved:

1. To date, approximately $5 million in overturned denials has been recouped as revenue for the organization. (This dollar amount reflects organizational cost.) In addition, follow-up for appeal of denials has been reorganized and centralized. Previously, denials went to various parts of the organization, making it difficult to tabulate a denial rate. A denial log has been placed on a shared computer drive so that the Strategic Development and Business Offices have access to this information.

2. Organized physician education was implemented to improve documentation related to the type of patient admission (i.e., acute admission status versus observation status) that affects reimbursement.

STAGES OF PROGRAM DEVELOPMENT FROM THE HUMAN PERSPECTIVE

Stage 1

As the program was implemented, weekly interdisciplinary meetings were held, consisting of nurse case managers, social workers, home care coordinators, and at times third-party payer case managers. At this point staff was working in dyads as teams, but true team behavior had not yet developed. Nurse case managers and social workers sat on opposite sides of the room, receiving information on the technical aspects and expectations of the new program. In-service training was provided on topics such as medical necessity and level of care criteria, high-risk screening, and Medicare and Medicaid regulations. Staff was learning their accountabilities, competency expectations, and the like. They listened but clearly had not yet internalized the process. Questions were basic and technical in nature and displayed a high level of anxiety. Questions about third-party payers were phrased to indicate staff viewed the third-party payer as the "bad guy." Staff did not yet display creativity in options for patients. Often they would advocate for whatever the physician had requested, not yet evaluating whether the request was appropriate or whether there were quality cost-effective alternatives. At the end of meetings, people left immediately without much interaction.

Stage 2

Staff began to implement the model and started to accept that they will have a partner. Beginning compliance with requirements appeared, but teams still required extensive one-on-one supervision. Next appeared the predictable power struggles over role definition. Although job descriptions delineated separate duties, there were some gray areas of responsibility, forcing each dyad to negotiate a working relationship. Most teams worked out acceptable arrangements without intervention; one or two required mediation. The individual personalities of team members caused each dyad to have a unique team personality. Most teams blended well and were able to demonstrate flexibility in working out role assignments.

Stage 3

Teams began to develop a consistent daily routine. The need for supervision on cases decreased to occasional supervision on complex cases. Teams began to consult with internal institutional resources, for example, consulting with the wound care nurse to help a patient improve faster or consulting with the pharmacy to enable a patient to obtain a drug on the correct insurance formulary. Less input from leadership was necessary. More creative planning for cases, incorporating benefit management, financial concerns, patient clinical needs, and psychosocial needs, began to appear. Teams now began to solicit input from all disciplines, such as physical or occupational therapy, speech, and respiratory therapy as well as the physician, and incorporate their input into the plan. However, at this stage, when they were presented with data about their team/unit, they were unclear as to how to utilize and analyze. "This is a nice report. Now what am I supposed to do with it?" was often the response.

Stage 4

Cooperation emerged within teams, and they began to function as true working partners, even completing some cross-training with each other. This was in sharp contrast to the initial stages, when staff members were territorial about their job duties. Teams now tolerated more shades of gray in role definition, allowing for greater cooperation. Most teams adapted to using the strengths of each partner. The comfort level of approaching physicians proactively for discharge plans versus waiting for a physician recommendation increased tremendously. Questions in meetings became more sophisticated, indicating a new level of knowledge and skill sets and demonstrating a broader system perspective.

Participants began to analyze their data for the purposes of improvements in contrast to the attitude, "I don't want this data to make me look bad." Data were presented to groups outside the team, for example, at a clinical pathway or medical staff quality meeting.

Stage 5 (Current)

As the insurance industry demands evolved, the need for a gradual metamorphosis of the model emerged. Continued evaluation of institutional and patient needs had become crucial. As the program evolved from the dyad to the triad model, the teams went back through the cycle of adjustment to change but at a higher level of expertise. Teams became healthier and stronger, and a staff-based self-governance committee was formed. The committee has been delegated responsibility for development of protocols for issues such as vacation leave coverage and case management documentation standards. Clearly, the model is beginning to expand from a program to a systemwide way of thinking, incorporating other key players in decision-making and development. Case management truly becomes not a person, but a process.

▎STRATEGIES FOR IMPLEMENTATION, OR "WHAT DID WE LEARN ALONG THE WAY?"

Any new program is a work in progress, and as much was learned along the way about what did not work as about what was successful.

What Did Not Work?

RAW DATA

In the early stages of database development, monthly reports were created that summarized all activity for each team. The lengthy data were not in a user-friendly format and were difficult to read, let alone interpret. Over time, the data were formatted into meaningful reports that each team could use to make improvements.

EXPECTING STAFF TO CHANGE PROCEDURES WITHOUT A BUILT-IN ACCOUNTABILITY PIECE

As the program developed, procedures, protocols, and expectations also developed. As a change in protocol became necessary, it would be reviewed with staff and they would indicate understanding verbally. It was assumed then that because we had laid out our expectations, staff would implement the changed protocol. Later it was discovered that staff actually had difficulty incorporating the changes into their routine unless there was a method of accountability. For example, staff was asked to orchestrate brief multidisciplinary conferences on all patients who stayed longer than 7 days. The purpose was for the team to develop a patient-specific plan to help move the patient to the next lower level of medical care as appropriate. Although staff agreed in theory that this was a good idea, as the day got busy, this task was often overlooked. It was not until we instituted a form for documentation that could also be used for auditing purposes that we began to see compliance. The meetings began to be held regularly, resulting in better team planning for patient care.

LONG PRESENTATIONS TO ADMINISTRATION

In the beginning, elaborate presentations were prepared that demonstrated detail on significant programmatic outcomes. Meetings at upper administrative levels are so tightly packed with agenda that the point of the presentation was rarely reached before the allotted time expired. We learned that the presentations needed to be short and to the point and to "pack a punch." Key outcomes were prepared for the presentation, with background information available only if asked.

What Did Work?

In retrospect, several strategies assisted administration to understand the validity and positive cost-effective program outcomes. There were also several that helped to break down the human barriers and resistance to change.

SELECTIVE USE OF E-MAIL

A summary email of important program outcomes sent to key administrators received more feedback than many other strategies. The e-mail listed in bullet form the specific program outcomes.

AWARDS LUNCHEONS

Twice a year, a luncheon was held to celebrate the successes of the program. Key administrators were invited, and awards were given for various team successes. Cases selected for recognition were complex, requiring teamwork, creativity, and skill to work toward a quality cost-effective patient outcome. Each team that received an award was given a certificate. In addition to providing recognition for a job well done, it provided a learning tool to demonstrate complex problem solving, as well as humor. For example, the "best travel agent" award was presented to the case manager who was able to negotiate with an employer for an airline ticket for a stroke patient who could not get home. A "Most Dollars and Days Saved" award was given to the neonatal case management team (physician, case manager, social worker, staff nurse, and parents) who worked with the payer in negotiating an early discharge for a premature baby. The payer was able to substitute additional home visits, allowing the parents to care for their baby at home instead of at the hospital. This saved 3 weeks of hospitalization and improved care for the baby by being at home.

SYSTEM ACCOUNTABILITY AND CONSISTENT STRUCTURE AND FEEDBACK

This was by far the most labor-intensive part of program startup. Assisting teams to learn the technical aspect of the job as well as make the internal changes necessary to work as a team proved to be a crucial aspect of program development. Setting up how staff team behaviors could be measured, rated, and audited was time consuming but helped change behavior most effectively. Management time was spent on lots of one-on-one supervision on difficult cases, chart audits, feedback and encouragement, and helping staff compare data on a month-to-month basis. Currently, management staff makes weekly rounds, reviewing charts and giving immediate feedback to the triad teams.

MODELING BEHAVIOR

At first, each team required leadership presence at their quarterly meetings to model how to analyze and present their data. Eventually the case managers were able to assume the leadership function.

Anticipated Further Development

The program began as unit-based dyad teams to get the system up and running and to ensure that all patients received services. The program then transitioned to a more population-based triad model that serves inpatients and outpatients, providing for better continuity of care. The logistics of such a model are difficult. How does one team provide inpatient and outpatient care when outpatient clinics are spread all over the city? How do patients receive services if they do not fit into one of the team case-managed populations? An additional sophistication in the use of data and outcomes is anticipated. The data were first used to change internal system issues. It was hoped that the case management program would partner with the business contract development office. The data should be useful in procuring contracts for the health care institution.

With each change in the model, it is anticipated that the teams will move back into the stages of resistance to change. However, although the process of resistance to change remains the same, staff should deal with it at a less traumatic level because they are at a more sophisticated stage of team development.

Key Factors in Program Success

1. Pay strong attention to the human dynamics, as they are as crucial to program success as the model you choose. Human dynamics are the most labor-intensive part of new program development. It took 6 to 9 months before consistent behavior change occurred on the part of the teams.
2. The model must include consistent ongoing structure, accountability, and feedback to staff. Newly hired staff must be brought up to the same skill level as experienced staff.
3. Personnel skilled in database design are crucial. At first, a full-time person was available to enter data, develop report formats, and analyze the data. As data collection matured, the program was able to partner with the Quality and Outcomes Department for reports and analysis.
4. Develop baseline data with measurable outcomes to justify program viability. This contributes to morale, allowing staff to measure their contribution.
5. Market your program to your administrators, as well as internal and external customers.
6. Celebrate your successes to administration and to staff.

And remember that case management is a process, not a person!

Reference

Riippi, L., & Jackson, S. (1997). Case management finds success in a university hospital. *QRC Advisor, 13*(10):7-9.

The University of Colorado Hospital Psychiatric Service Health Case Management Model

An Innovative Approach to Client-Centered Care

Bari K. Platter
Bonnie Cox Young
Kay Vaughn

CHAPTER OVERVIEW

The emphasis of managed care on providing rapid reintegration of psychiatric clients into the community has forced psychiatric programs to develop more efficient care delivery systems. Although University of Colorado Hospital (UCH) faculty members have written extensively about the provision of inpatient psychiatric treatment in the age of managed care, the body of knowledge concerning brief, cost-effective psychiatric hospital treatment is extremely limited. Furthermore, literature regarding the development of inpatient psychiatric case management models is practically nonexistent.

This chapter discusses how the University of Colorado Hospital Psychiatric Service (UCHPS) has successfully navigated today's complex managed care and economic environment while maintaining high-quality care. Ethical considerations, philosophical and theoretical approaches, orientation and training, variance issues, and customer satisfaction are reviewed. Thoughtful integration of brief therapy approaches, family preservation techniques, and assertive community treatment combined with our strong belief that client input is essential to successful treatment has led to the development of a comprehensive, holistic model of case management.

INTRODUCTION

Although ideas regarding the concept of case management have been present for decades (Tahan, 1998; Floersch, 2002), the advent of managed care in the 1980s has been a catalyst for the development of case management models (Baker & Giese, 1992; Sulman et al., 2001). In this era of managed care oversight, mental health systems have had to respond with major reform (RESPONSE, 1998; Sulman et al., 2001). The literature regarding psychiatric case management is scant and does not outline a comprehensive model that addresses the complexity of psychiatric clients (Baker & Giese, 1992; Forchuk et al., 2002; Sulman et al., 2001; Tempier et al., 2002; Thomas, Dubovsky, & Cox-Young, 1996; Thomas et al., 1996).

Because of managed care's insistence that clients be quickly reintegrated into the community, inpatient psychiatric staff can no longer exclusively focus on the microsystem of the hospital (Bedell et al., 2000; Krmpotic, 1992). Development of effective relapse and discharge plans has been one step toward addressing length-of-stay and quality-of-care issues. Another important piece has been the development and use of a treatment plan that drives forward treatment and helps emphasize variances in clinical care (Forchuk et al., 2002; Goode, 1995; Sulman et al., 2001).

Historically, economic concerns and societal views about the environment in which psychiatric clients should be treated have influenced the delivery of mental health services (Anthony et al., 2000; Bedell, 2000). Currently, the emphasis of mental health treatment is in keeping the client in the community and avoiding the restrictive and costly environment of the hospital. Because mental health systems have not clearly articulated an inpatient case management model, a comprehensive model includes orientation, training opportunities, and the development of professional standards (Forchuk et al., 2002; Sulman et al., 2001). In addition, competency demonstration, continuum of care design, and treatment plan development are equally important (Forchuk et al., 2002; Thomas et al., 1995). The literature advocates for input from consumers regarding evolution of the case management model (Samele et al., 2002; Tempier et al., 2002). Incorporation of customer satisfaction data is a component of addressing the need for frequent and continual evaluation of newly developing case management models (Vaughn, Cox-Young, Webster, & Thomas, 1997; Vaughn, Webster, Orahood, & Cox-Young, 1995; Webster, Vaughn, Webb, & Playter, 1995).

Recent literature also notes the need to discuss theoretical models of case management (Cohen & Cesta, 2001; Koenig, 2001; Michaels & Cohen, 2001). Nursing theory emphasizes the relationship between the caregiver and the client and adds a therapeutic element that can be incorporated into a successful case management model. Thoughtful decision-making concerning the underpinnings of theory that guide clinical practice must address the client, as central. Montgomery and Webster (1994) believe that brief forms of psychiatric care are congruent with nursing's metaparadigm. Brief therapy theories, assertive community treatment models, and family-centered interventions form the theoretical base of a holistic case management model. Ethical dilemmas of managing care must be addressed when developing a case management model. Basing clinical decisions solely on cost containment is unethical. Case managers (CMs) must position themselves to advocate for quality-of-care issues while speaking the language of business concerns of managed care companies. This type of treatment must be highly individualized so the client and family are actively involved in the treatment planning process (Anthony et al., 2000; Bedell et al., 2000; Samele et al., 2002; Tempier et al., 2002; Vaughn et al., 1997).

The UCHPS includes a philosophy in which the provision of efficacious and quality care is provided within the framework of not a day too long and not a day too short. This chapter outlines an innovative model of inpatient psychiatric case management that bridges the gap between the hospital and the community. This model specifically addresses the scope of practice, training, orientation, support, communication skills, treatment plan development, and macromanagement of the larger, real world environment of clients. Thoughtful integration of brief therapy approaches, family preservation techniques, and assertive community treatment models are deliberately combined to articulate a theoretical conceptualization of the UCHPS Case Management Model (Berg, 1991; De Shazar, 1991; Stein & Test, 1980; Test, 1992).

▋ EVOLUTION OF THE UCHPS CASE MANAGEMENT MODEL

Early on, UCHPS recognized the need to respond to the demands of third party providers to offer efficient hospitalization (Webster et al., 1995). With the demand for cost-effective treatment, UCHPS leadership realized that we would have to make changes in our philosophy and purpose and the roles of interdisciplinary team members (Forchuk et al., 2002; Vaughn et al., 1995). The ethical dilemma we faced was to provide efficient care without sacrificing quality. As other psychiatric programs struggled to shorten lengths of stay while continuing to use longer-term therapy modalities, we, on the other hand, explored theories that envisioned the client as the center of clinical decision-making. By reviewing the literature, we ascertained that solution-focused therapy, assertive community treatment, and family preservation models were most congruent with treating the client by focusing on their strengths and real world concerns (Berg, 1991; Stein & Test, 1980; Vaughn et al., 1997). In developing our continuum of care model, we applied principles of solution-focused therapy, assertive community treatment, and family preservation models to acute inpatient services (Vaughn et al., 1997). As length of stay continued to decrease and acuity increased, we quickly realized that close clinical coordination was essential to successful outcomes (Baker & Giese, 1992; Thomas et al., 1996). The role of the CM was developed: a clinical coordinator, responsible for driving treatment forward, maintaining a solution-focused approach with clients and their families, efficiently involving ancillary providers in treatment, documenting treatment plans and progress, and developing and maintaining close working relationships with third-party providers (Figure 10-1).

Due to fragmentation of the mental health system and the complexity of many of our clients, we developed a guideline by which to assign CMs to work with specific patients. This guideline describes

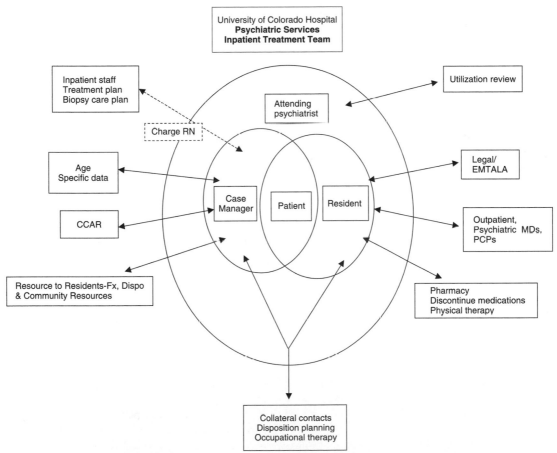

FIGURE **10-1**   University of Colorado Hospital case management model.

patient conditions, psychosocial problems, and complex treatment issues that are seen as being highest risk. Decisions regarding development of this guideline were made after a review of the current literature (Bedell et al., 2000; Forchuk et al., 2002; King et al., 2002; Mehr, 2001, 2002; Sulman et al., 2001; Ziguras et al., 2002). This tool also assists the attending psychiatrist in identifying which patients will be followed by a CM.

The UCHPS Case Management Model was structured to ensure that the CM is able to smoothly guide the client and family through the care continuum (Vaughn et al., 1997). Unlike other case management models, we visualized the scope of this role as encompassing both internal inpatient and outpatient treatment as well as external community systems of care (Figure 10-2). Consistent with the assumptions of brief therapy, the UCHPS continuum of care includes the value of identifying the client's highest level of functioning, establishing treatment goals that incorporate what is working in the client's life, and, most important, returning the client to the community as the paramount goal of hospitalization.

When the UCHPS Case Management Model was first conceptualized, leadership discussed the parameters of the CM job description. Issues that led to development of the CM role included inconsistencies in the quality of treatment plans and a breakdown of communication between the treatment team and line staff. Because nurses are trained in the formulation of psychosocial/biomedical treatment plans and have direct knowledge of formal and informal communication patterns on inpatient psychiatric unit, we determined that a nurse would best fill the role of CM. Social workers were also determined to be important members of the treatment team, coordinating family work and discharge planning. Therefore, when the UCHPS Case Management Model was first implemented in 1990, each treatment team consisted of a nurse CM, a social worker, and an attending psychiatrist. The caseload of one treatment team included approximately five to eight inpatients. Nurse CMs and social workers managed two treatment teams, responsible for the care of a total of 10 to 16 patients.

The nurse CM's role included development of the treatment plans and implementation with the line staff; communication with ancillary services, such as occupational therapy, physical therapy, and pharmacy; coordination of follow-up appointments for medical problems; and utilization management (UM). The social worker's role was limited to providing family intervention and coordinating discharge planning. Social workers were discouraged from participating in discussions of milieu issues, and nurse CMs did

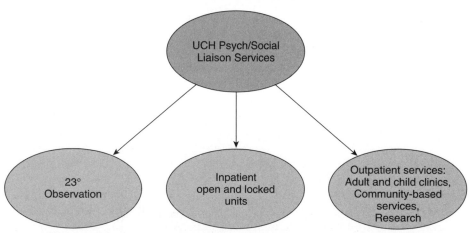

FIGURE **10-2**   University of Colorado Hospital continuum of care model.

not discuss family systems issues. The nurse CM and the social worker met several times each day for clinical updates. Although there was consistency in the provision of care in this model, both the nurse CMs and the social workers were dissatisfied, seeing the model as fragmented and compartmentalized. The social workers complained that because they did not know many important details of the patient's treatment, it was difficult to keep the family and outpatient providers updated about the patient's progress. Nurse CMs felt left out of discussions about family and support system issues. As the psychiatric and medical acuity continued to increase, both groups experienced the system as inefficient and unsatisfactory.

To increase efficiency, positive outcomes, and job satisfaction, UCHPS leadership asked the nurse CMs and the social workers to make a list of job responsibilities. It quickly became apparent that the social worker's scope of practice was limited. The social workers, all experienced in inpatient psychiatry, were quite capable of competently performing many of the duties of the nurse CMs. Conversely, many of the nurse CMs had extensive experience with family and support system work. After many months of negotiating responsibilities, leadership decided that the roles of the nurse CM and the social worker could be combined to form the role of psychiatric CM. In this way, each psychiatric CM would have expanded responsibility for one treatment team (five to eight patients and their families) instead of two teams, as in the previous model.

To ensure a smooth transition from a model with the team consisting of a nurse CM, social worker, and attending psychiatrist to the new model of a psychiatric CM and an attending psychiatrist, both nurses and social workers met weekly over several months. In these meetings, members of each discipline exchanged detailed information about their own duties/responsibilities. When the CMs and leadership felt comfortable with the transition, new teams were formed. Each discipline made a commitment to be available to the other for professional consultation.

Having successfully negotiated this transition in provision of case management services, UCHPS faced a new challenge in 2002: balancing the fiscal concerns regarding case management with the need to provide structure and support for significantly ill patients. To achieve this balance, UCHPS leadership decided to assign case management by outlier, using a tool to assist in identification of high-risk and complex patients.

Although this chapter focuses on the provision of CM services in the inpatient setting, it is important to recognize that UCH has been able to adapt the UCHPS case management model to community settings. The UCHPS Community Service provides outpatient case management, which incorporates brief therapy, family preservation, and assertive community models. This team was developed in response to requests from public managed care systems to provide intensive home-based services for their clients. Team members work with families in their homes, providing case management, psychotherapy, and parenting education. The CMs in this setting, all licensed clinicians, work independently to provide care delivery. Formal group clinical supervision occurs once a week for 2 hours with a psychiatrist and a licensed marriage and family therapist. Clinicians also receive frequent formal and informal individual clinical supervision.

As the UCHPS continuum of care model evolved, so did the role of the CM. Because we conceptualized the CM role to be flexible and dynamic, resistance to change thus far has been minimized (Baker & Giese, 1992; Thomas et al., 1995). Leadership recognized that the complexity of this model could lead to role dissatisfaction and poor treatment outcomes. Thoughtful discussions concerning the educational needs of the CM led to the development of a competency-based orientation to the role, continued education and training, and development of ongoing clinical supervision. Although costly to our organization, orientation, training, and supervision programs are strongly supported by our administration. In the next section of this chapter, we discuss the six components of a successful case management model.

COMPONENTS OF A SUCCESSFUL CASE MANAGEMENT MODEL

Orientation

The process of clinical orientation at UCH is multidimensional. CMs participate in a competency-based, hospitalwide, department- and unit-specific orientation that includes didactic learning experiences and clinical orientation with a trained preceptor. Because CMs are responsible for both communicating the plan of care to the line staff and guiding treatment forward, they must have an understanding of the responsibilities of the line staff and an ability to develop treatment plans that clearly articulate line staff interventions for their patients. To clearly understand the role of line staff, CMs are oriented to milieu management and mental health worker and clinical nurse responsibilities.

Classroom orientation consists of 2 full days of lecture and didactic learning. An overview of UCH patient services programs and our performance improvement model is presented. A clinical nurse specialist with prescriptive authority teaches a 2-hour course about psychotropic medications and administers a competency performance examination to participants. The clinical nurse specialist/educator conducts a 1-hour risk assessment course and a 5-hour brief therapy course (Webster et al., 1995). A mental health worker with more than 15 years of inpatient psychiatry experience teaches a course about lower-level interventions in the milieu and behavior management. CMs must demonstrate competency in risk assessment, brief therapy approaches, and behavioral management before orientation is completed.

The clinical nurse specialist/educator meets with each CM orientee before the first clinical orientation day. CM orientees are given a packet called the "Competency Performance Orientation Checklist" (see Appendix 10-1). This packet includes competencies, both knowledge and skill based, that the CM must either understand or demonstrate before the end of the orientation period. The clinical nurse specialist/educator updates the checklist annually in response to changes in clinical practice and role responsibilities. Areas of competency reviewed in the checklist include utilization of brief therapy approaches, interdisciplinary communication, discharge/disposition planning, group and family therapy, therapeutic relationships, milieu management, policies and procedures, documentation guidelines, and mandatory safety procedures. All of the competencies are reviewed formally in classroom orientation and reinforced in clinical orientation with the assigned clinical preceptor.

The clinical nurse specialist/educator assigns a trained clinical preceptor to provide clinical orientation. During clinical orientation, which lasts 3 to 4 weeks, CM orientees first observe the clinical preceptor on the unit. The clinical preceptor reviews the Competency Orientation Performance Checklist with the CM orientee each morning, developing daily and weekly goals for clinical orientation. Typically, CM orientees begin some independent practice by the end of the first week of clinical orientation. At the end of the clinical orientation, the clinical nurse specialist/educator reviews each section of the completed Competency Orientation Performance Checklist with the CM orientee to ensure that the CM orientee feels comfortable to begin managing a caseload. If the CM orientee or the clinical nurse specialist/educator identifies deficits that must be addressed immediately, the clinical nurse specialist/educator can either choose to work directly with the orientee or ask the clinical preceptor to continue clinical orientation. Because the role of CM is so complex, leadership staff expects that most CMs will work approximately 6 months before they feel a sense of mastery in the position. This expectation is reinforced to new CMs, as many have stated that they feel pressure to "know it all" when clinical orientation ends. To allow new CMs to flourish in this complicated and multifaceted role, UCHPS leadership has organized extensive clinical supervision for this group.

Clinical Supervision

Because the CM's role as the hub of the treatment team is crucial for effective treatment, clinical supervision becomes essential for positive treatment outcomes. Historically, patient services staff have not received intense, ongoing clinical supervision, nor has this modality been valued (Forchuk et al., 2002; Sulman et al., 2001). Clarity of the supervision model to reinforce competency-based orientation came as leadership recognized the need to provide several modalities of supervision for CMs. Currently CMs participate in many formal and informal supervision activities. Professional role development, family supervision, and "behind the mirror" supervision are discussed.

PROFESSIONAL ROLE DEVELOPMENT

To support new CMs in integrating with treatment team members, they meet weekly with the Clinical Nurse Specialist/Educator to discuss role development issues. New CMs have struggled to successfully function in this complicated system and have voiced a need to meet with a knowledgeable mentor to discuss emerging role development issues. Areas of discussion include the UCHPS Case Management Model, UCHPS continuum of care model, high-risk cases, patient advocacy issues, and customer relations. Because the facilitator of this group is not a direct supervisor, new CMs are more apt to openly discuss barriers to role development. UCH leadership supports this costly intervention, because not to do so causes role ambiguity and may lead to implementation of incongruent philosophies of care. This group meets weekly for 1 hour.

FAMILY SUPERVISION

A key role of the CM is the provision of family and support system intervention. Level of competency in systems interventions varied, depending on the prior training and experience of the CM. Discrepancy in functional levels of the CM led to the need to have formalized supervision that acknowledged the expertise CMs brought to the role, while recognizing that deficits did exist. Because the training needs varied between disciplines, the clinical nurse specialist/educator and the lead social worker met to discuss the goals and format of the supervision.

In the family supervision "Case Presentation Outline" (Box 10-1), the CM's role is structured both to develop a professional case presentation and to facilitate a peer discussion. In the monthly family supervision meetings, CMs have presented a wide variety of cases. Issues have included transcultural intervention, multisystem coordination, countertransference issues, complex medical comorbidity, substance-abusing patients and family members, and how to successfully intervene with families with special needs. Initially, CMs were hesitant to give feedback to their peers. Because clinical supervision has not been consistently valued in inpatient psychiatric settings (Bedell et al., 2000; Forchuk et al., 2002), many CMs were not comfortable with and did not understand the concept of giving and receiving peer feedback regarding clinical performance. To model acceptable ways of giving and receiving feedback, the clinical nurse specialist/educator and the lead social worker presented the first two cases in family supervision.

BEHIND-THE-MIRROR SUPERVISION

Because brief therapy philosophy includes rapid mobilization of client's resources, supervision supporting this philosophy becomes essential in short-term hospitalization. The CM needs expertise in directing clinical care with families, support systems, and inpatient/outpatient staff. Behind-the-mirror supervision is a process by which CMs are able to receive immediate feedback from their peers and supervisors (Vaughn et al., in press). In behind-the-mirror supervision, CMs conduct individual interviews with patients and/or families using brief therapy modalities. The literature concerning clinical supervision suggests that the model should reflect the philosophy of patient care delivery

---

BOX 10-1 ▶ UNIVERSITY OF COLORADO HOSPITAL, PSYCHIATRIC SERVICES

Family Supervision—Case Presentation Outline

The family supervision presentation is a 30-minute formal presentation followed by a 20-minute peer discussion. The case presentation is to include the following:

1. Warm up
   Why are you presenting this case?
   - Difficult
   - Interesting
   - Negative outcome
   - Positive outcome
2. Literature review
   Present at least one article/book/chapter pertinent to this case.
   Include the following in your presentation:
   - Theoretical framework
   - Main points for the article/book/chapter
3. Analysis of the case
   - Precipitants
   - Goals of the patient, family and support system
   - Clinical assessment
   - Treatment plan and interventions
   - Evaluation
   - Any change in patient, family, or support system goals resulting from the outcomes of the case
   - What went well
   - What you would do differently

During the 20-minute peer discussion, participants will
1. Discuss whether you've dealt with a similar patient, family, or support system.
2. Talk about what approach you took with that family.
3. Describe whether you had a similar or dissimilar outcome.
4. Discuss any feedback you have for the presenter.

Courtesy of University of Colorado Hospital, Denver, Colorado.

(Vaughn et al., in press). Therefore supervision is a parallel process whereby the supervision team provides the CM with feedback in the same structured format as used by the CM to give feedback to the patient/family. This process has been described in detail in previous articles (Vaughn et al., unpublished manuscript).

Interdisciplinary Team

Traditionally, inpatient psychiatric treatment has been coordinated by psychiatrists (Thomas et al., 1995). As third-party providers and other external systems have demanded shorter lengths of stay and more consistent communication of the patient's progression, psychiatrists have realized that it is imperative to share and delegate clinical and organizational functions (Baker & Giese, 1992; Thomas et al., 1995, 1996; Vaughn et al., 1997). Development and implementation of the UCHPS Case Management

Model would not have been successful if the medical staff had not first agreed to change the model of patient care delivery. Thomas et al. (1995) describe the process of redefinition of multidisciplinary team roles. They acknowledge that both attending psychiatrists and trainees initially had difficulty with the transition from a more traditional model of care delivery to the UCHPS Case Management Model. Their stance, however, is that clear role definition of the CM ensures "clinical efficiency" and will ultimately "optimize the use of the psychiatrist's time." Attending psychiatrists are oriented to the UCHPS Case Management Model by their peers. Support of the model is reinforced when new attending psychiatrists begin working on the units and see the positive effects of collaborative interdisciplinary working relationships. Residents in training and medical students are oriented to the UCHPS Case Management Model by senior CMs at the beginning of their clinical rotation. Attending psychiatrists and CMs formally and informally reinforce both the CM and resident roles with the residents and medical students during interdisciplinary meetings.

Treatment Plan

Clinical information is formally reviewed with the treatment team in daily multidisciplinary rounds and twice-weekly treatment planning meetings. The CM contacts treatment team members informally if there is new clinical information that must be reviewed immediately. The CM is responsible for leading treatment planning meetings and for integrating and documenting all clinical information in the patient's treatment plan. The purpose of treatment planning meetings is to review new clinical information and to revise the plan of care. All of the treatment team's patients are presented in 1 hour, giving the treatment team approximately 10 minutes to revise the plan of care for each patient. In-depth discussion regarding the psychodynamic formulation of the case is completed outside of the treatment plan meeting (Baker & Giese, 1992; Thomas et al., 1995).

CMs contact external providers to negotiate how clinical information will be exchanged. Telephone conferences, treatment update meetings, and discharge meetings are coordinated at the beginning of hospitalization, ensuring external provider participation. Examples of external treatment provider participation include outpatient CMs, group home staff, probation and parole officers, social services technicians, and clergy. The CM is responsible for establishing and maintaining contact with family and community supports of assigned patients. Family input is considered essential to successful treatment. Issues that appear to be part of the precipitating events of hospitalization are addressed in family meetings. Patient services staff meet every shift with the client to establish treatment goals and interventions. At the end of each shift, patient services staff document progress toward goal attainment and response to interventions. If the client cannot participate in problem solving because of cognitive impairment, the treatment team works with the family and community supports to develop goals to expedite restabilization. Patient services staff attend and participate in the treatment planning meeting, bringing up-to-date clinical information.

Treatment plans are structured to provide clear interventions for line staff and the multidisciplinary team. A performance improvement team reviews the treatment plans annually and makes appropriate revisions. This team is chaired by the Clinical Nurse Specialist/Educator, and group participants include an attending psychiatrist, patient services managers, a CM, a charge nurse, and a mental health worker.

An example of one of the UCH treatment plans is the "Suicide Attempt/Ideation" treatment plan (see Appendix 10-2). In the treatment planning meeting, the CM and the charge nurse are responsible for completing this form. The first part of the plan includes a brief formulation of the case and the psychiatric and medical diagnoses. The second section of the treatment plan documents measurable goals. Goals are developed with input from the treatment team, line staff, patient, family, and support system (Webster et al., 1994). Next, interventions are addressed. Interventions associated with providing safety (risk assessment and suicide precautions) for the patient and the milieu are listed first. Other interventions include laboratory testing and consultation, medication regimen and administration, medication and illness education, group participation, family and support system interventions, discharge planning issues, and treatment of acute medical issues. The last section of the treatment plan is the outcome section. In this section the treatment team identifies what the functioning level of the patient must be before the patient is discharged.

After the treatment planning meeting is completed, the CM and charge nurse are responsible for ensuring that the line staff implements the interventions outlined in the newly revised plan. Other treatment plan forms that the CM may use to develop a complete plan of care include the "Behavioral Care Plan" and "Take Care of Yourself" (see Appendix 10-3). The Behavioral Care Plan guides the line staff in behavioral interventions aimed at providing the patient with the external structure he or she needs to stay in behavioral control on the unit. The Take Care of Yourself form is completed by the CM with input from the outpatient provider. The outpatient provider gives the CM information about the client's cognitive and functional ability to complete activities of daily living (ADLs). With this information the CM completes the form, giving the line staff detailed information about level of assistance with ADLs and how often ADLs should be completed. Because it is often difficult to assess the client's cognitive and functional ability during a short hospital stay, it is important to provide care that is consistent with the care provided in the community setting. If the level of assistance provided is consistent between inpatient and outpatient providers, the client is less likely to demonstrate symptoms of regression after discharge.

Use of treatment plans is not a new concept; most medical inpatient units use critical pathways and/or care maps to structure clinical intervention and to provide standardized outcome measures (Cohen & Cesta, 2001; Goode, 1995). In psychiatry, where complex psychosocial and environmental variables influence the client's clinical progress, measuring outcomes and accounting for variances in length of stay are challenging and have not been well documented (Baker & Giese, 1992; Thomas, Dubovsky, & Cox-Young, 1996; Thomas et al., 1996, 1997).

Variance tracking within mental health systems is sadly at a rudimentary stage of development. UCHPS has contributed to the development of variance tracking by collecting both inpatient and outpatient outcomes data in conjunction with managed care companies (Baker & Giese, 1992; Thomas, Dubovsky, & Cox-Young, 1996; Thomas et al., 1996, 1997).

In the infancy of psychiatric managed care, CMs partnered with managed care providers to develop UM tools that measured length of stay, recidivism, successful suicides, and readmission within 24 hours (Baker & Giese, 1992; Thomas, Dubovsky, & Cox-Young, 1996; Thomas et al., 1996, 1997). As we developed partnerships with an increasing number of managed care companies, the time expenditure required of CMs to perform UM duties began to take away from important clinical responsibilities.

Utilization Management

In June 1999 a social worker was hired for the specific purpose of completing inpatient UM processes. Before this time, CMs were responsible for all authorizations for clients on their caseload. It became evident that the focus of client care was being negatively affected by this UM function. As the UM process became more complicated, it also became more time consuming; CMs had an increasingly difficult time completing other clinical duties. UM inherently involves a great deal of telephone work; unless the CM is readily available to answer telephone calls, an inordinate amount of time is spent brokering authorizations for continued treatment. Before changing our UM system, the rate of successful authorization for treatment was 50%. Lack of authorizations for treatment created difficulty in

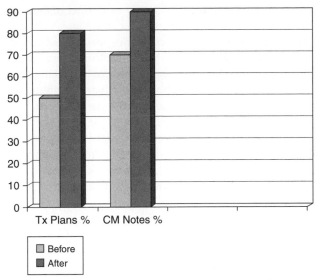

FIGURE **10-3**   Comparison of completion rates of treatment plans and case management progress notes before and after utilization review was separated from case management responsibilities.

hospital billing and collections. On the clinical front, the quality of CM documentation decreased and quality of treatment plans was insufficient, secondary to emphasis on the time-consuming task of UM (Figure 10-3).

The decision to allocate resources to UM has had several positive outcomes. The rate of successful authorization improved dramatically. There is increased flexibility in the CM's schedule. The UM process now interfaces with finance and billing departments. There is an organized, careful review and response to denials. The UM staff member generally works independently but consults with CMs when there are complex clinical issues that require additional input for authorization for treatment. The UM/utilization review staff member reviews all cases regardless of health care coverage using InterQual standards (McKesson, 2002). All cases with a length of stay greater than 14 days are reviewed with the interdisciplinary treatment team. Any identified quality concerns are reported to the program manager. The UM position works closely with the Admissions Department to recommend benefits acquisition, financial counseling, and assistance with gathering insurance information.

Customer Satisfaction

Customer satisfaction has long been viewed as an important indicator of quality of care (Anthony et al., 2000; Caslyn et al., 2002; Goode, 1995; Samele et al., 2002; Tempier et al., 2002). In this age of increased managed care, third-party providers, and regulatory agency oversight, customer satisfaction data carry more weight (Baker & Giese, 1992). At UCH, we have always maintained that patient satisfaction is the most important indicator of our clinical success. Valuing customer satisfaction meshes solution-focused philosophy with our model of care delivery. In solution-focused therapy, core concepts include the belief that clients have the best answers for their problems and that they should always be involved with formulating treatment goals and evaluating treatment outcomes

(Vaughn et al., 1997). We firmly believe that successful evolution of our model depends on client input.

In 1990 we began to gather customer satisfaction data. We used these data to determine educational needs for line staff and program redesign. In 1996 we began to participate in a national patient satisfaction benchmarking program, RESPONSE Healthcare Information Management, Inc. This enabled us to compare our customer satisfaction data with similar psychiatric facilities across the nation. UCHPS data indicate that across categories we met or exceeded the national benchmark (RESPONSE, 1998) (Figure 10-4).

As indicated in Figure 10-4, the areas of greatest customer satisfaction were in teamwork among staff, respect shown and dignity maintained, overall quality of care and services, outcome of care, discharge instructions, and coordination of care after discharge. In completing the customer satisfaction questionnaire, clients are encouraged to provide comments regarding their treatment.

"I realize that most of what needs to be done to help myself needs to come from me." UCHPS inpatient, 1998

Clients frequently note how useful the treatment experience has been for them, that the staff gave them confidence to succeed, and that they were involved with treatment decisions.

Currently UCH participates in a national benchmarking program by Press, Ganey Associates, Inc. (2003). Current results from this national program are available online and are regularly reviewed with all staff. This process allows CMs to receive feedback about their role and gives them an opportunity to participate in the dynamic process of performance improvement.

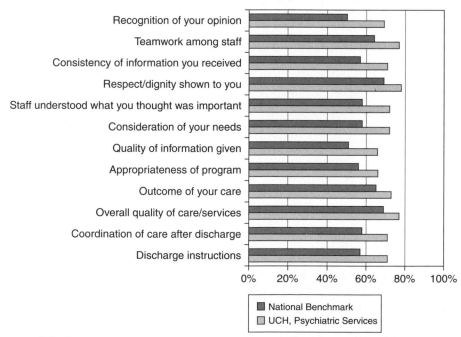

FIGURE **10-4**   Percentage of responses from the "very good" to the "excellent" range.
Data were compiled from *National Benchmark Report, Psychiatric Hospitals (1998)* and *RESPONSE (1998).*

SUMMARY

In this chapter, we have outlined an innovative psychiatric case management model. We hope that our model adds to the paucity of information currently available regarding psychiatric case management models. Part of our success has been attributable to the support of UCHPS leadership, who back expensive orientation, training, and supervision aspects. Theoretical underpinnings that hold the client as central to successful treatment have remained the cornerstone of our success. Evolving treatment plans and UM processes reflect our desire to address our rapidly changing health care system. It remains important to evaluate new and innovative approaches in case management (Bedell, et al., 2000). Emerging programs include self-case management (Liberman & Kopelowicz, 2002) and new approaches in case management of patients who have borderline personality disorder (Nehls, 2001).

Changes in clinical systems are occurring so rapidly that they outstrip the meager empirical data used to make changes in health care delivery models. Our hope is that psychiatric programs will band together to collect essential data regarding clinical variance, clinical outcomes, lengths of stay, and diagnosis-specific critical pathways. Outcome measures are particularly critical because psychiatric inpatient case management is new and relatively unstudied. Formal research projects are required to address the specific needs of various psychiatric populations.

References

Anthony, W.A., Cohen, M., Farkas, M., & Cohen, B.F. (2000). Clinical care update: The chronically mentally ill case management—more than a response to a dysfunctional system. *Community Mental Health Journal, 36*(1), 97-106.

Baker, N.J., & Giese, A.A. (1992). Reorganization of a private psychiatric unit to promote collaboration with managed care. *Hospital and Community Psychiatry, 43*(11), 126-129.

Bedell, J.R., Cohen, N.K., & Sullivan, A. (2000). Case management: The current best practices and the next generation of innovation. *Community Mental Health Journal, 36*(2), 179-194.

Berg, I.K. (1991). *Family preservation: A brief therapy workbook.* London: BT Press.

Caslyn, R., Morse, G.A., Klinkenberg, W.D., Yonker, R.D., & Trusty, M.L. (2002). Moderators and mediators of client satisfaction in case management programs for clients with severe mental illness. *Mental Health Services Research, 4*(4), 267-275.

Cohen, E.L., & Cesta, T.G. (2001). Within-the-walls case management: A acute care-based nursing case management model. In *Nursing case management from essentials to advanced practice applications,* 3rd edition, St. Louis: Mosby.

De Shazer, S. (1991). *Patterns of brief family therapy.* New York: Guilford Press.

Floersch, J. (2002). *Meds, Money, and Manners: The Case Management of Severe Mental Illness.* New York: Columbia University Press.

Forchuk, C., Ouwerkerk, A., Yamashita, M., & Martin, M. (2002). Mental health case management in Canada: job description analyses. *Issues in Mental Health Nursing, 23,* 477-496.

Goode, C. (1995). Impact of a care map and case management on patient satisfaction, and staff satisfaction, collaboration and autonomy. *Nursing Economic, 13*(6), 337-348.

King, R., Yellowlees, P., Nurcombe, B., Spooner, D., Sturk, H., Spence, S., & LeBas, J. (2002). Psychologists as mental health case managers. *Australian Psychologist, 37*(2), 118-122.

Koenig, E. (2001). Collaborative models of case management. In E.L. Cohen & T.G. Cesta (Eds.), *Nursing case management from essentials to advanced practice applications,* 3rd edition, St. Louis: Mosby.

Krmpotic, D. (1992). Successful implementation of case management. *Nursing Connections, 5*(2), 49-50.

Liberman, R.P., & Kopelowicz, A. (2002). Rehab rounds: Teaching persons with severe mental disabilities to be their own case managers. *Psychiatric Services, 53,* 1377-1379.

McKesson Health Solutions, LLC. (2002). *InterQual Level of Care Criteria.* Marlborough, Mass.: McKesson Health Solutions, LLC.

Mehr, J. (2001). Case management: A review with implications for services for concurrent severe mental illness and alcoholism or substance abuse. *Psychiatric Rehabilitation Skills, 5*(1), 80-107.

Michaels, C., & Cohen, E.L. (2001). Two strategies for managing care: Care management and case management. In E.L. Cohen & T.G. Cesta (Eds.), *Nursing Case Management from essentials to advanced practice applications*, 3rd edition, St. Louis: Mosby.

Montgomery, C., & Webster, D. (1993). Care and nursing's metaparadigm: Can they survive in the era of managed care? *Perspectives in Psychiatric Nursing, 29*(4), 5-12.

Montgomery, C., & Webster, D. (1994). Caring, curing and brief therapy: A model for nurse-psychotherapy. *Archives of Psychiatric Nursing, 8*(5), 291-297.

Nehls, N. (2001). What is a case manager? The perspective of persons with borderline personality disorder. *Journal of the American Psychiatric Nurse's Association, 7*(1), 4-12.

Patient Satisfaction Survey (1998). RESPONSE. Baltimore, Md.: Healthcare Information Management, Inc.

Press, Ganey Satisfaction Measurement (2003). South Bend, Indo: Press, Ganey Associates, Inc.

Samele, C., Gilvarry, C., Walsh, E., Manley, C., van Os, J., & Murray, R. (2002). Patient's perceptions of intensive case management. *Psychiatric Services, 53*, 1432-1437.

Stein, L.I., & Test, M.A. (1980). Alternative to mental hospital treatment. I: Conceptual model, treatment program, and clinical evaluation, *Archives of General Psychiatry, 37*, 392-397.

Sulman, J., Savage, D., & Way, S. (2001). Retooling social work practice for high volume, short stay. *Social Work Health and Mental Health, 34*(3-4), 315-332.

Tahan, H. (1998). Case management: A heritage more than a century old. *Nursing Case Management, 3*(2), 55-60.

Tempier, R., Pawliuk, N., Perreault, M., & Steiner, W. (2002). International report. Satisfaction with clinical case management services of patients with long-term psychoses. *Community Mental Health Journal, 38*(1), 51-59.

Test, M.A. (1992). Training in community living. In R.P. Lieberman (Ed.), *Handbook of psychiatric rehabilitation.* New York: Macmillan.

Thomas, M.R., Dubovsky, S.L., & Cox-Young, B. (1996). Impact of external versus internal case managers on hospital utilization. *Psychiatric Services, 47*(6), 593-595.

Thomas, M.R., House, R., Shore, J., & Cox Young, B. (1995). The impact of economic and health care delivery changes on psychiatric residency training. Adapting to the new realities for clinical services and residency education in managed care. *Proceedings of the AACPD/RTD Conferences*, Baltimore, Md.: Deparment of Psychiatry, University of Maryland School of Medicine.

Thomas, M.R., Kassner, C.T., Fryer, G.E., Giese, A.A., Rosenberg, S.A., & Dubovsky, S.L. (1997). Impact of shorter lengths of stay on status at discharge in bipolar mania. *Annals of Clinical Psychiatry, 9*(3), 139-143.

Thomas, M.R., Rosenberg, S.A., Giese, A.A., Dubovsky, S.L., & Shore, J.H. (1996). Shortening length of stay without increasing recidivism on a university-affiliated inpatient unit. *Psychiatric Services, 47*(9), 996-998.

Vaughn, K., Cox-Young, B., Webster, D.C., & Thomas, M.R. (1997). Solution-focused work in the hospital. A continuum-of-care model for inpatient psychiatric treatment. In S.D. Miller, M.A. Hubble, & B.L. Duncan (eds.). *Handbook of solution-focused brief therapy*. San Francisco: Jossey-Bass Publishers.

Vaughn, K., Hastings-Guerrero, S., & Kassner, C. (1996). Solution-oriented inpatient group therapy. *Journal of Systemic Therapies, 15*(3), 1-13.

Vaughn, K., Webster, D.C., Orahood, S., & Cox-Young, B. (1995). Brief inpatient psychiatric treatment: Finding solutions. *Issues in Mental Health Nursing, 16*, 519-531.

Vaughn, K., Webster, D.C., Platter, B., Playter, A., & Webb, M. (Unpublished manuscript.). Solution oriented hospital practice and supervision: Building psychiatric nursing competencies. *Perspectives in Psychiatric Care.*

Webster, D.C., Vaughn, K., & Martinez, R. (1994). Introducing solution-focused approaches to staff in inpatient psychiatric settings. *Archives of Psychiatric Nursing, 8*(4), 254-261.

Webster, D.C., Vaughn, K., Webb, M., & Playter, A. (1995). Modeling the client's world through solution-focused therapy. *Issues in Mental Health Nursing, 16*(6), 505-518.

Ziguras, S.J., Steuart, G.W., & Jackson, A.C. (2002). Assessing the evidence on case management. *The British Journal of Psychiatry, 181*, 17-21.

Appendix 10-1

University of Colorado Hospital Psychiatric Services

Competency Performance Orientation Checklist–Psychiatric Case Manager

Name:

Competency: Utilizes brief therapy in individual, group, family, and milieu therapy

Evaluation Criteria

1. Verbalizes value system of long- and short-term therapist.
2. States the assumptions of solution-oriented therapy.
3. Verbalizes obstacles and pitfalls to avoid in brief therapy.
4. Reads brief therapy manual.
5. Has 1:1 interactions with patients, families, and support systems using solution-focused therapy and other brief therapy approaches.
6. States factors that contribute to regression in hospitalized patients.
7. Demonstrates use of reframing techniques.
8. States types of interviewing techniques used in solution-focused therapy and other brief therapy approaches.
9. Sets goal with patients, families, and support systems that are client centered, achievable, and measurable.
10. Attends solution-focused therapy and change theory orientation class and demonstrates competency through passing post-test with score of 80% or greater.
11. Attends monthly "behind the mirror" supervision sessions, participating as the clinician and as part of the supervision team.

Preceptor/Educator			Comments	I Have Satisfactorily Performed the Above Competency

Taught	Performed with assistance	Performed independently		**Orientee**
				    Date
				
				Preceptor
				    Date

Courtesy University of Colorado Hospital, Denver, Colorado.

University of Colorado Hospital Psychiatric Services

COMPETENCY PERFORMANCE ORIENTATION CHECKLIST–PSYCHIATRIC CASE MANAGER

Name:

Competency: Complies with hospital policies outlining documentation requirements

Evaluation Criteria

1. Completes treatment plan and ensures patient services implementation of treatment plan (including biophysical, psychosocial, and environmental realms).
2. Completes "Behavior Plan" with patient services staff input when applicable; used to address behavioral issues of assigned patients.
3. Completes "Take Care of Yourself" with patient services staff input when applicable; used to address self-care issues of assigned patients.
4. Documentation on the patient record is legible, accurate, and concise.
5. Completes 2-hour RN/LSCW reassessment forms in compliance with "Psychiatric Use of Seclusion and Restraint" policy.
6. Completes risk assessment on the Suicide Risk Assessment and Violence Risk Assessment forms, documents clearly in the chart, and communicates results with treatment team. Repeats this process as indicated, based on patient presentation.
7. Completes case manager section of the discharge plan form. Ensures that an RN has completed the RN section of the form before the patient is discharged.
8. Completes or describes the AMA discharge procedure.
9. Ensures completion of patient teaching standards for medication, diagnosis, and other educational issues.
10. Completes case manager progress note, minimum of 1 per week.

Ensures completion of psychosocial data base (childhood and developmental history, cultural issues, living arrangements, military history sections) and signs encounter form signature log.

Preceptor/Educator			Comments	I Have Satisfactorily Performed the Above Competency
Taught	Performed with assistance	Performed independently		**Orientee** Date **Preceptor** Date

Courtesy University of Colorado Hospital, Denver, Colorado.

University of Colorado Hospital Psychiatric Services

COMPETENCY PERFORMANCE ORIENTATION CHECKLIST–PSYCHIATRIC CASE MANAGER

Name:

Competency: Discharge planning

Evaluation Criteria

1. Ensures appropriate transportation is arranged for patient.
2. Clarifies patient's ability to take passes and makes necessary arrangements.
3. Coordinates/leads staffings with outpatient providers.
4. Arranges appropriate psychiatric/medical and other outpatient follow-up.
5. Coordinates/secures appropriate housing at discharge.
6. Educates patient, family, and support system about patient's current medication regimen and ensures that all understand the information presented.
7. Educates patient, family, and support system about how to secure financial resources.
8. Arranges facility transfers as indicated: coordinates completion of EMTALA forms.
9. Ensures completion of paperwork for nursing home placement.
10. Coordinates legal issues, such as legal status on the unit and legal issues in the community.
11. Is a liaison for community resources.

Preceptor/Educator			Comments	I Have Satisfactorily Performed the Above Competency
Taught	Performed with assistance	Performed independently		**Orientee** Date **Preceptor** Date

Courtesy University of Colorado Hospital, Denver, Colorado.

University of Colorado Hospital Psychiatric Services

COMPETENCY PERFORMANCE ORIENTATION CHECKLIST–PSYCHIATRIC CASE MANAGER

Name:

Competency: Interdisciplinary communication

Evaluation Criteria

1. Demonstrates interdisciplinary communication and coordination with medical staff, students, line staff, occupational therapy pharmacy, family medicine, internal and external consultants, patient representative, and others.
2. Demonstrates and documents appropriate sign-out of cases for planned absences from the unit.
3. Demonstrates appropriate sign-out of cases for unplanned absences.
4. Demonstrates ability to manage complaints related to assigned patients and involves the use of appropriate resources.

Preceptor/Educator			Comments	I Have Satisfactorily Performed the Above Competency

Taught	Performed with assistance	Performed independently		**Orientee**
				      Date
				
				Preceptor
				      Date

Courtesy University of Colorado Hospital, Denver, Colorado.

University of Colorado Hospital Psychiatric Services

COMPETENCY PERFORMANCE ORIENTATION CHECKLIST–PSYCHIATRIC CASE MANAGER

Name:

Competency: Establishes therapeutic relationships with patients and families

Evaluation Criteria

1. Reads and signs policy on confidentiality and therapeutic relationships.
2. States principles of therapeutic interactions.
3. Verbalizes difference between therapeutic and social relationships.
4. Reads policy on therapeutic relationships.
5. Reads guideline for staff/patient and family interactions.
6. States how age, race, gender, and culture of patient and family may affect therapeutic relationship.
7. States importance of terminating the therapeutic relationship with the patient and the family when the patient is discharged.
8. Reads adolescent and geriatric manuals and provides age-appropriate care.
9. Attends and participates in monthly family supervision meetings.

Preceptor/Educator			Comments	I Have Satisfactorily Performed the Above Competency
Taught	Performed with assistance	Performed independently		**Orientee** Date **Preceptor** Date

Courtesy University of Colorado Hospital, Denver, Colorado.

University of Colorado Hospital Psychiatric Services

Competency Performance Orientation Checklist–Psychiatric Case Manager

Name:

Competency: Provides and maintains a safe therapeutic environment

Evaluation Criteria

1. States five therapeutic aspects of milieu treatment.
2. Verbalizes difference between traditional inpatient milieu therapy and brief milieu therapy.
3. Verbalizes safety issues in the milieu.
4. Verbalizes hierarchy of interventions in the milieu.
5. Demonstrates use of lower level interventions in the milieu.
6. Verbalizes age-appropriate limit setting in the milieu.
7. Initiates search procedures as indicated.
8. States procedure when patients go AWOL.
9. Attends behavior management class and demonstrates competency by passing the seclusion/restraint test and the behavior management test with scores of 80% or better.
10. Demonstrates safe application of mechanical restraints.
11. Communicates with family and support system about the criteria/procedures for seclusion/restraint and maintenance of a safe milieu.
12. Supports family and support system by maintaining close contact with clinical updates and reassurance when patient is in seclusion/restraint.

Preceptor/Educator			Comments	I Have Satisfactorily Performed the Above Competency

Taught	Performed with assistance	Performed independently		**Orientee**
				        Date
				
				Preceptor
				        Date

Courtesy University of Colorado Hospital, Denver, Colorado.

University of Colorado Hospital Psychiatric Services

COMPETENCY PERFORMANCE ORIENTATION CHECKLIST–PSYCHIATRIC CASE MANAGER

Name:

Competency: Co-leads group therapy/family therapy/case conferences

Evaluation Criteria

1. Able to assess and address family dynamics and intervene using brief therapy and systems theory interventions.
2. Formulates the psychosocial focus of the acute care episode with the treatment team.
3. Educates the family and support system about the patient's medications, illness, and treatment needs.
4. Negotiates treatment goals and follow-up plans with the patient, family, and support system.
5. Applies new knowledge in family and support system intervention from monthly family supervision group to clinical practice.
6. Understands expectation of participation in ongoing educational activities that address family and support system intervention.
7. Verbalizes difference between group process and content.
8. Reads guideline on co-therapist before and after group conference.
9. Verbalizes effective and ineffective group therapist language and behavior.
10. Reads group therapy manual.

Preceptor/Educator			Comments	I Have Satisfactorily Performed the Above Competency
Taught	Performed with assistance	Performed independently		**Orientee** 　　Date **Preceptor** 　　Date

Courtesy University of Colorado Hospital, Denver, Colorado.

University of Colorado Hospital Psychiatric Services

Competency Performance Orientation Checklist—Psychiatric Case Manager

Name:
Competency: Complies with standards of job description
Evaluation Criteria
1. Verbalizes the three missions of UCH and vision statement.
2. Reviews the UCH organizational chart.
3. Reviews the UCH quality management plan and participates in performance improvement projects.
4. Reads and signs job description.
5. Participates in weekly professional role development group with the clinical nurse specialist/educator.

Preceptor/Educator			Comments	I Have Satisfactorily Performed the Above Competency
Taught	Performed with assistance	Performed independently		**Orientee** Date **Preceptor** Date

Courtesy University of Colorado Hospital, Denver, Colorado.

Multidisciplinary Treatment Plan

Suicide: Attempt/Ideation

DATE _____   Next Staffing _____

Privileges _____   **Legal status** _____   **ELOS** _____

DIAGNOSIS _____

Focus: Behavior Management: Self-Harm Related to:

☐ Psychosis   ☐ Depression   ☐ Panic   ☐ Hopelessness   ☐ Chronic illness
☐ Terminal illness   ☐ Altered cognitive status   ☐ Grief/loss _____
☐ Psychoactive substances   ☐ _____   ☐ _____

Illustrated by:

☐ Suicidal ideation with a plan _____
☐ Suicide attempt _____
☐ _____
☐ _____

Goals (must be measurable):

☐ Patient will demonstrate ability to manage symptoms.
☐ _____
☐ _____

Interventions

☐ 1. Risk assessment (discipline responsible/frequency) _____
☐ 2. SUICIDE PRECAUTIONS
    • Assess and document suicidal ideation every shift • Must be RTW and on escape precautions • 15-minute safety checks • Patient searched and placed in hospital gowns • Patient to remain in public areas on the unit during waking • MD note daily regarding continued suicide risk • Controlled items with staff supervision only
☐ 3. Labs/Procedures/Medical Consults:

_____   _____   _____

☐ 4. Medications prescribed (list medications and dosages):

_____   _____
_____   _____
_____   _____
_____   _____

☐ 5. Administer medications as prescribed and document response
☐ 6. Medication education (as tolerated) to:
    ☐ Patient   ☐ Family   ☐ Outpatient providers   ☐ _____

Courtesy University of Colorado Hospital, Psychiatric Services.

☐ 7. Patient to receive education or instruction on:
   ☐ Diagnosis   ☐ Symptom management   ☐ Substance abuse
   ☐ Stress management   ☐ _____

☐ 8. Assess/scale current level of hopefulness

☐ 9. Patient to identify ways to increase hopefulness
   ☐ Symptom management plan   ☐ Continue to scale hopefulness
   ☐ _____   ☐ _____

☐ 10. Patient to attend groups as appropriate (list groups):
   ☐ _____   ☐ _____
   ☐ _____   ☐ _____

☐ 11. Administer assessment tools (indicate frequency/discipline responsible):
   ☐ MMSE _____   ☐ _____
   ☐ Beck _____

☐ 12. Assess and document symptoms of psychosis (include confusion, disorganization)

☐ 13. OT consultation (indicate type): _____

☐ 14. Case manager or designee to:
   ☐ Gather collateral data
   ☐ Communicate with outpatient system regarding patient progress and discharge planning
   ☐ Assess and document level of family involvement
   ☐ Document discharge staffing/discharge family meeting
   ☐ _____
   ☐ _____

☐ 15. Diet _____

☐ 16. Acute medical issues and interventions _____

☐ _____
☐ _____
☐ _____
☐ _____

Outcomes

The patient demonstrates increased ability to maintain safety, as evidenced by:

☐ Decreased Beck score
☐ Increased GAF
☐ Symptom management plan in place
☐ Increased hopefulness
☐ _____
☐ _____

I have discussed the above treatment plan with my treatment team

_____   _____

Patient signature   **Staff signature**

Behavioral Care Plan

Date _____

Warning signs:

Expectations of behavior:

Interventions:

Positive reinforcers:

_____   _____

Patient signature   **Date**

_____   _____

Staff signature   **Date**

University of Colorado Hospital
Psychiatric Services
MR#1500.222
6/02 BP

Date: _____

Take Care of Yourself

Levels
1—Independent
2—Prompting
3—With assistance
4—Need 2 for assistance
5—Total care

Level of Assistance

	Frequency	**Levels of Assistance**	**Explanation/Re-Evaluation**
Shower			
Meals & fluids			
Deodorant			
Dress			
Mouth care			
Hair care			
Make bed			
Laundry			
Tidy room			
1:1			
Meds			
Group			
Other			

Behavioral Plan:
I understand that I am in the hospital to focus on _____
_____

I agree to do these things to achieve my goal _____
_____

Staff agrees to help me by _____
_____

Patient signature _____   **Staff signature** _____
_____
_____
_____

Courtesy of the University of Colorado Hospital Psychiatric Services

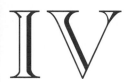

IV

CONTEMPORARY MODELS OF CASE MANAGEMENT

Beyond-the-Walls Case Management

In response to the shift to primary health care interventions and the convergence of wellness and prevention modalities, community-based nursing case management models have literally exploded onto the health care scene. The hallmark of these models is an integrated approach to continuous and seamless health care delivery. Unit IV presents several models that exemplify the care of individuals and communities. These models offer challenges and future ways to make the health care system more effective and to enhance the practice of the nurse case manager.

Beyond-the-Walls Case Management

CHAPTER OVERVIEW

Nursing case management approaches have grown in sophistication and diversity as evidenced by their emergence in community-based programs and capitated system arrangements. A beyond-the-walls program offers magnificent opportunities for professional nursing to control and manage health care resources and quality of patient care. Such a program also provides multiple advantages for the coordination and integration of outcomes and costs. The nursing profession's emphasis on the patient strengthens its power base and reconfirms its professional commitment to society.

Beyond-the-walls case management represents yet another example of the versatility and applicability of the case management model. This community-based approach has and continues to demonstrate great promise in reshaping nursing practice and health care management. Examples of some of the more prominent models are presented in this unit.

COMPELLING FORERUNNER: NURSING CASE MANAGEMENT ACROSS CARONDELET'S CONTINUUM OF CARE

Cathy Michaels and Gerri Lamb
(adapted for this edition by Elaine Cohen)

Carondelet Health Care: A Network of Nurse Partnerships and Care Coordination Strategies

During the past 10 years, nursing case management and other nursing partnerships have evolved that prepared Carondelet St. Mary's Hospital & Health Center, Tucson, Arizona, for the managed care environment. In 1985, at the onset of nursing case management beyond the walls of Carondelet, this facility began developing nurse partnerships to assist people at varying levels of risk to manage their health care. Initially, nurse case managers partnered across time and across health care settings with people at high risk. Then nurse practitioners, together with other nurses and staff from other disciplines, partnered with people at moderate risk in nurse-managed and neighborhood-accessible community health centers.

Based on Carondelet's experience of creating and maintaining integrated services of nursing case management and home health, respite, and home infusion therapy (Burns, Lamb, & Wholey, 1996; Michaels, 1991), Carondelet was selected as one of the four national demonstration sites for the Health Care Financing Administration (HCFA)–funded Community Nursing Organization, a risk-adjusted, capitated, nurse-managed ambulatory system of care. In this research program, Carondelet provided nurse partnerships and nurse-authorized services to Medicare enrollees at high, moderate, and low risk. Carondelet offered a system of care coordination and case management.

Evolution

Carondelet's model of professional nursing case management evolved from a decentralized home care program and nursing network that provided a multitude of services in a variety of settings (Ethridge, 1987, 1991; Ethridge & Lamb, 1989). The services available in the original system included acute or inpatient care, long-term extended care, home health care, and hospice, rehabilitation, primary prevention, and ambulatory care (Ethridge, 1991; Ethridge & Lamb, 1989). Nursing case management reduced the fragmentation associated with preadmission assessment, discharge planning, postdischarge follow-up, and hospital readmission (Health Care Advisory Board, 1990). The foundation for this work was partnership based on mutual respect. By helping people to understand the relationship between the choices they made and the consequences of their actions, nurse case managers not only translated the illness experience into learning about self and others but also acknowledged the patient as responsible for outcomes and the nurse for facilitating the process. In this regard, Carondelet nursing case management was one of the first models to relate practice to nursing theory, specifically Newman's Health as Expanding Consciousness (Newman, Lamb, & Michaels, 1991).

Two areas of evaluation predominated: the benefit of partnership and the impact of that partnership on use of hospital services. Qualitative findings supported a strong base in the nurse case manager–client relationship (Lamb & Stempel, 1994; Newman et al., 1991). Quantitative evaluation demonstrated reduced hospital use. The nursing case management process of assessing, coordinating, planning, and monitoring through partnership reflected appropriate use of medical intervention technology, reduced severity of illness when hospitalization was required, subsequent decreases in bed days, and increased accessibility to hospital alternatives (Ethridge, 1991; Ethridge & Lamb, 1989; Health Care Advisory Board, 1990).

Building on the success of this service, Carondelet established a nursing health maintenance organization (HMO) to provide health care and support services to elderly, chronically ill, and disabled individuals within a Medicare Senior Plan Contract (Ethridge, 1991; Michaels, 1991, 1992). If considered high risk, enrollees in this senior plan received integrated, community-focused nursing services, specifically, nursing case management and home health, respite, and home infusion therapy. Enrollees who did not match the high-risk profile were often referred to the Carondelet Community Health Centers for health monitoring, teaching, and care coordination. Overall, hospital bed days for the high-risk senior enrollees were significantly reduced (Burns et al., 1996), and enrollees served expressed high levels of satisfaction.

In 1992 Carondelet was selected as one of the four national sites to establish a Community Nursing Organization. A 3-year program funded by HCFA, the Community Nursing Organization is a research program based on experimental design. Indeed, the first outcome for this program was meeting the enrollment targets of 2000 in the experimental program called the Healthy Seniors Program and 1000 in the control group.

Carondelet's initial nursing HMO experience focused on people at high risk for managing their health care; the Healthy Seniors Program offers enrollment to Medicare beneficiaries whatever their risk for managing their health. Hence, nurse partnerships were established for enrollees at low, moderate, and high risk. Building even further on Carondelet's nursing HMO experience, the Healthy Seniors Program is based on a broader array of integrated ambulatory services: community health center, respite, home health, outpatient behavioral health and rehabilitation services, prosthetics, durable medical equipment, respiratory therapy, medical supplies, and ambulance services. This risk-adjusted, capitated, nurse-managed ambulatory system of care for Medicare beneficiaries ended in December 1996 (Lamb, 1995).

In 1997 Tucson was one of the most heavily penetrated managed care markets in the nation. To provide case management services and other nurse partnerships across Carondelet's full continuum of care, a system of case management evolved to coordinate care for those at high risk. Community-focused or continuum nurse case managers partnered with people at high risk to manage their health concerns across the continuum of care and over time. In general, the people who were served faced life-threatening chronic illness, such as congestive heart failure and end-stage chronic obstructive pulmonary disease. The community-focused nurse case managers linked with clinical nurse case managers within the hospital (Mahn, 1993). Clinical nurse case managers served patients at high risk during hospitalization, and, like clinical nurse specialists, they had a specialty focus.

Social workers were also available as consultants or as the primary case manager for clients whose situations were confounded by complex shelter, financial, legal, or behavioral issues. Finally, case managers for behavioral health and rehabilitation also offered services to clients needing their specialized continuum of care.

Except for behavioral health, payment for case management services came from the global capitation rate that covered hospitalization and that was negotiated in the contract. Behavioral health services were also capitated but were contracted for separately.

Transition

> "Changing times are invitations for participation."
> — *Anne Wilson Schaef*

Carondelet's model of professional nursing case management has transitioned to fully participate in the many changes occurring in its environment. The pioneers of this model led by example and envisioned a probable future.

It was envisioned that Carondelet would fully implement a risk identification process recently piloted to evaluate a person's risk for managing his or her health care as people shifted into Carondelet's integrated delivery network. Through risk screening and identification of modifiable risk factors, people at high, moderate, and low risk would be identified earlier. Then there would be targeted interventions, framed in terms of primary, secondary, and tertiary prevention and health promotion and based on Carondelet's nurse partnerships, care coordination strategies, practice guidelines, and system of case management. As in the past, Carondelet's goal was to offer service that people believed improved their health and well-being or that brought a peaceful death.

The future will also call for increased integration with primary care providers. For people at moderate risk, especially at the high end, the primary care site was accessible during teachable moments. Targeted intervention may enable people, through partnerships with physicians and nurses and staff from other disciplines, to stop progression to a higher risk status. As the future builds on experience from the past and the practices of today, Carondelet's goal was constant: through partnership, to offer health services that people believed improved their health and well-being or that facilitated a peaceful death.

Although the practice setting has changed, the principles that Carondelet's model of professional case management imbued have become the foundation and wisdom for the continued development and growth of case management well into the millennium. A more personal and compelling account of the evolution of this model is presented later in the book. The challenges and lessons bear repeating.

References

Burns, R., Lamb, G., & Wholey D. (1996). Impact of integrated community nursing services on hospital utilization and costs in a Medicare risk plan. *Inquiry, 16*(1), 1, 30 41.

Ethridge, P. (1987). Building successful nursing care delivery systems for the future. In National Commission on Nursing Implementation Project. *Post-conference papers second invitational conference* (pp. 91-99). Milwaukee: W.K. Kellogg Foundation,.

Ethridge, P. (1991). A nursing home: Carondelet St. Mary's experience. *Nursing Management, 22*(7), 22-27.

Ethridge, P., & Lamb, G.S. (1989). Professional nurse case management improves quality, access and costs. *Nursing Management, 20*(3), 30-35.

Health Care Advisory Board (1990). Tactic #6 "home-based" case management. Superlative clinical quality: Special review of pathbreaking ideas. *Clinical quality* (pp. 71-74). Washington, D.C.: The Advisory Board Company, vol 1.

Lamb, G.S. (1995). Case management. *Annual Review of Nursing Research, 13*, 117-136.

Lamb, G.S., & Stempel, J. (1994, Jan./Feb.). Nurse case management from the client's view: Growing as insider-expert. *Nursing Outlook,* 7-13.

Lamb, G.S. (1992). Conceptual and methodological issues in nurse case management research. *Advances in Nursing Science, 15*(2), 16-24.

Mahn, V. (1993). Clinical nurse case management: A service line approach. *Nursing Management, 24*(9), 48-50.

Michaels, C. (1991). A nursing HMO—10 Months with Carondelet St. Mary's hospital-based nurse case management. *Aspen's Advisor for Nurse Executives, 6*(11), 1.3-4.

Michaels, C. (1992). Carondelet St. Mary's nursing enterprise. *Nursing Clinics of North America, 27*(1), 77-86.

Newman, M., Lamb, G., & Michaels, C. (1991). Nurse case management: The coming together of theory and practice. *Nursing & Health Care, 12*, 404-408.

Wilson Schaef, A. (1995, Jul. 23) *Native wisdom for white minds.* New York: Ballantine Books.

Outcomes of Community-Based Nurse Case Management Programs

Jill Scott
Michal Boyd

CHAPTER OVERVIEW

Community-based nurse case management has been effective for individuals with chronic illness. However, measuring success within this complex, relationship-centered delivery model is challenging. Success of the intervention relates to the development of an insider–expert relationship and, hence, the self-management skills. Considering the complexity of this relationship, its influence on the chronically ill person may be enhanced with the use of a health care utilization framework as a means to integrate the multidimensional outcomes that need to be considered as success is evaluated. This chapter considers models of community-based case management, their outcomes, and challenges of measuring the complexities of the insider–expert relationship.

THE CHALLENGE FOR COMMUNITY-BASED CASE MANAGEMENT: THE CHRONICALLY ILL

Chronic illness continues to challenge an acute care–oriented health delivery and payment system (Throne & Robinson, 1989). With the advent of "managed lives," there was hope that concerns related to the health and well-being of the large cohort of chronically ill Americans would be addressed. Capitated systems were heralded as the payment strategy that would direct health care delivery systems to function more holistically to decrease costs related to acute health care use (Stahl, 1998; Williams, 1995). The idealistic provider saw opportunity from changes in payment structures. It was hoped that this would include a new means to motivate health care organizations to focus on health promotion and prevention as well as facilitation of self-management skills. Self-management skills that are facilitated by community-based nurse case managers are designed to decrease the wide variability present within the chronic illness trajectories of many (Scott & Rantz, 1997).

Evaluation of managed care contracts, such as those established in many states by Medicaid, indicates that long-term commitment between payer, providers, and patient continues to put management of chronic illness and promotion of healthful practices as a low priority. Many states have no structured relationships with payers, providers, and patients to facilitate commitment to chronically ill persons for the period of time necessary for the investment to be financially productive for the payer. Development and investment in health care delivery models, such as community-based nurse case management of the chronically ill, require longitudinal commitment for the "payoff" to occur.

Ironically, particularly within Medicaid contracts, individuals covered may inadvertently sabotage their opportunity for community-based nurse case management by continually changing providers.

This behavior undermines the potential for longitudinal relationships so necessary for community-based nurse case management to be successful (Lamb & Stempel, 1994).

Therefore continued examination of the outcomes and populations that community-based nurse case management can and does serve is required. Understanding what should, and does, motivate creation of health care delivery models that enhance self-management skills, such as community-based nurse case management, is essential as the population continues to shift to a larger numbers of elderly and as those with chronic conditions live longer.

This chapter considers the issues of measurement and determination of success in the community-based care of the chronically ill at an aggregate level and a disease-specific level. In addition, the chapter considers how historical models and their outcome measures have enhanced our understanding of care of the chronically ill, how community-based nurse case management models have evolved in their delivery of care and the measurement of the outcomes of care, and how we must evaluate and demonstrate success in the care of the chronically ill in the future.

CHRONIC ILLNESS

Chronic illnesses are present across age cohorts. Within each age cohort trajectories and resulting consequences differ. The psychological and physical development and socioeconomic realities of sustained illness have a unique effect on each age cohort. Typical consequences discussed among cohorts relate to psychological and physical development and socioeconomic realities of sustained illness (Lancaster, 1988; Woods & Lewis, 1995). Common chronic illness diagnoses reported in the literature include cancer, diabetes mellitus, cardiovascular disease, chronic obstructive pulmonary disease, renal disease, arthritis, and neuromuscular disorders (Anderson-Loftin, Wood, & Whitfield, 1995; Hwu, 1995). Also not typically considered are children with long-term sequelae from prematurity, birth defects, and poor prenatal care.

Chronic illnesses are slow, insidious, irreversible pathological changes. These illnesses require vigilance by the chronically ill person, significant others, and key health care providers to confront the long-term impact on health care, emotional, functional, and financial needs. The effects of chronic illness influence all of human existence (Lancaster, 1988). Lifelong treatment and behavior changes are required for the management of the chronic illness over time. Thus the person with a chronic illness must be active in the self-management of his or her chronic illness, further underlining the importance of key health care providers, such as nurse case managers, supporting the chronically ill within community-based models.

Chronic illnesses have courses that vary and change over time (Corbin & Strauss, 1984, 1988, 1991). According to Corbin and Strauss (1988), the unfolding of any chronic illness may be thought of as traveling a course. It is the trajectory of that course that community-based nurse case management attempts to alter. The course described by Corbin and Strauss (1984, 1989, 1991) is a probable path that the disease progression is predicted to follow. The influences of a chronically ill person's predisposing and enabling attributes directly affects progression of their chronic illness and need for health care resources, particularly community-based health care resources.

Distinctions between the course of a chronic illness and the trajectories of the illness are central to understanding the essence of chronic illnesses and the needs of the patient. Consideration of the trajectory of illness refers not only to physiological unfolding of chronic illness but also to the total organization of work or self-management and the attributes influencing this work (Strauss, 1975; Strauss et al., 1984). Community-based nurse case management models influence health care utilization through the nurse case manager's influence of the work and self-management required by the chronic illness. Community-based nurse case managers influence and shape the course of chronic illnesses through the building of insider–expert relationships with patients (Lamb & Stempel, 1994; Scott & Rantz, 1997).

Lamb and Stempel (1994) investigated the relationship of the nurse case manager and patient, identifying and describing growing together as insider-experts. The process develops through the affective, cognitive, and behavioral changes brought about by development of a strong, trusting nurse–patient relationship. The result of this relationship is the ability of the nurse case manager to have influence on the chronically ill person and the management of their chronic illness. The interpersonal phases of the relationship have been identified as bonding, working, and changing (Lamb & Stempel, 1994). This evolving relationship supports the development of self-management skills to influence the variability of a chronic illness trajectory.

Use by Chronically Ill Persons of Health Care Resources

Evaluation of those with progressing chronic illnesses as a cohort requiring substantial amounts of health care strongly suggests that the relationship of the person who is chronically ill, and the health care system must be considered in the context of a utilization framework. In analyzing the trajectories of the chronically ill, it is critical to consider how and when the health care system is accessed. How and when health care is accessed are key outcomes for consideration in the success of community-based models.

A framework providing integration of key elements related to the population at risk, their attributes, and actual utilization patterns of health care resources provides a context for studying this cohort over time within the context of the larger health care system and all the many variables that influence the delivery of care. Anderson's Framework of Health Care Utilization considers population attributes, health care delivery system attributes, the actual utilization of health care resources, and consumer perception (Aday & Anderson, 1974).

Chronic illness involves complex sets of relationships and structures to support them such as community-based nurse case management. Anderson's Framework of Health Care Utilization facilitates further understanding of the complex relationships among predisposing, enabling, and need attributes within a complex group of patients. Interrelationships among key variables noted above are displayed in Figure 12-1.

Chronically ill persons have a propensity for utilization of health care resources. Predisposing attributes are an abstraction of this concept to the individual level. These propensities are thought to be predictable from individual characteristics before an illness or periods of exacerbation. Many attributes predispose the chronically ill person to utilization of health care resources and can be used within a community-based model to predict those most likely to benefit from nursing case management. Predisposing attributes should be considered as predictor variables of health care utilization (Scott, 1998).

Enabling attributes are abstracted from the proposition that although individuals may be predisposed to the use of health care resources, they must have some means of obtaining resources. Factors typically considered relate to access and economic components of health care (Aday & Anderson, 1974; Wolinsky & Johnson, 1991).

Community-based care models using nurse case managers have proved to be key enablers of care for those who are chronically ill. Community-based nurse case management has demonstrated key outcomes of success related to enabling care with more cost-effective health care utilization. However, many payment models still do not consistently facilitate access to these types of services.

Predisposing and enabling factors are considered the present reality of the chronically ill person. Predisposing attributes are considered unchangeable. Enabling attributes may be unchangeable, depending on health care resources and financing available to the chronically ill person. Predisposing and enabling attributes are not sufficient in and of themselves to require engagement with the health care system.

The chronically ill person must "need" to access the health care system. "Need" typically relates to an inability to self-manage the course of the chronic illness and the certain variability that will be present throughout its progression. Therefore evaluation of the chronically ill and the successful management of

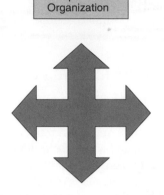
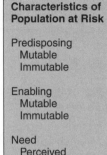

Health Policy

Financing
Education
Manpower
Organization

**Characteristics of
Health Delivery
Systems**

Resources
  Volume
  Distribution

Organization
  Entry
  Structure

**Characteristics of
Population at Risk**

Predisposing
  Mutable
  Immutable

Enabling
  Mutable
  Immutable

Need
  Perceived
  Real

**Utilization of
Health Services**

Type
Site
Purpose
Time interval

**Consumer
Satisfaction**

Quality
Convenience
Costs
Coordination
Information

FIGURE **12-1**   An adaptation of Anderson's framework of health care utilization.

their care must evaluate what predisposing, enabling, and need factors exist within and around the chronically ill person and community-based nurse case manager dyad. These attributes are highlighted in Table 12-1 (Aday & Newman).

Need ultimately creates the immediate cause for accessing the health care system (Wolinsky & Johnson, 1991). Examination of who has historically demonstrated need and how success has and should be measured using community-based nurse case management is considered through the remainder of the chapter.

Understanding how predisposing, enabling, and need factors relate to health care resource utilization provides insight for the community-based nurse case manager on how to influence these attributes within the context of shaping and managing chronic illness. Conceptualizing chronic illnesses as a trajectory captures the temporal orientation of chronic illness and the interplay of predisposing, enabling, and need factors. The interplay results in, and places influence on, the use of health care resources, which is a critical outcome measure for community-based models and nurse case management models. Consideration of chronic illness as a trajectory creates rationales for similarity across chronic illnesses so that evaluating the management and measurement of the multidimensional outcomes can be generalized within the population as it relates to decreasing the variability of the progression of the illness.

Outcomes related to management of the chronically ill are multidimensional. Quality, cost, and access are often cited as the standard for health measurement and are noted within the Anderson model in

TABLE 12-1	INDIVIDUAL ATTRIBUTES OR DETERMINANTS OF HEALTH CARE UTILIZATION	
Predisposing	**Enabling**	**Need**
Demographic	Income	Perceived
Age	Health insurance	Disability
Gender		Symptoms
Marital status	Community	Diagnosis
Past illness	Ratio of health care providers and facilities to population	General state
Social structure	Type of regular source of health care	Evaluated
Education	Accessibility of health care	Symptoms
Race	Compatibility of health care to need	Diagnosis
Occupation	Presence of community-based services	
Family size		Progression
Religion	Price of health care services	
Residential mobility	Region of country	Trajectory
	Urban-rural residence characteristics	
Beliefs		
Values concerning health and illness		
Attitudes toward health care services		

Figure 12-1. The following discussion of different models of community-based case management demonstrates that nurse case management improves quality of care, effectively manages costs, and enhances access (Bower & Falk, 1996).

Although the studies noted demonstrate many outcomes related to the changes in how resources are used, much is still to be studied related to the qualitative measures of success such as patient and family value related to the support of the management of the chronic illness (Papenhausen, 1996) and the value of the development of the insider-expert relationship as it relates to the reduction of stress on the health care team (Scott & Rantz, 1997).

A HISTORICAL REVIEW OF COMMUNITY-BASED CASE MANAGEMENT

Community-based case management can be traced to nursing's early roots in the 1890s, when Lillian Wald became one of the first nurses to manage patients in a community setting. She and her colleagues autonomously provided direct patient care and, in addition, organized and mobilized family and community resources. Lillian Wald started the Visiting Nurses Association (VNA) in partnership with the Metropolitan Life Insurance Company. The partnership provided an early measure of success in community-based nursing by demonstrating decreased health care utilization. By 1925 community-based nurse case management provided by the VNA had saved an estimated $43 million (Kersbergen, 1996).

NATIONAL LONG-TERM CARE DEMONSTRATION PROJECTS: "CHANNELING"

During the early 1980s, the federal government initiated the National Long-Term Care Demonstration, funded through the Health Care Financing Administration. The demonstration included the Channeling and On Lok programs (Kemper, Applebaum, & Harigan, 1987). Experts in the fields of behavioral health, social work, and health services research initiated this demonstration.

At the time, and still today, these demonstration projects represent some of the most comprehensive assessments of community-based care. The goal of the evaluation was to demonstrate cost containment for the rapidly increasing costs of long-term care with the use of community-based interventions. Although the demonstration projects are considered classic work, because of methodological issues results were not conclusive. However, many valuable lessons were learned for later projects (Christianson et al., 1988; Phillips, Kemper, & Applebaum, 1988).

Of the 10 demonstration projects initiated, five projects focused on measurement related to medical system difficulties because of ineffective or absent information and lack of coordination of services. The interventions within these five projects did not relate to the introduction of case management but focused on improving information flow and coordination of services, basic case management, and existing community services.

The remaining five demonstration projects provided the same information and coordination of services but added access to more community resources with additional funding from Medicare and Medicaid. The additional services included such critical elements as in-home care.

The results of these demonstration projects are difficult to interpret because of several issues. First, inconsistent definition of the population and other measures created concerns about generalizability of the findings. Second, case management interventions were poorly defined, and inconsistencies were noted with regard to who was considered the population most likely to benefit from the intervention. Third, inconsistency in group composition was noted. Finally, the studies did not use outcome measures that were keenly sensitive to elucidate the unique contribution of the intervention. These indicators were often defined as the tasks performed, without specific definitions of the clients served, the setting in which they resided, and the distinct services provided by the case managers (Kemper, Applebaum, & Harigan, 1987; Lamb, 1995; Phillips et al., 1988).

One study performed within the Channeling demonstration project did illustrate the impact of case management. Distinct differences were explored between the community-based case management models' function and caseload characteristics. This study (Eggert et al., 1991) noted that community-based case management models that used a more hands-on approach and smaller caseloads did have a reduction in health care expenditures.

EVOLVING MODELS OF COMMUNITY-BASED CASE MANAGEMENT

Community-based case management has been expanding in recent years and is used for a variety of patient populations. These programs have evolved to address client needs and increase quality of care in a changing reimbursement environment. Several different models are presented. Outcome measures are considered within each model as they relate to demonstrating success in the care of the chronically ill.

One of the first community-based nurse case management systems originating from a hospital was the Carondelet St. Mary's Hospital & Health Center, Tucson, Arizona, Professional Nurse Case Management (PNCM) program. This model was developed to decrease hospital lengths of stay in response to Medicare Prospective Payment, which was initiated in 1984. The PNCM worked with individuals in the community along with nurse practitioners based in a system of 20 wellness centers that were located in retirement complexes. Professional nurse case managers bridged the gap between health care settings and followed patients through the hospital, in long-term care facilities, and in their homes. This program was successful in reducing costs through decreased hospital admissions, decreased hospital acuity, and the resulting decreased length of stay, and set the tone for what and how to measure success for the intervention (Ethridge, 1997; Ethridge & Lamb, 1989).

Since the inception of the Carondelet St. Mary's PNCM model, many other hospitals around the country have used it as a prototype for the development of their own community-based care programs. Many of the interventions were borrowed from the original Carondelet St. Mary's model and implemented with some adjustment for a particular setting. However, lack of funding and poor reimbursement resulted in an inability of many pilot programs to implement the vast network of wellness clinics and integrated care achieved by Carondelet St. Mary's (Berenson, & Horvath, 2003). Despite the struggles to operationalize community-based case management, many programs achieved impressive outcomes (Boyd, Fisher, Ward-Davidson, & Neilsen, 1996; Rogers, Riordan & Swindle, 1991). Sund and Sveningson (1998) found that an integrated delivery system incorporating community-based nurse case management as an intervention reduced overall health care costs. This single-group preintervention and postintervention study demonstrated the following outcomes: a substantial decrease in hospitalizations (54%), decreased clinic and physician visits (31% decrease), and decreased clinic charges (43% decrease). In another study it was found that community care management reduced institutional days by 42% and found a 53% reduction of acute care hospitalization (Quinn, Prybylo, & Pannone, 1999).

Other models of noteworthiness include the Carle Clinic Community–based Case Management Model and the Cooperative Health Clinic. The Carle Clinic Association refers to the nurse case manager as a nurse partner (Schraeder & Britt, 1997). These nurses work closely with physicians in the clinic to manage high-risk individuals in the community setting. This model is efficient because the physician and nurse partnership function as a team in daily contact. The Carle Clinic model provides opportunities for nurse partners to guide the care of individuals across the continuum of health care settings, including ambulatory care, acute care, long-term care, and care in the home.

The model supports coordinated medical intervention and mentoring for the development of self-management skills. Nurses within the model have been creative in their use of the capitated dollar. The nurse partners are able to authorize home repair, transportation, respite services, and home-delivered meals. Availability of these services would be limited in traditional fee-for-service reimbursement systems.

The benefits of integration of care across the continuum have been demonstrated by the controlled/experimental clinical trial of comprehensive discharge planning with home follow-up for hospitalized elders. In this landmark study, Naylor et al. (1999) used advanced practice nurses (APNs) to perform the discharge planning of at-risk elders in the hospital and then followed these individuals in the community for 4 weeks after discharge. These APNs replaced usual visiting nurses during the first month after hospital discharge. The outcomes of this care included significant reduction in hospital readmissions at 6 and 24 weeks postdischarge by the group receiving the intervention by the APNs. Other findings included a significantly lower number of total hospital days and reduced mean length of stay by the intervention group compared with the control group at 24 weeks postdischarge. The authors attribute the success of this intervention to integrated primary health care that includes care for co-morbidities and the other social and health issues that are common in chronically ill older adults rather than focusing on the management of a single disease.

The Cooperative Health Care Clinic of Kaiser Permanente of Colorado implemented a group outpatient visit model providing comprehensive care through an interdisciplinary team approach. This intervention is an efficient method for using an interdisciplinary team. Although this model is mainly used for medical management of the chronically ill, it provides a model in which nurses could easily introduce community-based case management as a supplement. The intervention provides group support, timely medical intervention, education, and information regarding resources. Additionally, longitudinal care needed by the chronically ill is provided. Outcome measures that have indicated success include a decrease in emergency department visits, a decrease in visits to specialists, and a decrease in hospitalization. In addition, the study notes that patients placed more telephone calls to the nurse, visited the nurse more frequently, and engaged with the physician less, providing an outcome measure of appropriate use of the nurse as chronic disease manager (Beck et al., 1997).

In addition to the general models of community-based nurse case management already noted, some models and studies have focused the intervention on a specific population. Many chronically ill populations present unique challenges for the health care team in the management of the trajectory of chronic illness and the development of self-management skills. These unique groups include the mentally ill, those with chronic physical diseases such as congestive heart failure and diabetes, and those with chronic, catastrophic, contagious diseases such as acquired immunodeficiency syndrome (AIDS).

Deinstitutionalization of the chronically mentally ill during the 1950s and 1960s shifted care from the hospital to the community. In response to the needs of this population, mental health professionals created community-based case management programs. An extensive outcome data base exists in the literature regarding the specific outcome measures indicating success as it relates to the care of the mentally ill in the community (Bedell, Cohen, & Sullivan, 2000).

The community-based case management systems that evolved placed the case manager primarily in the role of brokering for community resources and coordinating care. As time progressed, data suggested that there was a need to integrate the clinical role for the provision of direct care in addition to the brokering and coordinating of care (Mueser et al., 1998).

Two models of community-based models have emerged to support the mentally ill: the Assertive Community Treatment Model and the Intensive Case Management Model. Both models incorporated low patient-to-staff ratios (10:1 rather than 30:1), services in the community rather than mental health centers, 24-hour availability of health care provider support, and the majority of services provided within the organization. Differences in the two models related to who managed the care. The Assertive Community Treatment Model used a team approach of nurses and psychiatrists sharing the caseload (Stein & Test, 1980). The Intensive Case Management Model did not share the caseload among team members, theoretically providing the opportunity for a strengthened relationship between case manager and client (Shern, Surles, & Waizer, 1989; Surles et al., 1992). Both models demonstrated decreased hospitalizations, decreased length of stay, improved housing stability, and independence. Outcomes of the studies also showed an improved quality of life for case-managed chronically mentally ill patients (Meuser et al., 1998; Ziguras & Stuart, 2000).

In addition to the chronically mentally ill, those with long-term chronic physical illness present challenges. The patient with congestive failure is a classic example of a population requiring frequent readmission into the acute care components of the health care system because of high variability within the progression of this chronic illness (Kegel, 1995). Many factors have been cited as contributing to rehospitalization of those with congestive heart failure, including a lack of understanding by the patient of the disease process, an inability to self-manage, and inconsistent follow-up care after hospitalization (Vinson et al., 1990). Many patients with congestive heart failure have high variability with the course of their chronic illness and would benefit from community-based case management. The nurse case manager can facilitate the development of self-management skills that decreases this variability.

Rich et al. (1995) used extensive patient assessment by a multidisciplinary team and comprehensive patient education for individuals with congestive heart failure. The intervention included follow-up in the home by nurses to increase the client's ability to self-manage through education and follow-up support. This randomized group-comparison study evaluated readmissions as an indicator of decreasing the wide swings in the variability of the illness. The study demonstrated a 33% reduction in hospital readmission compared with the control group (Rich et al., 1995). Mixed results were found in a study of care management of a heterogeneous group of congestive heart failure patients (Laramee, et al., 2003). Two factors that were shown to influence the effectiveness of the intervention were (1) the close working relationship between the case manager and the physician and (2) whether the patient had ready access to the physician and case manager.

Another chronically ill group that demonstrates a high variability within the trajectory of their illness is the person with diabetes. Not only is variability a challenge, but also the long-term sequelae from inaction to the illness early on may have profound consequences. The traditional health care system has been inconsistent in providing the disease management required. Programs are needed that increase monitoring and follow-up to identify potential problems early to reduce the severity of the resulting complications.

Individuals in the community have used an automated voice messaging system to improve the management of diabetes. Patients are identified with poor glucose control or other problems that require more intensive follow-up. An automated voice messaging system calls the patients at their homes and inquires about glucose control and other diabetes-related symptoms to determine what patient education should be provided.

Diabetes nurse educators monitor responses to the calls, and calls are returned to those individuals who require intervention. Preliminary results of enhanced glucose control, early intervention for complications, and acceptance of this technology by patients suggest this is a feasible and innovative alternative to ongoing evaluation and support of patients with diabetes (Piette, 1997).

The need for chronic care of individuals with human immunodeficiency virus (HIV) infection and AIDS has been heightened dramatically by the enhanced availability of drug therapies that have greatly increased life expectancy and the widespread expansion in the number of people infected with HIV. The care of people with AIDS is moving to an integrated system that focuses on health and wellness rather than on acute care (Mitchell, & Anderson, 2000; Morrison, 1993). Because of the complex physical needs of these individuals, nurse case management has been recommended rather than case management from other disciplines (Green et al., 1987).

In a Robert Wood Johnson demonstration project of case management for people with AIDS, individuals with case management were more likely to report service needs being met than were clients without case management (Fleishman, Mr, & Piette, 1991). Outcomes within the study also suggest improved survival for those who were case managed. The results related to mortality were inconclusive, because medical treatment regimens did vary between comparison groups (Sowell et al., 1992).

A second study, the Denver Nursing Project in Human Caring (Schroeder, 1993), provided a nurse-managed outpatient clinic for people with AIDS. Clients of the clinic could elect to enter into a nurse care partnership. This nursing intervention provided care across clinical settings and was particularly helpful when the client was hospitalized. The nurse care partner was a valuable member of the health care team, providing information about the client's wishes and needs. Outcomes from this project demonstrated improved access to cost-effective and high-quality care. Outcomes measured indicating health care savings included decreased hospitalizations, decreased length of stay, decreased cost of outpatient procedures, and increased home care during the dying process (Schroeder, 1993).

COMMUNITY-BASED NURSE CASE MANAGEMENT'S FUTURE: MEASURING SUCCESS

Community-based nurse case management outcomes need additional qualitative and quantitative measurement to provide the multidimensional view required to capture the true impact of the insider–expert relationship. More research is needed on how this relationship affects self-management skills and the subsequent ability to decrease the variability of an individual's trajectory of chronic illness. Qualitative research is providing insight into patients' and families' values. Papenhausen (1996) found through interviews that these values include decreased physical disability, increased perception of social satisfaction, improved symptom management, decreased severity of illness, and increased general self-efficacy. More studies are required to enhance our understanding of what is valuable to patients and families and how their roles can be enhanced in the management of chronic illnesses (Watt, 2001).

Quantitative measures must continue to be refined to more accurately reflect the impact of the ability of nurse case management to decrease the variability of those with wide swings within their trajectory of chronic illness. Large-scale data-mining efforts are needed within national databases, such as the Centers for Medicare & Medicaid billing data, to facilitate additional understanding of what key predisposing, enabling, and need factors best predict wide variability within those chronic illnesses. This understanding will facilitate more effective targeting of the chronically ill persons who would most benefit from community-based nurse care management interventions.

Finally, triangulation studies related to community-based case management are required to understand the interplay of reducing health care consumption, improving reported well-being and satisfaction of chronically ill persons and their families, and measuring consistent demonstrations of self-management skills that stabilize the variability of the chronic illness progression. Studies should also consider the influence of community-based case management on the functioning and satisfaction of the health care team (Scott & Rantz, 1997). Community-based case management can and does make a difference. What is the challenge? To prove it!

References

Aday, L.A., & Anderson, R. (1974). A framework for the study of access to medical care. *Health Services Research, 9*(3), 208-220.

Anderson, R., & Newman, J. (1973). Societal and individual determinants of medical care utilization in the United States. *Millbank Quarterly, 51*(1), 95-124.

Anderson-Loftin, W., Wood, D., & Whitfield, L. (1995). A case study of nursing case management in the rural hospital. *Nursing Administrative Quarterly, 19*(3), 33-40.

Beck, A., Scott, J., Williams, P., Robertson, B., Jackson, D., Gade, G., & Cowan, P. (1997). A randomized trial of group outpatient visits for chronically ill older HMO members: The cooperative health care clinic. *Journal of the American Geriatrics Society, 45*, 543-549.

Bedell, J.R., Cohen, N.L., & Sullivan, A. (2000). Case management: The current best practices and the next generation of innovation. *Community Mental Health Journal, 36*(2), 179-194.

Berenson, R.A., & Horvath, J. (2003). Confronting the barriers to chronic care management in Medicare. *Health Affairs, 22*(2), 11.

Bower, K.A., & Falk, C.D. (1996). Case management as a response to quality, cost, and access imperatives. In E.L. Cohen (Ed.), *Nurse case management in the 21st century*. St Louis: Mosby.

Boyd, M.L., Fisher, B., Davidson, A.W., & Neilsen, C.A. (1996). Community-based case management for chronically ill older adults: A comparison study. *Nursing Management, 27*(11), 31-32.

Christianson, J.B., Applebaum, R., Carcagno, G., & Phillips, B. (1988). Organizing and delivering case management services: Lessons from the national long term care demonstration. *Home Health Care Services Quarterly, 9*(1), 7-27.

Corbin, J.M., & Strauss, A. (1984). Collaboration: Couples working together to manage chronic illness. *Image: Journal of Nursing Scholarship, 26*(4), 109-115.

Corbin, J.M., & Strauss, A. (1988). *Unending work and care*. San Francisco: Jossey-Bass Publishers.

Corbin, J.M., & Strauss, A. (1991). A nursing model for chronic illness management based upon the trajectory framework. *Scholarly Inquiry for Nursing Practice: An International Journal, 5*(3), 156-174.

Eggert, G.M., Zimmer, J.G., Hall, W.J., & Friedman, B. (1991). Case management: A randomized controlled study comparing a neighborhood team and a centralized individual model. *Health Services Research, 26*(4), 471-505.

Ethridge, P. (1997). The Carondelet experience. *Nursing Management, 28*(3), 26-28.

Ethridge, P., & Lamb, G. (1989). Professional nursing case management improves quality, access and costs. *Nursing Management, 20*(3), 30-35.

Fleishman, J.A., Mr, V., & Piette, J. (1991). AIDS case management: The client's perspective. *Health Services Research, 26*, 447-469.

Green, J., Singer, M., Wintfeld, N., Schulman, K., & Passman, L. (1987). Projecting the impact of AIDS on hospitals. *Health Affairs, 6*, 19-31.

Hwu, Y.J. (1995). The impact of chronic illness on patients. *Rehabilitation Nursing, 20*(4), 221-225.

Kegel, L.M. (1995). Advanced practice nurses can refine the management of heart failure. *Clinical Nurse Specialist, 9*(2), 76-81.

Kemper, P., Applebaum, R., & Harigan, M. (1987). Community care demonstrations: What have we learned. *Health Care Financing Review, 8*(4), 87-100.

Kersbergen, A.L. (1996). Case management: A rich history of coordinating care to control costs. *Nursing Outlook, 44*, 169-172.

Lamb, G.S. (1995). Case management. *Annual Review of Nursing Research, 13*, 117-135.

Lamb, G.S., & Stempel, J.E. (1994). Nurse case management from the client's view: Growing as the insider-expert, *Nursing Outlook, 42*(1), 7-13.

Lancaster, L.E. (1988). Impact of chronic illness over the life span. *American Nephrology Nurses Association, 15*(3), 164-168.

Laramee, A.S., Levinsky, S.K., Sargent, J., Ross, R., & Callas, P. (2003). Case Management in a heterogeneous congestive heart failure population: A randomized controlled trial. *Archives of Internal Medicine, 163*, 809-817.

Mitchell, J.M., & Anderson, K.H. (2000). Effects of case management and new drugs on Medicaid AIDS spending. *Health Affairs, 19*(4), 233-243.

Muescr, K.T., Bond, G.R., Drake, R.E., & Resnick, S.G. (1998). Models of community care for severe mental illness: A review of research on case management. *Schizophrenia Bulletin, 24*(1), 37-74.

Morrison, C. (1993). Delivery systems for the care of persons with HIV infection and AIDS. *Advances in Nursing Research, 28*(2), 317-333.

Naylor, M.D., Brooten, D., Campbell, R., Jacobsen, B.S., Mezey, M.D., Pauly, M.V., & Schwartz, J.S. (1999). Comprehensive discharge planning and home follow-up of hospitalized elders: A randomized clinical trial. *Journal of the American Medical Association, 281*(7), 613-620.

Papenhausen, J.L. (1996). Discovering and achieving client outcomes. In E.L. Cohen (Ed.), *Nurse case management in the 21st century*. St. Louis: Mosby.

Phillips, B.R., Kemper, P., & Applebaum, R.A. (1988). The evaluation of the National Long Term Care Demonstration. *Health Services Research, 23*(1), 67-81.

Piette, J.D. (1997). Moving diabetes management from clinic to community: Development of a prototype based on automated voice messaging. *Diabetes Educator, 23*(6), 672-680.

Quinn, J.L., Prybylo, M., & Pannone, P. (1999). Community care management across the continuum: study results from a Medicare health maintenance plan. *Care Management Journal, 1*(4), 223-231.

Rich, M.W., Beckham, V., Wittenberg, C., Leven, C.L., Freedland, K.E., & Carney, R.M. (1995). A multidisciplinary intervention to prevent the readmission of elderly patients with congestive heart failure. *The New England Journal of Medicine, 333*(18), 1190-1195.

Rogers, M., Riordan, J., & Swindle, D. (1991). Community-based nursing case management pays off. *Nursing Management, 22*(3), 31-34.

Schraeder, C., & Britt, T. (1997). The Carle Clinic. *Nursing Management, 28*(3), 32-34.

Schroeder, C. (1993). Nursing's response to the crisis of access, costs, and quality in health care. *Advances in Nursing Science, 16*(1):1-20.

Schroeder, C., & Maeve, K. (1992). Nursing response to the crisis of costs and quality in health care. *Advances in Nursing Science, 16*(11), 1-20.

Scott, J. (1998). A study of health care utilization among chronically ill rural older adults. In review.

Scott, J., & Rantz, M. (1997). Managing the chronically ill in the midst of the health care revolution, *Nursing Administrative Quarterly, 21*(2), 55-64.

Shern, D.L., Surles, R.C., & Waizer, J. (1989). Designing community treatment systems for the most seriously mentally ill: A state administrative perspective. *Journal of Social Issues, 45*, 105-117.

Sowell, R.L., Gueldner, S.H., Killen, M.R., Lowenstein, A., Fuszard, B., & Swansburg, R. (1992). Impact of case management on hospital charges of PWAs in Georgia. *Journal of the Association of Nurses in AIDS Care, 3*, 24-31.

Stahl, D.A. (1998). Growth through capitation and physician practice management. *Nursing Management, 29*(1), 14-16.

Stein, L.I., & Test, M.A. (1980). Alternative to mental hospital treatment: I. Conceptual model, treatment program, and clinical evaluation. *Archives of General Psychiatry, 37*, 392-397.

Strauss, A. (1975). *Chronic illness and the quality of life.* St. Louis: Mosby.

Strauss, A., Corbin, J., Fagerhaugh, S., Glaser, B.G., Maines, D., Suczek, B., & Wiener, C.L. (1984). *Chronic illness and the quality of life,* 2nd edition. St. Louis: Mosby.

Sund, J., & Sveningson, L. (1998). Case management in an integrated delivery system. *Nursing Management, 29*(1), 24-25.

Surles, R.C., Blanch, A.K., Shern, D.L., & Donahue, S.A. (1992). Case management as a strategy for systems change. *Health Affairs, 11*, 151-163.

Throne, S.E., & Robinson, C.A. (1989). Guarded alliance: Health care relationships in chronic illness. *Image: Journal of Nursing Scholarship, 21*(3), 153-157.

Vinson, J.M., Rich, M.W., Sperry, J.C., Shah, A.S., & McNamara, T. (1990). Early readmission of the elderly patients with congestive heart failure. *Journal of the American Geriatrics Society, 38*(12), 1290-1295.

Watt, H.M. (2001). Community-based case management: a model for outcome-based research for non-institutionalized elderly. *Home Health Care Services Quarterly, 20*(1), 39-65.

Williams, D.B. (1995). Case management without walls: Breaking down traditional barriers among organizations. *Inside Case Management, 1*(10), 1-3.

Wolinsky, F.D., & Johnson, R.J. (1991). The use of health services by older adults. *Journal of Gerontology, 46*(6), S345-S357.

Woods, N.F., & Lewis, F.M. (1995). Women with chronic illness: Their views of their families' adaptation. *Health Care for Women International, 16*, 135-148.

Ziguars, S.J., & Stuart, G.W. (2000). A meta-analysis of the effectiveness of mental health case management over 20 years. *Psychiatric Services, 51*(11), 1410-1421.

Integrated Case Management Model

Mary Lu Gerke

CHAPTER OVERVIEW

Nursing case management is a patient delivery system that evolved out of the primary nursing model. The focus of case management is to use the professional nurse as the agent who integrates care, cost, and quality (Zander, 1985). Like an amoeba, environmental pressure influences nursing case management to change composition, shape, and structure. The ever-changing patient needs, professional roles, and health care systems create space for nursing case management to flow into unexplored territories. Mergers, downsizing, and reengineering have created an opportunity to strategically position nursing case management as the mechanism to ensure care to all patients across the continuum. The external force of redesign and integration influenced the evolving form of the Differentiated Case Management Model at Gundersen Lutheran.

The core of nursing case management at Gundersen Lutheran was based on the work of two projects: "Facilitating ADN Competency Development" and "Defining and Differentiating ADN and BSN Competencies." The outcome of these two projects was the Differentiated Case Management Model, operationalized in 1990 at the acute care setting, Lutheran Hospital. The model continued to evolve in the acute care setting but was not extended to the ambulatory or home care settings until 1997, when Gundersen Clinic and Lutheran Hospital began the integration process.

This process enabled our organization to clearly see the possibility of providing nursing case management across the continuum. Up to this point, few of the acute care case managers actualized care planning across the continuum. Many of them dreamed of providing a continuum care plan for patients, but physical walls and governing structures impeded their attempts. The clinic and home care systems did not have a case management model in place but instead practiced in the team or total patient care model.

Integration of systems, models, and people, although difficult in many ways, provides an opportunity to use diverse eyes for seeing new ways of creating and evolving. The merger promoted the evaluation of case management in all three settings: acute care, ambulatory care, and home care. Additionally, it opened the opportunity to build the differentiated case management model across all systems and settings. Weaving new relationships and partnerships, nursing case management is nurtured by integration, growing, changing, and strengthening.

DIFFERENTIATED CASE MANAGEMENT MODEL

National Development

Differentiated case management was developed through the work of two major projects sponsored by the Midwest Alliance in Nursing (MAIN) and funded by the W.K. Kellogg Foundation: "Facilitating ADN Competency Development" and "Defining and Differentiating ADN and BSN Competencies." These two studies developed between 1980 and 1984. Service and education together developed a differentiated scope of practice for the BSN and the ADN through competency statements. Dr. Peggy Primm led the task force toward defining competencies in three major areas of care: provision of care, communication, and management of care. Job descriptions were then formatted and several sites selected to test the model (Primm, 1986). In the differentiated case management model, there are two roles established for professional nursing staff: the case manager role and the case associate role. The case manager role is designed to be accountable for the independent scope of practice and focused on health and human response. The case associate role is designed to be accountable for the dependent scope of nursing practice and focused on the technical aspects of care. Together the two roles deliver the full scope of nursing practice to each patient. Each role holds the essence and the full scope of practice of professional nursing. Therefore both participate in all aspects of care, such as admission assessment and preparation for discharge. The difference lies in the focus and depth of each role. The case manager focus is integration and orchestration of the health care team throughout the hospital length of stay, and the case associate focus is on the day-to-day patient assessment, care, teaching, and evaluation.

Application Of Differentiated Case Management

In 1988 Lutheran Hospital embarked on a journey of redesign. With the advent of rapid changes in social structures, technology, and health care, the primary nursing model lacked the depth and breadth to meet the changing needs of patients and systems. We hoped we would be able to discover a new patient care delivery model that would support the new consumer of health care and at the same time maintain financial strength.

> "With health, human response, and quality of life as new imperatives to integrate into each individual's care, the way in which nursing care was organized and delivered clearly required a fundamental change."
>
> —*Johnson, Friend, & MacDonald, 1997*

Professional colleagues and literature searches helped the organization to commit to the differentiated case management model. The underlying belief of the differentiated nursing model is that "each nurse is expert in their role, each role is mutually valued, and collaborative practice utilizing both roles is the whole of nursing" (Larson, 1992). These beliefs fit with the vision of the Lutheran Hospital nursing department.

Differentiating the roles meant redesigning the professional nursing framework. A task force of grassroots staff and leadership participated in developing professional nursing job descriptions and performance appraisals for two registered nurse (RN) roles. This was no small task, because the existing clinical ladder consisted of four levels of RN staff. Therefore eight complete job descriptions and performance appraisals were developed. Countless hours of inservice training and educational sessions were scheduled for 700 RNs as well as licensed practical nurses (LPNs), nursing assistance, and ancillary services staff. After the educational sessions, the RNs were asked to complete a factoring tool that assisted them and their nursing directors to dialogue and decide which role, case manager or case associate, best matched their practice. Physicians were educated through their noon conferences and in a one-to-one dialogue. By the end of 1990, Lutheran Hospital practiced in a differentiated case management model.

By 1992, experience with differentiated case management highlighted areas of clarification and strengthening. The rehabilitation unit put into place a pilot th the two roles of case manager and case associate. In the original model, profes a case manager with some of the patients and as case associate with other pati This led to confusion and lack of clarity in both roles. The pilot placed profe a case manager or a case associate role that they would practice 100% of th manager was no longer given a patient assignment for direct care, the case associates we patients with an LPN or a nursing assistant colleague to attend to the daily care of the patients. Thu case managers to attend to the individualized care planning for patients. Further change required further education in the areas of delegation and teamwork. Trust and respect for each other's work became core to successfully meeting the needs of patients and families. The case managers primarily work day and evening hours and meet with other health care providers daily to discuss the individual needs of their patients for the acute care stay and the discharge plan. Over a 2-year period, this variation of the differentiated case management model spread to all patient care areas of the hospital. With the job descriptions updated, professional nurses were refactored into a case manager or case associate role. Some patient care units required few case managers, whereas other patient care units needed several. The decision on the number of case managers required is determined by data such as length of stay, patient populations, and severity of illness on the specific unit.

The case managers meet monthly to discuss practice issues, development of their role, and barriers to their work. Some of the case managers managed the patient care from unit to unit. However, this was not standard practice, inconsistencies became apparent, and, as in any evolutionary system, evaluating and revising are the norm.

Implementation of a Professional Roles Model

In 1996 a task force was formed to evaluate and revise the clinical ladder system at Lutheran Hospital. After a brief review, the task force decided to move from a clinical ladder system to a professional roles model. The new model used Patricia Benner's 1984 work, *From Novice to Expert*, as a resource and guide. The task force decided to change the title of case manager to care manager and case associate to care associate. Three job descriptions and performance evaluations were developed for the care associate: essential (beginner), proficient, and expert/leader. The care manager job description and performance evaluation were similar in the communication and leadership criteria to the case associate expert/leader criteria but differed in the patient/family criteria. The care associate's focus continues to be the standard technical care, and the care manager continues to focus on the independent individual patient care plan across the episode of illness. (See Appendix 13-1 for job descriptions and competencies of the care manager and care associate.)

The professional role model moved the nursing department to a new way of seeing work. Benner's theory helped the nursing staff understand that differences in practice can and do enrich the care provided for patient and family. Nurses wrote three exemplars reflecting their practice as professionals. With guidance from Benner, Tanner, and Chelsa's book, *Expertise in Nursing Practice—Caring Clinical Judgment and Ethics*, the exemplar assists in assessing the practice level of the nurses. Each nurse presented the exemplars along with the performance appraisal to the unit's peer review committee. This session served as a means to discover, with the individual nurse, where practice has evolved to on the continuum from novice to expert. The process of moving from a clinical ladder system to a professional roles model assisted in evaluating the role of the care manager and raising questions about the purpose and meaning of nursing care management across the continuum. From the very beginning, there was good intent to work across the continuum, but concerns and barriers continued to block the success of delivery care across the systems.

Barriers to Integrate Nursing Case Management Across the Continuum

There are several models of nursing case management. However, few models have successfully been able to stretch across the ambulatory, acute, and home care settings. Some barriers to building a structure for integrating nursing case management are as follows:

- A perspective by health care providers and society that health care and disease management are owned by the provider, not a mutual partnership between patient and provider
- Health care institutions not governed as a integrated system with poor articulation between the providers of acute care, ambulatory care, and home care
- Different reimbursement and regulations dependent on the location of the treatment or service and which provider is delivering the treatment or service
- Educational curriculums segregated according to ambulatory, acute, or home care settings instead of the focus on primary, secondary, and tertiary care in any setting
- Management structures that place managers leading only a section of the continuum because of physical or economic barriers
- Inability of staffing patterns, budgets, and numerous structures to span the continuum

INTEGRATION OF A CLINIC, HOSPITAL, AND HOME CARE AGENCY

In 1998 Gundersen Clinic and Lutheran Hospital merged. The Lutheran Home Care agency was a branch of Lutheran Hospital and therefore part of the system. The merger brought forth a system composed of regional clinics; regional hospitals and affiliated hospitals, a home care agency, a main clinic (280 physicians), and a 400-bed acute care hospital. The merging and integration of organizations and systems are now common around the world, yet we still deal with coping issues and with rebuilding new relationships and organizations from these mergers.

In their book A *Simpler Way*, Margaret Wheatley and Myron Kellner-Rogers state, "Systems are fluid relationships that we observe as rigid structures. They are webby, wandering, nonlinear, entangled messes . . . systems create pathways, communication flows, causal loops" (Wheatley & Kellner-Rogers, 1996). The work of integration has indeed been a tangled web. Nevertheless, out of the chaos there blooms the opportunity to reach a wholeness we have not been able to grasp or even dream about in the old structures.

Defining Integration

Integration means "to form, coordinate or blend into a functioning or unified whole, to unite with something else, to incorporate into a larger unit and to end the segregation of and bring into common and equal membership in society or an organization" (Webster, 1988). This definition should strike at the core of nurses, because one tenet of the essence of nursing is the persistence and passion to promote the wellness and *wholeness* of human beings. Therefore, in seeking wholeness, integration of nursing case management across the continuum is a natural evolution. Nursing has always integrated the body, mind, and spirit into a holistic approach. Now it is our path to integrate that whole human system throughout the manmade acute, ambulatory, and home care systems.

In reading Florence Nightingale's *Notes on Nursing*, many things have changed but some things have not. Nightingale fought the battle of educating others to understand that nursing is a distinct profession, separate but connected to medicine. More important, Nightingale wanted nurses and others to understand the sacredness and importance of the nurse–patient relationship. Her definition of nursing—"Nursing creates an environment to assure that the patients not only be well, but to use well all of their being"—was a call to nursing to integrate the parts and to understand the importance of the patient's wholeness. We have reached into our humanism and understood that humankind is an integral part of the whole and that the environment and all creation affect each other. One element cannot exist separately, for we are all connected; we are all the same stuff. Complementary and alternative therapy is a manifestation of that concept and intent. As nurses we embrace these concepts and appreciate them. Application of our values and beliefs work toward integrating patient care to wholeness.

Another level of integration is now our challenge—the work of integrating the care by a nurse for the same patient over the continuum. Nursing can stop the segregation of the patient's health care. Patient care often has different care standards depending on the setting in which care is delivered: ambulatory, acute, or home care. We are the link between these settings, not solely by a paper trail but also by our sacred connectedness and relationships with our patients. We can manifest the essence of nursing embracing a new and different society, a health-centered society with wellness as the core. Collaborating with the mechanistic illness models avails us the opportunity to create a system that provides a holistic care system.

Bringing Two Models Together

Hospital and clinic systems integration started in 1997. It is vital to *understand* that the practice models of team and total patient care gave birth to primary nursing and case management models and that bringing the models together is the goal. Current health care systems have moved toward a case management model. This urges the organization to use the good components of the models currently in the clinic and hospital but also to move beyond what either one has in place. The differentiated case management model in the hospital is evolutionary and needs to expand beyond the walls of the acute care setting.

Establishing trust and respect is the grounding for *understanding* to be a priority. "Understanding takes time. Understanding is a process, not an event, and it is not possible unless we are willing to take the time and effort to stay with it" (Schaef, 1998). The seeking to understand each other as we co-create the new case management model takes patience and persistence. Implementing a new patient care model causes structures, job descriptions, and roles to change to support the model. The clinic and hospital structures, job descriptions, roles, and a multitude of support frameworks change as a result of different patient needs and environments.

A task force composed of both ambulatory nurses and hospital care managers was developed to work on building a differentiated case management model that spans all settings. The establishment of a position for director of case management promotes the work of building nursing care management across the continuum. This individual heads the task force and works with numerous subgroup specialties to build an integrated patient care model. The first work of the main task force is to look at all the roles of professional nurses in all settings. Many roles exist, and this work indeed requires understanding and patience.

The work is in progress, but some areas have already moved toward successful integration. One such department is the obstetrics service line. Hospital care managers and clinic nurses have developed a care management role that starts with seeing the mother in the clinic three times, continues through the hospital event, and then ends after two follow-up telephone calls and at least one follow-up clinic visit. During the prenatal visits, the care manager works with the parents to complete the individualized care path for the birth. These care paths are provided online so they are readily available in the clinic and hospital. Patient satisfaction has always been very good in this area but has been even more positive since the integration of the hospital and clinic care managers became a reality.

In the general surgery department of the clinic, a care manager follows all patients with breast cancer through the ambulatory, acute, and home care settings. The patients develop a relationship with the nurse that is built on trust and partnering. This alleviates some of the fear and anxiety, establishes a consistent care plan, reduces duplication of baseline assessments, and creates a patient advocate to help navigate a complex health care system.

An area of care management new to Gundersen Lutheran is in the area of infusion therapy. One care manager shares her exemplar:

I was asked to place a midline catheter in a hospice patient. On arriving at the home of the patient to place the catheter, the husband smiled with delight to discover that I was going to place the catheter. He reminded me that I had put an intravenous line in his wife when she was in the hospital. He was grateful that someone with that level of expertise was able to come to their home. The placement of the catheter proceeded without any complications, and both the patient and her husband were content when I left their home. I found out later that the patient had died the next day; it was a good feeling for me to know that her last day had been a comfortable, peaceful day.

Many areas in the clinic are just starting the process of integration. Some of the interesting obstacles to overcome are as follows:

- Nursing roles that are attached to a physician care provider
- Confusion of nursing assessment responsibilities versus technical skills that could be delegated to medical assistance
- Information systems that are not adapted to facilitate integrated documentation and communication links
- Resistance to implementing a new way without having the model and system completely defined and tested
- Merging a primarily day operation with a 24-hour operation
- Personnel structures of pay and benefits that are not completely integrated
- Need for further education regarding each other's settings and operations

BUILDING RELATIONSHIPS AND PARTNERSHIPS

Nursing case management builds on the partnership and relationship principles of trust, respect, support, communication, and commitment. These principles can be used to build all types of partnerships, not only partnerships with our patients. "Forming a partnership relationship requires time and effort. It means spending time with each other, sharing feelings and perceptions, discussing important values, putting into place the structure for the relationship" (Manion, Sieg, & Watson, 1998). When dealing with an integrated nursing case management system, dual application of these principles occurs, involving the patient and family partnership with the health care provider and the health care provider with the remainder of the health care team.

Trust

The element of trust is core to successful partnership development. The patient and family develop trust in the care provider through dialogue and being present with the care provider. When the care manager is not fully present and rushes through the appointment, the patient and family lose the opportunity to establish a trusting relationship with a care provider. The care manager must provide the component of patient's advocate. To accomplish that measure, time and trust go hand in hand. The care managers working across the continuum need to be expert in establishing trust. Self-reflection on one's own integrity and trust in the team must be part of partnership building, as must a firm belief that each member of the team has the ultimate goal of quality patient care.

Respect

Mutual respect for each other is key in all relationships and partnerships. Lack of respect breeds misunderstanding, leads to poor communication, and inhibits growth and creativity. Respecting the diversity of each individual creates a sense of collective individualism. This element is not easy to attain, because it calls for each person to fully listen and seek to understand the other person's point of view. Frequently, the health care provider sees the patient's viewpoint as less important or valuable than his or her own. The health care provider might believe the patient lacks the scientific knowledge to make complex decisions. The patient brings the expertise of knowing "self." The patient is the only expert on what values and beliefs are key to his or her recovery or coping of an illness; he or she is the only expert who can bring wholeness and health. Many of us have witnessed the relation of the patient's point of view and attitude to the outcome of a health care event. Who knows better the needs of an individual than the individual himself or herself? We are guides to offer the alternatives and options to the patient but not to make the health care decision for him. The importance of understanding diversity and respect is paramount to successful integration and partnership relations.

Support

Offering support for each other authentically creates an environment of caring. Supportive behaviors and communication are vital, in the easy times as well as the times of conflict and confusion. In the role of patient advocate, a nurse offering a caring and understanding ear is sometimes all that is necessary. With colleagues, this is just as important because it fosters the establishment of the oneness of the health care team. Frequently, the hectic pace we have set builds a maze in front of us, causing confusion and frustration for both provider and patient. Being too busy is an excuse for short, irritated responses and poor listening. Sadly, we all use this excuse and intimately feel the ramifications of a complex world. When this atmosphere is present, there is little or no support offered to either patients or colleagues. By embracing the importance of spending time with each individual, we can improve efficiency and effectiveness and meet the patient's demands.

Communication

Of all the elements of partnership and relationships, communication stands as the cornerstone. No element can build a strong, honest, and whole relationship more than good communication. The art of dialogue needs practice and patience. Honest, authentic messages and fully present listening are essential elements in patient and family care. It is vital to use communication skills that strengthen our connectedness to each other, to our patients, and to their families. Without strong communication, we get lost in the overabundance of information we have available about health care and about our patients. The information and data we collect are useless without connecting the information to each individual's uniqueness and values. Information and data may be our greatest tools or our greatest burdens.

Commitment

Being fully passionate and persistent in developing a partnership relationship with patients and families across the continuum requires a commitment to the human community. Obstacles and barriers—some built by our own egos, by other health care colleagues, or by government structures, rules, and agencies—get in the way. Without commitment to the patient and family, nursing lacks the integrity to follow through on the promise as a profession to provide care to society.

SUMMARY

Developing nursing case management is a process, not an outcome. It is a model that creates structures, tools, standards, and paths to accomplish the goal of healing and promoting wholeness. I see no end to the evolution of nursing case management. The amoebic motion of nursing case management continues growing and constricting as societal pressures and forces affect the model. Integration of this model across the continuum is well on its way, but is the next step in the creation of a patient management model that establishes the nurse as a steward and integrator for the health care community? Maybe so.

References

Benner, P. (1984). *From novice to expert.* Menlo Park, Calif.: Addison-Wesley Publishing Co.

Benner, P., Tanner, C., & Chelsa, C. (1996). *Expertise in nursing practice—caring clinical judgment and ethics.* New York: Springer Publishing Co.

Johnson, B., Friend, S., & MacDonald, J. (1997). Nurses' changing and emerging roles with use of unlicensed assistive personnel. In S. Moorehead (Ed.), *Nursing roles evolving or recycled?* Thousand Oaks, Calif.: Sage Publications.

Larson, J. (1992). The healing we: A transformative model for nursing. *Nursing & Health Care, 13,* 5.

Manion, J., Sieg, M.J., & Watson, P. (1998). Managerial partnerships: The wave of the future, *Journal of Nursing Administration, 28,* 4.

Nightingale, F. (1992). *Notes on nursing.* Philadelphia: J.B. Lippincott.

Primm, P.L. (1986). Entry into practice: Competency statements for BSN and ADNs. *Nursing Outlook, 34,* 3.

Schaef, A.W. (1998). *Living in process.* New York: Ballantine Publishing Group.

Webster, M. (1988). *Webster's ninth new collegiate dictionary.* Springfield, Mass., Merriam-Webster Inc. Publishers.

Wheatley, M.J., & Kellner-Rogers, M. (1996). *A simpler way.* San Francisco: Berrett-Koehler Publishers.

Zander, K. (1985). Second generation primary nursing: A new agenda, *Journal of Nursing Administration, 15,* 3.

Job Descriptions and Competencies of the Care Manager and Care Associate

REGISTERED NURSE CARE MANAGER			
	Self-Awareness	**Patient/Family Care**	**Relationships**
VALUE Remains respectful of and committed to:	■ Role ■ Own abilities ■ Experience ■ Knowledge/learning ■ Professional practice ■ Self-confidence ■ Motivation ■ Growth and development ■ Humility	■ Profession of nursing ■ Care delivery continuum ■ Potential power within patient/family ■ Patient's own healing power ■ Patients' health continuum ■ Patient/family interpretation for their own quality of life ■ Patients rights ■ Ethical care	■ Mission ■ Effective teamwork ■ Expertise of others ■ Integrity of individuals/teams ■ Multiple perspectives ■ Ongoing education, change, and growth ■ Mentoring ■ Proactive communication
KNOWLEDGE Demonstrates consistent understanding of:	■ Self ■ When to involve others ■ Importance of self-care ■ Boundaries/limitations ■ Presence ■ Impact of attitude	■ The nursing process ■ Family dynamics ■ Teaching theory ■ Motivation for patients ■ Impact of patient/family on community ■ Health care options/trends and resource management ■ The unexpected and the big picture ■ Patient/family response to health status ■ Empathy, compassion, and presence ■ Coping mechanisms ■ Systems theory ■ Assumes responsibility for the assessment and care of patients appropriate to the age of the patients served in the assigned service area	■ Change process ■ Group process ■ Learning styles ■ When to risk ■ Potential impact of attitude on the team ■ Roles/resources for information/problem solving ■ Boundaries of individuals and the team ■ Mentoring ■ Capacities of team members, when greater expertise may be required

Continued

REGISTERED NURSE CARE MANAGER—CONT'D

	Self-Awareness	Patient/Family Care	Relationships

SKILL
Consistently and intuitively demonstrates:
	■ Self-direction and motivation
	■ Open and objective perceptions
	■ Integration of past/present experiences
	■ Accountability for decisions
	■ Self-care
	■ Time management
	■ Independent thinking
	■ Self-reflection
		■ Resource utilization for optimal, cost-effective care
		■ Active listening, connecting, and communicating in patient terms
		■ Advocacy
		■ Nursing process:
		  ■ Assess functional health status
		  ■ Develop mutual goals
		  ■ Individualize care planning
		  ■ Evaluate response to care plan
		  ■ Assess individuals' learning needs
		  ■ Implement teaching strategies
		  ■ Plan and coordinate discharge needs
		  ■ Assess need for follow-up
		■ Response to ethical challenges
		■ Reasoning based on experience
		■ Management of multiple tasks simultaneously
		■ Resourcefulness—accessible—available—aware
		■ Comforting, distracting, being with, relieving pain
		■ Obtains and interprets information in terms of the patient's needs that are age specific and carries out treatments
		■ Demonstrates a knowledge of normal growth and development
			■ Active listening
			■ Open dialogue
			■ Conflict resolution
			■ Utilization of others' expertise
			■ Application of knowledge from one situation to another
			■ Accountability
			■ Flexibility and objectivity
			■ Focusing energy in a positive constructive direction
			■ Commitment to follow through
			■ Risk taking
			  ■ Negotiation—stepping in/back as the situation demands
			  ■ Assertiveness
			  ■ Persistence
			  ■ Persuasion
			■ Facilitation of learning for others
			■ Investigation of alternatives and shared rationale

REGISTERED NURSE CARE ASSOCIATE (ESSENTIAL)

	Self-Awareness	Patient/Family Care	Relationships	Communication
VALUE Remains respectful of:	■ Growth and exploration ■ Self-perception ■ Own value clarification	■ Essence of nursing ■ Care delivery system ■ Patient vulnerability, rights, and choices	■ Team concept ■ Expertise of other disciplines ■ Multidisciplinary approach ■ Differentiation in nursing practice ■ Mission of unit	■ Effective communication ■ Being open and non-judgmental
KNOWLEDGE Demonstrates increasing understanding of:	■ Self-care ■ The importance of others' perceptions ■ Objective feedback ■ Knowing self and why you are here ■ Importance of not projecting own value system ■ Personal/professional limits	■ Core nursing skills and practice ■ Pathophysiology of disease ■ Concepts of family dynamics ■ The need for empathy and compassion ■ Differentiated nursing roles ■ Assumes responsibility for the assessment and care of patients appropriate to the age of the patients served in the assigned service area	■ The elements of a team ■ The importance of being an effective team member ■ The roles of other disciplines ■ The nursing role within the patient care delivery system ■ Mission of nursing department and organization	■ The elements of facilitative communication ■ Nonverbal language

Continued

REGISTERED NURSE CARE ASSOCIATE (ESSENTIAL)—CONT'D

	Self-Awareness	Patient/Family Care	Relationships	Communication
SKILL Progressively demonstrates ability to:	■ Accept and listen to feedback on feelings/behaviors and reactions to situations ■ Share knowledge ■ Question the unknown ■ Understand and accept values of self and others	■ Perform core nursing process and skills ■ Organize and prioritize patient needs ■ Function in the team and assist patients in achieving mutual goals ■ Evaluate and give feedback on patient's response ■ Manage time ■ Teach ■ Obtains and interprets information in terms of the patient's needs that are age specific and carries out treatments ■ Demonstrates a knowledge of normal growth and development	■ Function in a team ■ Know when and how to recognize and use appropriate disciplines ■ Delegate	■ Recognizes self and others' perceptions and their impact ■ Exhibit effective listening, verbal, nonverbal, and written skills: ■ Non-blaming ■ Respectful ■ Honest ■ Courteous ■ Good eye contact ■ Clear messages ■ Provide concise reports and documentation

REGISTERED NURSE CARE ASSOCIATE (LEADER/EXPERT)

	Self-Awareness	Patient/Family Care	Relationships
VALUE Remains respectful of and committed to:	■ Own abilities—relies on clinical judgment for decisions ■ Experience ■ Knowledge/learning ■ Professional practice ■ Concern for patient as a person as central to practice ■ Self-confidence and self-responsibility ■ Humility ■ Motivation ■ Growth and development	■ Profession of nursing ■ Care delivery continuum ■ Moral and caring practices—doing things for the right reason ■ Potential power within patient/family ■ Patient's own self-healing power ■ Patient's interpretation for own quality of life ■ Ethical resource utilization	■ Change and growth ■ Expertise of others ■ Mission of the nursing department/organization ■ Integrity of individuals/teams ■ Multiple perspectives ■ Mentoring ■ Proactive communication
KNOWLEDGE Demonstrates consistent understanding of:	■ Self ■ Others' skills and knowledge ■ Boundaries ■ Presence ■ Impact of attitude	■ Nursing process, caring, and teaching theory ■ Practical knowledge of particular patient population ■ Warning signs, subtle changes ■ The unexpected and the big picture ■ Different roles of differentiated case management ■ Patient response to pathophysiology of disease ■ When technology has become excessive and intervenes appropriately ■ Empathy, compassion, and presence ■ The ongoing need for health and well-being ■ Coping mechanisms ■ Assumes responsibility for the assessment and care of patients appropriate to the age of the patients served in the assigned service area	■ Change process ■ Group process ■ Learning styles—strengths and weaknesses of others ■ When to risk ■ Resources for problem solving ■ Capacities of team members, when greater expertise may be required ■ Timing and pace of whole unit ■ Stepping in and stepping back as the situation demands ■ Boundaries of individuals and the team ■ Mentoring ■ Creating an environment for effective teamwork

Continued

REGISTERED NURSE CARE ASSOCIATE (LEADER/EXPERT)—CONT'D

	Self-Awareness	Patient/Family Care	Relationships
SKILL Consistently and intuitively demonstrates:	■ Self-direction and inner motivation ■ Awareness of personal limits ■ Open and objective perceptions ■ Integration of past/present experiences ■ Accountability for decisions ■ Self-care ■ Time management ■ Independent thinking ■ Self-reflection	■ Nursing process—skilled, innovative performance linked with judgment, timing, and anticipation of future events ■ Practical reasoning based on experience ■ Organization, prioritization, analysis of data to meet individual needs ■ Management of multiple tasks simultaneously ■ Thinking in action ■ Fluid, seamless performance of difficult tasks under time pressure ■ Resourcefulness for patient/family: accessible—available—aware ■ Reading patient's response, adjusting for individual needs, desires, wants in both clinical and human dimensions ■ Comforting, distracting, being with, relieving pain ■ Allowing patient/family to explore care options and respectfully advocates for their decisions; guided by patient response and desired outcomes ■ Ability to identify moral issues and to foresee ethical implications of clinical interventions and seek organizational response ■ Ability to design systems to support caring practices and create supportive space ■ Connecting and communicating in patient terms ■ Resource utilization for cost-effective care ■ Obtains and interprets information in terms of the patient's needs that are age specific and carries out treatments ■ Demonstrates a knowledge of normal growth and development	■ Respect, dignity, personhood, the integrity of close relationships ■ Advocacy ■ Caring relationships guided by patient response ■ Openness to exceptions in the usual level of involvement to allow vital caring work to occur ■ Utilizing expertise of others—working with others so no one is overburdened and all resources are used ■ Resourcefulness—for—unit/organization: available—aware—accessible ■ Application of knowledge from one situation to another ■ Accountability ■ Flexibility and objectivity ■ Response to ethical challenges (able to take strong positions with health team to get what patient needs) ■ Focusing energy in a positive constructive direction ■ Active listening ■ Commitment to follow through ■ Risk taking: negotiation—assertiveness—persistence—persuasion ■ Facilitation of learning for others ■ Investigation of alternatives and shared rationale ■ Open dialogue ■ Conflict resolution

REGISTERED NURSE CARE ASSOCIATE (PROFICIENT)

	Self-Awareness	Patient/Family Care	Relationships	Communication

VALUE
Remains respectful of and committed to:
	■ Self
	■ Personal/Professional limits
	■ Diversity
	■ Own philosophy regarding quality of life/ethical issues
	■ Reflective learning
	■ Learning from others
		■ Essence of nursing
		■ Quality individualized care
		■ Care delivery system
		■ Patients rights and choices
		■ Alleviation of pain and suffering
		■ Caring
		■ Cost-effective care
			■ Mutual respect of team members
			■ Expertise of all disciplines
			■ Team working as a whole
			■ Mentoring
				■ Process of facilitative communication:
				  ■ Truth
				  ■ Openness
				  ■ Productive outcomes
				  ■ Respect of others
				  ■ Understanding

KNOWLEDGE Demonstrates consistent understanding of:	■ Self as a resource ■ How self is perceived ■ Personal limits ■ Own emotions & internal reactions ■ Self-motivation ■ Personality traits ■ Response to diversity ■ Advocacy ■ Self-care	■ Nursing Code of Ethics & Practice Act ■ Roles in differentiated case management ■ Broad range of nursing skills ■ Significance of signs and symptoms ■ Complexities of patient's condition ■ Typical progression of illness and recovery ■ Pathophysiology of disease process ■ Family dynamics and importance of support people in healing process ■ Empathy and compassion ■ Ongoing need for health and well-being ■ Assumes responsibility for the assessment and care of patients appropriate to the age of the patients served in the assigned service area	■ Various roles of the team members ■ Limits within the team ■ Mutual goals and plan of care established with patient ■ Mission of nursing department and organization ■ Ongoing need for change and growth ■ Impact of attitude on team	■ Elements of facilitative communication ■ Variety of learning styles

Continued

REGISTERED NURSE CARE ASSOCIATE (PROFICIENT)—CONT'D

	Self-Awareness	Patient/Family Care	Relationships	Communication

SKILL
Consistently and effectively demonstrates:
	■ Independence in practice
	■ Attentiveness
	■ Sensitivity to own feelings and external elements that affect those feelings
	■ Active role in advocating and collaborating for quality of life issues
	■ Self-care
	■ Time management
		■ Nursing process:
		  ■ Accurate assessment and problem identification
		  ■ Planning/anticipating likely events
		  ■ Mastery of difficult technical tasks and multiple demands
		  ■ Combining standardization with professional judgment
		  ■ Data interpretation to identify complex needs
		  ■ Competent clinical judgment
		  ■ Organizing, prioritizing, analyzing data to meet needs
		  ■ Evaluation and feedback on response, adjusted for individual needs
		■ Teaching
		■ Advocacy
		■ Collaboration
		■ Obtains and interprets information in terms of the patient's needs that are age specific and carries out treatments
		■ Demonstrates a knowledge of normal growth and development
			■ Team collaboration
			■ Utilization of team members (consults/refers)
			■ Delegation of responsibility
			■ Integrity
			■ Flexibility
			■ Adaptability
			■ Commitment
			■ Professional behavior
			■ Preceptorship
				■ Communication in understandable language
				■ Listening and allowing input
				■ Sharing and teaching ideas
				■ Conflict management
				■ Manner that is approachable, interactive, sees both sides, positive, assertive
				■ Nonjudgmental interaction

A Faculty Case Management Practice Based in a College of Nursing

Mary Allen Carey
Margo MacRobert

CHAPTER OVERVIEW

Since 1995 the University of Oklahoma Health Sciences College of Nursing has been an accredited case management (CM) provider to the state of Oklahoma. As a result of community interest and requests from private pay sources for CM, private CM was developed and implemented in 2001. As far as we know, we are the only university to have such a form of faculty practice. In this chapter we describe the process by which we identified and instituted this service, our use of it for faculty practice and student learning, and the ongoing and emerging issues that mark its continuance.

THE ORIGIN OF THE CASE MANAGEMENT SERVICE

The faculty of the University of Oklahoma College of Nursing (OUCN) made major curriculum revisions in the mid-1990s to better prepare students for the evolving changes in the profession and the health care job market. Our deliberations supported the need for four significant changes. First, students needed more experiences in the community and clients' homes and with the aged, the chronically ill, and the disabled. Second, students needed greater familiarity with managed care, Medicare, and Medicaid and more active involvement in the wise use of limited resources. Third, they needed more experience working in interdisciplinary teams and with the management of care across sites and levels of acuity. Fourth, they needed more consistent integration of research and health promotion into their learning in relation to emerging trends in health care and nursing practice (Jacobson et al., 1998).

Achieving general faculty support for these principles was relatively easy. Determining how the needed experiences could be provided and in what proportions was much more difficult. Student data indicated a strong desire for more, not less, practice in acute care settings and strong resistance to more experience with the elderly and the chronically ill. Many faculty members expressed a lack of personal experience in the community with elderly or chronically ill populations and with managed care systems and voiced concern about their ability to guide students in these areas. A perennial community barrier was the shortage of sufficient practice sites with nursing role models and nursing control to provide the desired learning.

Portions of this chapter were adapted from Jacobson, S.F., McRobert, M., Leon, C., & McKennon, E. (1998). A faculty case management practice integrating teaching, service, and research. *Nursing Health and Perspectives, 19*(5), 220-223. Used with permission.

A concurrent, contextual faculty issue was the nature and importance of faculty practice. Although OUCN was an early leader in defining faculty practice as part of faculty workload and in defining a practice plan for compensation (Smith, 1980), historically only about 10% of faculty (mostly psychiatric nurses) engaged in what would be consistent with contemporary views of faculty practice as linked to revenue generation and student experience. However, the advent of certification and its accompanying need for practice, the start of a nurse practitioner program, the expectations by university administration that faculty would generate revenue, and the burgeoning literature on nursing centers and clinics revived interest in faculty practice at OUCN and its potential for student experience.

A possible solution to our curriculum and practice debates came with the state's entry into managed care. In 1995 the state legislature created the ADvantage Program, a Medicaid-funded program providing home- and community-based services to frail elders and adults over age 21 years (to be managed by the Long Term Care Authority of Tulsa [LTCA]). Analysis of the ADvantage Program philosophy by a core of faculty members found it to emphasize involvement of clients in service planning, interagency and interdisciplinary collaboration, health promotion and maintenance, use of family and community resources to supplement state funds, and separation of case management from provision of actual health care. These themes were highly compatible with our nursing values and needs for new student experiences and faculty practice. In September 1995, after faculty deliberation and the creation of a business plan, the college became an accredited case management provider to the Oklahoma ADvantage Program. Our goals were to provide a quality, visible nursing service to Oklahomans, a nurse-controlled experience for futuristic undergraduate and graduate education, a needed site for faculty practice and learning, a source of revenue for the college, and, eventually, a site for research, thus integrating the missions of the university (Jacobson et al., 1998).

THE ADVANTAGE PROGRAM OF OKLAHOMA

The ADvantage Program was developed to implement Oklahoma's 2176 Medicaid waiver. Its goal is to assist, in a cost-effective manner, clients with nursing home–level needs to remain in their homes with the formal services needed to do so. These services include case management, skilled nursing, personal care, homemaking, specialized medical equipment and supplies, prescription medications, home-delivered meals, environmental modifications to make the home safe and accessible, adult day care, various therapies, and respite for family caregivers. There were six original case management (CM) providers to ADvantage, including Eldercare, for-profit home health agencies, a community mental health center, and OUCN. We were the only provider based in a university, with all registered nurse (RN) case managers (CMs), and with all RNs holding master's or doctoral degrees. Within the conceptualization of case management models proposed by Conti (1999), our service is most closely related to the broker model. In Austin's typology of case management (Austin, 1992), our service is closest to the service management model, as we operate within clearly specified fiscal limits and purchase services on our clients' behalf.

In the beginning years of the program, the training of CMs began with 7 days of instruction by ADvantage Program staff. Presently, the instruction by ADvantage Program staff is 5 days long. The case management agency now assumes more responsibility for the training and orientation of new CMs. During the 5 days of instruction by program staff, CMs first become educated in the use of the client assessment tool that is completed by state Department of Human Services nurses before client selection of a CM provider. Next they work through the entire CM philosophy and process using lecture, discussion, and role late, additional change from indexed playing. After satisfactory completion of the 5-day instruction, the CMs are eligible to continue orientation at the specific case management agency. The OUCN orientation consists of management of at least five full cases under the guidance of a preceptor and successful completion of a quality improvement (QI) audit.

The actual CM process begins when ADvantage Program staff notifies the CM provider that a new client has been screened for eligibility and has selected us as the CM provider. CMs are assigned to cases by the CM director or may volunteer for cases according to their expertise. The CM then contacts the client and makes a home visit to validate or update the original client assessment. Next, the CM schedules an interdisciplinary team meeting with the client, family, key informal support persons, an RN from the home health agency, and other formal providers, such as physicians or Medicare. At this meeting participants discuss and agree on the general plan of care. The CM then develops a service plan with goals, action steps, outcomes, and an expenditure plan that is considered to be cost effective and less than nursing home placement. After the plan is approved by the client and the ADvantage staff, the CM implements the plan with the interdisciplinary team, monitors the client throughout the year, and evaluates and modifies the plan as needed.

Launching the Faculty Case Management Venture

Despite commitment to curricular redesign and faculty practice in some form, many faculty were not enthusiastic about the college becoming a full-time service provider to a state agency. Full-time faculty attitudes regarding clinical practice and the perceived role strain have been documented in the literature (Steele, 1991; Richmond, Mossberg, & Rahr, 2001). The 24-hour, 7-day-a-week responsibility to clients and an external employer represented a major discontinuity with the traditional rhythm of academic life and traditional faculty practice. Dissenting faculty pointed out, quite correctly, that few descriptions of faculty practice in the literature involved everyday, round-the-clock service and that 24-hour coverage was not the norm for existing CM services. (In 1998 Mullahy [1998] identified 24-hour coverage as a trend but still not common.) How, faculty asked, could such coverage be provided when CM activities were to be performed in addition to regular teaching responsibilities? The fear that the CM venture would devalue acute care skills for students or the faculty teaching in critical care resurfaced. Concerns about job security and issues of academic freedom were raised for faculty who were unwilling or unable to acquire experience in this practice arena. Questions about the relative emphasis on the need for a new form of student experience versus the need for revenue generation and whether students would be exploited if they participated in an activity for which faculty received additional pay circulated overtly and covertly. Nevertheless, a core of seven graduate and undergraduate faculty volunteered to be trained as CMs and to develop student learning experiences in the program. The director of research also completed the training as an aid to future development of research on case management.

Dr. Patricia Forni, Dean of the College of Nursing, provided strong administrative support for the program. The approach to incorporating the faculty case management practice activities within the College of Nursing offsets the difficulties frequently faced by managed care markets attempting to import faculty practice (Culbertson, 1997). Supporters of the approach taken by the College of Nursing continue to make a case for a college-based case management practice (Barger, 2000).

A faculty member with experience in administration, community health, and managed care was designated as the CM coordinator. Her visibility and legitimacy were enhanced by her appointment to the College Administrative Council and the Partnerships and Innovative Care Models Council. Secretarial support, office space, and equipment were provided. Teaching assistants were hired to relieve faculty taking CM training, and faculty were reimbursed for travel to training sites. A portion of the college's reimbursement from LTCA was used to pay CMs for mileage, in addition to their hourly rate. Faculty CMs also received merit points for service at their annual evaluations.

The period of training faculty as CMs and launching the service was neither smooth nor short. The CM coordinator position had to be filled three times in the first year. Turnover of faculty CMs was high initially because of dislike of the activity, frustration with the state bureaucracy, or competing demands from teaching assignments. Of 21 faculty trained as CMs in the first year, only 10 continued. Twice in the early months of the program we were unable to accept clients because of a shortage of CMs. Additionally, QI audits consistently demonstrated that faculty with extremely small client loads performed less satisfactorily. We now emphasize that CM training is a practice commitment to the college and we require faculty CMs to carry at least 20 clients.

Maintenance of Faculty Practice at Distance Education Sites

The University of Oklahoma College of Nursing currently offers selected components of the baccalaureate and graduate programs at four major sites across the state of Oklahoma. Several factors influence whether distance education site faculty can negotiate a faculty CM practice. These factors are the (1) total size of the full-time teaching faculty resources; (2) workload distribution among teaching, research/scholarly achievement activities, and professional service; (3) availability of clinical services and agencies to geographically support the ADvantage Program; and (4) availability of office space to house the case managers and client records.

With the decision to require faculty CMs to carry at least 20 clients, many faculty decided they could not maintain the commitment to the practice and to their teaching responsibilities. Presently, only three faculty practice as CMs.

The CM director prepared a business plan to propose the hiring of salaried registered nurses (RNs) to meet the client/case management staffing standard. As of 2003, the practice has three practice sites in the state of Oklahoma. The practice employs one director who is also a faculty member, three RN site coordinators, two QI coordinators, four secretaries, and 47 full-time case managers. The practice provides CM to 1600 ADvantage program recipients in 23 Oklahoma counties.

THE PRIVATE CM PROGRAM

The private CM venture began when families of patients who were not qualified for the ADvantage program heard about the OUCN CM program by word of mouth. These families desired similar assistance in caring for their elderly family member. A proposal and business plan were developed. Standards of practice were adopted and the CM process was refined to meet the needs of private pay clients. A master's-prepared clinical nurse specialist in gerontology was selected to provide CM for these clients.

Use of the CM Program for Student Learning

Student experience in the CM program started in fall 1997, the second anniversary of the CM service. Two faculty members offered 16 weeks of CM experience as a community clinical option for seniors; six responded. In spring 1998, 14 undergraduates chose case management for their leadership experience. To date, 48 undergraduates have had CM experience. We currently offer clinical experience in case management to senior students in the community; they are required to follow one of the CM clients throughout the junior year.

Seven graduate students have also had learning experiences in case management. Five in the gerontology clinical specialist track chose it as a clinical practicum site and worked with the CM coordinator to develop a quality management program, a fall management program for the elderly, and a diabetic learning module for CMs. Two from the administration/management track carried out required synthesis projects in case management, such as preparing a business plan for comprehensive case management, defined as a combination of case management and home health.

Student learning has exceeded all faculty expectations: "They see teams and coordination like they've never seen it before with the nurse CM as the linchpin. They are accomplished users of the telephone. They know the nature and cost of all the assistive equipment. They see the patient's physical environment and get steps repaired and ramps built. They've internalized the roles of advocate, planner, and coordinator far more than I've seen them do in the hospital" (Jacobson et al., 1998).

The effects of the CM experience continue when students return to inpatient settings. They are vocal about explaining how patients' needs could be adequately met in the community "without using up all their Medicare days." Their hospital discharge planning reflects much greater awareness of what is needed at home and what is available through the community. They recognize opportunities for health promotion among the chronically ill and disabled and that there are dynamic and critical episodes within chronicity (Jacobson et al., 1998).

Faculty also noted positive effects on the student-teacher relationship. In contrast to teaching in agencies where the faculty and students were guests and outsiders, "In CM, the students see me, a nurse, working in a college-controlled nursing setting. I perform in front of them and with them. I get more respect and more collegiality with students than I've ever known before" (Jacobson et al., 1998).

A graduate faculty member in the administration/management track reported: "This is exactly the type of clinical exposure administration students need—not site or specialty-bound and not hierarchically organized. It's good for them to be reminded of just how cost-effective expert nursing is . . . to think about what background is really needed for good case management and what's worth paying for. And this program and role are still so fluid yet, they get a real sense of grappling with the future" (Jacobson et al., 1998).

Faculty Experiences With the Case Management Program

PERSONAL SATISFACTION AND PROFESSIONAL GROWTH

Faculty CMs report great personal satisfaction with their work. They can see that their efforts have made important differences in client lives; simply keeping patients in their homes where they wish to be is immensely satisfying. The case manager have had dramatic successes with clients on whom other CM agencies had given up, such as a young quadriplegic Indian man who overcame depression and alcoholism, obtained his GED, and enrolled in college.

Development of their interviewing, negotiating, and telephone skills has been gratifying. Getting clients what they really need within the budgeting constraints of ADvantage or advocating successfully to override the budget limits in a particular case is both a personal and a professional triumph. Faculty without prior knowledge of community resources, managed care, and reimbursement systems now feel confident about their ability to guide student learning in these areas.

INTERACTIONS WITH PHYSICIANS

Despite fears that physicians would view CMs as threats to their autonomy, faculty interactions with physicians have been almost entirely positive. Physicians in general and rural physicians in particular have been appreciative of what CMs are doing for their patients and have been willing to learn about community resources. They have expressed pleasure at working with nursing faculty as CMs because they believe that their patients are getting the benefits of the latest nursing knowledge. Some CMs state that they and the nursing profession experience more respect from physicians in the CM context than they have been awarded in acute care settings.

ETHICAL ISSUES IN CASE MANAGEMENT

Long-term case management has been characterized as an "ethical minefield" in which issues of quality and cost, regulation and personal and professional integrity, and ethical theories or perspectives clash (Barnett & Taylor, 1999; McAuley, Teaster, & Safewright, 1999). During the third year of the case management service, the frequency and complexity of ethical issues facing CMs led to the creation of a case management ethics committee. The membership consisted of the director of case management, two senior CMs, and faculty members who teach ethics courses. The committee meets on an ad hoc basis to deal with very complex situations with no apparent or optimal solution. These situations most frequently involve suspected mental illness of the client or family members providing informal support, suspected abuse or neglect, situations where the CM believes the client must be removed from the home but neither the client nor the family will agree, or a combination of these circumstances. The committee has also dealt with cases where clients have had multiple case management providers and multiple CMs from within provider agencies and who have pushed us—the last available CM provider—to the point where the CM wishes to discuss the option of discontinuing services to the client. The ethics committee meetings have also served as a site for student learning for students in the policy and ethics course in the graduate program.

In regard to the perennial tension between client advocacy and gatekeeping responsibilities, a recent article (McAuley et al., 1999) contrasting regulatory system approaches and feminist ethics has been helpful. Briefly, the regulatory system approach used by social service agencies and programs originated in organizations designed to produce products. It values uniformity, order, certainty, and logical reasoning leading to reduction of case (human) circumstances to checklists and tallies. Circumstances that do not fit the official instrument or plan are ignored or considered irrelevant in the interests of values-neutral decision-making, unbiased application of the rules, and accountability to the organization. In contrast, the feminist ethics that underlie nursing emphasize listening to all voices in decision-making, the importance of caring and of meeting needs in an individualized manner, and acceptance of emotion and intuition as elements of decision-making in addition to logical reasoning. Both models are, and should be, visible in CMs to varying degrees, as total reliance on one model would bring its faults into bold relief. We agree with the authors that the critical needs in case management are achieving a respected voice for feminist ethics in public programs and establishing an appropriate and flexible balance between the two approaches. At stake is the *care* in managed care.

INTEGRATION OF SOCIAL WORKERS AND ADVANCED PRACTICE NURSES

We began to see that many of the clients had specialized care issues. Although the clients were all elderly, it became apparent that some had diagnosed mental health and substance abuse problems. Additionally, some clients had suffered abuse and neglect. Many CMs voiced concern about working with some of these clients because they thought that they did not possess the knowledge or skill to be effective in these areas. It became increasingly clear to us that these clients required specialized case management.

Based on these observations, the practice hired a psychiatric/mental health clinical nurse specialist for the purpose of providing case management to clients with mental health and substance abuse issues. The supervisor assigned these clients to the advanced practice nurse if the diagnoses were related to mental health or substance abuse. Because the supervisor reviewed the comprehensive assessment of each new client before assignment to a CM, clients with a potential for mental health issues were also identified and assigned to the advanced practice nurse. The practice also hired social workers to work with clients with the potential for abuse and neglect. These social workers provided the practice knowledge about community-based social service resources, were readily able to access these resources, and worked with the client and family members in these situations.

EDUCATIONAL AND EXPERIENTIAL PREPARATION FOR CASE MANAGEMENT

Our experience with case management has provided much opportunity to reflect on the educational and experiential background that makes a good CM. We realize that people of diverse backgrounds are functioning successfully as CMs, that certifying standards exist for CMs of many origins, and that interdisciplinary partnerships can work well (Mullahy, 1998).

Our clients, by their very eligibility for the ADvantage Program, are of very low income (an average of $513 per month), have at least two primary diagnoses (including HIV/AIDS and actual or potential mental health problems), and already meet the standards for admission to nursing homes, as shown by a mean risk assessment score of 108.6, where 106 indicates high risk for institutionalization (LTCA, 1999). Co-morbidities and polypharmacy predispose them to rapid change and decline. Their medical problems and needs for monitoring are so complex that the lack of a nursing knowledge base is detrimental to most of them. All CMs can supply examples of walking in on clients in acute medical or psychiatric emergencies or clients in whom subtle changes, which only a nurse would recognize, required immediate care. The scarcity of, or distance to, inpatient and emergency services for our rural clients makes the ability to make a prompt nursing judgment even more essential. It is far easier for nurses to acquire knowledge of community resources and reimbursement guidelines than for non-nurses to obtain the necessary clinical knowledge themselves or to secure timely consultation. We also believe that client needs require a minimum of baccalaureate preparation in nursing and that master's preparation in a clinical specialty is optimal and should become the standard. Furthermore, RNs with advanced preparation and faculty appointments have internalized the concept of lifelong learning and readily see the need for continuing education, which Mullahy (1998) identifies as a deficiency for some CMs.

Desirable experience for nurses before case management can best be described as broad. Ideally, prospective case managers should have several years of experience in more than one clinical area, in more than one type of treatment facility, and with clients of all ages. Experience in home health or community health is a major asset. At least some CMs in a service require knowledge of Medicare and Medicaid regulations and home health procedure and the ability to impart that knowledge to CMs without it. Superior oral and written communication skills and the ability to adapt them for different people or circumstances are essential. Because the family dynamics issues that CMs encounter are very draining and because conflicts between the client and team or between team members are inevitable, CMs need exceptional physical and emotional stamina.

Our best CMs are able to work in situations that are ambiguous, where there are no black-and-white answers or perfect solutions, and where there is often a need to switch mental gears and change plans and activities quickly. Novice nurses are usually unable to do this or are not comfortable doing this.

Of course CMs with ideal backgrounds are scarce, and CM supervisors, like those in acute care facilities, must develop less experienced or more narrowly experienced nurses as CMs. Our director has observed some common difficulties faced by new CMs. One circumstance that shocks people with experience only in hospitals is that the equipment and supplies always available in the hospital must be *found* in the CM situation. The role transition from being the person who gives the hands-on care to being a consultant, advisor, and facilitator of care is a major adjustment for some. Finally, a full appreciation of the autonomy of the client in the CM situation is a novel experience for many.

The CM supervisor also makes the CMs aware that burnout is a job hazard in this specialty. One advantage of the faculty case management service is that our CMs are not isolated, and observation by or interaction with sympathetic or knowledgeable others is always available. The faculty CMs also report that, after gaining a sense of proficiency in the CM role, their teaching responsibilities actually provide a buffer from the intense involvement with some clients.

CASE MANAGEMENT IN RURAL SETTINGS

Our clients are located in both rural and urban counties, giving us an opportunity to reflect on this dimension of case management. Demographically rural CM clients have been described as elderly, extremely hardy individuals who delay seeking health care longer than urban residents and are therefore sicker on entry into the CM system. They tend to be poorer than urban clients, to be more isolated, and to live in dilapidated housing, sometimes without electricity, telephones, or indoor plumbing. Their independence and self-reliance may predispose them to resist assistance from outsiders, making case management a sensitive issue for them. Service providers are fewer in rural areas, but informal support systems for neighbors are often more common (Parker et al., 1991). In addition, other successful models of case management in rural settings do exist (Reel, Morgan-Judge, Peros, & Abraham, 2002).

These characteristics are often true of our rural clients. However, the statewide publicity given to the ADvantage program and the fact that it aims to keep people in their homes as long as possible have worked to desensitize case management as an issue. Also, nurses are highly respected in rural areas, and we have benefited by being members of this trusted profession. At times, not being from the immediate community has been an advantage in that we are seen as safe confidants and not as people who will gossip about clients. Therefore we have not encountered the suspicion or distrust of urban health professionals described as characteristic of rural clients (Parker et al., 1991). If anything, our rural clients are more appreciative of our efforts and services than are our urban clients.

Although there are fewer service providers from which to choose, the stability and commitment to clients among home health aides from rural agencies have actually been higher than that among aides from urban agencies. Perhaps in the rural counties jobs are scarcer, so aides have fewer job alternatives and therefore tend to do better work and be more dependable.

Distance and mileage to clients' homes are time and money issues for our service. Our CMs drive 400 to 800 miles per month just in their CM responsibilities. Also, we often spend considerable time locating pharmacies that will deliver orders free to rural clients.

LOOKING BACK AND AHEAD

Adjusting to the demands of the case management service on the faculty has often been more a game of catch-up than of anticipation. After a slow start we experienced explosive growth in our client load caused by the death of two of the original CM providers. In just 3 months, our caseload soared from 180 to 325 clients. As we end the seventh year of our contract, our caseload is 1600 clients. The need to meet client needs immediately meant that the CMs coped without having time to think about how to adjust faculty assignments as the practice volume increased. This increased client base, plus the inability to enlist sufficient numbers of faculty CMs, led to another change in the original structure of our service. We hired 39 nonfaculty CMs (5 are social workers and 34 are RNs). Five of the RNs had masters' degrees. Of the 34 RNs, 6 had managerial responsibility in one of the three office sites, and 1 maintained responsibility for the quality improvement program. We are no longer entirely a staff of *faculty* CMs.

A CM Track in the Graduate Program

In the fall of 1999, OUCN offered a CM focus within the clinical nurse specialist (CNS) track. Students desiring CM preparation take the course in financial management currently taken by students in administration/management. This course includes content on the financing of managed care approaches. The core course, "Policy and Ethics in Health Care," and the concepts courses in the CNS track added content relevant to case management. One of two required clinical practicum courses is devoted entirely to case management and provides 288 hours of CM practice.

SUMMARY

Although the current faculty CMs are devoted to the program and wish to continue it, we realize that it will not have the faculty-wide support for which we had originally hoped, either for faculty practice or for student experience. Although some faculty have been impressed by the national interest in the service, the program is likely to remain controversial. We are heartened, however, by the quickness with which most students recognize the advantages of CM experience to them. Their comments about really understanding continuity of care, integrating all of their nursing knowledge just before writing the NCLEX, CM as a showcase for professional and advanced practice, and CM as an area for entrepreneurship are extremely reinforcing.

Above all, the ADvantage program is maintaining indigent elderly and disabled Oklahomans in their homes and is saving Oklahoma taxpayers money—approximately $32 million per year in 1998 (LTCA, 1999). We are very proud that we have helped to bring the benefits of CM and the resources of the College of Nursing to our citizens.

References

Austin, C.D. (1992). Have we oversold case management as a "quick fix" for our long-term term-care system? *Journal of Case Management, 1*, 61 65.

Barnett, R.J., & Taylor, C. (1999). The ethics of case management: Communication challenges. In E.L. Cohen & V. De Back (Eds.), *The outcomes mandate: Case management in health care today* (pp. 328-338). St. Louis: Mosby.

Barger, S.E. (2000). Making the case for a college-run case management practice. *Journal of Professional Nursing, 16*(4), 187.

Conti, R.M. (1999). The broker model of case management. In E.L. Cohen & V. De Back (Eds.), *The outcomes mandate: Case management in health care today* (pp. 122-131). St. Louis: Mosby.

Culbertson, R.A. (1997). Academic faculty practices: issues for viability in competitive managed care markets. *Journal of Health Politics and Policy Law, 22*(6), 1359-1383.

Jacobson, S.F., et al. (1998). A faculty case management practice: Integrating teaching, service, and research. *Nurse Health Care Perspectives, 19*, 220-223.

Long Term Care Authority of Tulsa (1999, Jan.). *ADvantage Waiver Status Report.* Tulsa: Author.

McAuley, W.J., Teaster, P.B., & Safewright, M.P. (1999). Incorporating feminist ethics into case management programs. *J Applied Gerontology, 18*, 3-23.

Mullahy, C.M. (1998). *The case manager's handbook*, 2nd edition. Gaithersburg, Md.: Aspen Publishers.

Parker, M., et al. (1991). Case management in rural areas: Definition, clients, financing, staffing, and service delivery issues. In A. Bushy (Ed.), *Rural nursing*, vol 2 (pp. 29-40). Newbury Park, Calif: Sage.

Reel, S.J., Morgan-Judge, R., Peros, D.S., & Abraham, I.L. (2002). School-based rural case management: A model to prevent and reduce risk. *Journal of American Academy of Nurse Practitioners, 14*(7), 291-296.

Richmond, S., Mossbert, K.A., & Rahr, R.R. (2001). Issues and dilemmas of developing a new faculty practice plan. *Journal of Allied Health, 30*(1), 26-29.

Smith, G.R. (1980). Compensating faculty for their clinical practice. *Nurse Outlook, 28*(11), 673-676.

Steele, R.L. (1991). Attitudes about faculty practice, perceptions of role and role strain. *Journal of Nursing Education, 30*(1), 15-22.

A Model of Emergency Department Case Management

Developing Strategies and Outcomes

Carolee Sherer Whitehill

CHAPTER OVERVIEW

The emerging role of emergency department case managers provides an opportunity to develop programs focused on the population needs and system issues of individual emergency departments. Organizing these programs into primary care, population programs, admission/discharge planning, and individual patient plans assists in developing processes with clear goals and outcomes. Expanding partnerships to the community and inpatient setting, linking with the public health agenda, and an awareness of issues effecting the provision of emergency care while expanding case management interventions will enhance patients' access to services and continuity of care.

A MODEL OF EMERGENCY DEPARTMENT CASE MANAGEMENT

Emergency Care Issues

The high volume of patients treated within emergency care facilities provides an opportunity not only to address acute clinical care but also to offer appropriate education, screening, and health care resources within the context of the patient's specific needs. Although overall goals of case management programs are similar, designing programs for the emergency department (ED) requires a unique approach. Unlike traditional hospital or community case management programs, which allow for thorough and repeat assessments, family contact, time for discharge planning, and the potential for long-term follow-up, the emergency environment is episodic and spontaneous. The patient contact involves rapid assessment, usually limited to the immediate event, appropriate acute interventions, and an expeditious disposition process. As ED case management programs evolve, it is important for the ED to identify its place in the continuum of care. What are patients' needs regarding clinical care, disposition, follow-up arrangements, education, and resources? Who are the partners the ED staff can contact to integrate patient services? Are the linkages made on an individual patient level or by developing system-wide programs? In addition, providers of emergency care need to develop outcome measurements to determine the impact of emergency treatment, risk screening, and cost effectiveness and quality of care (Cairns et al., 1998).

Finding a Focus

Surrounded by a multitude of fragmented health delivery systems while treating high volumes of patients who often have complex needs, it may be difficult to initiate a clear plan of action in developing a case management program for the ED. Programs should be developed that address the specific needs of the patient population and system issues of the department. Start by asking questions regarding patients, systems, and caregivers. This process may help focus on priority concerns.

Does the department have high-acuity, high-cost patients? A significant chronic care population? Quality of care issues? High volume of nonurgent patients? Patients who have difficulty accessing health care resources? Significant uninsured population? Recurrent ED patients? Individual patients with special needs? Patients who are noncompliant with discharge instructions? Clear expectations among the ED team? How does the department compare with ED benchmarking data? Efficient coordination of services between inpatient and outpatient sites? Adequate communication with primary care providers? Reimbursement denials? A need to search for cost savings? A growing capitated payer population? Patient satisfaction that needs improving? Long patient length of stay?

Although this is just a sampling of potential case management issues, together they affect quality of care, efficient and cost-effective use of resources, access to care, and integration of services. When addressed, they may improve continuity of care and the health status of patients, which are the ultimate goals of ED case management programs.

A Model of Emergency Department Case Management

Current and evolving ED case management programs may be organized into four prominent areas (Figure 15-1):

Primary care programs
Population-based programs
Admission and discharge planning
Individual patient plans

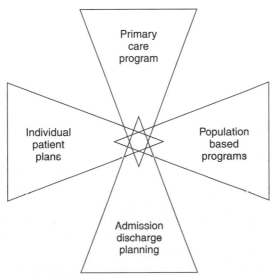

FIGURE **15-1**   Emergency department case management.
Courtesy of © 1999, Carolee Whitehill.

This model serves as a tool to assist in program design and to identify issues, goals, strategies, and outcomes within the context of each area. The center star represents goals that are potentially shared among the programs and patients who may benefit from more than one program. Case managers should develop programs based on the priority issues within their facility and the distinctive needs of their patient population. ED case management programs are not developed in isolation but rather by building alliances with providers in and out of the hospital setting. During the development or expansion of ED case management programs, role definitions for the ED case manager, social work, and utilization management is important, as well as coordinating programs with ED providers and administrators.

Frustration regarding frequent or recurrent ED patients is common among ED staff. As a group these patients have very diverse needs, access to resources, and reasons for using the ED. It is recommended that recidivism be evaluated within each program area to analyze and develop options appropriate to the specific patient or group of patients.

PRIMARY CARE PROGRAMS

Issues

Significant public health issues affect the provision of services in the ED: restrictions in access to health care, the growing uninsured population, financial limitations, overcrowding, and staffing constraints. Although estimates for patients presenting to the ED with nonurgent needs vary considerably, the Centers for Disease Control and Prevention (CDC) released the National Hospital Ambulatory Medical Care Survey: 2001 Emergency Department Summary, which identifies the following triage assessments: emergent accounted for 19.2%; urgent, 31.7%; semiurgent, 16.3%; and nonurgent, 9.1%, with 23.6% of the patients not identified at triage or unknown urgency (McCaig & Burt, 2003).

A variety of circumstances lead patients to use the ED for primary care conditions. Even patients with an identified primary care provider may not be able to access the provider's office for urgent issues because of busy provider schedules. Patients may be told to wait a day or days or to seek care in an ED or urgent care clinic. Some patients use the ED for convenience; it is available 24 hours a day, 7 days a week without appointments. Many patients lack the flexibility with work schedules to attend appointments during weekday hours. EDs continue to provide a health care safety net for the medically underserved in the United States, and they are the only source of care for some patients.

In a study of 1190 ambulatory patients in an urban public hospital, the majority of whom were uninsured, patients were asked if they needed to be seen immediately, with 89% responding in the affirmative. However, according to a physician acuteness rating, 56% did not require care within 24 hours (Baker, Stevens, & Brook, 1995). In examining factors that lead patients to use the ED for nonurgent care, Padgett and Brodsky (1992) found the most common reason was that patients reported no other care was available. In addition to lack of primary care resources, the authors report that psychiatric co-morbidities, socioeconomic stressors, and lack of social support influence patients' decision-making. This reliance on the ED as a "safety net" for patients has been described as providing "almshouse" services, such as warmth, rest, clothing, food, shelter, and relief from social distress (Malone, 1998).

EDs operate predominantly on a fixed budget based on historical workloads. Providers are available 24 hours a day, 7 days a week. Historically, most have believed that diverting nonurgent patients from EDs to physician offices would result in significant cost savings. However, Williams (1996) reports the marginal costs, defined as the extra costs of an additional ED visit, as $25 for a nonurgent visit. Diverting patients to a physician office would result in relatively low savings. Actual charges for the visits are often higher to compensate for overall poor reimbursements of care provided (Williams, 1996). It is also widely assumed that emergency care consumes a large portion of the health care dollar. Data suggest that less than 2% of national health expenditures occurred in EDs, and limiting access to this care would not result in substantial cost savings (Tyrance, Himmelsteine, & Woolhandler, 1996).

However, the effort to link patients to primary care services is beneficial for patients to receive screening and maintenance care that is not provided in an emergency setting. It is hoped that the effect will impact the number of patients presenting with nonurgent needs, diminish overcrowding, and allow ED providers to focus on more emergent cases.

Goals

Although significant barriers exist, the goal for primary care programs is to encourage patients to use appropriate primary care and community resources rather than continued reliance on the ED for non-emergent care. These resources are offered with respect to insurance benefits with sliding-scale or lower-cost options for the uninsured. Case management goals for primary care programs might include the following:

- Identify and maintain current resources for primary care services, health screenings, dental care, health education, psychosocial assistance, and community resources; match patient needs to available resources to improve the patient's health status.
- Decrease patient reliance on the ED for primary care needs.
- Act as a liaison to improve communication between the ED and primary care providers.
- Ensure that primary care provider receives communication regarding a patient's ED visit.
- Decrease overcrowding, minimize waiting time, and increase patient satisfaction.

Strategies and Outcomes

RESOURCES AND EDUCATION

Primary care service needs of the ED patient population should be assessed. *What percent of the population is without primary care services? What resources are available for the insured and uninsured? Are the patients with primary care services knowledgeable about access and appropriate use? Do primary care providers receive summary notes of their patient's ED treatment?* Once the patient's needs and available resources are identified, patient and staff education becomes the priority.

Many patients need education regarding the benefits of primary care services that are not routinely provided in the ED: disease screening, health education and maintenance, prevention services, chronic disease management, medication monitoring, consistency and continuity of the provider, and extended follow-up. In addition, patients need access education: encouragement to call the provider 24 hours a day for health care advice, to keep appointments even if feeling well, and to call after the ED visit for a follow-up or new appointment.

Not all patients perceive the need for primary care services. It is important to determine the needs of the patients regarding ongoing continuity of care and the patient's incentive for compliance. There are several subgroups of patients whose resources might be more individualized. Patients with chronic illnesses or conditions should be strongly encouraged to obtain primary care services because their health status and quality of life can be improved and their disease more successfully managed through regular primary care. Patients who have significant psychosocial stresses, such as poverty, homelessness, mental illness, substance abuse, or domestic violence, often use the ED because their needs are not being met elsewhere. Although primary care may be indicated for a medical condition, arranging social service intervention, counseling, addiction services, financial assistance, and community resources are also priority concerns.

There remains a subgroup of patients who are generally young or middle aged and healthy who use the ED for urgent health care needs. Some of these patients do not perceive a benefit of primary care and access health care only when they are ill or injured and prefer the convenience of the ED. These patients would benefit from education regarding the recommended disease screenings (i.e., Pap smear, mammography, prostate, colon cancer, cholesterol, etc.). Patients without insurance should be offered resources for low-cost, sliding-scale services available in the area.

Outcomes regarding the success of patients obtaining primary care access, compliance with follow-up appointments, and feedback regarding appointment availability can be helpful in adjusting resource education. In addition, monitoring the efficiency of forwarding ED visit documentation to primary care providers is an appropriate outcome measurement. If significant programs are developed with the goal of decreasing the nonurgent patient volume in the ED, decreases in the low-acuity triage categories would be useful as an outcome measurement.

HOSPITAL-BASED CLINICS

Many EDs have initiated fast track or urgent care clinics to assist with patient flow in the department. These clinics are focused on providing efficient care to nonurgent and stable urgent patients with the goals of decreasing wait time and overcrowding of the ED and on improving patient satisfaction. If there are limited resources for the medically underserved in the area and the ED is the regular provider of care for the uninsured population, it may be beneficial to develop a hospital-based primary care clinic.

POPULATION-BASED PROGRAMS

Issues

As health care policy evolves, there is an increased emphasis on managing the health needs of populations rather than of individuals. Among the most innovative ED programs are those focused on targeted population groups. Disease management programs evaluate health care needs of patients with a specific chronic condition or shared indicator such as age and develop a plan of care that addresses clinical needs, health maintenance and educational needs, resource utilization, and continuity of care with the purpose of improving the patient's health status. Although the primary focus of the ED is and will continue to be to provide emergent/urgent clinical care, by extending relationships with other providers, emergency caregivers are offered a great opportunity to expand the integration of health care services for targeted patient populations. Strengthening partnerships between the ED and primary care providers, acute care services, specialists, social services, health educators, pharmacists, hospital case managers, community resources, home care agencies, extended care facilities, alternative medicine providers, and payers will allow a more integrated, efficient, and resourceful health care delivery system to evolve.

Estimates suggest that 10% to 15% of ED patient visits result from exacerbations of chronic illnesses. Managing chronic care patients is often cited as the most successful method to decrease costs of preventable care in the ED (Advisory Board Company, 1993). In addition to acute care services to treat illness exacerbations, patients need information for accessing primary care services and education resources for managing their own disease.

One might select a patient group that accounts for a high volume or high cost to the institution, significant readmission rate, or a population that receives inconsistent care. Examples of conditions or diseases of population-based groups appropriate for disease or group management programs in the ED are as follows:
- Diabetes
- Asthma

- Chronic heart failure
- High blood pressure
- Trauma
- Chest pain
- Chronic obstructive pulmonary disease
- Sickle cell disease
- Human immunodeficiency virus (HIV) infection/acquired immune deficiency syndrome (AIDS)
- Elderly
- Pediatrics
- Chronic nonmalignant pain

Goals

The goals for population-based programs involve patient issues beyond the immediate ED visit; therefore some of the goals are attained in conjunction with interventions from other providers.

- Coordinate services to provide patient access to appropriate and cost-effective primary and specialty outpatient care, health education, and community resources.
- Improve quality of life indicators and patient's health status.
- Decrease repeat ED visits of targeted population because of a decrease in number of illness exacerbations.
- Provide an organized, efficient, and consistent multidisciplinary approach to care for a targeted population.
- Decrease hospital or ED length of stay.
- Decrease cost of care.

An excellent resource for defining goals in conjunction with the public health agenda is Healthy People 2010 (U.S. Department of Health and Human Services, 2000). Linking to goals such as increasing the number of patients who receive asthma self-management education are pertinent to ED case management interventions.

Strategies and Outcomes

RISK ASSESSMENT

One approach to developing a population-based program is initiating risk assessments to identify patients who are at risk for high service utilization and who might benefit from selective services. In the CDC's report *The Burden of Chronic Diseases and Their Risk Factors* (U.S. Department of Health and Human Services, 2002), the risk factors of cigarette smoking, lack of physical activity, overweight, poor nutrition, and lack of health care insurance were among those described to have significant effects on the development and screening of chronic illnesses.

The elderly population is having an ever-increasing impact on emergency services. During 1992 to 1999, ED visits by patients 65 years and older increased by 8% to a total of 15.2% of the ED volume (Burt & McCaig, 2001). During 2001, patients 75 years and older demonstrated the highest ED visit rate of any other age group, at 59.7 visits per 100 persons (McCaig & Burt, 2003). McCusker et al. (2000) developed a screening tool, Identification of Seniors at Risk (ISAR), to predict elders who will experience adverse health outcomes and high hospital resources during the 6 months after an ED visit. Items included are the need for regular assistance at home, hospitalization during the past 6 months, diminished vision and memory, and taking more than two different medications every day. Meldon et al. (2003) developed a five-item triage risk screening tool (TRST) completed by ED nurses to identify patients who were higher risk for hospital admission, subsequent ED visits, and nursing home admission. The assessment includes difficulty walking or transferring or recent falls, taking five or more medications, cognitive impairment, an ED visit within 30 days or hospitalization within the past 90 days, and registered nurse concern regarding elder neglect or abuse, ability to perform activities of daily living, or medication noncompliance.

Lowenstein et al. (1998) studied 923 patients to determine the prevalence of chronic disease risk factors and injury-prone behaviors among an ED population. Examples of the results are as follows:

- Of women over the age of 50 years, 42% had no Pap smear performed in the previous 2 years and 14% had never had a mammogram.
- Of the 923 patients, 23% had positive CAGE screens for problem drinking.
- Of the 923 patients, 38% reported no access to primary health care services.
- Of the 923 patients, 53% reported they did not wear seat belts regularly.
- Of the 923 patients, 20% had contemplated or planned suicide at least once in their lives.
- Of the female patients, 17% had been assaulted at least once in the preceding year.

The researchers suggest ED providers use screening data to target patients in need of counseling, prevention, and referral services.

A risk assessment program was initiated at University of Colorado Hospital in Denver in the ED for patients with diabetes. The purpose of the program was to identify patients in need of (1) primary care services, 2) diabetes self-care education, (3) specialty care (eye, endocrine, podiatry, or vascular), or (4) social service or home health care. The primary goal was to advocate patient access to appropriate and cost-effective primary and specialty outpatient care, health education, and community resources. In addition, outcome goals to be evaluated were to improve the health status of targeted population (hospital-wide goal) and to decrease ED/urgent care clinic visits of the targeted population with a corresponding decrease in costs related to that care.

The target population was patients who identified a medical history or new diagnosis of diabetes. A convenience sample of 114 patients was contacted by telephone during August through November 1997 and, as part of a courtesy follow-up call, asked additional risk assessment questions. Resource and referral information was provided as indicated as well as education on accessing and using primary care services.

Visits to the ED and urgent care clinic for the population group during the prior 12 months were calculated. ED and urgent care visits for the 12 months following the risk assessment were tracked, indicating a decreased visit rate of 46% overall. Based on average direct costs for the diabetic patients in the ED, the cost avoidance for the decrease in repeat visits was calculated at $13,300 for avoided outpatient ED visits and $135,087 for avoided admissions. It is important to note that with the exception of supply costs, most of the ED costs are "fixed." Unless programs result in a significant decrease in ED volume, personnel costs will not vary. Therefore it may be more appropriate to consider the savings a "cost diversion" for staff to focus on critical patients, improvement of patient flow, decreased wait time, and improvement of patient satisfaction.

The program has continued in a revised format; patients waiting discharge are given a one-page risk assessment form to complete that is returned to the case manager for follow-up. Patients are discharged with primary care physician resources, information regarding education programs, and self-management information. During 2002, 36 patients were screened, most of whom did not have a primary care provider and relied on the ED for care. Collectively, these patients had 76 visits to the ED in the prior 6 months. After case management intervention, these patients had a total of 10 visits to the ED, demonstrating an 87% drop in repeat visits.

Similar programs have been initiated for patients with asthma and high blood pressure. Intermittently, pharmacists have been available to provide education and assist in enrolling low-income patients into Medication Assistance Programs sponsored by pharmaceutical companies.

Clinical Pathways

An alternative approach for population-based programs is developing clinical pathways to provide an organized method to manage an acute episode of illness or injury. Clinical pathways assist in identifying and attaining outcomes-based, efficient, and consistent care to a targeted population. They are an evolution of protocols, algorithms, and standards of care that have been in existence for a number of years. What makes clinical pathways inherently unique from past management tools are that they:

- Are interdisciplinary *(identify who, does what, when)*
- Contain a time component *(hours or phases; for example, triage, assessment, intervention, disposition)*
- Measure specific outcomes *(clinical, functional, system process, financial, patient satisfaction)*
- Monitor variances to the outcomes *(patient/family, caregiver, internal system, external system)*

Outcomes may be measurements of reference points along the process of patient care, not just at the end point. Clinical pathways are not standing orders, but rather guides, that should be varied when indicated. Inpatient hospital pathways are generally focused on a specific diagnosis or an elective procedure. In the ED, focusing on presenting signs and symptoms (i.e., abdominal pain, chest pain, altered mental status) or systems process (i.e., criteria for laboratory and radiology testing) may be more appropriate. A mechanism that may improve compliance with clinical pathways is to develop the pathway as a documentation tool.

ADMISSION AND DISCHARGE PLANNING

Issues

The traditional admission and discharge planning responsibilities of the case manager in an acute hospital setting may be extended into the ED. This role allows for early assessment and intervention for selected patients. Broader system concerns may also be addressed by the case manager.

Goals

The goals for admission and discharge programs might be to

- Act as a liaison for hospital and community case managers to improve continuity of care
- Ensure and expedite appropriate patient disposition: evaluate admission criteria, level of care, and alternative placements
- Coordinate appropriate and efficient use of services and resources
- Evaluate systems concerning admission and discharge processes to ensure compliance with regulations, efficiency, and integration of resources

Strategies and Outcomes

INDIVIDUAL PATIENT APPROACH

If the department has case management resources available during the times of heavy ED volume, attention to individual patients is greatly beneficial. For patients destined for admission to the hospital, one can:

- Address admission to appropriate level of care, inpatient versus observation status, admission versus transfer to rehabilitation or extended care (long-term acute care [LTAC] of Tulsa or skilled nursing facility [SNF]), or discharge the patient with home care services.
- Contact the primary care provider to improve continuity of care.
- Determine if the patient qualifies for an inpatient clinical pathway or research protocol.

- Expedite plan for hospital case manager or social worker.
- Provide family support.
- Initiate insurance notification and out-of-network issues.
- Provide resources for health care insurance and financial assistance.

Brewer and Jackson (1997) reported a savings of $20,000 over 6 months as a result of deferred inpatient admissions for patients whose care was manageable with home care assistance. Perhaps when an ED case manager is not available to assess an admitted patient, the ED charge nurse or primary nurse could contact the appropriate inpatient case manager or social worker with specific concerns.

For those patients who will be discharged from the department, the case manager might:

- Evaluate options for follow-up plan: home care, community services, primary and specialty care, transportation, and medical equipment with respect to benefits.
- Ensure compliance with transfer policies.
- Determine if patient qualifies for outpatient clinical pathway or research protocol.
- Contact primary care provider.
- Monitor compliance of follow-up care arranged.
- Complete laboratory and radiology follow-up.
- Provide financial assistance.
- Provide family support.

Traditionally, these interventions represent short-term patient involvement after an episode of acute illness. For those selected patients who may benefit from long-term follow-up, a more formal individualized plan may be indicated along with expanded monitoring.

Dubay (1997) described a unique referral nurse role that followed up on selected discharged patients from a level II trauma center. Outcome goals were to improve continuity of care and decrease unnecessary repeat visits to the ED. From 30 to 50 patients were identified daily and contacted after discharge. Selection criteria included those with a questionable discharge diagnosis and home health referrals, as well as contacting patients to monitor compliance with physician follow-up. Patients could also call the referral nurse to clarify discharge instructions. In addition, this nurse screened laboratory results and radiology discrepancies.

SYSTEMS APPROACH

If the staff in the ED currently fulfill admission and discharge functions, or if case management services are limited, perhaps a more pertinent approach may be to focus on systems issues. The following questions should be asked:

- How well has the organization integrated inpatient and outpatient services to ensure continuity of care?
- Is capacity management or patient throughput a concern?
- What are the causes of ED overcrowding, holding admissions, and ED divert?
- Is the ED linked to inpatient clinical pathways?
- What are the eligibility criteria for observation status, and what is the compliance?
- What is the denial rate from payers for charges?
- Are denials due to level of service decisions or documentation issues?
- Is the department compliant with Emergency Medical Treatment and Labor Act (EMTALA) and Health Insurance Portability and Accountability Act (HIPPA) regulations?
- What are the trends with frequent readmissions?
- Is patient "choice" in postdischarge service arrangements being offered and documented?
- Can the uninsured population access care recommended in the discharge instructions, including primary and specialty care follow-up?
- Does the uninsured population have access to financial assistance?

- Does the cost of care for a particular patient group "match" with the contracts negotiated by the business office?

These issues are system-wide concerns, and it is imperative that the ED is represented during their resolution.

At the University of Colorado Hospital, approximately 50% of the ED population is uninsured. Many of these patients do not have a primary care physician; in the past it was common for 10% to 15% of the ED population to be referred to a specialty clinic for follow-up. It became apparent as the outpatient specialty clinics were limiting access to uninsured patients due to financial constraints, the ED patients referred to those clinics were not consistently gaining access. It was determined that a process pathway to expedite access to specialty care was needed. A more vigilant assessment for identifying the need of *urgent* specialty care verses *routine* specialty care was initiated. The decision to recommend follow-up care by a specialty service is now made jointly by the ED provider and the specialist provider on call, regardless of the patient's insurance status. This recommendation for *urgent* follow-up is based on a clinical need not typically managed by a primary care provider that needs to be addressed in a relatively short time. An "Urgent Follow Up" form sent via fax from the ED to the appropriate clinic appointment personnel is key for the patient to receive priority in scheduling. Although this expedites communication for an appointment for patients with managed care, this process does not replace the need for an insurance referral from the primary care physician if required. All other *routine* specialty care needs are not arranged through the ED; rather patients are discharged to their primary care physician or with primary care physician resources and instructed to arrange specialty care access through the primary care physician. During the past 3 years, an average of 2.5% of the total ED volume is referred for specialty care follow-up directly from the ED.

INDIVIDUAL PATIENT PLANS

Issues

There are patients who "fall out" of the previously described programs and who may benefit from individualized recommendations for ED care. These patients may have specialized clinical needs for which ED visits are expected, or they may possess significant psychosocial stresses such as substance abuse, homelessness, poverty, mental illness, or domestic violence that contribute to a pattern of noncompliance with follow-up arrangement, frequent ED visits, or both. The presence of these patients often causes distress among the staff because of the inability to provide an efficient resolution.

Goals

Goals for individual patient plans might be to:
- Develop guidelines to provide consistent emergency care to identified patients by integrating information from all involved providers
- Improve communication among providers to increase continuity of care
- Advocate access and appropriate use of primary care and community resources
- Decrease unnecessary use of the ED by patients who are recurrent visitors
- Improve quality-of-life indicators

These are general goals and will not pertain to every patient's plan. For example, a patient with significant clinical pathology may continue to have frequent ED visits; the goal would be to provide consistent care for that patient.

Strategies and Outcomes

REFERRALS

At University of Colorado Hospital in Denver, Colorado, individual patient referrals are forwarded to the nurse case manager by nurses and physicians. The patient's records are reviewed, including past 12-month ED visit history and hospital admission rate; current providers of care are contacted for advice; the emergency psychiatric/social services and inpatient and community case managers or social workers are contacted as indicated; and a discussion with the patient occurs.

The plan may be as simple as more individualized patient/family education in accessing health care resources and completing follow-up telephone calls to encourage compliance. If indicated, a clinical guideline is developed in conjunction with providers of care to ensure continuity and a consistent approach to the patient in the ED. These guidelines are not standing orders but are recommendations for ED care and will be adjusted according to the patient's presentation and response. The guidelines are reviewed and revised at least once a year. Although the goal of decreasing ED visits may or may not be a part of the plan, patient visits are monitored and primary care providers receive dictated ED notes. Often the providers of patients who have been frequent visitors will be more flexible in accommodating the patient for unscheduled, urgent events. Based on a 6-month visit history before and after case management intervention, there has been a 55% to 65% decrease in repeat ED visits of the patients for whom that was a goal. Cost avoidance can be calculated using average ED cost per patient.

As a note of caution, occasionally a primary care provider has requested that the ED staff "refuse" to see a patient. These providers need to be educated that all EDs must provide at minimum a medical screening examination as dictated by EMTALA regulations and that refusal to examine a patient is not a legal option.

PARTNERSHIPS WITH COMMUNITY CASE MANAGERS

Developing partnerships among case managers and social workers within the hospital and in other health care settings may improve the continuity of care. A community case management program followed 21 adult patients who were identified with frequent ED visits and hospital admissions and with difficulty managing a chronic illness. Reported outcomes at 6 months indicated a 52% decrease in hospital admissions and 30% decrease in costs (Sund & Sveningson, 1998). San Francisco General Hospital found a decrease in ED and inpatient costs, homelessness, drug use, and increased access to a primary care physician after intensive case management of 53 patients with a history of frequent visits to the ED (Okin et al., 2000).

■ CHALLENGES AND OPPORTUNITIES

ED case managers are on the horizon of a great opportunity to expand outreach to the inpatient and community setting. The health care market is increasingly difficult for patients to manage; ED staff have the ability to assist large volumes of patients with access to care, public health education, and individualized resources. Partnerships must be developed within health care delivery systems to share resources and information, avoid duplication of services, and improve continuity of care (Smith & Brooks, 1999). Any of the strategies and outcomes related to enhancing the delivery of care to patients or system improvements would be recognized as continuous quality improvement programs. The emerging roles of ED case managers will encompass many responsibilities and processes: access, advocacy, compliance, continuum of care, education of staff and patients, ethics, resource identification, liaison, outcomes, program design, quality, and partnerships.

References

Advisory Board Company (1993). *Redefining the emergency department; Five strategies for reducing unnecessary visits.* Washington, D.C.

Baker, D., Stevens, C., & Brook, R. (1995, Mar.). Determinates of emergency department use by ambulatory patients at an urban public hospital. *Annals of Emergency Medicine, 25*(3), 311-316.

Brewer, B., & Jackson, L. (1997, Dec.). A case management model for the emergency department. *Journal of Emergency Nursing, 23*(6), 618-621.

Burt, C., & McCaig, L. (2001). *Trends in emergency department utilization: United States, 1992-1999.* Washington, D.C.: US Department of Health and Human Services, National Center for Health Statistics, Vital and Health Statistics.

Cairns, C., et al. (1998). Development of new methods to assess the outcomes of emergency care. *Annals of Emergency Medicine, 31*(2), 166-171.

Dubay, D. (1997, Oct.). Emergency center follow-up program. *Journal of Emergency Nursing, 23*(5), 455-456.

Lowenstein, S., et al. (1998, Aug.). Behavioral risk factors in emergency department patients: A multi-site survey. *Academic Emergency Medicine, 5*(8), 781-787.

McCaig, L., & Burt, C. (2003). *National Hospital Ambulatory Medical Care Survey: 2001 emergency department summary. Advance data.* Washington, D.C.: U.S. Department of Health and Human Services, National Center for Health Statistics, Vital and Health Statistics.

McCusker, J., et al. (2000, Nov.). Prediction of hospital utilization among elderly patients in the 6 months after an emergency department visit. *Annals of Emergency Medicine, 36*(5), 438-445.

Malone, R. (1998, Oct.). Wither the almshouse? Over-utilization and the role of the emergency department. *Journal of Health Politics, Policy and Law, 23*(5), 795-832.

Meldon, S., et al. (2003, Mar.). A brief risk-stratification tool to predict repeat emergency department visits and hospitalizations in older patients discharged from the emergency department. *Academic Emergency Medicine, 10*(3), 224-232.

Okin, R., et al. (2000, Sept.). The effects of clinical case management on hospital service use among ED frequent users. *American Journal of Emergency Medicine, 18*(5), 603-608.

Padgett, D., & Brodsky, B. (1992). Psychosocial factors influencing non-urgent use of the emergency room. *Social Science Medicine, 35*(9), 1189-1197.

Smith, T., & Brooks, A.M. (1999). Redefining quality. In E. Cohen (Ed.), *The outcomes mandate: Case management in health care today* (pp. 198-206). St. Louis: Mosby–Year Book, Inc.

Sund, J., & Sveningson, L. (1998, Jan.). Case management in an integrated delivery system. *Nursing Management, 29*(1), 24-25.

Tyrance, P., Himmelsteine, D., & Woolhandler, S. (1996, Nov.). U.S. emergency department costs: No emergency. *American Journal of Public Health, 86*(11), 1527-1531.

U.S. Department of Health and Human Services (2000). *Healthy people 2010.* McLean, Va.: International Medical Publishing, Inc.

U.S. Department of Health and Human Services, Centers for Disease Control and Prevention (2002). *The burden of chronic diseases and their risk factors.* Available at: www.cdc.gov.

Williams, R. (1996, Mar.). The costs of visits to emergency departments. *The New England Journal of Medicine, 334*(10), 642-646.

V

ADDRESSING HEALTH CARE DELIVERY THROUGH CASE MANAGEMENT

Public Policy Implications

The day-to-day work of the case manager is greatly affected by public policy, particularly at the federal and state levels. Conversely, case managers are in a position to affect public policy as it has an impact on health care legislation and the delivery of patient care services. Up-to-date knowledge of legislative changes can assist case managers in their role as patient advocate. Unit V provides a framework for understanding current legislative issues in terms of their broad effects on health care reimbursement and their application at the patient level. Knowledge of both perspectives is imperative for the successful case manager.

Patient Demographics Affecting Health Care

CHAPTER OVERVIEW

Shifts in the nation's demographics are causing substantial changes in the delivery of health care. Both the growing elderly population and the acquired immunodeficiency syndrome (AIDS) epidemic have prompted health care workers to look for alternatives to the traditional approaches of acute patient care and have fostered the growth of integrative models such as case management. The prevalence of chronic illness and disability associated with demographic changes is also influencing public health policy as we shift our resources from acute to chronic care.

Enacted legislation has provided for the civil rights and liberties of individuals with chronic illness and has supported much-needed community-based, long-term health care delivery systems. Many businesses and corporations have developed programs and services that will help them adapt to the long-range social, economic, and health care implications of the growing number of elderly and those with AIDS.

AGING PATIENT POPULATION

The U.S. Department of Health and Human Services (DHHS) (1990) predicts that by 2020, 7 million Americans will be older than 85 years. Estimates reveal that by 2050, one in four Americans will be 65 years or older and will make up 18.5% of the U.S. population by 2025 (Freudenheim, 1996; U.S. Census Bureau, 2000). There is no doubt that the older adult group represents the fastest growing section of the U.S. population. This increase in the number and percentage of older individuals primarily results from advances in research, technology, and preventive treatments that have markedly reduced the mortality associated with cancer, cardiovascular disease, diabetes, stroke, and hypertension (Hospitals & Health Networks, 2003; National Center for Health Statistics, 1985; Olshansky, 1985).

Rogers, Rogers, and Belanger (1989) found a correlation between dependency and age. Their study indicates that with an increase in age there is a corresponding rise in functional dependency related to basic activities of daily living. Furthermore, once dependency sets in, the likelihood of returning to an independent status decreases. An example of this is that although women have a longer life expectancy than men, much of that time is spent in dependent situations, which increases the morbidity of this population group (Manton, 1988; Schneider & Brody, 1983).

The DHHS estimates of years of healthy life showed a decline in health-related quality of life despite increases in life expectancy (U.S. Department of Health and Human Services, 1995a). Statistical projections show that by 2044, 7.3 million people will have dependent lifestyles (Rogers et al., 1989). Another projection indicates that by 2040, the elderly population will account for 45% of health care expenditures (Callahan, 1987).

State and federal health budgets will be profoundly affected as health care options increase for the elderly. In a statistical analysis of the future health care environment, Hospitals & Health Networks/IDX (2003) revealed that the elderly consume a disproportionate share of health care products and services. In 1999, they accounted for 12% of the U.S. population but used 25% of health care products and services. By 2025, they are expected to consume one third of health care resources.

With advanced age, there is also a proportionate growth in the incidence of chronic diseases, mental disability, and degenerative illnesses. Chronicity represents the fastest growing, most expensive segment in health care today. Eighty percent of people over age 65 have one or more chronic conditions, and one in every three over age 65 have an activity limitation due to a chronic condition. More than 50% of present-day costs of acute care medicine are incurred to treat chronicity. These factors, along with increased dependency and disability, intensify the need and demand for health care services (Freudenheim, 1996; Goldsmith, 1989; Guralnik, Yanagishita, & Schneider, 1988; Shi & Singh, 1998a).

It is estimated that by 2040, 2.8 million people, age 85 years and older, will require institutional care (Guralnik et al., 1988; Hing, 1987). These data indicate that the aging population will have a significant effect on long-term and skilled nursing care.

Increased longevity and its concomitant effects have encouraged new approaches to the delivery of health care services and the development of noninstitutional systems of care. Nursing case management, managed care programs, community-based home care, and chronic care networks that include hospitals, nursing homes, residential community services, and care management (White, 1999) are some examples of alternative approaches to meeting the health care needs of the elderly. These approaches lend themselves to scrutiny and analysis related to cost-effectiveness and the value and quality of services delivered.

In an extensive review of home- and community-based long-term care programs, Weissert, Cready, and Pawelak (1988) found that there were greater total expenditures and no statistically significant cost savings related to home- and community-based care. In fact, an analysis of the effectiveness of various programs showed that even though there were reductions in admissions to institutional care settings, these findings were significant for only a small group of patients who had an obvious need for home-based care. This group consisted of the disabled, chronically ill, and frail elderly.

The study showed, however, that within this patient population, preadmission assessment and screening of those individuals at risk for institutionalization effectively reduced nursing home use. This finding was supported in studies that evaluated the effectiveness of community-based programs in preventing hospitalization. It is known that more specific identification and evaluation of patient requirements of care decrease the need for and length of inpatient treatment and hospitalization (Eggert & Friedman, 1988; Potthoff, Kane, & Franco, 1997).

A study conducted by Naylor et al. (1999) demonstrated that focused discharge planning and care management of hospitalized elderly patients helped reduce readmissions, increased time spent out of the hospital, and decreased cost of care. Success factors highlighted by the authors of this study pointed to clinical interventions by advanced practice nurses on patient care–related events the move beyond disease management models and look at primary health problems, comorbidity, and other health and social issues that are common in the elderly patient population (Boling, 1999; Naylor et al., 1999).

One major benefit of community- and home-based care was found in its beneficial and significant effect on the psychosocial well-being and satisfaction of patients and care providers. The community- or home-based care proved better at meeting the patients' needs for physical and social activities as well as medical, mental health, and educational requirements (Weissert, 1985). In an extensive study conducted by Burns, Lamb, and Wholey (1996), the value of integrated community nursing services for elderly people in a health maintenance organization (HMO) was substantiated. The result showed that this integrated community program was associated with reduced hospital costs, preventable admissions, and intensive care visits. Services provided included continuity of care, management of patients across organizational settings, and high-risk screening and identification (Burns et al., 1996).

Another study, conducted by Roos, Shapiro, and Tate (1989), indicated that only 5% of the elderly are extensive users of health care in the inpatient acute care and nursing home settings. The expenditures associated with this care are higher during the individual's last year of life. However, 45% of the elderly population make large demands on the health care system, and these demands entail greater expenditures.

One recommendation for decreasing the chance of hospitalization is to provide the elderly with a geriatric specialist. Early assessment and evaluation by such a specialist might help reduce the incidence of hospitalization, which in turn decreases costs. In addition, continuous monitoring of discharged patients through home care, community-based care, long-term care, and primary preventive services can be cost-effective and aid in the transition to a more independent lifestyle (Stuck et al., 1995).

It is clear that to plan effectively for future health care needs of the elderly and disabled population, changes in the delivery of health care services and benefits are needed. Resources are now being shifted from acute care and long-term institutional care to home care, community-based services, respite centers, nurse-run HMOs and care centers, case management, and rehabilitation programs (Dimond, 1989; Hollinger & Brugler, 1991; Manninen & Baines, 1998; Maraldo & Solomon, 1987; Marshall, 1999; Shi & Singh, 1998a). Many alternatives to nursing home services have become available for older people who require long-term care. Popular choices include home care, congregate housing, assisted living, continuing care retirement communities, and adult day care (Booth, 1999; Greenwald, 1999; Shi & Singh, 1998a). In addition, some nursing homes have engaged in transforming themselves to improve the quality of life and care for their residents (Drew & Brooke, 1999). As advocated by Shi and Singh (1998a), long-term care must be integrated within the entire health care delivery system to maintain a seamless transition between different types of health care settings and services.

To maintain control of some of the long-range economic and social implications, major business groups and corporations have developed and offered resources and referral services to employees who have caretaking responsibilities for elderly and dependent family members (Buchsbaum, 1991; Peterson, 1992). Called *eldercare*, these programs provide a range of services, including counseling, family leave plans, position reinstatement, flexible work schedules, automated office arrangements that make it possible for employees to work at home, subsidized health care benefits, and reimbursement for adult day care. Websites have also been developed that provide information and assistance regarding funding for care referral sources, provider lists, and research findings (Field, 1999).

The benefits of such an approach include decreased work-related conflicts; lowered costs associated with recruitment, training, and absenteeism of personnel; and increased productivity, loyalty, and commitment to the organization. Referral services have also helped decrease the costs of health services associated with deferred spending, out-of-pocket expenses, lost time, and stress (Buchsbaum, 1991; Peterson, 1992).

Increasing costs, aging baby boomers, and new government regulation and legislation have raised challenges with regard to the solvency of Medicare. Estimates show that by 2030, the projected Medicare eligibility will approach 20% of the U.S. population, with an increase in the number of Medicare beneficiaries of 69 million by 2025 (Leone, 1997; Urban Institute, 2003). By 2012, Medicare Part A spending will increase 85.4%, reaching $267 billion, and Medicare Part B spending will grow 110%, reaching $216 billion. Additionally, Medicare Part A spending on home health services will increase 217%, whereas Medicare Part B spending for home health will rise by more than 333%. Part A spending on skilled nursing will also increase 136% (Hospital & Health Networks, 2003). More daunting statistics show that Medicare and Medicaid will also experience large increases in prescription drug expenditures from 2001 to 2011, with a projected rise for Medicare of 95.7% and an increase of 232% for Medicaid (Centers for Medicare & Medicaid Services, 2003).

By 2010, the average cost of a prescription for the elderly will rise by more than 72%. Another astounding but heartbreaking statistic is more than one third of the 38 million people covered by Medicare have no prescription coverage, leaving some of them no alternative but to choose between food, rent, and medication (Hospitals & Health Networks, 2003).

Although strategies abound in saving Medicare from further spending reductions in the wake of the Balanced Budget Act (BBA) of 1997, the provision of health insurance and prescription drug coverage for the elderly and the privatization of Medicare into HMOs have become the key issues in many political arenas. These challenges will have reverberations well into this century and involve measures aimed at offering long-term care (LTC) insurance policies as employee benefits, making LTC premiums fully tax deductible, and implementing a prescription drug discount program for seniors (Deloitte & Touche, 2002; Gleckman, 1999; Hospitals & Health Networks, 2003). Other initiatives include prescription drug subsidies and allowances for transportation and housekeeping services to keep individuals in their home environment (Garrett, 1999; Shapiro, 1999).

HUMAN IMMUNODEFICIENCY VIRUS (HIV) INFECTION

Surveillance data from the Centers for Disease Control and Prevention show that more than 500,000 Americans have contracted AIDS and that 62% of these persons have died. HIV infection is currently considered the leading cause of death in men age 25 to 44 years and the third leading cause of death in women of the same age group (U.S. Department of Health and Human Services, 1995b).

There is substantial evidence that the rapid spread of HIV will increase hospitalizations and the use of more complex health care resources.

Federal spending for HIV is in medical care, education and prevention, research, and assistance programs (Shi & Singh, 1998b). Current estimates place the total medical care costs of HIV at $119,000 per person (Aday, 1993). This estimate includes the cost of hospitalization, home health care, hospice, and outpatient care as well as costs related to disability and chronicity.

Studies show the initial length of hospitalization averages 30 to 60 days, with cumulative acute care treatment lasting up to 170 days (Hardy et al., 1986; Sedaka & O'Reilly, 1986). On average, a person with AIDS is hospitalized three or four times. These hospitalizations occur in the early and late stages of illness (Scitovsky, Cline, & Lee, 1986).

Because AIDS is chronic, debilitating, and terminal, it places a substantial burden on the health care system (Benjamin, 1988). Continuum of care approaches that provide home care, community-based services, hospice, disease management, and case management are alternatives to hospitalization (Case Management Advisor, 1998; Shi & Singh, 1998b).

Various strategies have been considered to improve accessibility to AIDS care settings. Hospitals have created designated AIDS units in which registered nurses coordinate, plan, and evaluate the delivery of care (Chow, 1989; Fox, Aiken, & Messikomer, 1990). Some institutions, such as the San Francisco General Hospital, have implemented comprehensive care programs through multidisciplinary, collaborative efforts with outpatient and community-based services and home care agencies (Volberding, 1985). These initiatives, along with improvement in treatment and management protocols, have worked toward decreasing the length of stay for AIDS patients, thereby affecting the overall care and cost-effectiveness of this group (Fox, 1986).

The effectiveness of ambulatory and community-based programs for AIDS care is being evaluated in many federal, state, and private foundation–sponsored projects (Benjamin, 1988; Fox, 1986). The programs could reduce cost by reducing the need for inpatient hospital care resources and services.

Hospice care is another promising alternative for AIDS treatment. Using a multidisciplinary team approach, the hospice setting provides for the psychosocial needs of both the patient and caregiver

(Benjamin, 1988). The emphasis of hospice care is on reducing time spent in institutional care and eliminating the need for acute medical intervention.

Studies by Mor and Kidder (1985) on the cost-effectiveness of hospice care show savings related to decreases in inpatient length of stay and use of hospital resources. Such decreases possibly result from the shift in caregiving responsibility to the patient's community, family, and significant others.

Case management presents an additional option for planning nonacute care services and interventions for individuals with AIDS. Capitman, Haskins, and Bernstein (1986) and Spitz (1987) demonstrated the effectiveness and efficiency of a well-integrated case management system. Their studies show that through comprehensive targeting and planning and integration of inpatient, ambulatory, and community-based services, the medical and social needs of AIDS patients can be met. Case management also provides flexibility in service options and reduces the inappropriateness, overuse, and inefficiency associated with hospital and medical care of the chronically ill (Schramm, 1990). Other hospital-based nursing case management models dedicated to AIDS care have also been effective in delivering less-expensive quality care (American Nurses Association, 1988).

Because AIDS presents enormous acute and long-term care needs, business firms have begun to develop and provide employee education and assistance programs, counseling services, nondiscriminatory employment policies, and flexible work schedules. Corporations have also begun to comply with federal, state, and local infection control guidelines (McDonald, 1990; Mello, 1991).

The passage of the Americans with Disabilities Act (ADA) in 1992 has also helped to ensure the rights of HIV-infected people and people with AIDS in the workplace. The benefits and entitlements under this act include opportunities for employment, access to public services, accessible transportation, and a mechanism of communication with employers to support nondiscriminatory policies, confidentiality, and ongoing education (Feldblum, 1991; LaPlante, 1991). The Medicaid waiver program and the Ryan White Comprehensive AIDS Resource Emergency (CARE) Act are additional initiatives that work toward providing treatment and care coordination for individuals with HIV and AIDS (Shi & Singh, 1998b; Summer, 1991).

Innovative case management models have emerged in developing countries such as East Africa to care for people with AIDS. These models are grounded in the principles of primary health care and have demonstrated enhanced individual and community health outcomes (Ivantic-Doucette & Maashao, 1999). These case management models serve as exemplars and point to the basic fact that attention to a community's primary health care needs of access to care and interventions driven from within communities and with community participation are crucial to success (Ivantic-Doucette & Maashao, 1999).

References

Aday, L. (1993). *At risk in America: The health and health care needs of vulnerable populations in the United States.* San Francisco: Jossey-Bass Publishers.

American Nurses Association (1988). *Nursing case management.* Kansas City, Mo.: ANA.

Benjamin, A.E. (1988). Long-term care and AIDS: Perspectives from experience with the elderly. *The Milbank Quarterly, 66*(3), 415-443.

Boling, P. (1999). The value of targeted case management during transitional care. *Journal of the American Medical Association, 281*(7), 656-657.

Booth, C. (1999, Aug. 30). Taking care of our aging parents. *Time*, 48-51.

Buchsbaum, S. (1991). Sending "care" packages to the workplace. *Business and Health, 9*(5), 56-69.

Burns, L.R., Lamb, G.S., & Wholey, D.R. (1996). Impact of integrated community nursing services on hospital utilization and costs in a Medicare risk plan. *Inquiry, 33*, 30-41.

Callahan, D. (1987). *Setting limits: Medical goals in an aging society.* New York: Simon and Schuster.

Capitman, J.A., Haskins, B., & Bernstein, J. (1986). Case management approaches in community oriented long-term care demonstrations. *Gerontologist, 26*, 398-404.

Case Management Advisor (1998, Oct.). Case management leads to success in HIV/AIDS managed care. *Case Management Advisor, 9*(10), 177-179.

Chow, M. (1989). "Nursing's response to the challenge of AIDS. *Nursing Outlook, 37*(2), 82-83.

Deloitte & Touche (2002). *The future of health care: An outlook from the perspective of hospital CEOs,* 9th edition. Chicago, Ill.: Deloitte & Touche LLP.

Dimond, M. (1989). Health care and the aging population. *Nursing Outlook, 37*(2), 76-77.

Drew, J.C., & Brooke, V. (1999). Changing a legacy: The Eden alternative nursing home. *Annals of Long-Term Care, 7*(3), 115-121.

Eggert, G., & Friedman, B. (1988). The need for special interventions for multiple hospital admission patients. *Health Care Financing Review,* (suppl.)57-67.

Feldblum, C. (1991). Employment protections. *The Milbank Quarterly, 69*(suppl. 1/2), 81-110.

Field, A. (1999, Nov. 22). The best old-age home may be at home. *Business Week,* 180-182.

Fox, D. (1986). AIDS and the American health policy: History and prospects of a crisis of authority. *The Milbank Quarterly, 64,* 7-33.

Fox, D. (1989). Policy and epidemiology: Financing health services for the chronically ill and disabled, 1930-1990. *The Milbank Quarterly, 67*(suppl. 2, part 2), 257-287.

Fox, R., Aiken, L., & Messikomer, C. (1990). The culture of caring: AIDS and the nursing profession. *The Milbank Quarterly, 68*(suppl. 2), 226-256.

Freudenheim, D. (1996). *Chronic care in American: A 21st century challenge.* Princeton, N.J.: Institute for Health and Aging.

Garrett, M. (1999, Nov. 22). Health divides the candidates. *U.S. News & World Report,* 24.

Gleckman, H. (1999, Mar. 29). A golden (years) opportunity. *Business Week,* 181-182.

Goldsmith, J. (1989). Radical prescription for hospitals. *Harvard Business Review, 89*(3), 104-111.

Greenwald. J. (1999, Aug. 30). Elder care: Making the right choice. *Time,* 52-56.

Guralnik, J., Yanagishita, M., & Schneider, E. (1988). Projecting the older population of the United States: Lessons from the past and prospects for the future. *The Milbank Quarterly, 66*(2), 283-308.

Hardy, A., Rauch, K., Echenberg, D., Morgan, W., & Curran, J.W. (1986). The economic impact of the first 10,000 cases of acquired immunodeficiency syndrome in the United States. *Journal of the American Medical Association, 225,* 209-211.

Hing, E. (1987). Use of nursing homes by the elderly, preliminary data from the 1985 National Nursing Home Survey. *Vital and Health Statistics,* no. 135. DHHS publication No. (PHS) 87-1250. Washington, D.C.: National Center for Health Statistics.

Hollinger, W., & Brugler, K. (1991). Managing resource use. *Healthcare Forum, 34*(6), 45-47.

Hospitals & Health Networks/IDX (2003). *Digest of health care's future.* Chicago, Ill.: Health Forum Inc.

Ivantic-Doucette, K. & Maashao, G. (1999). Huduma Kwa Wagonjwa: An African perspective on case management. In E. Cohen & V. De Back (Eds.), *The outcomes mandate: Case management in health care today* (pp. 276-285). St. Louis: Mosby, Inc.

LaPlante, M. (1991). The demographics of disability. *The Milbank Quarterly, 69*(suppl. 1/2), 55-77.

Leone, R. (1997). Why boomers don't spell bust. *The American Prospect, 30*(1), 68-72.

Manninen, R., & Baines, B. (1998). Medical management in the Medicare population. In P.R. Kongstvedt & D.W. Plocher (Eds.), *Best practices in medical management* (pp. 623-636). Gaithersburg, Md.: Aspen Publications.

Manton, K.G. (1988). A longitudinal study of functional change and mortality in the United States. *Journal of Gerontology, 43*(5), 153-161.

Maraldo, P., & Solomon, S. (1987). Nursing's window of opportunity. *Image, 19*(2), 8386.

Marhsall, B.S. (1999, Nov./Dec.). Case management of the elderly in a health maintenance organization: The implications for program administration under managed care. *Journal of Healthcare Management, 44*(6), 477-493.

McDonald, M. (1990). How to deal with AIDS in the workplace. *Business and Health, 8*(7), 12-22.

Mello, J. (1991, Sept.). Getting to know about AIDS. *Business and Health, 9*(9), 88-89.

Mor, V., & Kidder, D. (1985). Cost savings in hospice: Final results of the National Hospice Study. *Health Services Research, 20,* 407-421.

National Center for Health Statistics (1985). *Vital Statistics of the United States, 1980.* 2(pt. A., mortality). DHHS publication No. (PHS) 85-1101. Washington, D.C.

Naylor, M., Brooten, D., Campbell, R., Jacobsen, B., Mezey, M., Pauly, M., & Schwartz, J. (1999). Comprehensive discharge planning and home follow-up of hospitalized elders: A randomized clinical trial. *Journal of American Medical Association, 28*(7), 613-620.

Olshansky, S.J. (1985). Pursuing longevity: Delay vs. elimination of degenerative diseases. *American Journal of Public Health, 75,* 754-757.

Peterson, H. (1992, Feb.). Eldercare: More than company kindness. *Business & Health, 10*(2), 54-57.

Potthoff, S., Kane, R., & Franco, S. (1997). Improving hospital discharge planning for elderly patients. *Health Care Financing Review, 19,* 47-72.

Rogers, R., Rogers, A., & Belanger, A. (1989). Active life among the elderly in the United States: Multistate Life-table estimates and population projections. *The Milbank Quarterly, 67*(3-4), 370-411.

Roos, N., Shapiro, E., & Tate, R. (1989). Does a small minority of elderly account for a majority of healthcare expenditures? A sixteen-year perspective. *The Milbank Quarterly, 67*(3-4), 347-369.

Schneider, E., & Brody, J. (1983). Aging, natural death, and the compression of morbidity: Another view. *New England Journal of Medicine, 309*(14), 854-855.

Schramm, C. (1990). Health care industry problems call for cooperative solutions. *Healthcare Financial Management,* 54-61.

Scitovsky, A.A., Cline, M., & Lee, P.R. (1986). Medical care costs of patients with AIDS in San Francisco. *Journal of the American Medical Association, 256,* 3103-3106.

Sedaka, S., & O'Reilly, M. (1986). The financial implications of AIDS. *Caring, 5*(6), 38-44.

Shapiro, J. (1999, Nov. 22). Giving doctors the final word. *U.S. News & World Report,* 20-24.

Shi, L., & Singh, D. (1998a). *Delivering health care in America: A systems approach.* Health services for special populations (Chapter 11) (pp. 426-440). Gaithersburg, Md.: Aspen Publications.

Shi, L., & Singh, D. (1998b). *Delivering health care in America: A systems approach.* Long term care (Chapter 10) (pp. 344-391). Gaithersburg, Md.: Aspen Publications.

Spitz, B. (1987). National survey of Medicaid case management. *Health Affairs, 6,* 61-70.

Stuck, A., Aronow, H., Steiner, A., et al. (1995). A trial of in-home comprehensive discharge assessments for elderly people living in the community. *New England Journal of Medicine, 333,* 1184-1189.

Summer, L. (1991). *Limited access: Health care for the rural poor.* Washington, D.C.: Center on Budget and Policy Priorities.

Urban Institute. (2003). Washington, D.C.

U.S. Census Bureau. (2000). Washington, D.C.

U.S. Department of Health and Human Services (2000). *Healthy People 2000.* Washington, D.C.: DHHS.

U.S. Department of Health and Human Services (1995a). *Healthy People 2000: Midcourse review and 1995 revisions* (p. 6). Washington, D.C.: DHHS.

U.S. Department of Health and Human Services, Centers for Disease Control and Prevention (1995b). *HIV/AIDS surveillance report: U.S. HIV and AIDS cases reported through December 1995, 7*(2), 1-39.

Volberding, P.A. (1985). The clinical spectrum of the acquired immunodeficiency syndrome: Implications for comprehensive patient care. *Annals of Internal Medicine, 103,* 729-732.

Weissert, W.G. (1985). Seven reasons why it is so difficult to make community-based long term care cost effective. *Health Services Research, 20*(4), 423-433.

Weissert, W.G., Cready, C., & Pawelak, J. (1988). The past and future of home- and community-based long term care. *The Milbank Quarterly, 66*(2), 309-388.

White, M. (1999). Eligibility in the ever-changing continuum of care. *Annals of Long-Term Care, 7*(3), 113-114.

The Business of Health Care and the Prospective Payment System

CHAPTER OVERVIEW

Shifts in consumer behavior, along with various government and private industry strategies, have brought major change to the health care delivery environment. Programs are being developed to increase access to care and to evaluate and monitor cost-effective outcomes. National health reform initiatives address universal access to care by working for changes in insurance coverage and benefits, reimbursement regulation, and alternative care arrangements. Quality and cost are also addressed through managed care and capitated payment approaches. Long-term care services are being sponsored both publicly and privately.

Collaboration among health care providers for policy formation and implementation, public and private support for health care planning and outcomes research, and further development of alternative care delivery and clinical resource models are among the crucial factors needed to develop an accessible, effective, and socially responsive health care system.

COST CONTAINMENT: THE ADVENT OF THE PROSPECTIVE PAYMENT SYSTEM

The incentives promoted by the prospective payment system not only affect the efficiency, safety, and quality of health care in the inpatient setting but also have a direct relationship to the cost-containment efforts present in managed care arrangements (Jones, 1989; Sloan, Morrisey, & Valvona, 1988). Increased enrollment in HMOs and other prepaid coordinated health care plans, restructuring of the physician fee and payment schedule to provide incentives for the delivery of primary care services, the national drive for health care reform, and competition among alternative delivery systems to improve cost-effectiveness and quality all influence prospective payment initiatives (Enthoven & Kronick, 1989a, 1989b; Ginsburg & Hackbarth, 1986; Swoap, 1984; Waldo, Levit, & Lazenby, 1986; Wilensky, 1991).

Prospective payment has also promoted a more efficient use of health care resources and encouraged the study of outcomes to evaluate accessibility, management, and economic effectiveness of care (Jones, 1989; Sloan et al., 1988).

The economic effect of rising health care costs has taken its toll on the private sector through increases in group health insurance premium rates and changes in the structure of employee health care benefits. Mullen (1988) and Traska (1989) reported that employers experienced rate increases of 15% to 29% in their efforts to cover health care costs. According to the Hewitt Associates' survey, the double-digit inflation was due to an estimated 21.5% increase by insurance carriers in medical benefit costs (Hewitt Associates, 1989). Increases in premiums were driven primarily by rises in the cost, volume, and variations in health services and were fostered by medical technological change, an inadequate reimbursement system, demographic changes of an aging population, care for persons with acquired immunodeficiency syndrome (AIDS), and care for persons with chronic illness (Kramon, 1989; Welling, 1990).

With national health care expenditures projected to grow to 17% of the gross domestic product at an estimated cost of $2.8 trillion in 2011, the issue of escalating health care costs has long been represented in both the political and economic arenas and has prompted furious debates in the public and private sectors over the provision of basic health care services (Hospitals, 1992; Hospitals & Health Networks, 2003). Public expenditures for health care (Medicare, Medicaid, state and local programs are examples) are expected to grow 103%, accounting for over $1 trillion in 2011. In 2011, federal spending is expected to grow 96.6% to almost $900 billion and state and local spending is projected at 117.8% to $425 billion. Expenditures on private health insurance are expected to increase 98.5% by 2011, with out-of-pocket expenses growing 88% over the same time period (Hospitals & Health Networks, 2003).

Advocates for a national health care policy have locked horns with those who support the rationing of health services. Attempts were made by Congress in the past to institute a national health insurance plan to ensure equal access to care (Altman & Rodmin, 1988; Reinhardt, 1987a, 1987b). Legislative mandates and congressional bills that would provide health care coverage have been introduced as a means of rationing care through regulation and achieving control over government expenditures. State-mandated benefit laws offer a broad range of service coverage and access to mental health and substance abuse care, prenatal care, mammography, cancer screening, and major organ transplantations (Brown, 1988; Davis, 1985; Dwyer and Garland, 1991; Eckholm, 1991; Frieden, 1991; Tallon, 1991; Thorpe, 1991; Traska, 1989).

Major health care reform for America began in 1993 with the introduction of the Health Security Act (HR3600, 1993), a President Clinton initiative. For almost a year, the administration sought information about the existing health care system through task forces, committees, and town meetings directed by the First Lady, Hillary Rodham Clinton. This data collection process stimulated discussions nationwide about the present and future health care systems. The momentum created by a national discussion on health care reform gave the change process a life of its own, separate from the administrative and legislative agendas. Health care providers, health care agencies, and state government agencies began to design new systems based on a shifting paradigm—even before federal laws were enacted. The basic premise of the new paradigm, which continues to unfold, is a focus on health and care replacing or augmenting the old paradigm of illness and cure (DeBack & Cohen, 1996).

Many special interest groups have joined forces to propose reform in the current health care system. One such group, the American Medical Association, supports an employer-based health care plan, and another group from organized nursing has endorsed a proposal titled "Nursing's Agenda for Health Care Reform." The latter plan supports a consumer partnership with the health care provider regarding decisions about care; access to primary health care services via community-based settings; allocation of more resources to chronic and long-term care; increased access to nonphysician providers, such as nurse practitioners; wellness and prevention classes; public and private sector review and financing of health care; and managed care and case management arrangements (National League for Nursing, 1991).

Changes in payment structure have taken place in almost every sector of the health care industry. Private corporations and insurance providers have adopted many different strategies aimed at cost containment. Various efforts have focused on the redesigning of health insurance plans and policies, shifting the direct financial burden of health care expenditures to the federal government and individual payers. This approach includes the following: a single-payer plan, which is a government-financed plan that insures all individuals; introduction of copayments and deductibles applied to health care services; cost sharing, in which employees share the costs of health care by paying for the care of convalescing patients and hospice care for the terminally ill; catastrophic health plans, which provide coverage for high-cost illnesses; second opinions for surgical interventions; and primary prevention and stress management programs aimed at controlling smoking, alcohol use, and hypertension (Brown, 1988; Frieden, 1991; Gilman & Bucco, 1987; Herzlinger & Calkins, 1986; Herzlinger & Schwartz, 1985; Peres, 1992).

As an effective strategy for controlling health care costs, major corporations have also encouraged participation in comprehensive, capitated rate plans, such as health maintenance organizations (HMOs) and preferred provider organizations (PPOs). In these managed care plans, providers set an amount to cover all of their enrollees" health care needs. A percentage of that payment is put into a risk pool as insurance against unexpected expenditures. Providers assume a certain element of risk in exchange for the opportunity to benefit from lower costs, an integrated care system, and management savings (Brown, 1988; Christensen, 1991; Hicks, Stallmeyer, & Coleman, 1992; O'Connor, 1991).

Another initiative, called *managed competition,* finances health insurance coverage through large businesses. The employer is required to purchase insurance or pay a payroll tax for a public (government) sponsor. This system promotes competition among private insurers and ensures quality improvement standards (Enthoven & Kronick, 1989a, 1989b; Garland, 1991). All of these health care delivery arrangements focus on both primary and secondary prevention, thereby increasing positive health outcomes and reducing costs (Hospitals, 1988; Luft, 1978, 1982; Rosenberg, Perlis, Lynne, & Leto, 1991; Sloss et al., 1987).

Another response to the problems of financing health care benefits is ensuring the employer's involvement in managing the delivery of health care services. Providers are developing and participating in corporate health care programs that monitor the cost and use of health care services. Those services that are monitored include preadmission testing, which has been shown to reduce inpatient stays; utilization review; monitoring of catastrophic illness and injury through medical case management programs; and mandatory employer-sponsored health insurance that would extend both private and public employer-sponsored health insurance coverage through various financial arrangements (Aaron, 1991; Brown, 1988; Dalton, 1987; Dentzer, 1991; Herzlinger, 1985; Herzlinger & Calkins, 1986; Herzlinger & Schwartz, 1985; Peres, 1992). Such monitoring programs have helped reduce and eliminate medical inefficiency and have improved the effectiveness of care delivery.

Businesses have also begun to form health care coalitions that purchase health care services and offer them at a discount to their members. These coalitions guarantee accessible health care services, cost-effective delivery, and quality care. Some of the services provided by the coalitions include Workers' Compensation, inpatient and outpatient programs, primary prevention and treatment, and case management services (Bell, 1991).

CONTEMPORARY APPROACHES TO COST CONTAINMENT

Regulatory attempts to contain health care costs continue to grow through various managed care strategies. The Health Care Financing Administration (now known as the Centers for Medicare & Medicaid Services [CMS]) initiated a reimbursement method for outpatient procedures called ambulatory patient groups (APGs). APGs are used in the ambulatory setting as diagnosis-related groups (DRGs) are used for inpatient services; they are used to reimburse the cost of providing outpatient procedures or visits. APGs reimbursement, however, does not cover the professional or physician cost elements (HCFA, 1996; Shi & Singh, 1998). Ambulatory payment classification (APC), an offshoot of APG's, is a more refined reimbursement strategy implemented by HCFA. Working as an encounter-based patient classification system, APCs attempt to predict the amount and type of resources used for a variety of types of ambulatory visits. The groups and payment rates are based on categories of services that are similar in cost and resource utilization (Cesta & Tahan, 2003). In addition, CMS has identified certain procedures as "inpatient only," which are operations that require more services than can be provided in an outpatient setting.

Other CMS initiatives include a prospective payment system for home care visits. Home health resource groups (HHRGs) rely on a nursing assessment as a driver for reimbursement and are based on data from the Outcome and Assessment Information Set (OASIS). Prospective payment for inpatient/acute rehabilitation uses the Inpatient Rehabilitation Facilities Patient Assessment Instrument (IRF-PAI) to collect outcomes and resource utilization data for reimbursement.

Skilled nursing facilities are also under a prospective payment system initiative. With resource utilization groups (RUGs), this approach mandated by the Balanced Budget Act (BBA) of 1997 uses the minimum data set (MDS) to differentiate nursing home patients by their levels of resource use—that is, principal diagnosis and activities of daily living (ADLs) (Cesta & Tahan, 2003; Shi & Singh, 1998). Prospective payment system (PPS) rates reimburse for routine, ancillary, and capital-related costs.

The Medicare program itself is predicted to become bankrupt by this century and is targeted for major cutback initiatives (Rabinowitz, 1996). The BBA is legislation that was initiated in 1997 to reduce payments to providers by $116 billion over a 5-year period starting in 1998 and extending to 2003. Its intent is to keep Medicare solvent through 2007.

The effects of BBA, however, have been devastating and have reached into the coffers of hospitals, physicians, home care, skilled nursing facilities, and Medicare beneficiaries (American Organization of Nurse Executives, 1999; McGinley, 1999). Some of the unintended consequences have resulted in closures of several home care facilities and nursing homes, making patient placements difficult. In addition, appropriate follow-up care has suffered, making access to continuum of care services problematic.

Relief in terms of a $16 billion Medicare bill was advocated. Overall, the provisions of the bill may give back funds to institutions affected by the Medicare payment reductions and, it is hoped, restore access to care (American Hospital Association, 1999).

NON-NURSING CASE MANAGEMENT MODELS

The primary focus of the case management model is to improve patient outcomes and control costs through the organization and coordination of health care services. The underlying economic premises of case management depend on the linkage to managed care strategies developed by the private sector and insurance provider groups. Managed care programs became popular when private corporations and industry affiliations took an active part in maintaining control over soaring health care expenditures (Federation of American Health Systems Review, 1988).

Medical case management has become an effective way for private industry groups to maintain control over the use and costs of health care and to develop effective management and intervention methods (Califano, 1987; Dentzer, 1991; Katz, 1991). Case management identifies procedures used excessively that involve extended hospital stays and evaluates uncoordinated health care delivery systems, which promote duplication and fragmentation of services. Medical case management controls both the demand for and the supply of health care by identifying potential high-cost cases (appropriate targeting); by coordinating and channeling the delivery of care among providers, patients, insurers, and agencies that may be involved; and by evaluating and managing the patient's existing benefits plan to cover needed services (Dentzer, 1991; Henderson, Bergman, Collard, Souder, & Wallack, 1987; Henderson & Collard, 1988).

Until recently, the cost-effectiveness of the case management method has not been implicitly justified. Past research investigations were concerned with process and structured measures of efficiency. Such investigations sought to discover whether the use of a physician as a case manager or an HMO as an insurer and provider of care actually reduced health care expenditures and increased quality assurance (Austin, 1983; Manning, Liebowitz, Goldberg, Rogers, & Newhouse, 1984).

In 1986, researchers at the Bigel Institute for Health Policy Studies at Brandeis University undertook a major study to evaluate medical case management for catastrophic illnesses. Funding from The Robert Wood Johnson Foundation (Henderson et al., 1987) supported this 2-year project. Specifically the project involved the evaluation of a case management program offered by a predominantly private insurance group and was representative of other case management arrangements offered by other major insurers (Henderson et al., 1987; Henderson & Collard, 1988; Henderson & Wallack, 1987).

Patient case load was identified by five diagnostic categories, which included the high-risk infant, head trauma, spinal cord injury, cancer, and AIDS (Henderson et al., 1987; Henderson & Wallack, 1987). Cost criteria were developed that incorporated the economic rationale of limiting inappropriate use of high-cost procedures and unnecessary ancillary resources. The factors contributing to high costs that were evaluated included patient length of stay that exceeded predefined limits, evidence of complications indicated by the primary and secondary diagnoses, a repeat admission within a set time frame, and total patient charges exceeding a certain limit (Henderson & Wallack, 1987).

Cost-effectiveness was determined when the case management program was initiated and implemented an alternative plan that decreased the patient's length of stay in the hospital, facilitated patient transfer to a less costly facility, and decreased expenditures associated with home care services (Henderson et al., 1987).

Case management responsibilities in this study were assigned to registered nurses who were accountable for the assessment, care planning, monitoring, and evaluation activities. A case management plan was developed that incorporated the input of the physician provider and used appropriate resources to meet the individual needs of the patient and family (Henderson & Collard, 1988). Henderson and Collard found that the successful implementation of the case management plan required the cooperation of the attending physician. For the most part, case management was seen as a comprehensive plan for ensuring patients would receive health care services that would not ordinarily be reimbursable.

The Brandeis study found that use of the medical case management model significantly reduced costs. Several factors contributed to the effectiveness of this classic program:

- Early patient identification and intervention ensure access to the most appropriate and least restrictive care.
- Appropriate resource use helps maintain cost-effective care.
- Alternative treatment programming and benefit management allow for flexibility in the payment structure.
- Directing of the case management approach to specific patient groups helps achieve significant gains from services.
- A cooperative and supportive relationship develops between the care provider and case recipients.
- Interpretable, standardized reporting mechanisms help relate program objectives to patient care delivery.
- Case management integrates the case planning process with resource allocation based on a patient classification system or DRG methodology.
- A computerized information system allows for continuous data monitoring and analysis (Henderson et al., 1987; Henderson & Collard, 1988; Weisman, 1987; White, 1986).

CASE MANAGEMENT AND CATASTROPHIC ILLNESS

The case management model used depends on the patient population it serves. Such adaptability makes it possible to match a particular patient's needs with the appropriate case management approach. For example, the primary care case management model, when used for treating chronically ill patients, may require the addition of medical or social case management services (Merrill, 1985).

Although no one model of case management is applicable in all circumstances, medical case management programs have been adapted for use in the management of care associated with catastrophic illness or injury (Brown, 1988; Henderson & Wallack, 1987). Traditionally, care of those with catastrophic illnesses has been expensive because of a lack of coordination and fragmentation of services. Duplication of patient services and failure to work out alternative care arrangements have also added to the cost of treating catastrophic illness (Henderson & Collard, 1987). The medical case management model focuses cost-containment efforts on a small percentage of the patient population that includes frequent users of hospital and medical technology services (Rosenbloom & Gertman, 1984; Zook & Moore, 1980). Zook and Moore identified two types of catastrophic cases that used a considerable amount of health care resources. The first group consisted of unanticipated illnesses such as spinal cord injury, head trauma, neonatal complications, cancer, cardiac disease, and stroke. The second type of catastrophic illness includes chronic medical or psychiatric conditions.

The rationale behind using the medical case management model with catastrophic illness is based on a study by the Health Data Institute of the medical care patterns of major businesses in the United States. This investigation showed that in more than 1 million episodes of hospital care between 1980 and 1983, there were consistent patterns of high-cost illness. This study revealed that a large proportion of health care costs were attributable to only 5% to 10% of health-insured individuals (Rosenbloom & Gertman, 1984). Because catastrophic illness occurs less frequently than ordinary ailments, cost-containment efforts should be directed to some of these high-cost illnesses. The Health Data Institute study indicates that medical, social, and financial consequences of catastrophic illness and injury can be controlled through a systematic effort characteristic of the case management approach.

References

Aaron, H. (1991). Choosing from the health care reform menu. *The Journal of American Health Policy, 1*(3), 23-27.

Altman, S.H., & Rodmin, M.A. (1988). Halfway competitive markets and ineffective regulation: The American health care system. *Journal of Health Politics, Policy and Law, 13*(2), 323-339.

American Hospital Association (1999, Nov.). *AHA News Wire.* AHA website: www.aha.org.

American Organization of Nurse Executives (1999, Aug.). AONE Policy Briefing: Balanced Budget Act Relief. Chicago: AONE.

Austin, C.D. (1983). Case management in long-term care: Options and opportunities. *Health and Social Work, 8*(1), 16-30.

Bell, N. (1991). From the trenches: Strategies that work. *Business and Health, 9*(5), 19-25.

Brown, R. (1988). Principles for a national health program: A framework for analysis and development. *The Milbank Quarterly, 66*(4), 573-617.

Califano, J. (1987). Guiding the forces of the health care revolution. *Nursing and Health Care 8*(7), 400-404.

Cesta, T.G., & Tahan, H.A. (2003). *The case manager's survival guide: Winning strategies for clinical practice,* 2nd edition, pp. 15-39. St. Louis: Mosby, Inc.

Christensen, L. (1991). The highs and lows of PPOs. *Business and Health, 9*(9), 72-77.

Dalton, J. (1987). Alternative delivery systems and employers. *Topics in Health Care Financing, 13*(3), 68-76.

Davis, R.G. (1985). Congress and the emergence of public health policy. *Health Care Management Review, 10*(1), 61-73.

DeBack, V., & Cohen, E. (1996). The new practice environment. In E. Cohen (Ed.), *Nurse case management in the 21st century* (pp. 3-9). St. Louis: Mosby.

Dentzer, S. (1991, Sept. 23). Agenda for business: How to fight killer health costs. *U.S. News and World Report*, 50-58.

Dwyer, P., & Garland, S. (1991, Nov. 25). A roar of discontent: Voters want health care reform now. *Business Week*, 28-30.

Eckholm, E. (1991, May 2). Rescuing health care. *The New York Times*, A 1, B 12.

Enthoven, A., & Kronick, R. (1989a). A consumer-choice health plan for the 1990s, part I. *New England Journal of Medicine, 320*(1), 29-37.

Enthoven, A., & Kronick, R. (1989b). A consumer-choice health plan for the 1990s, part II. *New England Journal of Medicine, 320*(2), 94-101.

Federation of American Health Systems Review (1988, July/Aug.). Special report: The facts of life about managed care. Author, 20-49.

Frieden, J. (1991). Many roads lead to health system reform. *Business and Health, 9*(11), 38-66.

Garland, S. (1991, Oct. 7). The health care crises: A prescription for reform. *Business Week*, 59-66.

Gilman, T., & Bucco, C. (1987). Alternate delivery systems: An overview. *Topics in Health Care Financing, 13*(3), 1-7.

Ginsburg, R.B., & Hackbarth, G.M. (1986). Alternative delivery systems and Medicare. *Health Affairs, 5*(1), 6-22.

Health Care Financing Administration (1996). Overview of the Medicare program. *Health Care Financing Review: Medicare and Medicaid Statistical Supplement 5.*

Henderson, M., Bergman, A., Collard, A., Souder, B., & Wallack, S. (Draft, May 1, 1987). *Private sector medical case management for high cost illness.* Waltham, Mass.: Brandeis University Heller Graduate School Health Policy Center.

Henderson, M.G., & Collard, A. (1988). Measuring quality in medical case management programs. *Quality Review Bulletin, 14*(2) 33-39.

Henderson, M.G., & Wallack, S.S. (1987). Evaluating case management for catastrophic illness. *Business and Health, 4*(3), 7-11.

Herzlinger, R.E. (1985). How companies tackle health care costs: Part II. *Harvard Business Review, 63*(5), 108-120.

Herzlinger, R.E., & Calkins, D. (1986). How companies tackle health care costs: Part III. *Harvard Business Review, 64*(1), 70-80.

Herzlinger, R.E., & Schwartz, J. (1985). How companies tackle health care costs: Part I. *Harvard Business Review, 63*(4), 68-81.

Hewitt Associates. (1989). *Salaried employee benefits provided by major U.S. employers.* Lincolnshire, Ill.: Hewitt Associates.

Hicks, L., Stallmeyer, J., & Coleman, J. (1992). Nursing challenges in managed care. *Nursing Economics, 10*(4), 265-275.

Hospitals (1988, April 5). Managed care: Whoever has the data wins the game. *Hospitals*, 50-55.

Hospitals (1992, Jan. 20). Health care reform a priority in the legislative years. *Hospitals*, 32-50.

Hospitals & Health Networks/IDX (2003). *Digest of health care's future.* Chicago, Ill.: Health Forum, Inc.

Jones, K. (1989). Evolution of the prospective payment system: Implications for nursing. *Nursing Economics, 7*(6), 299-305.

Katz, F. (1991). Making a case for case management. *Business and Health, 9*(4), 75-77.

Kramon, G. (1989, Jan. 8). Taking a scalpel to health costs. *The New York Times*, pp. 1, 9.

Luft, H.S. (1978). How do health maintenance organizations achieve their savings? Rhetoric and evidence. *The New England Journal of Medicine, 298*(11), 1336-1343.

Luft, H.S. (1982). Health maintenance organizations and the rationing of medical care. *The Milbank Quarterly, 60*(2), 268-306.

Manning, W.G., Leibowitz, A., Goldberg, G., Rogers, W., & Newhouse, J. (1984). A controlled trial of the effect of a prepaid group practice on the use of services. *The New England Journal of Medicine, 310*(23), 1505-1510.

McGinley, L. (1999, May 26). As nursing homes say "no," hospitals feel pain. *The Wall Street Journal*, B1-B4.

Merrill, J.C. (1985). Defining case management. *Business and Health, 3*(5-9), 5-9.

Mullen, P. (1988, Dec. 27). Big increase in health premiums. *Health Week, 2*(26), 1, 26.

National League for Nursing (1991). *Nursing's agenda for health care reform.* New York: NLN.

O'Connor, K. (1991). Risky business: HMOs and managed care. *Business and Health, 9*(6), 30-34.

Peres, A. (1992). Business must act now to shape reform. *Business and Health, 10*(1), 72.

Rabinowitz, H. (1996). Health policy and the future of health care reform. *Journal of the American Board of Family Practice, 9*(1), 37-40.

Reinhardt, U.E. (1987a, Jan. 11). Toward a fail-safe health-insurance system. *The Wall Street Journal.*

Reinhardt, U.E. (1987b). Health insurance for the nation's poor. *Health Affairs, 6*(1), 101-102.

Rosenberg, S., Perlis, H., Lynne, D., & Leto, L. (1991). A second look at second surgical opinions. *Business and Health, 9*(2), 14-28.

Rosenbloom, D., & Gertman, P. (1984). An intervention strategy for controlling costly care. *Business and Health, 1*(8), 17-21.

Shi, L., & Singh, D. (1998). *Delivering health care in America: A systems approach.* Cost, access, quality, Chap. 12, pp. 443-488. Gaithersburg, Md.: Aspen Publications.

Sloan, F., Morrisey, M., & Valvona, J. (1988). Effects of the Medicare prospective payment system on hospital cost containment: An early appraisal. *The Milbank Quarterly, 66*(2), 191-220.

Sloss, E.M., Keeler, E.B., Brook, R.H., Operskalski, B.H., Goldberg, G.A., & Newhouse, J.P. (1987). Effect of a health maintenance organization on physiologic health. *Annals of Internal Medicine, 106*(1), 130-138.

Swoap, D. (1984). Beyond DRGs: Shifting the risk to providers. *Health Affairs, 3*(4), 117-121.

Tallon, J.R. (1991). A report from the front line: Policy and politics in health reform. *The Journal of American Health Policy, 1*(1), 47-50.

Thorpe, K. (1991). The national health insurance conundrum: Shifting paradigms and potential solutions. *The Journal of American Health Policy, 1*(1), 17-22.

Traska, M.R. (1989). What 1989 holds for health benefits. *Business and Health, 1*(1), 22-30.

Waldo, D.R., Levit, J.R., & Lazenby, H. (1986). National health expenditures, 1985. *Health Care Financing Review, 8*(1), 1-21.

Weisman, E. (1987). Practical approaches for developing a case management program. *Quality Review Bulletin, 13*(11), 380-382.

Welling, K. (1990, June 11). The sickening spiral: Health-care costs continue to grow at an alarming rate. *Barron's,* 8.

White, M. (1986). Case management. In G.L. Maddox (Ed.), *The encyclopedia of aging* (pp. 92-96). New York: Springer Publishing.

Wilensky, G. (1991). Treat the causes, not the symptoms of the health care cost problem. *The Journal of American Health Policy, 1*(2), 15-17.

Zook, C.V., & Moore, F.D. (1980). High-cost users of medical care. *New England Journal of Medicine, 302*(18), 996-1002.

Patient Mix and Cost Related to Length of Hospital Stay

CHAPTER OVERVIEW

Prospective payment systems have influenced the development of innovative care delivery models by placing limits on the use of hospital resources. Because the length of time an individual spends in the hospital affects the appropriation of services and costs involved in that care, the number of hospitalized days becomes an important variable in assessing and measuring the institution's financial outcome.

The effects of care delivery models on health care services provided an important strategy for evaluating system effectiveness, efficiency, and quality. The coordination and integration required for case management are two reasons why such a health care delivery model maximizes the use and allocation of available resources and services.

Nursing case management methods provide indicators that help assess the effectiveness of patient care delivery. By focusing on the coordination and integration of inpatient services, nursing case management can affect the patient length of stay (LOS) while keeping it within medically appropriate boundaries.

With the implementation of diagnosis-related group (DRG) strategies, patient LOS has become an overall indicator of a hospital's financial performance and cost-effectiveness. Numerous variables that have an effect on the cost and LOS have been identified. This chapter reviews and analyzes studies related to patient LOS variables.

The chapter is divided into three general categories: (1) patient demographics, such as age and gender variables; (2) related variables, such as diagnosis and comorbidity, discharge planning, patient care delivery systems, and nursing intensity and workload (a critique of the nursing intensity and workload studies is provided); and (3) nonclinical variables that affect patient LOS, such as day-of-the-week admission (weekday versus weekend) and organizational factors.

PATIENT DEMOGRAPHICS

Certain patient characteristics, such as age, were reported to be important in judging the postoperative recovery time of patients undergoing surgical procedures, such as a hernia repair or a cholecystectomy (Kolouch, 1965). Although the reasons for a correlation between age and length of surgical convalescent time were not provided, the finding was anticipated because of the close association among age, chronicity, hospital-induced infections, age-related risk factors, patient dependency needs, and increased time required for postoperative healing.

In this study, however, age did not account for all the variations in average LOS reported by surgical case mix. Other variables existed that were not subject to control, such as postoperative surgical complications, patient rehabilitation time, method of payment (i.e., third-party, Blue Cross, or charity), and type of hospital (i.e., teaching or nonteaching).

In another study by Marchette and Holloman (1986), age was the significant variable in prolonging the LOS of cerebrovascular accident (CVA) patients. On average the CVA patients were older and had the longest hospital stays. Again, as in the Kolouch (1965) study, age did not account for all of the diversity attributed to LOS. Other intervening variables, such as severity of illness, discharge planning, and social consults, also affected the average LOS of the hospitalized patients.

Posner and Lin (1975) studied the age variable in association with predicted LOS for medical patients. In this study, age was evaluated in terms of its effects on comparable diagnoses. The study also evaluated the effect of various hospital settings (voluntary or municipal) on the patient LOS. It was found that the hospital LOS was not exclusively affected by the age of the patient. Wide variations were found in LOS within age groups even when diagnostic categories and hospital variables were controlled.

The unreliability of age as a predictor of hospital LOS was confirmed in another study by Lave and Leinhardt (1976). This study placed emphasis on case-mix factors and variables that related to the patient's medical condition and that contributed to changes in the patient's LOS.

Both Lave and Leinhardt (1976) and Marchette and Holloman (1986) looked at the effect of gender on patient LOS. Findings showed that male patients have shorter hospital LOSs than female patients and that single women have the longest stays. Several explanations of these findings were offered. First, because women live longer than men, women will experience more hospitalizations. Second, single women have longer stays because they less often have adult family members available to care for them. Although all these findings are associated with longer than average hospital stays, the effect of patient gender could not be validated. Lave and Leinhardt (1976) advised that although patient demographic variables may be statistically significant in some situations, such variables may have minimal effect on the overall variability of the patient's LOS.

CLINICALLY RELATED VARIABLES

The patient's primary diagnosis, number of surgical procedures, and number of secondary diagnoses were factors that had a significant effect on patient LOS (Lave & Leinhardt, 1976; Lew, 1966; McCorkle, 1970; Ro, 1969). These variables were found to account for 38% of the variation in LOS, with primary diagnosis alone accounting for 27% of the variability in patient LOS (Lave & Leinhardt, 1976). Patients diagnosed with acute myocardial infarction had the longest hospital stays, whereas patients with hyperplasia of the prostate had shorter LOSs. The findings indicate that patients with urgent or emergent status had longer hospital stays. In addition, the poor health of such patients on admission and the unscheduled nature of these admissions resulted in delays and inefficient mobilization of hospital services.

In two earlier studies, Riedel and Fitzpatrick (1964) and Mughrabi (1976) concluded that the primary diagnosis and the concomitant levels of severity are the most important factors contributing to the length of a patient's hospitalization. Additional studies indicated that comorbidity and related complications resulted in significantly longer LOSs (Berki, Ashcraft, & Newbrander, 1984; Grau & Kovner, 1986).

In an investigation conducted by Marchette and Holloman (1986), discharge planning (that of nurses and of social workers) was found to affect patient LOS. This study demonstrated a decrease of 0.8 day of hospitalization for those patients who received discharge planning early in their hospital stays. Conversely, the LOS increased by 0.8 day for those patients who received discharge planning later in their hospitalization. In addition, a decrease of 2 days of hospitalization was shown because of nurses' discharge planning activities with patients diagnosed with CVA. This finding demonstrates that the effect of discharge planning is indicative of individual patient diagnoses (Cable & Mayers, 1983).

Timely social service planning and early referral programs were shown to shorten a patient's LOS. Factors associated with changes in patient Medicaid status, a lack of alternate care resources, failure of medical staff to complete transfer and referral forms, and other confounding variables delayed patient discharge (Altman, 1965; Boone, Coulton, & Keller, 1981; Schrager, Halman, Myers, Nichols, & Rosenblum, 1978; Schuman, Ostfeld, & Willard, 1976; Zimmer, 1974).

The nursing case management model for patient care delivery has been recognized for its significant effect on decreasing patient LOS (Zander, 1988). Through the coordination and monitoring of resources needed for patient care, ischemic stroke patients' LOS was reduced by 29%, and adult leukemia patients' LOS decreased from an average of 6 to 8 weeks to 32 days.

Rogers (1992) makes a distinction between the way that beyond-the-walls (BTW) and within-the-walls (WTW) models affect LOS:

Both models involve nurses in relatively autonomous positions that use a holistic nursing approach, "system savvy," collaboration to coordinate professional care team functions, and individualized care planning to achieve reductions in resource utilization while enhancing actual, as well as perceived, quality of care. The reduction in patient anxiety and increased patient compliance when they are more involved in the process and assured that someone they know is watching over things is attested to almost daily. These translate to reduced demands on nursing time during a given stay and in reductions in the actual LOS.

Beyond this, our experience has been that enhanced transit through the course of a stay and improved discharge planning, particularly with acute cases, takes days off of the end of the stay. This phenomenon is a hallmark of the WTW model.

On the other hand, the forte of the BTW models is care of the chronically ill. The impact of these models on LOS tends to be on the beginning of the stay. This occurs because the BTW nurse case managers know their patients' patterns and disease processes very well. They tend to get these patients into the hospital earlier in an exacerbation than they previously were. Being admitted "less sick" tends to keep these patients out of high-cost emergency and critical care departments and keep the overall LOS down. This phenomenon was noted by Ethridge and Lamb (1989) and alluded to by Rogers, Riordan, and Swindle (1991). St. Joseph Medical Center in Wichita, in an unpublished internal management analysis, has since documented an overall reduction in the admission acuity for their BTW patients.

A major problem with studies relating to patient care delivery systems is the lack of uniformity and sophistication in defining costs. Variations exist as to what factors should be included in direct and indirect cost categories. Some studies included supplies and equipment, whereas other investigations allocated costs based on overhead expenses from ancillary and support services and general hospital operations. In some studies, nursing costs included the professional services of registered nurses. In other studies, nursing costs included all of the costs of providing nursing care to hospitalized patients (Edwardson & Giovannetti, 1987). Further research is needed to determine the applicability of cost accounting approaches to nursing models of care with the expected clinical and financial outcomes.

Nursing intensity, which is the amount of nursing care provided per patient day, along with various nursing interventions and staffing levels, was cited as reducing LOS and costs associated with hospitalization. In an investigation done by Halloran (1983a, 1983b), nursing diagnoses were used to classify patients according to their nursing care requirements and to describe the time spent by professional nurses in caring for patients. Nursing diagnoses describe patient conditions and problems that require nursing intervention. It was found that a predominantly registered nurse staff, versus a staffing mix of registered nurses, licensed practical nurses, and nursing attendants, decreased costs associated with patient care. The investigation showed that an all–registered nurse staff would be more likely to deal with total patient needs than would a staff composed of various skill mixes. Halloran also proposed that nursing care costs should be identified and defined according to nursing diagnoses (unit of service) instead of the medical DRG currently in use.

In another study, Halloran and Kiley (1984) proposed a nursing information system model that allocated staffing and resources using nursing diagnoses. This process was based on a nursing workload unit of analysis that calculated costs using a patient classification system for staffing. The reason for using a patient classification system was that such a system made it possible to measure the nursing workload and allocate costs to distinguish the costs of nursing care services from the cost of the hospital's room and board rate.

As outlined by Edwardson and Giovannetti (1987), the patient classification system makes it possible to calculate the hours of care used during a patient's hospitalization. Once the number of patient care hours is identified, this number is translated into a dollar amount. Patients are then classified into DRG categories, and nursing care costs for patients are aggregated and analyzed.

Although patient classification systems offer a more reliable representation than traditional methods of identifying the nursing care needs of patients (i.e., global averages, such as the average amount of care required per day by the typical patient), there are still some inherent problems. As identified by Giovannetti (1972) and Edwardson and Giovannetti (1987), the problems associated with this system include the inadvisability of comparing a patient classification system developed in one hospital with that in another because of the differences in treatment modalities, architectural structure and design of the inpatient units, and standards and policies of the institution. Some of the factors used to weigh the categories are subjective, which results in problems of reliability. Furthermore, methods of validating the system and workload indexes are not transferable. Despite these difficulties, the method of staffing by workload index has been generally accepted by health care institutions across the country.

An investigation done by Halloran and Halloran (1985) found that nursing diagnoses were accurate for predicting nursing workload and quantity of nursing care. In addition, nursing diagnoses contributed to some of the variation in patient LOS. It was suggested that nursing instead of medical needs kept patients in the hospital. Nursing diagnoses that dealt with the patient's psychosocial needs and self-care requirements were significant in increasing nursing workload. In another study, nursing workload activities correlated with 77% of the patient's length of hospitalization. These findings imply that variations in LOS within specific DRG categories can be explained by the clinical management of patient care by nurses (Halloran & Kiley, 1986).

Ventura, Young, Feldman, Pastore, Pikula, and Yates (1985) found that nursing interventions associated with health protection activities for patients with peripheral vascular disease significantly decreased the patient's LOS and lowered hospitalization costs, which were based on a fixed per diem rate. Mumford, Schlesinger, and Glass (1982) and Devine and Cook (1983) demonstrated that psychological and educational interventions (i.e., patient teaching related to pain prevention and complications) with postsurgical patients reduced the LOS and improved patient recovery time.

Flood and Diers (1988) identified the effect of professional nurse staffing levels on LOS. According to the study, decreased nurse staffing levels could lead to a reduction in productivity and inadequate patient care, resulting in longer hospitalization. Patients whose case mixes included gastrointestinal hemorrhages and CVAs and who had been located on a unit with significant staffing shortages were found to have longer LOS intervals, 3.8 and 4.14 days, respectively, when compared with patients on a unit that had adequate staffing levels. The increase in LOS was attributed to patient-related complications and nosocomial infections and resulted in the use of high levels of nursing care resources.

However, the findings of the Flood and Diers study are speculative because many of the variables associated with patient LOS, for example, primary diagnosis, comorbidity, medical complications, and discharge planning factors, had not been controlled. Because these variables were not controlled, the study is not adequate for showing a significant correlation between nurse staffing levels and LOS.

The results of the nursing intensity and workload investigations support the premise that patient care requirements, nursing interventions, and level of staff affect the delivery of care. However, other variables that have a profound effect on the delivery of nursing care services were not accounted for. Some of these variables were identified by Edwardson and Giovannetti (1987) and include service standards of the institution, physician practice patterns, nature and extent of support services, adequacy of the physical plant, and quality-of-care indexes. The last variable would have to be studied with various mixes of staffing personnel to determine the efficacy of patient care delivery.

The general findings of the nursing intensity and workload studies take on a different perspective when viewed in light of the investigations done by the Prospective Payment Assessment Commission (ProPAC). ProPAC was established as an independent advisory board to the Department of Health and Human Services (DHHS) and Congress to report on issues surrounding the impact of the prospective payment system on health care delivery and finance. ProPAC's responsibilities include annual recommendations to DHHS regarding appropriate changes in Medicare payments for inpatient hospital care and changes in the relative weights of DRGs. ProPAC is also required to report to Congress its evaluation of any adjustments made to DRG classifications and weights (Price & Lake, 1988).

ProPAC focused its research efforts on the DRG allocation method as it related to the intensity of nursing care. The nursing intensity and workload studies done over the last few years established that inaccuracies existed in the allocation of DRG weights to nursing costs. In the past, nursing service in health care institutions was calculated as part of the room and board rate and did not directly affect patient charges. Variations in the patient's nursing care and attributable costs were strictly related to the patient's LOS and routine and intensive care levels (Cromwell & Price, 1988; Young, 1986).

Accounting for the amount of time spent and for the type of care delivered by nursing is one problem generated by the nature of the services offered. Defining nursing care through a patient classification system became one way of alleviating this difficulty. Matching the type of care a patient will need with a specific category on the patient classification instrument and then determining the amount of nursing resources needed for that patient category provided the foundation for establishing the costs of nursing services and developing a basis for charges to patients. The patient classification system was used as an instrument to measure the severity level of patients (in terms of nursing workload) as well as variations in nursing care. However, studies have shown that because of systematic errors (i.e., quantity of care and level of care are both objective and subjective estimates), a lack of cross-institutional comparability and generalizability, and lack of ongoing validity and reliability, patient classification systems were not accurate resources for determining the cost of nursing services (Dijkers & Paradise, 1986). In addition, the wide variations in the methods used in the numerous nursing intensity studies bring into question the appropriateness and applicability of using nursing patient classification systems to account for DRG-specific nursing intensity values (Price & Lake, 1988).

In view of these limitations, a major research effort directed by ProPAC to provide national adjustments of DRG weights based on nursing intensity variations was abandoned (Cromwell & Price, 1988; Price & Lake, 1988). Recommendations from ProPAC for further research included the following:

- Developing nursing intensity adjustments for selected DRGs on a case-by-case basis
- Documenting nursing intensity variation with DRGs over a patient's LOS by identifying factors related to patient complexity, changes in staff volume, and skill mix
- Establishing uniformity among patient classification systems
- Establishing the cost base used to allocate DRG weights

ProPAC also said that the effects of nursing intensity on DRG weights would be greater if applied to all routine and department costs rather than just direct nursing care (Cromwell & Price, 1988; Price & Lake, 1988).

A study by Blegen, Goode, and Reed (1998) demonstrated that the total hours of care from nursing personnel were associated directly with medication errors, incidence of decubitus, patient complaints, and mortality. The study indicated that as the proportion of registered nurses to patients increased, rates of unfavorable outcomes decreased. Two most recent investigations, those of Needleman et al. (2002) and Aiken et al. (2002), linked registered nurse staffing to the care of hospitalized patients and rate of adverse outcomes. All these research activities validate that the relation of nurse staffing ratios to patient outcomes is another dimension of quality care that affects LOS.

NONCLINICAL VARIABLES

Lew (1966) studied how the day of the week that a patient was admitted affected the average LOS. Patients who came in for medical admissions on Sunday had the lowest average LOS (10.83 days), and those admitted on Friday had the highest average LOS (13.81 days). For surgical patients, those admitted on Wednesday had the lowest average LOS (9.88 days), and those admitted on Friday had the highest average LOS (11.85 days). When medical and surgical admissions were combined, those patients admitted on Friday had the highest average LOS and those admitted on Sunday had the lowest average LOS. Reasons for the variations in the weekday LOSs were attributed to the availability of resources—such as personnel, operating rooms, equipment, and procedures—and services needed for the care of the patient.

Day-of-the-week variables were found significant in studies conducted by Lave and Leinhardt (1976) and Mughrabi (1976). However, these variables did not account for a large portion of the variation in average LOS.

Institutional practices related to management, patient care delivery, and use of facility resources (e.g., laboratory, radiology) were among the many variables that affected LOS. Becker, Shortell, and Neuhouser (1980) identified managerial and organizational factors that had significant effects on over-all patient LOS. In this study, reductions in patient LOS and increases in the quality and efficiency of services were attributable to the following variables:

- Administrative and clinical managers' awareness of traditional outcome measurements of patient care (i.e., LOS, infection and mortality indexes, and preventable complications) compared with other hospitals
- Degree of professional autonomy related to hospital operations and clinical decision making
- Interdisciplinary as well as interdepartmental collaboration and accountability for the efficient use, coordination, and monitoring of hospital resources, including nursing services, radiology, and laboratory

Decreased hospital LOS facilitated by interdepartmental coordination and integration of patient services was achieved by regularly scheduled meetings among radiology, nursing service, and laboratory personnel.

Another study, conducted by Berki, Ashcraft, and Newbrander (1984), showed that with certain DRG classifications, patient LOS variations were related to use and consumption of hospital services. Increases in laboratory and radiology services were found to be associated with longer LOS periods in those DRG categories, such as diabetes and arthritis, that required intensive use of ancillary services. Other DRG categories, for example, eye disease, which requires reattachment of the retina and repair of the cornea, increased nursing service intensity and resulted in decreased patient LOS.

References

Aiken, L., Clarke, S., Sloane, D., Sochalski, J., & Silber, J. (2002, October). Hospital nurse staffing and patient mortality, nurse burnout, and job dissatisfaction. *Journal of the American Medical Association, 288*(16), 1, 987-991, 993.

Altman, I. (1965). Some factors affecting hospital length of stay. *Hospitals, 39*(7), 68-176.

Becker, S., Shortell, S., & Neuhouser, D. (1980). Management practices and hospital length of stay. *Inquiry, 17*, 318-330.

Berki, S., Ashcraft, M., & Newbrander, W. (1984). Length of stay variations within ICDA-8 diagnosis related groups. *Medical Care, 22*(2), 126-142.

Blegen, M., Goode, C., & Reed, L. (1998, Jan./Feb.). Nurse staffing and patient outcomes. *Nursing Research*, 43-50.

Boone, C., Coulton, C., & Keller, S. (1981). The impact of early and comprehensive social work services on length of stay. *Social Work in Health Care, 7*(1), 1-9.

Cable E., & Mayers, S. (1983). Discharge planning effect on length of hospital stay. *Archives of Physical Medicine and Rehabilitation, 64*(2), 57-60.

Cromwell, J., & Price, K. (1988). The sensitivity of DRG weights to variation in nursing intensity. *Nursing Economics, 6*(1), 18-26.

Devine, E., & Cook, T. (1983). A meta-analytic analysis of effects of psychoeducational interventions on length of postsurgical hospital stay. *Nursing Research, 32*(5), 267-274.

Dijkers, M., & Paradise, T. (1986). PCS: One system for both staffing and costing. Do services rendered match need estimates? *Nursing Management, 17*(1), 25-34.

Edwardson, S., & Giovannetti, P. (1987). A review of cost accounting methods for nursing services. *Nursing Economics, 5*(3), 107-117.

Ethridge, P., & Lamb, G. (1989). Professional nursing case management improves quality, access and costs. *Nursing Management, 20*(3), 30-35.

Flood, S., & Diers, D. (1988). Nurse staffing, patient outcome and cost. *Nursing Management, 19*(5), 34-43.

Giovannetti, P. (May 1972). *Measurement of patient's requirements for nursing services.* Paper presented to the National Institute of Health Conference, Virginia.

Grau, L., & Kovnor, C. (1986). Comorbidity one length of stay: A case study. In F.A. Shaffer (Ed.), *Patients and purse strings: Patient classification and case management* (pp. 233-242). New York: National League for Nursing.

Halloran, E. (1983a). Staffing assignment: By task or by patient. *Nursing Management, 14*(8), 16-18.

Halloran, E. (1983b). RN staffing: More care, less cost. *Nursing Management, 14*(9), 18-22.

Halloran, E., & Halloran, D. (1985). Exploring the DRG/nursing equation. *American Journal of Nursing, 85*(10), 1093-1095.

Halloran, E., & Kiley, M. (1984). Case mix management. *Nursing Management, 15*(2), 39-45.

Halloran, E., & Kiley, M.L. (1986). The nurse's role and length of stay. *Medical Care, 23*(9), 1122-1124.

Kolouch, F. (1965). Computer shows how patient stays vary. *The Modern Hospital, 105*(5), 130-134.

Lave, J., & Leinhardt, S. (1976). The cost and length of a hospital stay. *Inquiry, 13*, 327-343.

Lew, I. (1966). Day of the week and other variables affecting hospital admissions, discharges and length of stay for patients in the Pittsburgh area. *Inquiry, 3*, 3-39.

Marchette, L., & Holloman, F. (1986). Length of stay variables. *Journal of Nursing Administration, 165*(3), 12-19.

McCorkle, L. (1970). Duration of hospitalization prior to surgery. *Health Services Research, 5*, 114-131.

Mughrabi, M.A. (1976). The effects of selected demographic and clinical variables on the length of hospital stay. *Hospital Administration in Canada, 18*, 82-88.

Mumford, E., Schlesinger, H., & Glass, G. (1982). The effects of psychological intervention on recovery from surgery and heart attacks: An analysis of the literature. *American Journal of Public Health, 72*(2), 141-151.

Needleman, J., Buerhaus, P., Mattke, S., Stewart, M., & Zelevinsky, K. (2002, May). Nurse-staffing levels and the quality of care in hospitals. *The New England Journal of Medicine, 346*(22), 1715-1722.

Posner, J., & Lin, H. (1975). Effects of age on length of hospital stay in a low income population. *Medical Care, 13*(10), 855-875.

Price, K., & Lake, E. (1988). ProPAC's assessment of DRGs and nursing intensity. *Nursing Economics, 6*(1), 10-16.

Riedel, D., & Fitzpatrick, T. (1964). *Patterns of patient care: A study of hospital use in six diagnosis.* Ann Arbor: The University of Michigan Graduate School of Business Administration.

Ro, K.K. (1969). Patient characteristics, hospital characteristics and hospital use. *Medical Care, 7*(4), 295-312.

Rogers, M. (Aug. 1992). Personal communication.

Rogers, M., Riordan, J., & Swindle, D. (1991). Community-based nursing case management pays off. *Nursing Management, 22*(3), 30-34.

Schrager, J., Halman, M., Myers, D., Nichols, R., & Rosenblum, L. (1978). Impediments to the course and effectiveness of discharge planning. *Social Work in Health Care, 4*(1), 65-79.

Schuman, J., Ostfeld, A., & Willard, H. (1976). Discharge planning in an acute hospital. *Archives of Physical Medicine and Rehabilitation, 57*(7), 343-347.

Ventura, M., Young, D., Feldman, M.J., Pastore, P., Pikula, S., & Yates, M.A. (1985). Cost savings as an indicator of successful nursing intervention. *Nursing Research, 34*(1), 50-53.

Young, D. (1986). ProPAC: Future Directions. *Nursing Economics, 4*(1), 12-15.

Zander, K. (1988). Nursing care management: Strategic management of cost and quality outcomes. *Journal of Nursing Administration, 18*(5), 23-30.

Zimmer, J. (1974). Length of stay and hospital bed misutilization. *Medical Care, 12*(5), 453-462.

19

Case Management Legislation

National Attempts to Provide Efficient Health Care

CHAPTER OVERVIEW

The prospective payment system gave hospitals the incentive to shorten length of stay, thereby encouraging strategies using case management to focus on postdischarge planning and community-based long-term care. Case management has also demonstrated its applicability as a resource in the development of health legislation and policy in regard to the delivery of patient care. The usefulness of case management is an integral part of the administration and management of health care and is also a vital quality and cost-containment measure.

HISTORICAL LEGISLATION

In 1992, 37 states had Medicaid provisions for case management. Legislation for governing the practices of case managers and for developing national certification and specific state requirements was also considered (National Case Management Task Force Steering Committee, 1991-1992; Sager, 1992).

Case management has been integrated into many of the federal and state policies associated with the delivery of health care and social support services. The overall goal is to reduce the use and costs of expensive treatments. Case management is used in these situations to reduce institutionalization, increase and monitor access of needed services, and expand alternative community resources such as home and long-term care (Boling, 1992; Capitman, 1986; Kane, 1985; Strickland, 1992).

Case management has also been a major component in several federally funded demonstration projects.

The Triage Demonstration Project provided case management and health care services outside the traditional Medicare benefits. These services include adult day care, companion homemaking services, counseling, transportation, pharmaceuticals, and access to residential care. To be eligible for these services, persons had to be age 65 years or older; had to have medical, social, and financial problems and a failing support system; and had to be at risk for institutionalization. Case management services were provided by a professional team consisting of registered nurses, physicians, and social workers (O'Rourke, Raisz, & Segal, 1982).

People eligible for the Wisconsin Community Care Organization included those individuals who were at risk for institutionalization as determined by the Geriatric Functional Rating Scale. This scale rated individuals' ability to perform functional and cognitive activities. Services included companion and home health aide services, medical supplies and equipment, transportation, respite care, and skilled nursing care (Applebaum, Seidl, & Austin, 1980; Seidl, Applebaum, Austin, & Mahoney, 1983).

The On Lok demonstration project provides case management to dependent and elderly individuals eligible for skilled nursing or intermediate nursing home care. This model, which was started more than 30 years ago, remains one of the most successful programs to promote community care for the elderly. Acute care services, including hospitalization, are provided in addition to other services, including adult and social day care, dental care, home health care, optometry, and occupational and pharmaceutical services. Case management is provided by an interdisciplinary team that includes registered nurses, physicians, social workers, physical and occupational therapists, geriatric aides, dietitians, and van drivers. Providers are linked by an integrated electronic medical records system to offer all-inclusive health care to this vulnerable population (Bodenheimer, 1999; Kimball, 2002; Zawadski, Shen, Yordi, & Hansen, 1984).

The On Lok model serves as a prototype for many community-based programs, most notably, PACE (Program of All Inclusive Care for the Elderly). Available in 14 states, PACE provides medical and social support in collaboration with local health centers and manages care through contract arrangements with community providers. Current data demonstrate decreased utilization of institutional care and medical specialists and improved mortality (Eng, 1997; Kimball, 2002).

The New York City Home Care program offered services to chronically ill and elderly individuals residing in the New York City area. The program provided homemaker and personal care, transportation assistance, and various medical therapies (Sainer et al., 1984).

The Long-Term Care Channeling Demonstration Project provided case management services to dependent and chronically ill individuals. Services included mental health counseling, homemaking, personal care, supportive services, such as adult foster care and day care, skilled nursing, transportation, medical therapies, and equipment (Applebaum, Harrigan, & Kemper, 1986; Kemper et al., 1986; Wooldridge & Schore, 1986).

Those who were eligible for Access, Medicare's long-term care demonstration project, included all individuals age 18 years or older and Medicare beneficiaries older than 65 years who needed long-term, skilled nursing care. Services included case management, skilled nursing and home care, and Medicaid-waived services. Waived services included community health nursing, home health aide, medical and nursing consultations and therapies, personal care, equipment and supplies, respite care, and transportation (Berkeley Planning Associates, 1987; Eggert, Bowlyow, & Nichols, 1980).

LEGISLATION SUPPORTING THE DELIVERY OF CASE MANAGEMENT SERVICES

Despite the defeat of health care reform measures proposed at the start of the Clinton administration, several legislation and health care reform proposals have pointed to principles of managed or coordinated care for providing a framework for cost-effective health care delivery. By focusing on case management and long-term care, an alternative to costly hospital and institutional care can be found. These legislative proposals have sought to reduce unneeded care and the use of expensive inpatient services through preventive and primary care interventions. They have also supported comprehensive community-based services and initiatives to improve overall health status and prevent inappropriate hospitalizations (Blankenau, 1992; Pollack, 1992; Strickland, 1992; Wagner, 1991).

Targeted populations included, among others, the chronically ill elderly, young and middle-age individuals with chronic illness and disabilities, the uninsured, and the impoverished. It was also suggested that resources be directed to reducing infant mortality and improving maternal health status (Darman, 1991; Hospitals, 1992a; Wagner, 1991).

Managed care has played a major role in proposals to expand Medicare and Medicaid. The social health maintenance organization (SHMO) is a national managed-care demonstration program initiated in 1985 to provide and finance long-term care services for the elderly. The program includes four nonprofit sites and was approved by Congress for six additional locations. Sponsored by the Health Care Financing Administration (HCFA) in cooperation with the Health Policy Center of Brandeis University, this initiative uses case management and integrated service delivery as key features at each of the demonstration sites. The SHMO is recognized as one of the only national demonstration projects to successfully integrate acute and chronic care using existing funding resources (Abrahams, 1990; Abrahams, Macko, & Grais, 1992; Paone, 1996; Yordi, 1988) and one in which such care can be delivered within a capitated system.

Managed Medicaid legislation, passed in 1987, makes recommendations for a flat payment for Medicaid beneficiaries in need of medical and long-term care. This plan reduces hospital stays and excessive use of services, increases affordable access, and strengthens community-based services and resources (Hospitals, 1992b; McNeil, 1991; "Medicaid-Mandated Managed Care," 1992).

Another example of how the concept of case managed care is used is with the legislation of the CHAMPUS (Civilian Health and Medical Program of the Uniformed Services) Reform Initiative (CRI). This plan extends coverage under a case-managed structure for military dependents and retirees younger than 65 years (Burke, 1992). It also helps reduce health care expenditures and increase access by encouraging the use of military medical services and facilities (Burke, 1992).

Tricare, introduced as an alternative to CHAMPUS, is structured to be a more efficient, cost-effective system of delivering care. It offers three options for medical care: 1) services can be obtained from a government-approved network, 2) users can choose their own medical providers, and 3) inpatient care can be obtained at an out-of-network facility (CHAMPUS, 1995).

Of the major reform plans introduced in the 102nd Congress, six addressed long-term care policies and legislation. It is important to note that these health reform proposals were ground-breaking legislation for case management.

The 1990 Pepper Commission Proposal, developed by the Bipartisan Commission on Health Care, suggested extending Medicare's long-term care initiatives to all disabled individuals. Under the proposal, which was introduced in the Senate by Senator Jay Rockefeller (D-W.Va.), eligibility would be determined by state, local, or federally funded agencies and based on standardized assessments of the beneficiary's resources and support systems.

It was proposed that case managers be used to evaluate and monitor the services provided. Benefits were to include comprehensive home- and community-based services that involve skilled nursing; physical, occupational, and speech therapies; personal care; homemaker services; adult and social day care; respite care for caregivers; hospital care; primary and preventive care; and support counseling (Darman, 1991; Harrington, 1990; Pepper Commission, 1990).

Coverage structure would have incorporated a play or pay plan requiring employers to provide health insurance to employees and their dependents or pay into a public tax plan. A provision was made in this plan for the phasing in of small businesses. Federal and state financing was to have been made available to cover home- and community-based care programs and nursing home care.

Quality-of-care issues were addressed through standardized practice guidelines, outcomes research, and peer review. Overall costs for this proposal included $24 billion for home care and $18.8 billion for nursing home care (Darman, 1991; Frieden, 1991).

The Long-Term Home Care Act (HR 2263), introduced by Senator Claude Pepper (D-Fla.), proposed to provide coverage for the chronically ill or disabled elderly and children younger than 19 with cognitive and functional impairments. It also included individuals with severe functional disabilities.

Benefits included skilled nursing care, homemaker and personal care services, physical, occupational, speech, and respiratory therapies, medical supplies and equipment, caregiver education, support and counseling, and adult day care. Eligibility determination was to be made by a long-term care management agency or private nonprofit agency along with the individual's physician.

Patient care management was to be provided through case management agencies that did not have affiliations or control interest in the referral facilities. Estimated costs for this plan were $8.9 billion (Darman, 1991).

The Elder Care Program (HR 3140), proposed by Representative Harry Waxman (D-Calif.), was to provide for Medicare beneficiaries and disabled individuals. Eligibility determination was to be made by community assessment and review agencies that were restricted in affiliation and ownership to community or nursing care facilities.

Home- and community-based services were to include adult day care, skilled nursing, homemaker, and personal care services, medical and social services, diagnostic tests, medical supplies and equipment, caregiver education and training, and physical and occupational therapy. Estimated costs ranged from $50 billion to $60 billion in 1992 (Darman, 1991; Hospitals, 1992a).

Life Care (S2163/HR4093), sponsored by Senator Edward Kennedy (D-Mass.) and Representative Edward Roybal (D-Calif.), proposed extending eligibility to the chronically ill older than 65 years or younger than 19 years, all disabled and dependent individuals, and people with a life expectancy of 1 year or less.

Federally funded case management agencies were to determine eligibility and provide patient management. Benefit coverage was to include up to the first 6 months of nursing home care with extended nursing home coverage provided through a federal long-term care insurance program.

Proposed financial structure included Medicaid and income-related subsidies. Services provided included skilled nursing, adult day care, primary and preventive care, transportation to health and social care facilities, respite care, institutional or noninstitutional care, nutrition and dietary counseling, and physical, occupational, and speech therapies. The estimated cost of such a program was $20 billion (Darman, 1991; Harrington, 1990; Hospitals, 1992a).

Similar to Life Care, the Comprehensive Health Care Plan (HR 4253), proposed providing for the chronically ill older than 65 or younger than 19. The plan also was to provide for Medicare-eligible disabled individuals of all ages and to insure those with a life expectancy of 1 year or less.

Eligibility and patient care were to be determined by federally funded case management agencies. Benefits were to include nursing home coverage and income assistance programs.

Home- and community-based services were to include skilled nursing; physical, occupational, and speech therapies; homemaker services; medical and social work care; transportation; adult day care and respite care; and counseling services. The estimated cost of this plan was $258 billion, which included universal health care and preventive and long-term care provisions (Darman, 1991).

MediPlan (HR 5300), sponsored by representative Pete Stark (D-Calif.), suggested that Medicare benefits be extended to chronically ill and disabled individuals of all ages. This plan also included primary and preventive care for children in addition to well-baby care.

It was proposed that eligibility determination and patient management be conducted by case management agencies, which were to have provider and ownership restrictions. A full range of home- and community-based services were to be provided, including skilled nursing; counseling services; medical supplies; adult day care; physical, occupational, and respiratory therapies; medical and social services; caregiver education and training; homemaker and personal care services; and prescription-drug coverage.

The plan's financing structure incorporated payroll tax increases and state contributions. The estimated cost of such a program was $120 billion, which included universal health care provisions and long-term care arrangements (Darman, 1991; Frieden, 1991; Hospitals, 1992a).

Additional legislative initiatives indicated case management as an integral component of health care delivery and policy formation. These plans serve as examples of several state assembly and senate bills developed in California that would have affected case management (Kowlsen, 1991). An overview of three such bills follows.

- California Assembly Bill 1341 was to provide for a 3-year demonstration project to provide case management to children at risk for abuse and neglect. Case management services were to be provided by public health nurses. The goal of this project was to reduce shelter or foster care placement and decrease emergency department visits and hospitalizations among children.
- California Senate Bill 1108 established the Primary Care Case Management Advisory Board as part of the California Department of Health Services. It also provided for the delivery of case management services for Medicaid-eligible individuals to promote and increase accessibility to affordable health care resources.
- California Assembly Bill 14 would have ratified primary health care coverage to all individuals. Cost-containment strategies were to include managed care principles such as case management.

References

Abrahams, R. (1990, Aug.). The social/HMO: Case management in an integrated acute and long-term care system. *Caring Magazine*, 30-40.

Abrahams, R., Macko, P., & Grais, M.I. (1992). Across the great divide: Integrating acute postacute, and long-term care. *Journal of Case Management, 1*(4), 124-134.

Applebaum, R., Seidl, F.W., & Austin, C.D. (1980). The Wisconsin community care organization: Preliminary findings from the Milwaukee experiment. *Gerontologist, 20*, 350-355.

Applebaum, R.A., Harrigan, M.N., & Kemper, P. (1986). *The evaluation of the national long-term care demonstration: Tables comparing channeling to other community care demonstrations.* Princeton, N.J.: Mathematica Policy Research, Inc.

Berkeley Planning Associates (1987). *Evaluation of the Access: Medicare long-term care demonstration project. Final Report.* Berkeley, Calif.

Blankenau, R. (1992, Jan. 6). Health-reform bills top 1992 agendas of Hill health leaders. *AHA News.*

Bodenheimer, T. (1999, October). Long term care for the frail elderly people: The On Lok model. *The New England Journal of Medicine, 34*(17), 1324-1328.

Boling, J. (1992). An American integrated health care system? Where are we now? *The Case Manager, 3*(3), 53-59.

Burke, M. (1992, Jan. 20). Armed services are marching toward managed care alternatives. *AHA News, 28*(3), 6.

Capitman, J.A. (1986). Community-based long-term care models, target groups, and impacts on service use. *Gerontologist, 26*(4), 389-397.

CHAMPUS (1995, Mar. 13). *CHAMPUS user's guide* (pp. 1-28). Author (special section to *Army Times, Navy Times,* and *Air Force Times*).

Darman, R. (1991, Oct. 10). *Comprehensive health reform: Observations about the problem and alternative approaches to solution. Presented to the House Committee on Ways and Means.* Washington, D.C.: Executive Office of the President, Office of Management and Budget.

Eggert, G., Bowlyow, J., & Nichols, C. (1980). Gaining control of the long-term care systems: First returns from the access experiment. *Gerontologist, 20*, 356-363.

Eng, C. (1997, Feb.). Program of all inclusive care for the elderly: An innovative model for integrated geriatric care and financing. *Models of Geriatric Practice, 45*(2), 223-232.

Frieden, J. (1991). Many roads lead to health system reform. *Business and Health, 9*(11), 38-66.

Harrington, C. (1990). Policy options for a national health care plan. *Nursing Outlook, 38*(5), 223-228.

Hospitals (1992a, Jan. 20). Health care reform a priority in the new legislative year. 32-50.

Hospitals (1992b, March 20). Managed care in the 1990s: Providers' new role for innovative health delivery. 26-34.

Kane, R. (1985). Case management in health care settings. In M. Weil & J. Karls (Eds.), *Case management in human service practice* (pp. 170-203). San Francisco: Jossey-Bass Publishing.

Kemper, P., et al. (1986). *The evolution of the national long-term care demonstration: Final report.* Princeton, N.J.: Mathematica Policy Research, Inc.

Kimball, B. (2002, Jul./Aug.). In step with On Lok. *Health Forum Journal,* 22-26.

Kowlsen, T. (1991, Oct.). California dreaming. *Washington Health Beat*, 28-29.

McNeil, D. (1991, Nov. 17). Washington tries to sort out health insurance proposals. *New York Times*, 2.

Medicaid-mandated managed care (1992, Jun.). *Nursing & Health Care, 13*(6), p. 288.

National Case Management Task Force Steering Committee (1991-1992, Feb. 9). *Work summary and survey of case management toward medical case manager certification*. Little Rock, Ark.: Systemedic Corporation.

O'Rourke, B., Raisz, H., & Segal, J. (1982). *Triage II: Coordinated delivery of services to the elderly: Final report*, vol 1-2. Plainville, Conn.: Triage, Inc.

Paone, D. (1996). Hospitals. In C.J. Evashwick (Ed.), *The continuum of long-term care: An integrated systems approach* (pp. 25-42). Albany, N.Y.: Delmar Publishers.

Pepper Commission (1990, Mar. 2). *Access to healthcare and long-term care for all Americans*. Washington, D.C.: U.S. Bipartisan Commission on Comprehensive Health.

Pollack, R. (1992, Jan. 13). Hospitals ready for reform of national health care system. *AHA News*.

Sager, O. (1992). Certification: From need to reality. *The Case Manager, 3*(3), 81-84.

Sainer, J.S., Brill, R.S., Horowitz, A., Weinstein, M., Dono, J.E., & Korniloff, N. (1984). *Delivery of medical and social services to the homebound elderly: A demonstration of intersystem coordination: Final report*. New York: New York City Department for the Aging.

Seidl, F.W., Applebaum, R., Austin, C., & Mahoney, K. (1983). *Delivering in-home services to the aged and disabled: The Wisconsin experiment*. Lexington, Mass.: Lexington Books.

Strickland, T. (1992, Apr., May, Jun.). Profile [interview with Gail R. Wilensky, Deputy Assistant to the President for Policy Development]. *The Case Manager, 3*(2), 72-81.

Wagner, L. (1991, Dec. 9). Cost containment: Carrot or the stick? *Modern Healthcare*, 36-40.

Wooldridge, J., & Schore, J. (1986). *Evaluation of the national long-term care demonstration: Channeling effects on hospital, nursing home, and other medical services*. Princeton, N.J.: Mathematica Policy Research, Inc.

Yordi, C. (1988). Case management in the social health maintenance organization demonstration. *Health Care Financing Review* (annual supplement), 83-88.

Zawadski, R.T., Shen, J., Yordi, C., & Hansen, J.C. (1984). *On Lok's community care organization for dependent adults: A research and development project (1978-1983): Final report*. San Francisco: On Lok Senior Health Services.

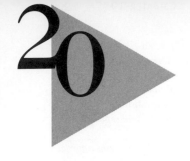

The Managed Care Market

Nurse Case Management as a Strategy for Success

Tina Gerardi

CHAPTER OVERVIEW

Managed care has become the primary health care policy in the United States. Coupled with *capitation*, fixed per member–per month payments, managed care is supposed to solve all of the U.S. health care problems, from rocketing health care costs to perceived shortcomings in health care quality. Remarkably there is little consensus, especially among the public, as to just what is managed care. Nurse case managers must understand managed care if they are to navigate the health care delivery system to meet the complex needs of their patients. This chapter describes the basics of managed care and interprets concepts as they relate to the current marketplace. The role of case management as a strategy for success in the managed care market is also discussed.

WHY MANAGED CARE?

Before World War I, hospitals were only for the most seriously ill patients. Babies were born at home, and family doctors made house calls. The center of care was the home, and financing was pay-as-you-go. Costs were relatively low, because medicine was not that sophisticated. Also, most people could not afford high fees. Only the very wealthy could afford a specialist.

After World War II, antibiotics made advanced surgery and long-term survival possible. New technologies made hospitals the centers of care, where patients came to see specialists. The federal government, through the Hill-Burton Act in 1946, subsidized hospital construction, which led to a hospital construction boom. With the passage of the Medicare and Medicaid bills in 1965, health care became an industry. The incentives were to fill beds and perform more procedures, and hospitals competed to have the best and most advanced facilities, creating a "technology race." Meanwhile, because most of the public were covered by some sort of indemnity insurance coverage, they were insulated from the true cost of care.

The traditional fee-for-service reimbursement system encouraged overutilization. With this type of reimbursement, hospitals and health care providers were reimbursed for each service provided; the more you ordered or provided, the more you were paid. In the 1960s, health industry leaders began to recognize the potential of prepaid group practice plans as mechanisms to contain the dramatic rise in health care costs. The federal government provided the impetus for expanding the number of prepaid health plans through legislation enacted in 1973. The term *health maintenance organization (HMO)* was coined during the Nixon administration.

Soaring insurance premiums in the 1980s caused businesses to reexamine the system for delivering and financing health care. Commercial insurance plans sought to protect their revenue base by writing narrower policies and raising group premiums based on the experience of one individual in the group. Use of services was discouraged by high deductibles and copayments. Staff were hired to review and approve individual cases to reduce inappropriate services. The diagnosis-related group (DRG)-based payment, a fixed rate for specific diagnoses or procedures, was also introduced as a means of controlling escalating health care costs. The utilization review programs and DRG system have been unsuccessful in reducing health care costs.

The predecessors of the HMO include organizations that mutualized costs and provided direct health care services for Venetian seaman in the thirteenth century, for British seamen in the sixteenth century, and for American merchant seamen in 1798. Kaiser-Permanente, the major prototype of the HMO, traces its origins to the 1930s. It developed from a system serving workers building the Los Angeles Aqueduct in 1933, construction workers and their families at the Grand Coulee Dam project in eastern Washington in 1938, and, on a larger scale, Kaiser shipyard employees in and around Portland, Oregon, and San Francisco, and employees of the Kaiser steel plant at Fontana, California, during World War II. The system was open to the public in 1945. Organized consumers formed the Group Health Cooperative of Puget Sound in 1946, and the Health Insurance Plan of Greater New York was organized in 1947.

Several advantages were identified as these organizations emerged:
- Ensured availability of and access to services through integrated group practices
- Evolution and creation of prepaid insurance plans
- Budgeting for provision of services
- Incentives for health maintenance and preventive health services
- Assurance of quality care through the group practice of physicians offering multiple specialties

To control escalating health care costs, payment systems and cost control measures have been discussed, and managed care programs have been reexamined by both the business community and health economists. Managed care is not a new idea, but it will definitely have new implications, particularly for nursing.

How Does Managed Care Work?

Patient care has somehow always been "managed." In many cases, human illness has been managed by the patient and family alone. At other times it has been managed for the patient and family by the health care professional (a gatekeeper) accountable for coordinating all patient health care services and supplying certain aspects of the patient's health services.

Managed care in its broadest form currently refers to any health care delivery system in which a party other than the health care giver or the patient influences the type of health care delivered. A managed care provider takes the risk for the patient's health care. In this way, rather than simply approving or denying the health benefit, the managed care provider intervenes to provide what it considers to be appropriate health care for the patient.

A montage of managed care organizations has evolved in response to the steady rise in health care costs as a percentage of the U.S. gross domestic product (GDP) (Figure 20-1). Health spending as a share of the GDP is estimated to increase from 13.6% to 16.6% from 1999 through 2007. Society has decided that the current growth of health care as a proportion of the GDP is more than it is willing to pay. Our average health benefits have increased in a similar vein. According to the Comparative Performance of U.S. Hospitals, the average cost per employee for annual health benefits in late 1998 was approximately $4000 compared with $600 in 1976. In the mid-late 1990s, managed care was viewed as an answer to the

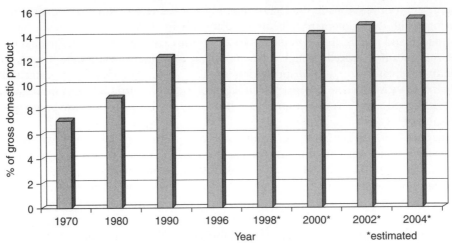

FIGURE **20-1**   The increase of health care expenses as a percentage of the gross domestic product. From *U.S. Department of Health and Human Services, 1997.*

problems of increasing price, decreasing access, and uncertain quality. In response to these escalating costs, purchasers of health plans, mainly local businesses, embraced the tenets of managed care and made arrangements with HMOs or independent managed care companies.

According to the Comparative Performance of U.S. Hospitals, the percentage of hospitals with arrangements with HMOs increased from 48% in 1986 to 98% in 1996. In traditional fee-for-service plans, an individual encounter between a covered individual and the health care system is compensated for by the insurer if the encounter represents a covered benefit of the patient's plan, subject to deductibles or other contractual reductions in benefits. If the patient does not have insurance coverage or the encounter is not a covered benefit, the patient is liable for the bill. The patient chooses the health care professional or hospital to provide the service based on his or her own criteria. On the other hand, the managed care organization generally presents the patient with a list of health care professionals from which to choose the one to supply a covered benefit. Many managed care plans have specified times during which patients can change health care professionals; therefore once a provider is chosen, it may be difficult to change. Depending on the plan, the patient may be required to see a primary care provider who will be responsible for making all assessments and determinations as to health care needs. Referrals must be initiated by the primary care provider. The patient is likely to have a fixed copayment or fee for every visit, regardless of its complexity, and will probably not need to file insurance papers or be responsible for any other payment. Hospitalizations are likely to be covered entirely with the exception of certain medically unnecessary amenities. Prevention visits such as immunizations, well-baby visits, Pap smears, and mammograms are likely to be covered benefits, with a copayment.

Traditionally, health care providers were physicians and hospitals. Physicians saw patients in their offices and in hospitals or clinics. Managed care has introduced a large number of additional people to the health care delivery system. Many managed care organizations have begun to depend on physician assistants and nurse practitioners to provide services, especially in the areas of primary care. In the "good old days," the choice of hospital was made predominantly by the physician. In a managed care environment, the choice is almost entirely made by the payor according to contractual arrangements negotiated for the entire plan. This makes the hospital a provider as well, because many of the covered benefits are provided as part of hospital services. These include home health nursing, pharmacy, physical and occupational therapy, respiratory therapy and ventilator management, and dietary counseling, to name a few.

To understand the cost control changes to the health care marketplace, we must first understand the traditional methods for managing health care costs and current managed care structures. Early managed care programs under the guidance of the professional standards review organizations (PSROs) attempted to control costs through cost sharing, education, second opinions for surgery, and incentives to use lower-cost sites of care such as ambulatory surgery. These early plans also assumed that physicians would modify their behavior based on information alone. Unfortunately, none of these early strategies controlled the continuing escalation of costs. However, the key characteristic of the most effective managed care plans was identified: control of cost and utilization. The cost, use, and appropriateness of services rendered by providers are tightly controlled. Providers are selected who are able to provide cost-effective care.

HMOs, preferred provider organizations (PPOs), and indemnity forms of insurance once were distinct products for providing health care benefits. Today the distinctions are disappearing as each product takes on characteristics of the other. Other common managed care structures include exclusive provider organizations (EPOs), independent practice associations (IPAs), and point-of-service (POS) plans. Definitions for each of these plans are provided in an attempt to clarify this managed care alphabet soup.

- HMOs are organized health care delivery systems responsible for both the financing and the delivery of health care services to an enrolled population. There are five common models of HMOs:
  1. In *staff model* HMOs, the physicians are employed by the HMO to provide covered services to the health plan enrollees. They are usually paid a salary with some bonus or incentive based on performance and productivity.
  2. In the *group practice model* HMO, the HMO contracts with a multispecialty physician group practice to provide all physician services to the HMO members. The physician group is technically independent but depends significantly on the HMO contracts for patients. An example of this type of model is the Permanente Medical Group under the Kaiser Foundation Health Plan.
  3. In a *network model*, a network contracts with more than one group practice to provide physician services to the HMO members. An example is the Health Insurance Plan (HIP) of Greater New York, which contracts with many multispecialty physician group practices in the New York City area.
  4. In the *IPA* model, the HMO contracts with an association of physicians to provide services to its members. Physicians are members of the IPA for purposes of the HMO contract but retain their practices separately and distinctly from each other.
  5. *Direct contract* models contract directly with individual physicians to provide services to their members. In direct contracting arrangements the employer contracts directly with the provider to provide health care services, thus eliminating the insurer.
- An IPA is an association of individual independent physicians or small physician group practices formed for the purpose of contracting with one or more managed health care organizations. The attractiveness of an IPA structure to HMOs and other managed care organizations is the ability of the IPA to provide a large panel of providers and to accept payment on a capitated basis.
- PPOs are entities through which employer health benefit plans and health insurance carriers contract to purchase health care services for covered beneficiaries from a selected group of participating providers. These providers may include hospitals, physicians, IPAs, or physician-hospital organizations. Most often PPOs negotiate on a basis of discounted fee-for-service charges, all-inclusive per diem rates, or payments based on DRGs. A major difference between PPOs and HMOs is the patient's

ability to choose a non-PPO member for covered services, subject to a higher level of deductible and copayment.

- EPOs are structured like PPOs but behave much like HMOs in their limitation of choice of providers. HMOs are carefully regulated by specific HMO statutes in the states in which they operate, whereas EPOs are insurance products subject to less rigorous insurance laws.
- POS plans contain features of PPO and HMO arrangements. Under POS plans, primary care physicians are reimbursed through fixed per member–per month payments (capitation) or other performance-based reimbursement methods. The primary care provider acts as a gatekeeper for referral and institutional medical services.

Health care providers are responding to the changing market and expansion of managed care products, which place greater emphasis on value, access, and quality of care. Responses to the market include provider's developing organizations that accommodate coordinated care and shared reimbursement. For example, an integrated health care delivery system provides coordinated care that allows participating providers, using economies of scale, to increase productivity, enhance the scope and quality of services, and reduce the administrative burden associated with those services. The goal of a mature, integrated health care delivery system is to become a provider organization that is seamless in its ability to deliver a broad range of health care services. Direct contracting is another financial arrangement that is gaining in popularity in the more mature markets. In direct contracting arrangements, the employer contracts directly with the provider to provide health care services, thus eliminating the insurer. The benefits to the provider in this type of arrangement are a known volume of beneficiaries and increased cash flow directly from the employer to the provider, generally on a monthly basis. The employer realizes decreased health care benefit costs and added value of working directly with the provider to realize specific services for their employee population.

RESPONSES TO MANAGED CARE

Provider responses to managed care varied from "bar the doors," to "respond only if pressured," to "let's reach out to the business community and begin strategic planning for these integrated services." The physician community appears to be most affected by the multiple changes in health care. Individual physicians have seen their autonomy and their often unique relationship with patients and families usurped by managed care companies. The individual physician in a solo practice cannot survive under either traditional managed care or any managed competition model. The cost of operating a small business is too high compared with the access to information and the discounted purchasing and discounted contracting provided by a managed care company or required by a health services purchasing cooperative. Managed care places new organizational demands on physicians, such as restricted referral and hospital panels, increased bureaucratic overhead from many types of plans, and an inability to refer out difficult patients. Many physicians view managed care with fear and loathing; loss of autonomy is the most common fear. As more nurse practitioners are becoming providers in the managed care environment, they may also experience these feelings of loss of autonomy. However, most nurses are experiencing increased opportunities in the managed care arena. Many managed care companies are seeing nurse practitioners and nurse midwives as cost-effective providers of primary care services and are increasing their provider panels to include these health professionals.

Physicians have led attempts to reduce medical costs since the introduction of PSROs in the 1960s. However, physician costs account for only about one fifth of the total health care dollar expenditure. They do, however, as gatekeepers, control the expenditure of many resources such as diagnostic tests and procedures. Until the late 1990s, physician income had not been greatly affected by health care reform.

As primary care providers increased their control of specialist care, however, physician income declined. In response to the pressure to reduce overall costs, physicians have organized into managed care organizations, have worked with hospitals in the development of clinical pathways, and have supported clinical case management in both the acute and community setting.

As 1998 came to a close, many managed care organizations were looking at the concept of the primary care provider as gatekeeper. Many organizations were rethinking the role of the specialist as gatekeeper for certain illnesses. They believed that certain diseases such as diabetes, asthma, and chronic pulmonary disease may be most cost-effectively managed by a specialist who is familiar with the effects of the disease on the entire body, rather than a primary care provider who may not be as knowledgeable of state-of-the-art treatments and medications. Although there is no consensus on the role of the primary care provider versus the specialist, the gatekeeper function may no longer be in the sole domain of the primary care provider.

Since the inception of DRGs in 1983, hospitals have been forced to focus on outcomes, utilization, and cost. For this reason, hospitals were better prepared than physicians for managed care. Physicians were not directly affected by DRGs because as private physicians they were reimbursed for services rendered in the hospital. Providers, such as hospitals, who accepted the managed care trend as reality, took a proactive approach to managed care. HMO contracting, network development, integrated service delivery, and the formation of independent managed care organizations have proliferated across the country. Resource allocation in the areas of inpatient care, outpatient care, and continuing care services are being evaluated and analyzed by individual providers as well as by networks. The goal is to be able to deliver seamless health care to specified populations. Inpatient utilization has dramatically decreased as managed care has penetrated certain markets.

Federal and state governments embraced the tenets of managed care and actively promoted Medicare and Medicaid managed care programs. Under these programs, Medicare and Medicaid recipients are enrolled in managed care programs in which they have a primary care provider from the managed care organization or HMO. In theory, they will receive the same access, quality, and cost that other members receive. This attempt by the government to reduce costs associated with caring for these distinct populations was under considerable scrutiny in late 1998-1999. The large for-profit health insurance companies and the Health Care Financing Administration (HCFA) found that many of the Medicare and Medicaid managed care programs were underfunded and unable to provide the services advertised to beneficiaries. In late 1998 several large companies withdrew from participating in Medicare and left many elderly individuals without health insurance. HCFA's total count as of October 1998 was that 507,727 Medicare beneficiaries would lose their current health plan coverage effective January 1999. The hardest hit state was Florida, followed by New York, California, Texas, Maryland, Washington, Ohio, Nevada, and Massachusetts.

These issues with managed Medicare and Medicaid bring to light other issues that are plaguing managed care providers as we begin the new millennium. There are increasing calls from grassroots consumer groups to hold managed care companies liable for bad outcomes of care, especially for individuals who are harmed by denials of care. The care issues being debated in 1998-1999 include the following:

- Liability of managed care providers
- Access questions, including choice of primary care provider, access to specialty care, and emergency care
- Timely claims decisions, including grievance and appeals provisions
- Privacy of medical information

Although there is an impact from managed care throughout the health care industry, there is specific impact on the operational areas of a facility. Providers have seen an increased need for discharge planning, social services, patient education, and a medical record that will follow the patient across multiple settings in a delivery system. The clinical impact has been evidenced by increased emphasis on length of stay reductions, evaluations of medical practice patterns with the purpose of reducing variation, the development of clinical pathways, and the implementation of case management. Although initially these clinical impact areas were mainly in the acute care institutions, the impact has spread to home care, sub-acute care, long-term care, and other continuing care services.

NURSE CASE MANAGEMENT IN A CHANGING ENVIRONMENT

Nurse case managers assist in creating and help to administer a network of services for their patients. The role of case manager was created solely to negotiate for, organize, and evaluate the need for using various resources for patient care. Traditionally case managers have operated between the realities of costs or covered services and the perceptions of patients' needs. The role of the case manager supports and embellishes the concepts of managed care.

Many professionals, as well as patients and families, can coordinate multiple services. The increased emphasis on discharge planning and social services highlights the need for professionals in these disciplines to coordinate these aspects of patient care both efficiently and effectively. However, the more complicated the services become or the more unable the patient or family becomes to coordinate care, the more an official case manager may be needed.

Nurse case managers traditionally have been based in conventional care settings (hospitals, hospices, clinics), dealing with episode-based management. Case managers sequence and organize services from many departments within the organization and are accountable for good financial and clinical outcomes. Nurse case management within the managed care environment has expanded to continuum-based case management in which accountability continues for good financial and clinical outcomes. The coordination of services and resources for the individual with complex needs continues indefinitely while the individual is covered by the managed care organization. In other words, the nurse case manager maintains a relationship with the individual after the disease or episode-specific problem has been resolved. In community health, nurses traditionally have practiced health promotion and disease prevention rather than cure and illness. This prevents the escalation of a person's health condition into a more serious condition. Community health nurses practice collaborative and comprehensive care rather than short-term intervention and episodic care. This integration of health services and health care delivery effects a more efficient use of health care services. Thus the community health care nurse can be an effective nurse case manager. In view of this, managed care programs have a unique opportunity to recognize the value of nursing both economically and in the provision of comprehensive care.

The nurse case manager must understand the contract the managed care organization or HMO has with the provider. This information is valuable in negotiating discharge and other care options for the patient. For example, if the managed care organization has a capitated or per diem financial arrangement with the provider, the organization is more willing to support less expensive settings for care delivery, such as home care, subacute care, or nursing home care. However, if the same provider has a DRG payment arrangement with the managed care organization, the organization may be less likely to support home care or a transitional care option until the patient has received inpatient services to cover the DRG prospective payment. In other words, home care may not be approved to expedite discharge, even though it is a covered benefit, until the patient has reached the DRG length of stay in the inpatient setting. In this instance the nurse case manager will need strong negotiation skills coupled with knowledge of the managed care financing system to advocate for the best quality care option for the patient.

As the nurse case manager identifies conflicts between managed care organization financing and quality-of-care issues, they should be brought to the attention of the provider administration. This information can be tracked and used in future contract negotiations with the managed care organization.

Nurse case managers are taking the lead in developing clinical pathways, practice guidelines, and outcomes measurements. Their knowledge of the health care environment and complex patient needs, coupled with their education and training, have given them the opportunity to lead multidisciplinary teams to develop cost-effective models of care that achieve positive patient outcomes and increased practitioner and patient satisfaction.

There are tremendous opportunities for nurse case managers in community-based practices where they assist individuals in managing both their health and their illnesses. Nurse case managers, who traditionally have dealt only with acute care, are now following up individuals beyond the walls of the facility into the clinic, home, and long-term care facility and assisting in coordinating services to keep them well. These practitioner-based models require sound financial and clinical judgment, as well as keen physical and psychosocial assessment skills. Some case management practices focus more on interaction with the individual by telephone rather than in person. Many managed care organizations prefer the telephone approach because of the decrease in overhead costs; however, it is impossible to measure the cost of losing the in-person interaction with the patient and family. Traditionally, nurse case managers believed that in identifying patient needs, nothing compares with the opportunity to use all of their senses in a complete face-to-face patient or family assessment. This assessment, coupled with sound financial and resource management of the individual's health benefits, results in the goals of managed care: high-quality, accessible care at the lowest possible cost. Nurse case management should never be considered a replacement for accountability in each professional discipline at the direct care level; for complex cases, however, there is no substitute for an effective nurse case management program.

Health care has seen a paradigm shift over the last decade of the 20th century. We are moving from a health care system built on a paradigm of unpredictable, acute simple disease to a focus on a paradigm of predictable, chronic complex illness that would favorably affect our ability to measure and manage quality care. According to the Centers for Disease Control and Prevention's National Center for Chronic Disease Prevention, chronic illness accounts for 90% of all illnesses and 70% of all deaths; it is the single most rapidly growing component of health care, and it is the greatest financial exposure for employers, business alliances, and managed care organizations. Case management may be moving toward an integrated lifetime care approach where a continuum of care is required that includes preventive, acute, psychological, rehabilitative, educational, and self-management interventions to meet both complex health and psychosocial needs of patients and families. This approach, again, supports the role of the nurse as the case manager. Nurses are educated to actively collaborate with individuals with complex, rare, or multiple risk factors. Nurses have a rich history in promoting preventive health and wellness services, with a focus on the patient's lifetime health care needs and concerns, as defined by the patient. As we look to the future, nurse case managers are well prepared and positioned to move into the role of the lifetime care manager.

Nurse case management also provides an excellent opportunity for the profession to increase public awareness of the role and image of nursing in the health care delivery system: to educate the consumer, the provider, and the payer as to the expertise of the nurse case manager, the registered professional nurse, and the advanced practice nurse. As one looks to the future, nursing research must validate the positive effect of nurse case management on health care costs, access to services, quality of services, and customer satisfaction.

References

Barth, S.M. (1997). Integrating payer and provider risk through capitation. *Managed Care Quarterly, 5*(1), 19-24.

Fuchs, V.R. (1990). The health sector's share of the gross national product. *Science, 247*, 534-538.

Garcia, L.B., Safriet, S., & Russell, D.C. (1998). *Healthcare financial management, 52*(7), 52-57.

Ginzberg, E. (1996). The potential and limits of competition in health care. *Bulletin of the New York Academy of Medicine, 73*, 224-236.

Grimaldi, P. (1998). Medicare's new capitation method. *Journal of Health Care Finance, 24*(4), 7-21.

Healthcare Underwriters Mutual, HUM Healthcare Systems, & PSS—Physician Sales & Service, Inc. (1996). *Managed care & capitation: Preparing for success.* Papers presented at a conference in Lake Placid, New York, May 9 & 10, 1996.

Kavaler, F., & Zavin, S. (1992). Health care for seamen in the port of New York. *New York State Journal of Medicine, 92*(8), 353-358.

Kennedy, K.M., & Merlino, D.J. (1998). Alternatives to traditional capitation in managed care agreements. *Healthcare Financial Management, 52*(4), 46-50.

Nelson, H. (1997). *Nonprofit & for-profit HMOs: Converging practices for different goals?* New York: Milbank Memorial Fund.

Phelps, C.E. (1997). *Health economics,* 2nd ed. Reading, Mass.: Addison Wesley Longman, Inc.

Reinhardt, U.E. (1995). Turning our gaze from bread and circus games. *Health Affairs, 14*(2), 33-36.

Bibliography

Blendon, R.J., et al. (1993). Physician's perspectives on caring for patients in the United States, Canada, and West Germany. *The New England Journal of Medicine, 328*(9), 621-627.

Deloitte & Touche, LLP and HCIA, Inc. (1995). *The comparative performance of U.S. hospitals: The sourcebook.* Baltimore: Author.

Gaynor, M., & Vogt, W.B. (1997). What does economics have to say about health policy anyway? A comment and correction on Evans and Rice (commentary). *Journal of Health Politics, Policy and Law, 22,* 475-496.

Kongstvedt, P.R. (Ed.). (1993). *The managed health care handbook,* 2nd ed. Gaithersburg, Md.: Aspen Publications.

Kongstvedt, P.R. (Ed.). (1995). *Essentials of managed care.* Gaithersburg, Md.: Aspen Publications.

Marmor, T.R. (1998). Forecasting American health care: How we got here and where we might be going. *Journal of Health Politics, Policy and Law, 23,* 551-571.

Menkin, H. (Ed.). (1997). *Handbook of managed care terminology.* Albany, N.Y.: CHPS Consulting.

Saward, E.W., & Fleming, S. (1980). Health maintenance organizations. *Scientific American, 243*(4), 47-53.

Sonnefeld, S.T., et al. (1991, Fall). Projections of the national health expenditures through the year 2000, *Health Care Financing.*

Financing Health Care in the United States

Economic and Policy Implications

Richard W. Redman

CHAPTER OVERVIEW

The financing of health care in the United States has evolved into a model unique among major industrialized countries in the world. The market-driven economy of the United States is clearly reflected in the way in which health care is paid for. In addition to these market features, the American value of individual rights prevailing over those of community good also is evident in health care. American citizens demand the right to choose their health care provider and the types of services they want in the same way that they make all other consumer choices. Although this "right to choose" has been challenged somewhat during the era of managed care, individuals still are willing to pay additional money where possible to maintain their freedom of choice. These unique American values have contributed to the way health care system financing has evolved.

This chapter provides an overview of how the major financing mechanisms in the United States have evolved as well as an examination of the total amount of national resources allocated for health care services. Issues and trends in the financing of health care delivery are also presented. As seen, the financing mechanisms and the projections for the future provide an excellent foundation for the role of the nurse case manager as the coordinator of resources for the delivery of quality health care services efficiently and effectively.

FINANCING MECHANISMS FOR HEALTH CARE

During the second half of the 20th century, the financing of the American health care system has undergone tremendous change. The fee-for-service payment mechanism, where purchasers of care paid for each health care service or product, has been replaced for the most part by managed care models with fixed payments and capitation. Even traditional indemnity insurance programs, such as Aetna and Metropolitan, and government insurance programs, such as Medicare and Medicaid, have adopted the principles and practices of managed care. These practices include programs such as second opinion, hospital precertification, and case management for groups with high-cost diseases and conditions.

"*Managed care*" refers to both an organization that coordinates the purchase and/or delivery of health care services and a set of techniques used to ensure the efficiency and effectiveness of the use of health care services. The health maintenance organization (HMO) is often seen as the prototype for a managed care organization, although in reality it is only one of many organizational forms. Managed care techniques, increasingly used by any type of health care provider or purchaser, include financial incentives for providers, health promotion and risk reduction programs, early identification of disease, disease management programs, and utilization management.

At the beginning of the 20th century, hospitals were not the center of the health care system. In fact, the ability of the health care system to meet the major challenges of the day, such as infectious diseases, was minimal. Most services were provided by physicians in their offices or to people in their homes at low cost. After World War II, the level of sophistication of health care interventions and technologies available began to gradually change. With that came increased cost of health services and an unrelenting demand on the part of the American public for whatever treatment the health care system could provide.

The payment mechanisms for health reflected this evolution and change in consumer demand throughout the century. From 1920 to 1950, different financing mechanisms developed to meet the needs of consumers for purchasing health care services. The first Blue Cross program was developed in 1929. Several HMOs were also developed during this period, primarily to meet the needs of various groups of industrial employees. These early HMOs are still evident today and include Kaiser (founded in 1937 in California), Group Health Association (founded in Washington, D.C., in 1937), and Group Health Cooperative of Puget Sound (founded in Washington State in 1947) (Fox, 1996).

The government became a major purchaser of health care when the Medicare program was implemented in 1965. This was followed shortly after by Medicaid, a program jointly funded by the federal and state governments. These programs enabled many who did not previously have access to health care services. This time period is often seen as the beginning of a 40-year period of unprecedented growth in health care, in terms of both the types of services and therapies available and the continual increase in costs to provide those services. As the third-party payment system evolved, the individual consumer was not directly responsible for payment of the health care services. This dynamic contributed to ever-increasing demand for services, often without awareness of their cost.

Until the early 1980s, most health care was paid for on a fee-for-service basis. It was referred to as retrospective payment because the bill for health care services was determined after all needed services were provided. This type of payment mechanism is now viewed as having served as an incentive for providers to deliver whatever the patient required or demanded, since it would be paid for by the purchaser, often an insurance company or governmental agency. During the 1970s, a period of high inflationary growth in all sectors of the American economy, health care costs skyrocketed. As a means to control health care inflation, several cost-containment and cost-limiting programs were introduced. First, voluntary mechanisms were employed; eventually they became mandated programs. These programs concentrated on the hospital sector because this increasingly was the most expensive component in the health care system. Eventually, the programs focused on physician services as well (Abbey, 1996; Fisher & Welch, 1999; Fox, 1996).

In the 1980s, a new payment mechanism was introduced. Prospective payment systems were implemented for hospital care. Diagnosis-related groups (DRGs) were implemented, first by Medicare and then quickly by other payer groups, with fixed payments attached for each DRG. This resulted in a major change in incentives for providers, which had become quite adept at functioning under the retrospective payment incentives. Under prospective payment, hospitals now had incentives to control the utilization of resources and the length of stay to minimize expenditures. If a hospital spent more to care for a patient than would be reimbursable under the fixed payment system, the hospital had to absorb the loss.

During the 1980s, the principles and techniques of managed care also began to be employed by indemnity insurance groups. Examples include the requirement of second opinion programs for elective surgery and the use of case management programs for high-cost diseases and conditions. Large employer groups also became much more involved in purchasing health care for the benefit packages of their employees. Often employers pointed out that the health care system was operating inefficiently and, as employers who provided health care benefits, they declined to absorb the annual inflation in health care services that they had to purchase for employees. Employers began to introduce utilization review programs. In addition, they became very interested in the competitive pricing available through managed care providers. The rapid growth in managed care throughout the United States is generally attributed to large employer groups, which turned rapidly to this form of health care financing as a cost-effective approach to meeting the health benefit needs of their employees.

Consumers have demonstrated their dissatisfaction with tightly controlled managed care programs, beginning in the late 1990s. Consumers prefer broader access to providers despite higher costs associated with that access. Enrollments in managed care options have been shifting from tightly controlled, lower cost HMO plans to more loosely managed, higher cost models, such as preferred provider options (PPO) and point of service (POS) plans. In addition, by 2001 the participation of Medicare enrollees in managed care programs declined by approximately 10% (Levit, Smith, Cowan, Lazenby, Sensenig, & Catlin, 2003). These indicators provide evidence that Americans continue to prefer freedom of choice even when it results in higher costs for their health care.

CURRENT LEVELS OF EXPENDITURES

The United States spent $1.42 trillion on health care in 2001—approximately $5,035 for each citizen. Private funding for health care comprised 54.8% of total expenditures ($778.1 billion); public or government sources paid for 45.2% ($658.8 billion) (Centers for Medicare & Medicaid Services, 2003). The sources of public and private funds and the types of goods and services they purchased can be seen in Table 21-1.

TABLE 21-1	HEALTH CARE EXPENDITURES IN THE UNITED STATES: 2001
Expenditure	**Percentage of Total**
SOURCES OF FUNDS	
Private insurance	34.8
Medicare	16.9
Medicaid	15.7
Other public sources	12.6
Out-of-pocket	14.4
Other private sources	5.3
DISTRIBUTION OF FUNDS	
Hospital care	32.8
Professional services	33.7
Nursing homes	7.2
Prescription drugs	10.2
Program administration costs	6.5
Other*	9.4

*Includes home health care, over-the-counter drugs and supplies, durable medical equipment, research, and public health programs.
Source: National Center for Health Statistics. Health United States, 2002.
Note: Numbers may not sum to totals because of rounding.

As the data illustrate, hospital and physician expenditures traditionally account for the majority of health care expenditures. However, growth in those categories has slowed in recent years. Expenditures for prescription drugs have increased dramatically because of the availability of new high-priced drugs, increased consumer demand for the drugs, and an increase in the number of prescriptions filled (Levit, Smith, Cowan, Lazenby, Sensenig, & Catlin, 2003).

Health insurance coverage is an important determinant of access to health care services. Individuals without either private or public health insurance coverage are more likely to report unmet needs for health care, less likely to have a usual source of health care, and less likely to receive preventive health care services (Peters, 1998).

The level of funding from public sources has led to debate about whether the U.S. health care system is private or public. In 1996, 43.1% of the U.S. population had health insurance paid for by private-sector employers. An additional 34% had publicly funded health insurance covered by Medicaid, Medicare, insurance resulting from former or current military service, or the Indian Health Service. Approximately 7% purchased their own insurance coverage, and nearly 18% were uninsured (Carrasquillo, Himmelstein, Woolhandler, & Bor, 1999). These data suggest that the U.S. system is still primarily a privately funded system, although the share of health care paid for by public sources is increasing. Private employers as purchasers of health insurance for employee benefit packages remain very influential in the health care marketplace.

ISSUES AND TRENDS

The evolution of the health care financing system and the interplay of the public and private sectors has shaped the health care delivery system as we know it today. Several issues and trends are noteworthy for the foreseeable future. These trends include continual increases in the cost of health care, system inequities, increasing potential for challenging decisions and ethical dilemmas, the increased importance of primary care providers, and renewed interest in population health outcomes.

Continuing Increases in Costs of Health Care

The annual increase in health care costs continues to outpace general inflation and the costs of other goods and services in society. In 2001, the growth in health care spending, an increase of 8.7% over the previous year, was the greatest in the past 10 years. The fastest growing category in health care expenses continues to be prescription drugs. In 2001, the costs for prescription drugs increased 15.7% over the previous year. Spending on prescription drugs grew almost twice as fast as that on all other health services, a pattern that has been evident in recent years. Hospital spending increases also continued to outpace inflation (Levit, Smith, Cowan, Lazenby, Sensenig, & Catlin, 2003).

Projections for spending on health care services through 2012 are expected to continue at an annual rate of 7.3%. Health care costs continue to outpace the general increases in costs of other goods and services. In 2002, the general consumer prices inflation rate for non-health care goods and services was approximately 1.1% (Heffler, Smith, Keehan, Clemens, Won, & Zizza, 2003). These continuing patterns place enormous pressures on society to try and deal with the seemingly uncontrollable cost of health care.

In 2000, a comparison with other industrial countries in the world revealed that the United States spent far more on health care than any other country. The U.S. level of expenditures for health care was 44% higher than that of Switzerland, the country with the next-highest level spending, and 83% higher than that of neighboring Canada. In that same time, U.S. spending was 134% higher than the median expenditures for the comparable industrial companies. Although the United States spends more on health care, the United States is below most measures of health service use compared with those other countries. The difference in spending appears to be due to the higher prices for health care goods and services in the United States (Anderson, Reinhardt, Hussey, & Petrosyan, 2003).

System Inequities and Disparities

The market-based financing for health care in the United States has contributed to many of the inequities that citizens experience with respect to access to quality health care services. The American system is often described as employer based because nearly all individuals who have access to private health insurance receive that insurance as part of employer benefits packages. In general, individuals who are not employed either depend on public sources of funding, such as Medicaid, or have no coverage.

In 1997, 18% of individuals between ages 18 and 64 years had no health insurance. Seventy-three percent of individuals had private insurance, 7% had Medicaid or some other type of public assistance, and Medicare covered 2%. Once an individual reaches age 65 years, Medicare coverage is available, so less than 1% of the elderly are uninsured (Amaradio, 1998; Health Care Financing Administration, 1999a).

The rapid diversification in the racial and ethnic composition of the United States is presenting new challenges to health care. Considerable inequities exist among different groups in society. There is growing evidence that racial and ethnic minorities receive lower quality of health care. The responsible factors are both historic and contemporary and include issues such as unequal access to health, differential treatment rates, discrimination, and racial bias (Smedley, Stith, & Nelson, 2003).

Major disparities are evident when the white population is compared with nonwhite populations, especially those who are black or Hispanic. These disparities are evident in infant mortality, life expectancy, homicide rates, motor vehicle–related injuries, suicide rates, and rates of many health conditions and diseases (National Center for Health Statistics, 2002).

Hispanic adults are much more likely to be uninsured than are white or black adults in the United States. In 1997, 34% of Hispanic adults lacked health insurance, more than twice the percent of non-Hispanic white persons without health insurance coverage and almost 60% more than the numbers of U.S. blacks without insurance coverage (Health Care Financing Administration, 1998, 1999a; Pamuk, Makuc, Heck, Reuben, & Lochner, 1998).

Lower socioeconomic level adults are much more likely to be uninsured regardless of race, ethnicity, or sex. Lower socioeconomic level white, black, or Hispanic men are 7 times as likely to be uninsured. Lower socioeconomic level white women are 8 times more likely than those with high incomes to be uninsured. At each level of income, Hispanics are more likely to be uninsured than either their white or black counterparts. Within most income categories, the numbers of blacks without insurance are either slightly higher or similar to whites without insurance. Lower socioeconomic level black women are less likely than lower socioeconomic level white women to be uninsured because of their higher levels of Medicaid coverage (Pamuk et al., 1998).

Unless a major change is made in the financing system for health care, it is unlikely that these inequities will change. In fact, they have continued to increase over the past two decades and will likely continue without some type of government intervention. It does not appear that Americans are willing to establish a nationalized health care system, especially if it would compromise choice. Given this fact, it does not appear that a resolution to the growing numbers of uninsured will be forthcoming in the short run.

Importance of the Primary Care Provider

The shift to managed care mechanisms has resulted in the dominance of primary care providers who have assumed responsibility for overseeing the allocation of resources in a managed care system. In a dramatic role reversal, primary care providers have generally risen above specialists in the health care hierarchy.

Primary care providers serve as gatekeepers who control access to services and specialty care in the managed care network. Many of these primary care providers are nurse practitioners who work in collaboration with large physician organizations or individual physician associations (IPAs). The functions performed by these primary care providers have been essential in managed care systems. In addition, they have given renewed interest within the medical care system to preventive and health promoting services, the hallmark of primary care providers.

Future Health Policy: Individuals versus Populations and Illness versus Wellness

The U.S. health care system is often criticized because of its overwhelming focus on illness and disease, especially given the amount of resources allocated to these types of services. A preferred approach would be to refocus services and incentives to promote health and reduce present or future risk for developing disease. While it is difficult currently to identify a clear national health policy in the United States, the focus on illness and disease is clear.

Peters (1998) states that U.S. health care policy has been built on a "clinical" model that has provided financial incentives for sophisticated technological excellence. Evidence of this includes the ongoing allocation of large amounts of the total health care dollar to hospital care and related treatments and interventions. Even in the managed care arena, it is often difficult to identify a focus or set of incentives directed toward health promotion. Often the cost savings in managed care are associated with the treatment of disease after it has developed, rather than examining cost savings associated with preventive services (Peters, 1998). An example of this would be the comparative study of breast cancer stage at diagnosis and treatment patterns for elderly women in HMO and fee-for-service settings. The results indicated that HMO enrollees are less likely to have breast cancer diagnosed at later stages than women in fee-for-service settings. While this evidence supports the importance of early detection in managed care environments, it also supports the observation that even managed care groups are often focused on cost-reducing treatments rather than extensive screening programs (Riley, Potosky, Klabunde, Warren, & Ballard-Barbash, 1999).

Kindig (1999) recommends that health policy must move beyond focusing on individuals and begin to emphasize population health as the desired outcome. In fee-for-service and capitated systems, incentives encourage providers to produce fewer hospital days and services along with lower unit prices. However, this focus on individuals fails to place individuals in a social context, ignoring the important contributions to health made by nonmedical factors such as socioeconomic status, the environment, and other societal factors. Given that the general indices of health in the United States, such as mortality rates, are still at unacceptable levels, policy needs to focus on the development of incentives and services that will contribute to the overall health of populations (Moskowitz, 1997).

A paradigm shift from individual to population is beginning to appear. Managed care concepts are compatible with this population focus, although the annual turnover in many HMO enrollee groups still operates against a population incentive in the long run. Given the large investment of public funds in purchasing health care, developing policies and programs that serve as incentives for increasing the health of populations will provide improved health outcomes per dollar invested.

Medicaid Challenges

In 2002, Medicaid provided services for one in every seven Americans. It is the largest purchaser of long-term care and care for individuals with human immunodeficiency virus infection/acquired immune deficiency syndrome; it lends major support to hospitals as a "safety-net" purchaser of care for those who do not have other types of insurance coverage; it pays for one third of all births in the United States; it is a major purchaser of care for those who have major mental disorders; and it covers the cost of early screening programs for eligible children. Yet, Medicaid is in jeopardy due to most states, and the federal government facing large budget deficits. The rapid decline in state funds coupled with the continual double-digit increases in health care expenditures are critical challenges for nearly all state-based Medicaid programs (Iglehart, 2003).

Medicaid spending, however, is projected to increase until at least 2012. This is due to the global economic recession and the difficulty in getting jobs, increased unemployment, and challenges for both skilled and unskilled workers (Heffler, Smith, Keehan, Clemens, Won, & Zizza, 2003). This projection is likely to continue to stress the Medicaid system, described as the "workhorse" of the U.S. health care system. It is uncertain how Medicaid will evolve under the increasing economic and social challenges (Weil, 2003). What is clear, however, is that without Medicaid, at least 51 million Americans, primarily poor women and their children, would be without health care coverage.

Implications of Slower Expansion in Future Health Care Expenditures

As mentioned previously, the U.S. health care system has undergone a 40-year expansion with continual growth and increased spending. This era is often referred to as the Golden Age of Health Care. However, recent statistics suggest that a plateau has been reached in the percentage of gross domestic product (GDP) allocated to health care in the United States. The share of GDP for health care had been increasing gradually over a 30-year period, reaching a high point of 13.6% for the years 1993 through 1996. In 1997, however, health spending as a share of GDP fell slightly to 13.5% (Fisher & Welch, 1999; Health Care Financing Administration, 1999a). By 2001, the health care share of the GDP was 14.1%. Although this is an increase over previous years, it is a much slower rate (National Center for Health Statistics, 2002). This plateau followed by a much slower rate of increase provides the first signs that the United States may no longer be able to sustain unlimited growth in expenditures for health care.

The gross indicators of morbidity and mortality are still at undesirably high levels, suggesting there is major room for improvement in the health care system. Yet, we are increasingly faced with difficult choices about how to allocate these fixed or declining resources for health care needs. The dynamics of public health care policy in a fixed state are projected to be very different from those when the health care economy was continually expanding. It is likely that the American public will face difficult decisions, including the possibility of rationing of health care. This type of decision-making has been unacceptable to the American public in the past. It also is likely to exaggerate the inequities and maldistribution of health care resources still seen today.

References

Abbey, F.B. (1996). Managed care and health care reform: Evolution or revolution? In P.R. Kongstvedt (Ed.), *The managed care handbook*, 3rd ed. Gaithersburg, Md.: Aspen Publications.

Amaradio, L. (Winter 1998). Financing long-term care for elderly persons: What are the options? *J Health Care Finance, 25*, 75-84.

Anderson, G.F., Reinhardt, U.W., Hussey, P.S., & Petrosyan, V. (2003). It's the prices, stupid: Why the United States is so different from other countries. *Health Affairs, 22*(3), 89-105.

Carrasquillo, O., Himmelstein, D.U., Woolhandler, S., & Bor, D.H. (1999, Jan. 14). A reappraisal of private employers' role in providing health insurance. *New England Journal of Medicine, 340*, 109-114.

Centers for Medicare & Medicaid Services (2003). *Highlights of health care expenditures.* Office of the Actuary, National Health Statistics Group. Available at: http://cms.hhs.gov.researchers/statsdata.asp.

Fisher, E.S., & Welch, H.G. (1999, Feb. 3). Avoiding the unintended consequences of growth in medical care: How might more be worse? *Journal of the American Medical Association, 281*, 446-453.

Fox, P.D. (1996). An overview of managed care. In P.R. Kongstvedt (Ed.), *The managed care handbook*, 3rd ed. Gaithersburg, Md.: Aspen Publications.

Health Care Financing Administration (1998). Statistical supplement. *Health Care Financing Review.* Washington, D.C.: HCFA.

Health Care Financing Administration (1999a). *Highlights: National health expenditures,* 1997. Washington, D.C.: HCFA.

Health Care Financing Administration (1999b). *Highlights of the national health expenditure projections, 1997-2007.* Washington, D.C.: HCFA.

Heffler, S., Smith, S., Keehan, S., Clemens, M.K., Won, G., & Zizza, M. (2003). Health spending projections for 2002-2012. *Health Affairs, WebExclusive: W3,* 54-65. Available at: http://www.healthaffairs.org/WebExclusives/Heffler_Web_Excl_020703.htm.

Iglehart, J.K. (2003). The dilemma of Medicaid. *New England Journal of Medicine, 348*(21), 2140-2148.

Kindig, D.A. (1999). Purchasing population health: Aligning financial incentives to improve health outcomes. *Nursing Outlook, 47,* 15-22.

Levit, K., Smith, C., Cowan, C., Lazenby, H., Sensenig, A., & Catlin, A. (2003). Trends in U.S. health care spending, 2001. *Health Affairs, 22*(1), 154-164.

Moskowitz, D.B. (Ed.). (1997). *Health care almanac & yearbook.* New York: Faulkner & Gray, Inc.

National Center for Health Statistics (2002). *Health, United States, 2002: With chartbook on trends in the health of Americans.* Hyattsville, Md.: NCHS. Available at: http://www.cdc.gov/nchs/products/pubs/pubd/hus/hus02.pdf.

Pamuk, E., Makuc, D., Heck, K., Reuben, C., Lochner, K. (Eds.) (1998). *Health, United States, 1998 with socioeconomic status and health chartbook.* Hyattsville, Md.: National Center for Health Statistics.

Peters, R.M. (1998). The negative effect of the clinical model of "health": Implications for health care policy. *J Health Care Finance, 25,* 78-92.

Riley, G.F., Potosky, A.L., Klabunde, C.N., Warren, J.L., Ballard-Barbash, R. (1999). Stage at diagnosis and treatment patterns among older women with breast cancer. *Journal of the American Medical Association, 281,* 720-726.

Smedley, B.D., Stith, A.Y., & Nelson, A.R. (Eds.) (2003). *Unequal treatment: Confronting racial and ethnic disparities in health care.* Institute of Medicine. Washington, D.C.: The National Academies Press.

Weil, A. (2003). There's something about Medicaid. *Health Affairs, 22*(1), 13-30.

22

Public Policy and Community-Based Case Management

*The Nurse-Family Partnership**

Patricia Moritz
Ruth A. O'Brien

CHAPTER OVERVIEW

This chapter traces the evolution of case management from the coordination of care for individuals with high-cost, high-volume illnesses to a community-based approach focused on health promotion and disease prevention at a population level. A salient factor contributing to the emergence of community-based models of case management is the increasing support to adopt more evidence-based programs as the cornerstone of public health practice. The Nurse-Family Partnership (NFP), an exemplar of community-based case management that uses an evidence-based approach in working with low-income, first-time parents from vulnerable populations, is described in depth. Finally, policy issues in the implementation of the NFP as a community-based case management strategy are enumerated.

PUBLIC HEALTH IN THE UNITED STATES: A PUBLIC POLICY TARGET IN THE TWENTY-FIRST CENTURY

Before 1900, infectious diseases represented the most serious threat to the health of populations throughout the world. Public health actions to prevent and control infectious diseases resulted in marked reductions in their incidence and prevalence in the United States by the early 1950s. Increasingly, attention shifted toward the prevention of morbidity and mortality arising from chronic illnesses, such as heart disease, cancer, stroke, diabetes, etc. Although early efforts in this arena were focused on screening and health education activities targeted toward at risk populations, gaps in the medical care system related to the care of indigent and uninsured populations and the availability of federal grant dollars to help fill those gaps gradually fostered the emergence of the provision of a wide array of personal health services by state and local public health entities.

In 1988, the Institute of Medicine (IOM) released a landmark report, *The Future of Public Health*, which reexamined the links between medical and public health practice. Based on extensive analysis of data collected through interviews and forums, the IOM concluded that "the system of public health activities had fallen into disarray" (p. 19) and that decision-making in public health was being driven by crises and the concerns of organized special interest groups, rather than by accurate data and continual assessment of community needs. The IOM report proposed to define the boundaries of public health by identifying three core functions: assessment, policy development, and assurance.

*Aspects of the work reported here are funded by the Robert Wood Johnson Foundation, No. 03569.

UNDERSTANDING THE CORE FUNCTIONS OF PUBLIC HEALTH

Clarity about the overall mission of public health is central to an understanding of the core functions. The IOM Committee affirmed that the primary aim of public health "is to generate organized community effort to address public concerns about health by applying scientific and technical knowledge to prevent disease and promote health." (p. 7). To accomplish this mission, public health services need to be population based. Practice aimed at a population addresses the overall health profile of the targeted group of people as opposed to treatment of individual needs. Typically, the interventions are aimed at risk factors that contribute to health problems and may focus on behavior, such as preventing tobacco use among pregnant women, or on environmental hazards, such as air pollution (Berkowitz, Dahl, Guirl, Kostelecky, McNeil, & Upenicks, 2001). The core functions provide a process for determining the services needed by a population.

Assessment

Assessment involves the regular collection, analysis, and interpretation of information about health conditions, risks, and resources in a community. Through the assessment function, trends in illness, injury, and death and the factors that may contribute to these events are identified and available services to address these issues are examined for adequacy, accessibility, and acceptability. Assessment results provide the foundation for policy development (Turnock, 2001).

Policy Development

Policy development involves prioritizing the health problems identified in the community, setting goals, and applying scientific knowledge in decision making about the best courses of action to address the problems. The process necessitates consideration of political, organizational, and community values to handle divergent views about what should be done and how resources should be allocated. Effective policy formulation incorporates broad information sharing, citizen participation, compromise, and consensus to nurture shared ownership of the policy decisions (Berkowitz et al., 2001; IOM, 1988).

Assurance

This function calls for state and local public health entities to assure their constituents that services necessary to achieve agreed upon goals are provided, either by encouraging actions by the private sector, by requiring such action through regulation, or by providing the services directly (Turnock, 2001). The assurance function also requires the monitoring of health services provided and evaluating whether the desired outcomes are attained (IOM, 1988).

CASE MANAGEMENT INTEGRAL TO PUBLIC HEALTH NURSING

Public health nursing has long had case management as an integral part of the repertoire of community-based strategies implemented with families and individuals within them. As nurses in public health practice evaluated the core functions for implementation recognition developed that these functions occur across three interacting levels—the community, health system, and family and individuals (Keller, Schaffer, Lia-Hoagberg, & Strohschein, 2002). The focus of nursing and its interventions occur within the core functions. Keller and colleagues (1998) identified 17 nursing interventions in public health nursing practice with *case management* defined as coordination of comprehensive care for individuals, families, and groups that require extensive services (p. 210). An important expansion of the definition notes that case management is "used to optimize self-care capabilities, promote efficient use of services, decrease fragmentation of care across settings, provide quality care in least restrictive environment, and promote cost containment."

Case management has evolved in public health practice as the health care requirements of the nation have changed, moving from a strict surveillance and quarantine mode when infectious diseases were rampant to today, when the emphasis is more on prevention, chronic disease management, and underserved populations. Public health nursing also has evolved as the sources of payment for their interventions have increasingly focused on the site and purpose of service, such as the home, clinic, or school (Keller et al., 1998). Among the interventions that nurses in public health integrate into their case management practice are surveillance and assessment, health teaching and counseling, referrals as needed and follow-up, delegated treatments, and advocacy.

STRENGTHENING POLICY DEVELOPMENT THROUGH EVIDENCE-BASED PUBLIC HEALTH PRACTICE

With increasing emphasis on the cost of health care and recognition of concerns about care quality and patient safety, health care systems began to change to a focus on managing individuals with high-cost, high-volume illnesses such as diabetes. As managed care evolved through the 1990s, health care organizations increased their emphasis on supporting interventions, therapies, and treatments with known effectiveness because of their responsibility for both care delivery and payment for that care within a structure of finite resources. The goal was to be able to predict health outcomes and lessen variation in practice that could not be explained by what was known. This approach came to be called *evidenced-based practice*, meaning that there was strong scientific evidence and informed clinical judgment underpinning decisions about therapeutic choices (Straus & Sackett, 1998; Sackett, Rosenberg, Gray, Haynes, & Richardson, 1996). Ingersoll (2000), building on the early developmental work for evidence-based medicine, addressed questions about evidence based practice being without a theoretical perspective and expanded the definitional components for such an approach in nursing practice. This work clarifies what the meanings of evidenced-based practice, administration, and education are within nursing.

The assessment of outcomes in health care practice is strengthened when there is evidence that shows what interventions and therapies are effective and which ones are not. Sidani and Braden (1998) have provided a strategy for outcomes assessment within nursing that bases such an approach on the theoretical and scientific knowledge of the interventions being implemented by nurses in practice. This approach gives outcomes assessment an important theoretical perspective.

Public health practice has been increasingly reviewed with the same vigor as is used in acute and primary care practice, but the study methods to attain strong evidence are different, the volume of evidence smaller, and the time between the delivery of the intervention and the effect on outcomes longer (Brownson et al., 2003). Evidence for public health practice is based on population-focused epidemiologic data in which intervention effects take time to occur, samples are large, and studies are costly to complete. These studies generally have no clear single 'gold standard' such as randomized controlled trials because studies of intervention effectiveness and efficiency are conducted when there is indication of efficacy, populations cannot be controlled in the same way as can be small clinical trial samples, and the cost of such trials are prohibitive.

Health policy is both informed by and informs public health practice and research. Brownson and colleagues (2003) note that the definition of *evidence-based public health* has been broadened to include a focus on practice, delivery systems, and policies. In responding to major national concern about quality in health care delivery, the Institute of Medicine of the National Academy of Sciences identified five core competencies and called for their implementation by all health professions, including nursing (Greiner & Knebel, 2003). Among these core competencies are the utilization of evidence-based practice, the provision of patient-centered care, and the application quality of improvement strategies.

Public health practice includes approaches for prevention, especially primary prevention, management of diseases and health problems in the community, application of behavioral science concepts and strategies, and recognition that social factors can inherently confound health. Recently, Lavis and colleagues (2003) described a framework for the effective transfer of knowledge to decision-makers active in health policy development and practice. Such a framework, when implemented as the guiding structure for informing decision-making by clinicians and policymakers, can facilitate both evidence-based practice and evidenced-based health policy.

THE NURSE-FAMILY PARTNERSHIP: AN EXEMPLAR OF COMMUNITY-BASED CASE MANAGEMENT

Program Description

The Nurse-Family Partnership (NFP) is an exemplar of community-based case management that uses an evidence-based approach to address identified community needs at a population level. Among the community needs addressed are rates of premature and low birth weight infants, child maltreatment and neglect, childhood injuries, family violence, school failure, antisocial behavior and juvenile crime. The NFP targets low-income first-time parents and their families during pregnancy and through the first 2 years of the child's life to accomplish three goals: (1) improve pregnancy outcomes by helping women alter their health-related behaviors, including reducing use of cigarettes, alcohol, and illegal drugs; (2) improve child health and development by helping parents provide more responsible and competent care for their children, and (3) improve families' economic self-sufficiency by helping parents develop a vision for their own future, plan future pregnancies, continue their education, and find work.

Bronfenbrenner's (1979, 1992) person-process-context model derived from human ecology theory, with the integration of human attachment (Bowlby, 1969) and self-efficacy theory (Bandura, 1982), provides a theoretical framework that guides the work of nurse home visitors with families. Although nurses have a structured set of visit-by-visit guidelines, they adapt them as needed to address the individual needs of families. On average, nurses visit weekly for the first month to establish a relationship and then every other week throughout pregnancy. Following the birth of the infant, weekly visits are resumed for the first 6 weeks postpartum and then decrease to every other week until the child is 21 months old. To facilitate termination of the relationship, nurses visit monthly thereafter through the child's second birthday.

The NFP approach to case management emphasizes primary prevention in that it focuses on an at-risk population of women and their families who have had no previous live births. Each full time nurse carries a caseload of 25 families. The early emphasis on beginning the intervention in pregnancy affords an opportunity to help women avoid unhealthy behaviors (cigarette smoking, alcohol consumption, and use of illegal drugs) that have the potential to result in neurodevelopmental impairment of the developing fetus, a significant factor in childhood behavioral problems and the later emergence of antisocial and criminal behavior. In providing support and guidance to young families while they are learning the parental role, it is reasoned that the skills and resources that parents develop to provide competent and responsible care of their first child will carry over to later children. And to the extent that the program is successful in helping parents plan for their futures, they are likely to have fewer unintended pregnancies and to develop the life skills (education, job training) necessary to enhance the material and social environment in which their children are raised (Olds, Kitzman, Cole & Robinson, 1997; Olds, Pettitt, et al., 1998).

Population-based practice has again emerged as the cornerstone of public health following the IOM report, but population-based interventions may be directed at entire populations within a community, the systems that affect the health of those populations, and/or the individuals and families within those populations known to be at risk (Keller et al., 2002). The NFP primarily intervenes at the individual/family level to change behavior and develop knowledge, skills and attitudes supportive of health, working with those families who are members of the designated population within a community that has been assessed as at-risk for adverse maternal and child outcomes. However, in working with families, nurse home visitors also advocate for changes in the policies of health and social service systems that serve them. A more detailed discussion of the varying roles that nurse home visitors use in their work with families follows.

Case Management Roles of the NFP Nurse Home Visitor

Central to the successful implementation of the NFP is the establishment of a trusting relationship with the family, referred to as the COACH Relationship Model (Hanks, Kitzman, & Milligan, 1995). The acronym COACH reflects the core ingredients of the relationship: *c*aring, *o*ngoing commitment, *a*ctive involvement of the family, *c*onsideration of family's culture and life situation, and *h*armony or congruence among the family's values, goals for change, and behaviors. Nurse home visitors use a strength-based approach directed toward optimizing the family's competence for self-care, that is, to develop their capabilities to take charge of their lives and make their own choices. Four strategies are intrinsic to building a family's competence for self-help: (1) listening to what families want and starting there; (2) believing that families are the experts on their own lives and are capable of making choices to attain desired goals; (3) expanding families' visions of options; and (4) helping families to set small and reasonable goals that when attained contribute to their growing sense of efficacy (O'Brien & Baca, 1997; Zerwekh, 1991). The latter necessitates that nurse home visitors assume multiple case management roles.

CLINICAL EXPERT
Nurse home visitors use their comprehensive knowledge of pregnancy and child health and development to identify the individual needs of each family relative to program's goals.

CHANGE AGENT
Much of the home visitor's interactions with women and their families focus on helping them to identify goals they want to attain for themselves. In this respect, nurses facilitate change by assisting families to identify what behaviors and actions are necessary to attain a desired goal, whether it involves quitting smoking, deferring a second pregnancy, or returning to school to obtain a high school diploma. Once the goal has been established, they support family members to initiate and maintain the behaviors needed to achieve it. Nurses are guided in this work through the use of Prochaska, Norcross, and DiClemente's stages of change (1994) and a series of "facilitators" (assessment tools) incorporated into the home visit guidelines.

EDUCATOR
Health teaching is central to any program, such as the NFP, that focuses on primary prevention. The home visit guidelines can be thought of as providing a map with multiple pathways for assisting families

toward program goals. Based on an assessment of learning readiness and reading level, home visitors provide information on a variety of such topics as nutrition, child health and development, home safety, and contraception. A parenting education curriculum, Partners in Parenting Education (PIPE) (Dolezol & Butterfield, 1994), is used by home visitors to engage parents in hands-on supervised interactions that facilitate the reading of infant cues and responding sensitively. For example, parents are taught how to use an interesting toy to distract infant/toddler from a prohibited activity in a nonthreatening way.

COORDINATOR OF CARE

Nurse home visitors routinely assess families' needs and then systematically help them make use of other needed services (Medicaid, Food Stamps, WIC, substance abuse counseling, and subsidized housing) in an attempt to reduce the situational stressors that many low-income families encounter. Another important aspect of coordination involves working with the families' primary care providers, clarifying and reinforcing recommendations made by such providers.

OUTREACH AND CASE FINDING

While the community organizations implementing the NFP usually have established referral processes with other health and human service providers, nurse home visitors at many sites frequently play an important role in early program implementation in educating referral sources about the program and the eligibility criteria. The NFP emphasis on primary prevention, rather than treatment of families with known problems such as child abuse, often requires frequent contact with referral sources to encourage identification of low-income pregnant women expecting their first child in the target population who might benefit from the program.

FAMILY ADVOCATE

Advocacy is an integral component of the nurse home visitor's role. Advocacy may occur at the individual/family level by helping a teenaged mother negotiate with her family a plan to return to school after the birth of the infant to complete her education. Or it may involve actions taken to improve the health and human service systems' responsiveness to family needs. For example, in the conduct of the Denver trial, nurses advocated with the local taxi company to install infant car seats so that parents using such transportation for clinic appointments could do so safely and in compliance with state law.

EVALUATOR

Nurse home visitors not only monitor each family's progress toward their own individual goals but also systematically collect data on all families in their caseload for input into a *clinical information system* that has been designed to track program implementation as a whole. The clinical information system includes a series of reports that nurses and supervisors may use to track local program implementation against benchmark standards based on the randomized clinical trials. In collaboration with the nursing supervisor, home visitors are encouraged to use such data for developing quality improvement strategies to strengthen local program performance, thereby enhancing the potential that program will indeed produce the outcomes attained in the clinical trials.

Evidence of the Effectiveness of the Program

Effectiveness of the NFP has been established through the conduct of three randomized clinical trials with diverse populations (white, black, Hispanic) in Elmira, New York, Memphis, Tennessee, and Denver, Colorado (Olds et al., 1997, 1998a, 1998b, 1998c, 2002). In each of the studies, pregnant women were randomly assigned to either the program model or comparison services and then were evaluated from the standpoint of the program's goals at completion of the program and over time (e.g., though adolescence). Key outcomes documented for nurse-visited families compared with control families include:

- Reduction in cigarette smoking during pregnancy
- Reduction in premature births among smokers at program entry
- Reduction in rates of children's health care encounters for injuries/ingestions
- Reduction in rates of child maltreatment
- Higher language skills for children at 21 months of age
- Reduction in subsequent pregnancies among unmarried women
- Reduction in use of welfare
- Reduction in long-term drug and alcohol problems among mothers in 15-year follow-up of Elmira sample
- Fewer arrests and convictions among adolescents in 15-year follow-up of Elmira sample

Although the sizes of beneficial program effects in Memphis and Denver were smaller than in Elmira for the same stage of the child's development, the program has produced statistically significant effects on its targeted outcome domains (women's prenatal health, infant health and development, maternal life course) across all studies. Furthermore, economic analyses support that the cost of the intervention is recovered by the child's fourth birthday (Olds, Henderson, Phelps, Kitzman, & Hanks, 1993) and that there is a 4-fold increase in savings over the cost of the intervention by the child's 15th birthday (Karoly et al., 1998).

Strategies for Effective Dissemination of the NFP

A critical issue in the translation of any experimental intervention into clinical practice is the extent to which the program is replicated with fidelity to the intervention tested in the randomized clinical trials. Strategies used by the NFP to foster effective dissemination of the research intervention include (1) site development with communities interested in possibly implementing the program, (2) design and use of home visit practice guidelines based on trial protocols, (3) training of public health nurses recruited to implement the intervention and their supervisors, (4) development of clinical data forms and an information system based on the trial measures and instruments translated for public health practice, and (5) agency access to and use of evaluation data for ongoing quality improvement.

SITE DEVELOPMENT

When prospective sites contact NFP staff with an inquiry about replicating the program, a collaborative process is initiated in which NFP staff work with key policy makers and administrators from the interested community (state, county, or city) to assist them in conducting an assessment to determine the fit of the program with their population needs and the availability of local resources (organizational entity to implement program, fiscal funding, and qualified nursing staff) needed to successfully implement the program. This process is analogous to the core public health function of assessment.

As part of the assessment process, community leaders also are encouraged to identify how the NFP will articulate with other maternal and child health programs provided in the community and to collaborate with representatives of these programs to reduce competition and resistance as planning for initiation of the NFP progresses. Because the NFP targets low-income, first-time parents only, policy development regarding how the program contributes to the community's overall plan for addressing diverse population needs is important. Such careful policy development not only facilitates appropriate referrals to the program but also is likely to help with fiscal decision-making when budget resources are limited. All too often when public dollars are constrained, lack of clarity about how different programs address varying population needs within a community result in premature closure of effective programs and the retention of less costly programs that have little evidence that they work.

TRAINING

Once a decision is reached with a community to move forward with implementation of the NFP, local program staff receive training by nurses from the national organization who have expertise in the program model. Selection of content for the training of program staff and the learning activities provided is guided by a competency-based approach and demonstration of expected performance standards as program implementation progresses. The latter is consistent with the emerging focus on competency-based education for all public health practitioners advocated by the Association of Schools of Public Health and the Association of State and Territorial Health Officials (Gebbie, Rosenstock, & Hernandez, 2003). The training occurs over the course of 1 year and involves face-to-face interactive sessions that bring new program staff from a variety of communities together as well as online modules and self-paced tutorials that staff completes at their work site. Ongoing consultation with training staff on issues encountered in the course of program implementation is available by telephone and through a list-serve. A complement to training is the visit-by-visit guidelines that have been developed based on trial protocols. Training of program staff and the provision of home visit guidelines complement the core public health function of assurance by maximizing the likelihood that program implementation will use clinical interventions with families comparable to those tested in the trials.

EVALUATION AND QUALITY IMPROVEMENT

Ongoing monitoring of health services provided and evaluating whether the desired outcomes are attained are other critical components of the core function of assurance. Local program staff complete a set of clinical data forms based on measures used in the trials that are entered into a Web-based clinical information system maintained by the national NFP organization. Nursing supervisors and administrators at the local program sites have access to a series of management reports produced by the clinical information system to assist them in monitoring the services provided to families and assessing whether established performance standards are being met. More detailed analytic reports on outcomes attained by program participants are produced for each site by evaluation staff at the national organization. Comparison of data for their site with benchmark standards derived from the clinical trials and Healthy People 2010 objectives (U.S. Department of Health and Human Services, 2000) enables local nursing supervisors to identify areas for quality improvement.

Policy Issues for the NFP as a Case Management Strategy

VALUING EVIDENCE-BASED PUBLIC HEALTH PROGRAMS

The concept of evidenced-based practice has become well accepted in many areas of health care as an important strategy to achieve appropriate and effective service delivery. Some have criticized this strategy as a cookbook approach that potentially compromises high-quality, individualized care. There is no prohibition to individualizing care when using an evidence-based approach. The emphasis is on knowing what is effective and acting on that knowledge. Evidence-based practice increasingly is recognized as one of the most effective ways to provide quality, safe, and efficient care in all health care settings. Public policy initiatives have begun to have requirements that interventions and therapies have strong evidence before there is expenditure of restrained public funds.

ARE NURSES REALLY ESSENTIAL FOR IMPLEMENTATION OF THE PROGRAM?

Due to limited fiscal resources in many public health settings, it is not uncommon for administrators and policy makers to question whether the program really needs to be implemented by nurses. In light of the nursing shortage, this question is likely to be raised with increasing frequency by those communities interested in the program model but who have difficulty in recruiting nurses. The evidence for the effectiveness of the program has been established only for nurses in the three randomized clinical trials. The most recent trial, conducted in Denver, did examine outcomes for participants visited by nurses and those visited by paraprofessionals (individuals with a high school education who came from a similar background as many of the participants). While the results supported that nurses produced significant effects on a wide range of maternal and child outcomes, paraprofessionals produced small effects that rarely achieved statistical or clinical significance (Olds et al., 2002). Given the consistency of significant effects for nurse-visited women compared to counterparts in control groups across the trials, the NFP is being disseminated only to sites that agree to use nurses as home visitors. However, many program sites have had to rely on nurses without baccalaureate preparation to implement the program. Lack of formal educational preparation in public health practice for professionals working in state and city/county health departments has emerged as a significant issue over the past two decades leading to the recent emphasis on competency-based education and attainment of performance standards rather than a specific degree requirement (Gebbie, Rosentstock & Hernandez, 2003).

SHOULD PUBLIC HEALTH NURSES HAVE ANY INDIVIDUAL CARE RESPONSIBILITIES?

Strong national and state emphasis on core public health functions has led some public health officials to make decisions that direct care services have no place in public health. With the historical public health approach to surveillance, case funding, and community-focused care coupled with the core function emphasis on community assessment and involvement, it is hard to see that all individualized care including case management should be abandoned. There is tension between the population focused prevention mission in public health and a strategy that works with families and the individuals within them to meet the prevention mission. Resolution in many agencies is toward evidenced-based programs and their added value to traditional services, and where this has occurred the agencies have considered the NFP program.

COMPETITION BETWEEN NATIONAL SECURITY AND THE HEALTH OF THE POPULATION

Who in the nation has not heard about bioterrorism? National security demands are of great importance, but at the same time they need to be balanced with the physical, mental, and social health demands of our nation. Major national threats more often than not drive public policy in ways that would not be considered under other circumstances. National health policy is being shaped to ensure that health initiatives are substantially focused on bioterrorism and other threats. Such a policy change leads to the need for hard choices and some dislocations, such as substantial change in state public health funding, or funding so narrowly targeted to specific topics that traditional public health programs are eliminated or considerably downsized. Choices are being made by states and counties about whether to continue funding for traditional public health programs, and these choices are controversial (May & Silverman, 2003). Intervention programs with strong evidence supporting effectiveness stand a better chance of continuing than those without such evidence when public agencies are setting their priorities.

FINANCING EVIDENCED-BASED PUBLIC HEALTH CASE MANAGEMENT

Even before public health resources were as constrained as they have been in the beginning of the twenty-first century, there has been tension between the public health ethic to provide at least some care to all of the involved population and more narrowly defining a specific subgroup at risk. When evidence-based interventions are implemented, they are focused on the part of the population with whom the intervention has demonstrated effectiveness and not the entire population. Case management has been valued in public health practice, and the NFP is an example of effective case management strategy. The segment of the population for which it is known to be effective is with those who are first-time mothers with risk factors such as low income and youth. Those at or near the poverty level are usually eligible for Medicaid services with Medicaid Targeted Case Management, one of the specific funding strategies used by agencies implementing the NFP. Other funding strategies have been Temporary Assistance for Needy Families (TANF), Title V Maternal and Child Health Block Grant, state and county general funds, state juvenile funds, and local programs, such as United Way, March of Dimes, and local foundations.

Is Primary Prevention Valued?

Prevention services rarely show an immediate effect, but their cost is immediate and their benefits occur at later time. There is an almost natural tension when making choices about providing resources for the provision of prevention services or treatment.

Prevention programs, especially those targeting well populations, such as the NFP, are easy targets to get set aside when resources are constrained because no one is ill and their lives obviously are not threatened. It can be very difficult for public health and local county agencies to fund primary prevention programs when the return on the investment of public funds occurs in the present and the rewards occur in the future. The NFP like many other prevention programs has savings in the future, sometimes the distant future of a decade or more. The public policy perspective is much more of the "here and now" primarily because public officials who are elected usually have terms of 2 to 4 years, and they will be held accountable for accomplishments for their constituents at election time. In addition, it can be hard for public health officials to support primary prevention services when the effect is not seen immediately. In reality, children and poor families have little influence at election time.

SUMMARY

Concerns over the rising cost of health care in the United States, quality of care delivered, and accountability for patient outcomes has prompted the emergence of a variety of case management models. In the search for solutions to these concerns, there has been increasing support for evidence-based practice as well as evidence-based health policy. Public health practice has been increasingly reviewed with the same vigor as acute and primary care practice, with a call to adopt more evidence-based programs. The NFP, an exemplar of community-based case management that uses an evidence-based approach to address community needs at a population level has been described and policy issues in the implementation of the NFP enumerated.

References

Bandura, A. (1982). Self-efficacy mechanism in human agency. *American Journal of Psychology, 37*, 122-147.

Berkowitz, B., Dahl, J., Guirl, K., Kostelecky, B.J., McNeil, C., & Valda, U. (2001). *Public health nursing leadership: A guide to managing the core functions.* Washington, D.C.: American Nurses Publishing.

Bowlby, J. (1969). *Attachment and loss: Volume I. Attachment.* New York: Basic Books.

Bronfenbrenner, U. (1979). *The ecology of human development: Experiments by nature and design.* Cambridge, Mass.: Harvard University Press.

Bronfenbrenner, U. (1992). *The process-person-context model in developmental research principles, applications, and implications.* Unpublished manuscript. Ithaca, N.Y.: Cornell University.

Brownson, R.C., Baker, E.A., Leet, T.L., & Gillespie, K.N. (2003). *Evidence-based public health.* New York: Oxford University Press, Inc.

Dolezol, S., & Butterfield, P.M. (1994). *Partners in parenting education.* Denver, Colo.: How to Read Your Baby.

Gebbie, K., Rosenstock, L., & Hernandez, L.M. (Eds.) (2003). *Who will keep the public healthy? Educating public health professionals for the 21st century.* Washington, D.C.: The National Academies Press.

Greiner, A.C., & Knebel, E. (2003). *Health professions education: A bridge to quality.* Washington, D.C.: National Academies Press.

Hanks, C., Kitzman, H., & Milligan, R. (1995). Implementing the COACH relationship model: Health promotion for mothers and children. *Advances in Nursing Science, 18*(2), 57-66.

Ingersoll, G.L. (2000). Evidence-based nursing: What it is and what it is not. *Nursing Outlook, 48*, 151-152.

Institute of Medicine. (1988). *The future of public health.* Washington, D.C.: National Academies Press.

Karoly, L.A., Greenwood, P.W., Everingham, S., Hoube, J., Kilburn, M.R., Rydell, C.P., Sanders, M., & Chiesa, J. (1998). *Investing in our children: What we know and don't know about the costs and benefits of early childhood interventions.* Santa Monica, Calif.: The RAND Corporation.

Keller, L.O., Schaffer, M.A., Lia-Hoagberg, B., & Strohschein, S. (2002). Assessment, program planning, and evaluation in population-based public health practice. *Journal of Public Health Management Practice, 6*(5), 30-43.

Keller, L.O., Strohschein, S., Lia-Hoagberg, B., & Schaffer, M. (1998). Population-based public health nursing interventions: A model from practice. *Public Health Nursing, 15*(3), 207-215.

Lavis, J.N., Robertson, D., Woodside, J.M., McLeod, C.B., Abelson, J., Knowledge Transfer Development Group (2003). How can research organizations more effectively transfer research knowledge to decision makers? *The Milbank Quarterly, 81*(2), 221-248.

May, T., Silverman, R. (2003). Bioterrorism defense priorities. *Science, 301*(5629), 17.

O'Brien, R.A., & Baca, P. (1997). Application of solution-focused interventions. *Journal of Community Psychology, 25*(1), 47-57.

Olds, D.L., Eckenrode, J., Henderson, C.R., Jr., Kitzman, H., Powers, J., Cole, R., Sidora, K., Morris, P., Pettitt, L.M., & Luckey, D. (1997). Long-term effects of nurse home visitation on maternal life course and child abuse and neglect: fifteen-year follow-up of a randomized trial. *Journal of American Medical Association, 278*, 637-643.

Olds, D., Henderson, C.R., Jr., Cole, R., Eckenrode, J., Kitzman, H., Luckey, D., Pettitt, L., Sidora, K., Morris, P., & Powers, J. (1998a). Long-term effects of nurse home visitation on children's criminal and antisocial behavior: 15-year follow-up of a randomized trial. *Journal of American Medical Association, 278*, 644-652.

Olds, D., Henderson, C., Jr., Kitzman, H., Eckenrode, J., Cole, R., & Tatelbaum, R. (1998b). The promise of home visitation. *Journal of Community Psychology, 26*, 5-21.

Olds, D., Henderson, C., Phelps, C., Kitzman, H., & Hanks, C. (1993). Effects of prenatal and infancy nurse home visitation on government spending. *Medical Care, 31*, 155-174.

Olds, D.L., Kitzman, H., Cole R., Robinson, J. (1997). Theoretical foundations of a program of home visitation for pregnant women and parents of young children. *Journal of Community Psychology, 25*(1), 9-25.

Olds, D.L., Pettitt, L.M., Robinson, J., Henderson, C., Econrode, J., Kitzman, H., Cole, B., & Powers, J. (1998c). Reducing risks for antisocial behavior with a program of prenatal and early childhood home visitation. *Journal of Community Psychology, 26*(1), 65-83.

Olds, D.L., Robinson, J.A., O'Brien, R., Luckey, D.W., Pettitt, L.M., Henderson, C.R., Jr., Ng, R.K., Sheff, K.L., Korfmacher, J., Hiatt, S., & Talmi, A. (2002). Home visiting by paraprofessionals and by nurses: A randomized, controlled trial. *Pediatrics, 110*, 486-496.

Prochaska, J.O., Norcross, J.C., & DiClemente, C.G. (1994). *Changing for good.* New York: Morrow.

Sackett, D.L., Rosenberg, W.M.C., Gray, J., Haynes, R.B., & Richardson, W.S. (1996). Evidenced based medicine: What it is and what it is not. *British Medical Journal, 312*, 71-72.

Sidani, S., & Braden, C.J. (1998). *Evaluating nursing interventions: A theory driven approach.* Thousand Oaks, Calif.: Sage Publications.

Straus, S.E., & Sackett, D.L. (1998). Using research findings in clinical practice. *British Medical Journal, 317*, 339-342.

Turnock, B.J. (2001). *Public health: What it is and how it works.* Gaithersburg, Md.: Aspen Publications.

U.S. Department of Health and Human Services (2000). *Healthy People 2010: Understanding and Improving Health,* 2nd edition. Washington, D.C.: U.S. Government Printing Office.

Zerwekh, J.V. (1991). A family caregiving model for public health nursing. *Nursing Outlook, 39*(5), 213-217.

VI

THE PLANNING PROCESS

Developing Collaborative Relationships

Relationships are the foundation of any organization and the building blocks of any successful change process. To develop successful partnerships within an organization, a commitment to planned change must be made. Unit VI outlines the assessment data needed to affect successful change to case management. The assessment process must include an analysis of the organization itself as well as the role functions of its members. With that information the change agent can begin to design and implement a successful case management system. A sound educational program will also assist the organization in planning for this change and should not be neglected during the planning process. Included in this section are design options for educational programs that can be applied to any learning organization.

23

Assessing the System and Creating an Environment for Change

CHAPTER OVERVIEW

Successful implementation of a case management system begins with a solid, well-conceived plan. The first step in creating the plan is to assess the system in which the case management model will be implemented. Human and financial resources should be reviewed. This information helps determine the degree of change that the organization can tolerate and the chances for a successful conversion.

Implementation involves a nine-step process. Target patient populations are identified and matched to nursing units, and the design structure for the units is decided. This new structure involves a change in the staff mix. The next step is the formation of interdisciplinary groups. These groups consist of the case manager, physician(s), social worker, and any other pertinent health care professionals. Benchmarks, which determine how the change will be monitored and evaluated over time, must be selected. Before implementation takes place, preimplementation data must be collected. The next step involves educating staff, physicians, and other professionals who will be affected by conversion to the case management model. At this stage, training is provided for the case managers. After managers are educated on how the model works, it can be implemented. Finally, evaluation should take place at predetermined intervals. Necessary changes should be made as quickly as possible.

FEASIBILITY OF THE MODEL

Converting to a case management model requires systematic planning. A solid plan that has been well thought out guarantees a higher rate of successful conversion. Without a plan, it is likely that the expected outcome of the model will be lost or that some important elements will be left out.

Administrators have always known that a plan is essential for change in any organization. This philosophy is no less true for nurses attempting to create a major change such as a conversion to a case management model. The first step in any planning process is to determine if the change is not only feasible but also worthwhile. The potential for success and the effect such a change will have on the organization must be evaluated from both a positive and negative perspective. Overall, the change should lead the organization in a positive direction.

ASSESSMENT OF RESOURCES

Assessing resources requires some homework. A thorough analysis of the organization, including its structure and financial status, must be done. Those implementing the change need to determine if the organization is strong enough to withstand the temporary instability that will accompany the change. As with any major change, errors will be made along the way. The complete support of all top administrators and a commitment to the long haul are absolutely necessary. In the beginning the road will be bumpy, and everyone concerned should be aware of this and ready to be supportive every step of the way.

THE COST OF IMPLEMENTATION

A case management system can be implemented with few additional personnel costs for the organization if the change is implemented carefully. For instance, good choices for the pilot program would be units that have current openings or units that have budgeted for an additional person. Such an opening can then be filled by someone qualified to be a case manager. In this way the new position will not incur any costs outside of those already budgeted. This is essential for a plan that must show success before it receives an allotment in the budget. Internal and preexisting resources can then be used for implementation.

If possible, the organization's budget should allow for certain expenditures needed for implementation. These expenditures will probably not be related to personnel costs unless the organization decides to hire a project manager. Costs may be incurred for documentation system changes or for data collection and statistical analysis necessary for measuring success. Additional resources needed include clerical support staff to perform such functions as faxing, photocopying, ordering durable medical equipment (DME), and providing transportation. The use of clerical staff can be an important adjunct to the professional staffing. In some cases the use of clerical support staff may mean that the professional staff can carry a higher caseload.

Today's contemporary case management departments also need to have computerized support in the form of databases, case management software programs, and hardware. Hardware may include laptops, hand- or palm-held computers, scanning capability, and variance collection and analysis capability (Favor & Ricks, 1996).

Both administrative and financial support must be obtained before switching over to a case management system.

INTERNAL MARKETING

Obtaining the support of those in senior management is relatively easy if the administrators already have some familiarity with the model. Senior management may have heard or read about the model and already have realized the need for such a change. Conversely, they may have misconceptions or may be misinformed about the model. Senior management might also object to the change solely because it comes at an inopportune time.

National managed care infiltration has now created an environment in which most forward-thinking organizations recognize that systems must be implemented that truly and consistently control cost and quality. Infiltration may be real or anticipated. In either case, senior administrators must support a conceptual and actual shift to case management. This process is much less difficult than it was even 10 years ago. Status quo is no longer an option, and each organization must determine what changes are needed to support a constantly changing health care environment.

Senior management support is a prerequisite for beginning the change process. The ways change may be attained are as diverse as the management styles of the individuals involved. Making sure that administrators are familiar with those initiating the change, and that they have positive working relationships with them, is essential for success.

Furthermore, the concept of the case management system should be introduced by someone who is familiar with the administrator, the president, the executive vice president of operations, and the chief financial officer. Essentially all executive staff of the organization should be included. Use of an outside consultant to introduce the concept may provide the catalyst the organization needs for change. The individual who introduces the concept to the administrator must have the facts of implementation readily available. Estimated cost, staffing needs, and time frames must be prepared for the first meeting. Expected outcomes, goals, and long-range plans should also be presented. A review of other organizations that have implemented the concept and have had positive results lends credibility to the proposed plan.

It may be necessary to explain the definition of case management from a care delivery perspective if the administrator has no previous knowledge of the model. Emphasis should be placed on how the model benefits all disciplines. Finally, but possibly most important, it is necessary to review the financial implications of conversion. An initiative whose goal is to reduce patient length of stay may be the best-selling feature in today's financial climate. An explanation as to why a nurse may be best suited to monitor this process may take some extra effort. Many people believe that social work, utilization review, or physicians themselves should be the facilitators and coordinators of the care plan. Other initiatives aimed at reducing length of stay may already have been attempted. The failure of these initiatives may help convince administrators to try a new approach. It is important to emphasize that although nursing drives the process, all disciplines must take part in achieving success. The input and participation of all health care providers are essential. The keys to case management's success are its nursing and interdisciplinary approaches.

Within the prospective payment system, length of stay can determine financial success or failure. However, in a discussion of how case management affects a reduction in length of stay, how length of stay affects quality should also be emphasized. The cost/quality ratio as it relates to case management must be reviewed. Any initiative that reduces length of stay without looking at quality and resources is doomed to fail the organization and the patients.

Although length of stay continues to be the clearest and most tangible way to measure financial success, other measures may add additional credibility. If available, a cost-accounting system helps identify reductions in the use or misuse of hospital resources. Other parallel reductions must also be seen. If the length of stay is reduced but the amount of resources is simply collapsed into fewer days, true financial savings are less likely.

In managed care reimbursement systems, shortened length of stay and overall cost reductions remain extremely important. Capitated or per diem managed care rates still require serious and consistent cost reductions.

The support of nursing administration is another vital component. Nurse managers and upper managers must support the concept fully to achieve success. Some suspicion may initially be felt as nursing roles change. The nurse manager may feel threatened by the introduction of another individual who is also managing care on the unit. Other departments most directly involved in the change process, and from whom support is needed, include social work, utilization management, and discharge planning. Initial and on-going support is essential here.

Before the advent of the prospective payment system, flex time, increased severity levels, and technology, the nurse manager carried out many of the role functions associated with case management, such as facilitation and coordination of patient care services. As the nurse manager's role expanded and became more administrative, the nurse had less time to focus on facilitating and coordinating the progression of patient care. It is necessary to emphasize that the new concept will allow the nurse manager to concentrate more on administrative functions, which will in turn mean patients receive a higher quality of care. Reducing the sense of personal threat is essential to effecting a positive change.

Downsizing and restructuring in health care organizations have in many cases eliminated the assistant director of nursing position. There often is no nursing administrator between the nurse manager and the director of nursing. Elimination of this position has placed a greater administrative responsibility on the nurse manager. Add accelerated hospital stays to the equation, and the result is a less-than-efficient system.

Case managers, if provided with the authority and accountability necessary, can become the clinical eyes and ears for the nurse manager. In addition, another fallout of the downsizing era has been elimination of many nurse educator positions. Perhaps among the most dangerous of reductions, removal of nurse educator positions has meant that unit-based staff development has suffered. This is particularly true for new staff nurses who need significant and consistent ongoing support. Although traditionally case managers have focused on patient and family education, in downsized environments they may need to incorporate staff education. This may take the form of case conferences or unit-based in-service training geared toward specific clinical issues.

STAFF INTEGRATION

If the nursing chief executive initiated the change to case management, then the staff might already accept the change. In this case, conversation with this group should concentrate on explaining the case management concept thoroughly and the changes it will bring.

The need to educate and fully enlist the support of staff nurses cannot be emphasized enough. If the organization has decided to create the case manager position as a staff position, then staff nurses must be fully aware of the role. The job expectations of the case manager should be clear. If available, the job description should be distributed and reviewed. The role of the case manager in relation to other nursing positions should be made as clear as possible.

As with the introduction of any new position, there may be some initial role blending, role conflict, or both. This can be minimized through open discussion and ongoing review of the role after implementation. Nurses should anticipate that roles and responsibilities will evolve over time. The fluid nature of the position means it can be improved and enhanced as a part of the evaluation process. Some role blending and confusion related to the changing roles of nursing and other disciplines, particularly social work and utilization management, can be expected. Job descriptions must be reviewed and amended to reflect the changing roles of all members of the health care team.

The collaborative nature of the model means that all disciplines must support it. At the top of this list are the physicians. Getting the involvement of both medical physicians and surgeons requires varying techniques, with emphasis placed on the outcomes achievable for their patients. Rogers says, "It is important to use nurses well known to the physicians, who have a history of solid communication, mutual trust, clinical experience, and an overall positive experiential record. This serves to gain the initial support of physicians who might otherwise be resistant" (M. Rogers, personal communication, 1992). For the surgeon who is reimbursed on a case basis, the incentive to discharge the patient more rapidly is a financial one because the discharge of one patient allows for the admission of the next. In addition, surgeons traditionally have treated patients in a protocol manner. In this setting, the applicability of the case management approach is easily understood and appreciated. Because the surgical patient generally runs a predictable course of recovery, care can be planned in an organized way. For this reason, surgeons are probably those most receptive to implementation of the concept.

The medical physician may pose a greater challenge. Within the prospective payment system and most managed care contracts, no financial incentives motivate these professionals to discharge patients more rapidly. Furthermore, it may be more difficult to predict the course of events for a particular medical diagnosis or condition. As the extent of managed care penetration has accelerated, some managed care organizations have begun to implement financial penalties on the physician for hospital days during which an acute care level of service was not rendered. Until recently, only the hospital received a denial of payment from the third party payer for days of service that were below the acute care level. By denying payment to the physician as well as the hospital, the managed care organization is producing incentives for the physician to be responsible and accountable for these nonreimbursable days.

Incentives motivating the medical physician toward an appreciation of the case management approach are probably not based on length of stay improvements unless these length of stay reductions are tied to quality issues. For example, are significant days added to the hospital stay during which little or nothing is being done for the patient? Emphasizing that improved quality of care will result may be one way to enlist physician support. Emphasis on the role of the case manager in ensuring, with the multidisciplinary action plan, that the physician's best plan is initiated and followed may also help enlist support.

In some cases, other initiatives may be useful. If the institution has several medical diagnoses whose lengths of stay are beyond state or federal averages, these should be targeted for initial intervention. In these cases, the chief physician may need to intervene. Essentially a practice guideline would be established that all physicians caring for a particular type of patient would be expected to follow. Whenever possible, active and positive participation is preferred.

Chart review and research are other techniques used to sell a treatment plan for a particular medical condition. Chart review often uncovers various ways to treat a medical problem. Each plan may not be equally effective, financially appropriate concerning resource use, or equally appropriate in terms of length of stay. By using chart review, inappropriate physician and nursing treatment interventions can be enhanced. The way other institutions treat particular types of problems can be used as a resource to determine the best possible treatment plan.

If the organization supports the notion that decreased variation in treatment will reduce costs and improve quality, more aggressive measures may be necessary. For example, if all admitted patients are to be treated under a particular case management plan, then a mandate from the president of the organization may be necessary. If there is a case management plan available for a particular case type, all patients admitted who match that case type should be treated consistently. Regardless of whether the patient is a service or private-pay patient or of whether the attending physician is in full agreement, that practice plan is initiated for that patient. This sort of global support may not be possible without a decree from a top administrator who has the power to demand uniform clinical management.

Standardized treatment plans are a great resource and asset for the resident or intern house staff. In addition, the case manager serves as a skilled resource for the new physician who is rotating through a particular nursing unit and is unfamiliar with the patient's present or past condition. In addition, the case manager helps the house officer elicit quick and accurate information. Ongoing dialogue between the two helps ensure that the best plan will be carried out.

Case management cannot be completely successful without the support and cooperation of ancillary departments. It is doubtful that an ancillary department will object to the model, although passive support is not enough to ensure success. To empower the case manager, a contact person in each department should be assigned to whom needs or concerns about patients can be referred.

Some areas play a bigger part than others. For example, the radiology department plays a key role in some length of stay issues. Appropriate scheduling of tests in terms of order and timeliness is crucial to an early diagnosis and treatment. Appropriate preparation also ensures that the patient's movement through the hospital is smooth.

Other ancillary departments, which play a key role in the case management model, are the admitting office, the medical records department, the pharmacy, the laboratory, and the emergency department. Failure to obtain the support and commitment of these departments will create problems during implementation and evaluation of the model.

Clearly, other direct care providers must be fully supportive and committed for the model to be most effective. Key areas for such support include social work, physical therapy, and nutrition. The patient problem or surgery determines the areas most vital at any particular time, but certainly each department should be fully educated and agreeable before implementation.

Most ancillary departments appreciate the opportunity to work collaboratively with other disciplines. Nursing is not the only discipline plagued by frustration because of the divergent directions taken by each group of providers.

PLANNED CHANGE

A plan for implementation provides the foundation for successful change. Each element outlined in this chapter should be evaluated and acted on if appropriate for the institution. Planning for implementation should be carefully thought out and choreographed. The nine-step plan for implementation outlined in Box 23-1 provides the foundation for the plan and identifies subsequent changes. This nine-step process provides a structure for planning any implementation program. Each element is reviewed and every aspect covered during the planning process. The ordering of each step may vary, depending on the institution, and certain steps may occur simultaneously.

Clearly the order is not as important as the actual carrying out of each step. This implementation process should be shared with everyone in the organization as the process is begun. The plan's steps for implementation, the ways in which those steps will be carried out, and the method of evaluation should be shared openly so that all those concerned have a chance to give input.

Because it will be advantageous to demonstrate some immediate success, selecting where to begin is important. A bad choice may mean failure or the cancellation of plans for adding units or teams to the model.

BOX 23-1   **NINE-STEP PLAN FOR IMPLEMENTATION**

1. Define target populations for case management.
2. Define target areas.
3. Agree on design structure for areas selected.
4. Form collaborative practice groups.
5. Choose benchmarks.
6. Collect preimplementation data.
7. Provide advanced skills and knowledge.
8. Implement model.
9. Evaluate model.

Step 1: Define Target Populations for Case Management

Target patient populations are selected based on the following factors:
- Volume of discharges
- Variance from length of stay standards
- Variance from length of stay at similar institutions
- Feasibility of developing case management plans
- Potential for control of resource consumption
- Opportunity for improvement in quality of care

If the organization's goal for implementation is to improve quality of care, this may be an additional factor to consider during the selection process. This determination can be made through chart reviews of targeted populations.

Step 2: Define Target Areas

Once the selection of patient populations has been made, these patients are matched to appropriate clinical areas. In some cases the type of patient group selected may not be found in one particular area of the hospital; therefore a *non–unit-based* case management team approach may be more appropriate. Some case management designs that are non–unit-based follow product lines, service lines, disease groups, populations, or across the continuum.

In other cases it will be possible to gather patients from a designated geographic area. The more homogeneous the patient population on a nursing unit, the fewer the resources are needed in terms of physicians and case management plans. Thus the model will positively affect a greater number of patients.

Step 3: Agree on Design Structure for Areas Selected

Once the nursing unit, geographic area, or patient type has been selected, the design structure is determined. If a *unit-based* model is being introduced, a determination must be made as to how many case managers will be on the unit. This decision is based on the number of patient beds, the severity of the patients' conditions, the average length of stay, and the available resources. If only one position is available for conversion, this may be the deciding factor. Additional factors to consider include the role functions of the case manager. The three common role functions of a hospital-based case manager include clinical coordination/facilitation, utilization management, and discharge planning. Beyond these core functions the case manager may be responsible for outcomes data collection or research, variance analysis, quality management, or patient education. The more functions that are combined in the role, the smaller will the caseload need to be.

If a *non–unit-based* case management model is being implemented, different factors are considered. Most case management teams have members from several disciplines. Therefore this type of team may require a greater number of resources for implementation. A physician, nurse, social worker, and others must be deployed, which may mean taking them away from other jobs or assignments, thereby requiring a greater financial commitment from the organization. The disciplines represented depend on the particular clinical type being followed by the team. For example, a diabetes team clearly needs a nutritionist and a social worker. Consultants with an affiliation to the team might include a podiatrist or an ophthalmologist.

An additional factor to consider during this step is the integration of beyond-the-walls clinical areas such as clinics, physician offices, and home care, among others. Relationships between the hospital-based case manager and these nonacute clinical areas must be considered in the design. Managed care areas, particularly those with capitated reimbursements, must allot time in the design phase to think about how case management might be structured in these areas (Swindle, Weyant, & Mar, 1994). More detailed information on community-based case management programs can be found in Unit IV.

Step 4: Form Collaborative Practice Groups

In the *unit-based* model the teams have a fluid structure, and the members of the team constantly change. The only constant member is the unit-based case manager. The patient, physician, social worker, and so on change as the professionals assigned to the patient change. For each new patient the case manager must gather a team, identify who is responsible for which aspects of the care plan, and ensure that everyone is working toward the same goals.

In the *non–unit-based* case management model, the professional team members remain constant, and the only changing member is the patient. In this model, the team members and their respective roles are clearly defined up front, so there is no need to bring the group together.

Step 5: Choose Benchmarks

As discussed in Unit VIII, choosing the outcome measures or benchmarks is an important step. Benchmarks must be selected as early as possible and certainly before implementation. The method of evaluation depends on the outcome measures chosen and the resources available for tracking the data.

Step 6: Collect Preimplementation Data

Once the benchmarks have been selected, the method for data collection is determined. The time frames are documented in advance and the individuals responsible for the various elements identified.

It may be necessary and appropriate to enlist the help of employees from other departments who have access to certain data. For example, a representative from the data support or the medical records department might be assigned the responsibility of monitoring and tracking the length of stay data. A representative from the quality improvement department might be recruited to track quality of care data on a quarterly basis. In some cases, it may even be possible to use students to assist with staff and patient questionnaires. A patient representative might be another good choice to help with patient satisfaction questionnaires.

Regardless of the data being evaluated, baseline data sets must be established before education or implementation of the model. If the staff is being tested via questionnaires, those questionnaires must be distributed and returned before implementation. Some of the data are retrospective; therefore the actual time when the data are pulled together is not as important.

Step 7: Provide Advanced Skills and Knowledge

In Chapter 24 the elements of a good educational program are reviewed and discussed. Employees from all departments must understand the general concepts of a case management system. To attain such understanding, an educational program may be offered, but the extent of such a program depends on the resources available.

The case managers should be provided with as extensive a program as possible. It cannot be assumed that an employee comes to the position with the skills and knowledge necessary to carry out the role effectively. An investment and commitment from the organization for providing advanced skills and knowledge help develop highly effective case managers. The need for education cannot be overemphasized.

To prevent contamination of subjects, educational preparation must follow any preimplementation data collection. This maintains the integrity of the study sample.

Step 8: Implement Model

Once all the previous steps have been accomplished, the model can be effectively implemented. The date for beginning is clearly communicated. The case management documentation system selected may or may not be in place; although it is desirable, it is not essential. The case manager can begin changing the system immediately after entering the position. Having the case manager begin the changes might be the only practical way because other employees do not have the time or advanced skills necessary to make this change.

The question is often asked, "How do we begin?" The answer to this question is simple—*by beginning*. The transition phase, or the time between announced implementation and a full integration of the change, may be as long as a year or more. Therefore, after completing all preimplementation steps, the case manager can work in the change gradually. It will take many months for all those involved to adjust to the system.

This time period requires communication with other members of the health care team, letting them know that the changeover has taken place and exactly what that means to them and to the organization. The more open and candid the communication, the more likely it is that the change will be accepted. The beginning is when many organizations falter because they expect much of the change to have already been made. This expectation, however, is not practical. Everyone must understand in advance that the bulk of the changes will be phased in slowly.

Step 9: Evaluate Model

Evaluation of the model involves rigorous data collection and analysis. Unit VIII covers the evaluation process in detail. The time frames for analysis are driven by the data elements themselves. Some data, such as length of stay, are collected and analyzed monthly. Other data, such as patient satisfaction, may need to be tracked only every 6 months. Annual tracking of staff satisfaction is sufficient.

In addition to this formal data collection and analysis, an informal evaluation should be ongoing. Those responsible for the model should never forget to query practitioners who work day by day within the model at the patient's bedside. Through discussions with the staff nurses and others, problem areas can be identified and corrective action taken. This ongoing dialogue may continue for 1 to 2 years while the change is being integrated. As the model expands, more and more employees will be affected. Barriers for successful integration continue to appear as the model expands in sophistication and sphere of influence.

References

Favor, G., & Ricks, R. (1996). Preparing to automate the case management process. *Nursing Case Management, 1*(3), 100-106.

Swindle, D.N., Weyant, J.L., & Mar, P.S. (1994). Nurse case management: Collaboration beyond the hospital walls. *Journal of Case Management, 3*(2), 51-52.

Case Management Education

Preparing for Successful Implementation

CHAPTER OVERVIEW

Education is an essential element in successful implementation of a case management model. This chapter reviews the two types of curricula required for implementation of a case management model. The first program, a general orientation to a case management model, is geared to a wide array of health care practitioners. The second program is a 3-day seminar designed to educate and train potential case managers. This chapter provides topical outlines and objectives for each program.

CURRICULUM DEVELOPMENT

Since case management's introduction to hospitals in 1985, implementation has often called for elaborate planning, meetings, time, and commitment. What has been lacking to this point is a formal means of educating the staff nurses, case managers, and other personnel who might be interacting with the case manager.

Although case management theory has been introduced into some undergraduate as well as graduate curricula, those employees already in the health care field probably have not been introduced to the concepts through formal education (American Association of Colleges of Nursing, 1997; Toran, 1998). Therefore education is a key element of success. The length of the institution's educational program will depend on the time that workers can take from their units to attend classroom instruction. For the most part the concepts of case management are relatively new to most employees, so didactic methods are important.

The amount of time set aside for instruction can range from 3 to 6 or more hours. However, the longer the program, the less likely it will be that employees from other disciplines can be included. Although it is crucial that all staff nurses and ancillary nursing personnel attend these introductory sessions, it is also important for members of other disciplines to participate. The number of hours that these employees can be present in the program will depend on the staffing patterns of their departments. Although other disciplines may be committed to the case management model, they may not have the financial or personnel resources to allow workers to leave their jobs for longer than 1 hour. For off-peak shifts, participation may be even less possible. It may be necessary to provide different programs of varying lengths to ensure that everyone can attend. The material is important here, not the length of the program.

250

The topical outline for an introduction to a case management program should contain the following essential elements. Development of the curriculum should reflect all elements and characteristics of the case management process (Fineman, 1996). Other topics might be added, depending on the needs of the organization. The more preparation and education provided to all members of the organization, the greater are the chances for success. Even those departments not directly involved with the program should be invited to attend. Although it may not be immediately obvious, switching to case management will eventually affect areas such as the pharmacy or the radiology department. At the very least, all administrators and executive management should be encouraged to attend. Those involved in operations in the hospital can provide valuable insight into elements required for successful functioning of the model. Other departments—such as medicine, social work, quality improvement, discharge planning, utilization review, the patient representative department, nutrition, medical records, and admitting—are vital to the success of a case management model. Even though some individuals in these departments may be familiar with the case management concept, it is still important to educate them on how case management will be implemented in their organization. Such instruction will help prevent misunderstandings.

MULTIDISCIPLINARY EDUCATION

The content of a program geared to a broad audience must be general enough to hold the attention of a wide range of health care providers, administrators, and operations personnel. This is no easy task. Specific examples of how case management might affect some of these workers will be helpful and should be included in the program.

Begin the presentation with an overview of case management, including the evolution of nursing delivery models, which provides the program's groundwork. Next, explain the relevance of case management in light of today's health care issues. Covering such topics will answer the "Why case management?" and "Why now?" questions. An understanding of the changes in health care reimbursement, downsizing and restructuring, changes in the current patient population, and other health care issues will help the audience see why case management is timely and essential for the continued success of most health care organizations. This framework for discussion will show that case management is not just a nursing project or a nursing problem. Case management needs them, and they need case management.

Empowering the Case Manager

Introducing the case manager and introducing the case management plans are the most essential changes in the implementation of a case management model. Although many, more subtle changes will occur, these are the changes from which all the others will come.

The case manager must be empowered, and one technique for empowering is ensuring that everyone in the organization knows what a case manager does and how the case manager fits into workers' daily routines. If a case manager calls to speak to the patient representative and the patient representative does not understand the case manager's role and function, problems arise.

Other disciplines' roles must be reviewed and clearly understood. Those who are most immediately affected are the social workers, utilization managers, discharge planners, and physicians. Some of these roles may be downsized, redesigned, or eliminated by the introduction of case management. If these changes have not occurred by the time the educational program begins, there may be resistance or hostility from those employees who fear being affected. Take care to engage these individuals, not alienate them.

Each discipline should understand and appreciate the other disciplines' roles and responsibilities. This mutual respect and understanding facilitates a smoother transition as role functions and responsibilities are reallocated.

Topical Outline

A curriculum that addresses a wide audience can cover an array of topics that are relevant to all employees (Table 24-1). The following is a list of possible topical objectives:

Reviewing the history of case management

Defining the concepts of case management

TABLE 24-1   GENERAL ORIENTATION PROGRAM CONTENT OUTLINE

Objectives	Content

Review the history of case management.	Overview
	    The beginnings of case management in the community
	    Case management transition across the continuum of care over the past 100 years

Define the concepts of case management.	Overview
	    A conceptual framework for case management
	    Evolution of nursing delivery models

Describe the role of the case manager.	Review
	    Job description
	    Job responsibilities
	    Daily operations
	    Relationship to other disciplines

Understand the changing roles of the health care team in case management.	Social work Discharge planning Utilization management Physicians

Explain the relationship between the prospective payment system and case management; explain the use of case management plans; review managed care reimbursement.	DRGs
	    Definition/changes in reimbursement including prospective payment in home care, ambulatory care, and acute rehabilitation/managed care
	    Relationship and link to case management
	    Use of case management plans and their relationship to DRGs/guidelines

Identify the case management outcomes for research.	Research outcomes
	    Improved registered nurse satisfaction
	    Decreased burnout
	    Decreased length of stay
	    Improved patient satisfaction
	    Improved quality of care
	    Improved cost per case/stay

Describing the role of the case manager

Understanding the changing roles of the health care team in case management

Defining the relationship between the prospective payment system and case management

Reviewing the managed care reimbursement systems

Understanding the use of the case management plan

Identifying the case management outcomes for evaluation or research

Defining the concepts of case management can be extensive or limited, depending on the audience. In the overview, include discussion of previous care delivery models, current health care crises, and health care reimbursement methods in reference to case management. An in-depth discussion of the prospective payment system and managed care reimbursements is essential.

Include also the evolution of the functional, team, and primary models and how these models relate to the case management model. After all, case management combines elements of team and primary nursing models.

Because institutions may implement a unit-based, free-floating, or combined case management model, the subtle variations should be explored and discussed. This discussion should include how the various versions are structured, organized, and implemented.

The changing role of each member of the health care team is an important element of the discussion. Discuss current role functions as well as how roles will change under case management.

Finally, offer a general overview of the expected outcomes of the case management model. The expected outcomes provide a relevant arena from which to set case management goals both for the organization and for individual workers.

A Conceptual Framework for Case Management

Any discussion of case management must take place in a context of cost and quality. Case management provides the process, structure, and outcomes that control the quality of care while reducing cost. An understanding of this framework and overall goals provides the context for the discussions that follow. A review of how case management as a contemporary and interdisciplinary care delivery system can enhance hospital revenues is essential.

Role of the Case Manager

During implementation, many false conceptions of the role of the case manager develop, usually because of a lack of understanding. Professionals from other disciplines may draw their own conclusions concerning what the case manager should or should not be doing. Although some role blending is necessary, education is the main way to avoid role confusion (Kahn et al., 1964).

Distribute the case manager job description during the educational sessions, or at least review it. This is the first step in distinguishing the roles and responsibilities of the case manager. Such steps help to ensure that other disciplines will respect the boundaries of the case manager's job description and will not expect the manager to function beyond those boundaries. Some workers may expect case managers to be less influential than their job descriptions indicate. Others may expect duties beyond the scope of their job descriptions. A clear description of the role set forth in the beginning will help minimize misunderstandings (Tahan, 1998).

A clear way in which to define and illustrate the job functions of the case manager is through a description of daily operations along with a description of what the case manager's typical day might be like. It is not uncommon to be asked, "What exactly does a case manager do?" Like many jobs of this nature, the specific tasks are often invisible, intangible, or both. Once again, emphasize the theoretic framework of the model and the expected outcomes.

Reviewing the Health Care Reimbursement Systems

The basic premise of case management is that expected outcomes of care can be achieved within appropriate time frames. A portion of the curriculum should be devoted to reviewing the present health care reimbursement systems. It is around these systems that much of case management is built (Cesta, Tahan, & Fink, 1998). Other points to be covered include how diagnosis-related groups (DRGs) work and how these predetermined lengths of stay determine reimbursement rates.

DRGs are one tool to help determine the goal length of stay for the case management plans. Other benchmarks used are national guidelines such as those of Schibanoff (1999). Define these relationships in detail. Also review other uses of case management plans, including how they are used to maintain quality in an accelerated health care system. Review the links between quality and cost in a case management environment. Finally, include an overview of the prospective payment systems that have been implemented in other settings, such as home care, ambulatory care, and acute rehabilitation medicine.

The effects of managed care infiltration should provide an additional context for case management. Whether the issue is capitated rates or per diem reimbursements, length of stay and resource allocation remain important. The processes applied through case management are applicable within the context of the prospective payment system or managed care. Include reviews of each in your discussions.

Projected Outcomes

The projected outcomes of the model can be covered next. Outline the general goals of any case management model and the specific goals of the organization. Include topics such as improved quality of care, improved caregiver satisfaction, improved patient satisfaction, decreased length of stay, and decreased resource utilization including reductions in cost/day/stay. Other projected outcomes might include reduction in insurance denials of payment, better turnaround time for tests, treatments, procedures and consults, and variance analysis methods.

Once again, the length and detail of this program must be determined by the audience and the amount of time that can be allotted by the various departments.

CASE MANAGER EDUCATION

Education of case managers requires several days to weeks. It cannot be assumed that nurses newly promoted to the role of case manager can function without training. Individual organizations must decide who is best qualified to provide this education. In some cases, outside consultants or experts in the field may be needed to provide this service.

In a 3-day program, 3 days are devoted to case management and related concepts. Nurses promoted to case management roles may have had no experience in either health care reimbursement, case management, leadership/management, or other related topics.

DAY 1
Explain the Differences Between Leadership and Management During the First Day (Table 24-2). Functioning as a Case Manager Requires the Use of Both Skills.

Some topics to be covered might be the qualities of a leader, the correlation between administrative style and the nursing process, contingency management theory, and accountability versus responsibility. Although the case manager role is not identifiable as a management position in the traditional sense, it is essential that the case manager understand these concepts and be able to use them to effect the changes necessary for achieving excellent outcomes.

TABLE 24-2 CASE MANAGER EDUCATION DAY 1 CONTENT OUTLINE	
Objectives	**Content**
Define leadership versus management.	Leadership versus management Definitions of leadership and management Qualities of a leader Difference between administrative process and nursing process Contingency management (situational management) Accountability versus responsibility

Describe power and its uses for a case manager.	Definition of power
	   Five sources of power
	   Constructive and destructive uses of power
	   Strategies to obtain power

Identify the change process.	Change theory
	   Three types of change
	      Technical
	      Structural
	      People oriented
	   Lewin's Phases of Change
	      Freezing
	      Moving
	      Exploring
	      Refreezing
	      Implementation
	Effecting positive change in management
	Ten conditions that make change acceptable
	Approaches to decreasing resistance to change

Relate the concepts of power and change.	Relationship between power and change
	   Empowerment
	   Change = empowerment: empowerment = change

Demonstrate effective communication techniques.	Communication
	   Do's and don'ts of effective communication
	   Active listening
	Assertive versus aggressive behavior
	   Conflict
	   Source
	   Resolutions
	   Problem-solving strategies

Describe the process of patient education.	Patient education
	   Adult learning principles
	   Strategies for effective teaching and learning

Continued

TABLE 24-2	CASE MANAGER EDUCATION DAY 1 CONTENT OUTLINE—CONT'D
Objectives	**Content**

State the legal rights of patients.	Legal rights of patients
	    Patient bill of rights
	    Health care proxy
	    Living will
	Do-not-resuscitate (DNR) laws
	Managed care legal issues
	Health care ethics
	Organizational ethics

Implement discharge planning process.	Discharge planning
	    Collaborative process
	    Assessment and planning
	    Referrals to provide continuity of care
	Balanced Budget Act

Review utilization management techniques.	Utilization management Assessment review Continued review Appeals process Using criteria

The case manager will, at the least, be managing patient care. This will be accomplished through the role's facilitation and coordination aspects. In addition, the case manager will be managing the health care team by ensuring that the interdisciplinary plan of care is in place and moving along in a timely fashion. These two elements of the role require excellent management skills. To be maximally effective, these management skills should be coupled with strong leadership skills.

The case manager must be empowered. A portion of this perceived empowerment must be inherent in the individual assuming the role. A working knowledge of the theories of power and their relationship to the case manager role should be included in the curriculum. Case managers should understand that their personal power sources are as related to their personal style as those found in the job description. Review strategies for obtaining as well as using power. A positive use of power will enhance self-esteem and bring more effectiveness to the role.

Implementation of a case management model involves both subtle and overt changes. It has been said that change is painful, but just how painful depends on the level of organizational support as well as individual support. Understanding the stages and processes of change can help decrease the difficulties associated with change. Whether the organization is large or small, complex or simple, change is never easy and seldom goes smoothly. If the case manager understands this in advance, difficulties can be lessened and ambiguities between case manager and other workers reduced.

The specific theory of change used by the instructor is not as important as conveying the message that the conversion to case management will be bumpy and that some days will not be productive or fulfilling. Nevertheless, the case manager should understand the techniques for effecting positive change and the conditions that make change more acceptable.

Implementation always involves some resistance. A portion of the organization will accept the change immediately; some will be resistant; and others will remain in the middle of the road, reserving judgment until they see the model in action. It will be impossible to win everyone over, and the case manager should understand this. Approaches to reducing resistance to change might be employed to help make the transition as smooth as possible.

Power and change are interrelated concepts. An empowered individual is in a better position to effect change. At the same time, the more change that is effected, the more empowered the individual becomes.

The effectiveness of any leader or manager depends on the styles of communication used. A substantial portion of the curriculum should be devoted to teaching effective communication techniques. One topic that can make a difference in the successful integration of the case manager role is the use of proper verbal and nonverbal communication styles, as well as proper techniques for listening. Active listening can result in positive communication interactions.

Integrated in this should be the technique for assertive communication versus the aggressive communication style, which has been shown to be less effective.

Finally, the case manager should be aware of the various sources of conflict that may come about as a result of the integration of this role and of the problem-solving strategies that should be used for resolving conflict.

Patient education is one of the three main role functions of the case manager. Therefore the principles of adult learning and strategies for effective teaching and learning should be included in the curriculum. Effective inpatient teaching is an aid to successful recovery at home.

The case manager must serve as a patient advocate, interacting on the patient's behalf with other departments and disciplines. This advocacy role is possibly more important than ever before. Include in the curriculum a discussion of do-not-resuscitate (DNR) laws, living wills, and health care proxy laws and the Balanced Budget Act, and any other relevant health care laws. Health care ethics and organizational ethics should be included. A lecturer with expertise in these areas should be recruited.

A portion of the curriculum should cover discharge planning, with an emphasis on collaboration. If the organization has a discharge planning department, the discharge planning process can be reviewed from this perspective. The role of the social worker is important in the discharge planning process, and a social worker should be enlisted to provide insights on how case manager and social worker roles can work together. Many disciplines share the responsibility of assessing and planning for discharge. Reaching out to the community is part of the discharge planning process. As much as possible, the case manager should be made aware of the various community resources available to address patient problems. Some of these referral sources will come to the case manager's attention once the manager begins working in the role, but giving the case manager an overview of some of the resources available is important. Utilization management education should include techniques for performing assessment and continued stay reviews as well as strategies for appealing third party payer denials. Finally, the use of criteria such as InterQual Criteria (1998) or those of Schibanoff (1999) should be explained in detail. The use of case studies here is helpful.

DAY 2

On the second day (Table 24-3), provide an overview and definition of case management. Review the relationship between cost and quality as they relate to case management along with the goals of a case management model. Also include an in-depth historical perspective of the evolution of nursing care delivery models. This will help to put today's case management model in perspective and give it relevance.

TABLE 24-3   CASE MANAGER EDUCATION DAY 2 CONTENT OUTLINE

Objectives	Content

Define the concepts of case management.	Overview of case management
	    Definition
	    Nine steps to case management
	    Goals of case management
	    Expected outcomes of case
	    management

Identify issues affecting health care delivery in the new millennium.	Health care crisis
	    Nursing shortage
	    Changes in reimbursement
	    Aging population
	    Chronicity
	    Increased technology

Explain the prospective payment reimbursement system.	Fiscal issues facing nursing
	    DRGs
	    Length of stay
	    Home care
	    Ambulatory care
	    Acute rehab medicine

Discuss managed care reimbursement.	Managed care
	    HMOs
	    PPOs
	    Capitation
	    Managed care contracts

State the role of case manager and other members of the health care team.	Professional image
	    Case manager job description
	    Collaborative roles
	        Nursing
	        Physicians
	        Social work

Define case management plans.	Case management plans
	    Design
	    Documentation
	    Relationship to length of stay
	    Collaborative tool
	    Education
	    Quality of care

Document accurately the changes in case management using the case management plan.	Changes
	    Length of stay
	    Patient/practitioner variances
	    Quality of care

TABLE 24-3	CASE MANAGER EDUCATION DAY 2 CONTENT OUTLINE—CONT'D
Objectives	**Content**
Identify appropriate strategies for measuring, evaluating, and assessing outcomes.	Quality improvement documentation Problem-solving techniques Tracking and trending: selection of population source data Development of monitoring tool Analysis of data Evaluation and follow-up

Case management is important as it relates to the past and present health care environment. There are numerous relevant health care crises, but some of the top ones might include the nursing shortage and how it affected the evolution of case management, changes in health care reimbursement as related to the prospective payment system, an aging patient population, chronicity, and increased technology in health care. Case management has evolved out of the current crises. Presenting case management from its historical perspective will lend relevance to the model.

Cover the prospective payment system in detail because it is this system of predetermined lengths of stay as related to the DRG system that has led to evolution of the concept of case management. Cover the system in its entirety including home care, ambulatory care, and acute rehabilitation reimbursement schemes. Discuss the differences between what the state calls an acceptable length of stay and what the federal government calls acceptable. Understand the varying expectations from managed care organizations and how these relate to the organization's managed care contracts. The case manager must understand the reimbursement system completely and must be fluent with the terms related to it. Guest lecturers who have expertise in this area or others should be invited to speak whenever possible.

Following this discussion should be one on managed care reimbursement systems. Case managers need to understand the finer points as they relate to case management in a managed care environment. Much of this discussion will relate back to the utilization management discussion.

Cover the role functions and responsibilities of the case manager, with a review of the case manager job description. Emphasis should be placed on the collaborative relationship between the case manager and all other disciplines. The specific responsibilities of the case manager can be covered during this time. These responsibilities include education, discharge planning, and facilitation of the patient's progress through the system.

The case management plan can be reviewed for form, content, and purpose. Possible topics to be covered in a discussion of case management plans include design, documentation, relationship to length of stay, use as a collaborative tool, and quality-of-care monitoring. Review case management plans in detail, as they are one of the more visible and tangible changes in case management. It is also important to review methods for writing the case management plan, especially how a case management plan can be used to track variances in care and quality data. Tracking and trending for selected patient problems or entire disease entities can be followed concurrently or retrospectively through the case management format.

DAY 3

On the third day (Table 24-4), review the roles and functions of the case manager. A "train the trainer" approach is useful at this time. If an experienced case manager is available, it is valuable for the new case

TABLE 24-4	CASE MANAGER EDUCATION DAY 3 CONTENT OUTLINE
Objectives	**Content**
Identify role of case manager.	Role functions 　　Planning and facilitation 　　Patient/family education 　　Discharge planning 　　Utilization management
Review the roles of the case management team.	Team members 　　Social work 　　Utilization 　　Discharge planning 　　Home care
Understand the in-depth roles of the case management team.	In-depth reviews 　　Discharge planning 　　Utilization management 　　Social work 　　Home care
Review case management assessment and documentation.	Assessment 　　On admission 　　Daily 　　Documentation 　　In-take assessment 　　On-going
Complete the case management plan.	Review plans, practice writing
Discuss variance analysis or outcomes.	Variances 　　Definition 　　Types 　　Monitoring Outcomes 　　Definition 　　Monitoring
Understand continuous quality improvement.	Continuous quality improvement 　　Definition 　　Relationship to case management
Discuss differentiated practice.	Relate differentiated practice to case management
Role play.	Relate to other disciplines in case manager role

manager to hear exactly how the role is carried out from someone already functioning in it. Provide a thorough review of how the case manager should collect data on patients. These data provide a framework from which the case manager can track the patients both while in the hospital and after discharge. Although each case manager will individualize the data collection process, some standard methods can be reviewed. In addition, walking the case manager through the day is helpful.

Review the roles of the case management team. If at all possible, representatives from each discipline should lecture on their role and on how their role relates to case management and to other members of the case management team. Include the social work, utilization management, discharge planning, and home care disciplines. This overview should be followed by in-depth discussions on discharge planning, utilization review and management, social work, and planning for home care.

A workshop dedicated to case management care plan writing is a must for the third day. Each case manager should be given the opportunity to write a managed care plan from beginning to end. Going through the process step by step helps identify areas of confusion or uncertainty.

Variance analysis is a unique opportunity provided by the case management model. A retrospective analysis of what did or did not happen and looking for patterns as well as causes of the variances can be used to justify changes in care (Cesta & Tahan, 2002). The case manager should be well versed in this process. In addition to providing the rationale for changes in care plans, variance analysis allows for future upgrading of the quality of care. It is much easier to track clinical outcomes with the variance analysis format. Include methods for identifying and monitoring outcomes. Outcomes can be identified as clinical and nonclinical, diagnosis specific, and generic. Also discuss continuous quality improvement (CQI) in relation to case management and case management plans.

Many case management programs use differentiated practice methods. Differentiated practice calls for the assignment of personnel based on employee level of education, experience, and expertise (American Hospital Association, 1990). An effective case management program should include a differentiated practice system so that optimal use can be made of the nurse's experience and education. One part of case management training should cover the levels of education for nurses, including a discussion of the strengths and weaknesses associated with each level.

Devote one part of the curriculum to role playing. This helps case managers by walking them through some of the situations they will encounter. One of the hardest areas for some new case managers is explaining to patients, physicians, and others exactly what the case manager role encompasses. Giving out business cards to patients is equally difficult because case managers are not familiar with such formalities. Practice with the card can address and solve these problems. This may seem rudimentary, but it is crucial that the case manager feel at ease with these tasks.

Role playing can also be used to practice how to confront and resolve conflicts that arise during the change process.

Time Allotments

An allotment of 3 days to this curriculum represents the absolute minimal amount needed. A highly desirable approach to take would be to expand the detail of the 3-day program and spend more time on each topic. In this way, the program might be 6 to 9 days long. The longer the time devoted to the program, the higher is the likelihood that the case managers will receive the complex didactic materials needed to function in this complex role.

In addition to this didactic portion, the case manager should be given the opportunity to precept with an experienced case manager and to apply the strategies and theories learned in the classroom.

References

American Association of Colleges of Nursing (1997). *A vision of baccalaureate and graduate education: The next decade.* Washington, DC: AACN.

American Hospital Association (1990). *Current issues and perspective on differentiated practice.* Chicago: American Organization of Nurse Executives.

Cesta, T.G., & Tahan, H.A. (2002). *The case manager's survival guide: Winning strategies for clinical practice.* St. Louis: Mosby.

Fineman, L. (1996). Developing a formal education program for case managers. *Journal of Case Management, 5*(4), 158-161.

InterQual, Inc. (1998). *System administrator's guide.* Mailborough, Mass.: InterQual.

Kahn, R.L., Wolfe, D.M., Quinn, R.P., Snoek, J.D., & Rosenthal, R.A. (1964). *Organizational stress: Studies in role conflict and ambiguity.* New York: Wiley.

Schibanoff, J.M., (Ed.), (1999). *Health care management guidelines,* New york: Milliman & Roberston.

Tahan, H.A. (1998, Nov.). *The case manager's excellence: Skills, traits and competencies.* Presented at the Medical Case Management Conference, Philadelphia.

Toran, M. (1998). Academic case management. *The Case Manager,* (1), 43-46.

25

The Competency Outcomes and Performance Assessment Model Applied to Nursing Case Management Systems

Carrie B. Lenburg

CHAPTER OVERVIEW

The roles, functions, and responsibilities of case managers continue to evolve and vary depending on setting, staffing, and other variables and thus specific competencies also vary. Despite inconsistencies, it is possible to develop a competency-based program for orientation and ongoing performance assessment that fits diverse positions and levels, conditions, and settings, whether institutional or community. The Competency Outcomes and Performance Assessment (COPA) model was created to promote competence in learning and evaluation to fit the needs across the spectrum of education and practice environments. The COPA approach provides a standardized, organizing framework of eight core competencies and a set of concepts and methods that can be used for multiple purposes. This chapter focuses on the constellation of core practice competencies and illustrates how they can apply to case management departments, programs, and personnel. The elegance of the model is its simultaneous universality and specificity.

The need for demonstrated competence in all areas of practice and education is essential and increasingly is being mandated by many regulatory, certification, and accreditation bodies. The multiple complex changes in society, health care, and nursing practice exert a profound influence on what nurses, including case managers, do and how well they are expected to do it. Although implementing a competency-based system has some unintended consequences, the benefits far outweigh them. Change is difficult for many and may impose threats to feelings about job security and ability. Thoughtful planning and collaboration, however, can allay most negative side effects and also provide opportunities for increased professional development (Bargagliotti, Luttrell, & Lenburg, 1999; Lenburg, 1991, 1999a, 2002).

In the context of changes in society and health care, it is even more important for case management departments, programs, and individuals to develop competency-based performance assessment protocols, despite diverse goals or functions and inconsistency in roles. The process of change essentially begins with developing or confirming the goals or outcomes for the department and individual case managers, ensuring the relevant fit with job descriptions, and defining competence consistent with the agency. The primary focus of the department determines the emphasis on competence in role performance. Thus, a department that focuses on clinical coordination will emphasize different components than one that targets utilization management and discharge planning. Regardless of the primary goals, case managers need to integrate clinical, interdisciplinary, economic, technological, cultural, and sociopolitical aspects of providing health care in complex, changing environments. Implementation of the new privacy regulations, under the Health Insurance Portability and Accountability Act (HIPAA) that became effective in April 2003, adds yet another major dimension to the challenge of contemporary and competent practice (HIPAA websites, 2001).

Continued

Case managers across the broad spectrum of practice may be required to assess their own practice and the competence of others, and so are challenged by the issues related to competency performance assessment. This presents an important rationale to improve competency assessment methods and programs. The ideas described in this chapter are intended to help case managers evaluate existing efforts and potentially apply a competency-based conceptual framework that is comprehensive and essentially universal in its application. As the role of case manager continues to evolve and be influenced by circumstances, the model described here allows for both flexibility and specificity. It is a guide for rethinking and determining which competencies define practice and, therefore, must be documented through relevant, effective and efficient assessment methods.

Among the many problems traditionally associated with performance evaluation is the use of multiple and seemingly unorganized checklists of tasks and activities for different levels of staff and types of units. In most settings these checklists use different organizing approaches, inconsistent language and procedures and, due to the persistent uncertainty about evaluation, they are modified often in an effort "to do it better." Duplication of effort on different units is frustrating and time consuming. An equally ineffective practice is *not* to change them due to lack of knowledge of how to improve the process. The situation becomes even more complex and troublesome with institutional mergers, staff shortages, and other related factors that increase workload and stress. Such circumstances have a negative influence on performance and the ability to develop and implement defensible competency assessment methods. Ironically, institutional accreditation depends on assessment of competence more than ever, at a time when it is more complex, time consuming, and difficult to validate with certainty. The COPA model helps to remedy some of these conditions and improve competence and performance assessment.

THE COMPETENCY OUTCOMES AND PERFORMANCE ASSESSMENT MODEL

The Competency Outcomes and Performance Assessment (COPA) model, developed by Lenburg over the past 15 years, offers a different perspective and approach to the evaluation of performance abilities of various levels of employees and students. Although initially developed for educational programs (academic and nonacademic), the model is applicable to those in practice across the continuum of diverse settings and various levels and types of personnel, including case managers. The COPA model provides a comprehensive framework for re-visioning and organizing performance expectations in actual practice; as such, it influences learning and assessment of abilities in the context of those expectations (Lenburg & Mitchell, 1991; Luttrell, Lenburg, Scherubel, Jacob, & Koch, 1999). It is flexible and comprehensive, yet it can be as specific as required for particular purposes.

The following concise description of the model reviews some of the primary components as a context for making decisions about its applicability in particular practice environments. At the outset, four essential questions are outlined to guide the process of development and implementation of a competency-based performance assessment program. They are sequential and each one is an essential component.

1. What competency outcomes are essential for actual practice? This question requires the identification of the broad performance-based competencies deemed mandatory for practice. They are the end results of learning and experience and collectively define practice in broad categories.

2. What specific practice skills and related actions or behaviors provide sufficient evidence to substantiate competence in each category? This question focuses on skills for particular personnel and units and the actions or inactions that must be observed to verify designated abilities. These skills and related critical elements define what competence looks like; when implemented, they provide objective evidence of actual abilities.

3. What are the most effective ways to learn these competencies (to upgrade, improve, and achieve them)? This question requires the integration of actual practice expectations and the use of related and effective learning strategies consistent with the characteristics of the learner (employee, orientee, student, etc.) and position description.

4. What are the most effective methods to assess achievement of designated skills? This question requires determination of specific assessment methods and related logistics, policies, and resources to be used to validate and document competence.

The COPA model reverses the typical process of development; the end result actually is the beginning. It requires that the preferred outcomes and the essential practice abilities be clearly specified and justified before determining how they can be achieved (learned) and evaluated. Unlike the commonly used approach of traditional objectives, which seem more like directions, activities, or procedures, competency outcomes focus on, and are stated as, the practice-oriented and performance-based expected results of such activities. The COPA outcomes approach is focused on the end results, the required byproduct of focused planning and effort. The set of outcomes is the destination; once that is clear, the map can be drawn for how to get there and how to know it is the right place. Learning and practice strategies are customized to promote the most effective and efficient methods to achieve the outcomes. Thereafter, specific methods of assessment are created to document achievement of actual performance. Thus, it is essential to begin with the competency outcomes, even those that often are considered too ambiguous to be assessed, like human caring relationships and critical thinking. (See Lenburg et al., 1995, regarding cultural competence.)

Outcome statements are worded precisely and in terms of what nurses *actually are expected to do* in practice, rather than what they *know about* practice. One example of the wording used for a comprehensive series of program outcomes is illustrated by those developed by the faculty of the University of Colorado Health Sciences Center School of Nursing (Redman, Lenburg, & Walker, 1999). Competency outcomes and related skills set the target for continued improvement and the basis for assessment. For example, contrast the wording of a typical objective with its edited version, wording as a competency outcome.

Typical objective: Describe the role of case manager in applying protocols for utilization review.

Competency outcome: Conduct utilization review according to established best practices.

Comment: In actual practice, nurses *conduct* utilization reviews according to standards, not *describe* the role.

The assessment component of the COPA model is effective and supportable because it is based on the integration of 10 psychometrically based concepts developed by Lenburg (1979, 1999b). These concepts include examination (as different from subjective evaluation), specified skills or dimensions of practice to be assessed, critical elements that define competence for each skill, level of acceptability, sampling, objectivity, comparability, consistency, flexibility, and systematized conditions. This constellation of concepts creates the framework for developing and implementing reliable and objective practice-based assessment instruments. All of them are required and interrelated, like 10 transparencies laid down over each other to create the "whole picture." These concepts applied to actual and simulation performance assessments are described by Lenburg (1979, 1999b) and Lenburg and Mitchell (1991).

THE EIGHT CORE PRACTICE COMPETENCIES

The practice competencies in the COPA model are derived from many years of analyzing the kinds of skills nurses are required to perform effectively in the context of diverse and multiple client needs in contemporary health care delivery. Over time, a long and unorganized list of skills was consolidated into eight categories, revised, refined, and tested for applicability and comprehensiveness in diverse situations. As developed in this model, all practice skills can be listed under one or more of these eight core competencies; all are required in practice, albeit to a different extent depending on various position descriptions and responsibilities, legal and regulatory requirements, and setting characteristics. The model makes it possible to use the same organizing framework for developing assessment instruments, logistics, and policies, regardless of these differences. This tends to promote consistency and objectivity across levels of employees (or learners) and settings (Bargagliotti et al., 1999; Lenburg, 1999b). Ultimately, after the initial components are developed, this model requires less time to develop additional skill checklists (or other instruments) or to revise existing ones and implement related processes. Typically, when employees are informed in advance, are subjected to similar performance expectations, and believe the process is fair, they are more willing to do their best and to feel more satisfied with the content and process of evaluation; in the COPA model evaluation is referred to as competency performance examinations (CPEs). The use of such objective assessment methods potentially helps staff to become more competent, efficient, and motivated to improve.

The model provides a standardized and comprehensive structure for developing specific skills under each category to correspond with different levels of staff and work environments. More typical approaches use a checklist of all procedures related to the job; when analyzed in the context of the core competencies, however, even long checklists may not include all of the core competencies required for the designated position. In contrast, the core practice competencies approach organizes essential skills into a consolidated and cohesive array and provides more assurance that all dimensions of practice are included, with emphasis on the most relevant skills for designated staff positions. Boyer (2002) described the application of the COPA model to a funded statewide nurse internship and preceptor project in Vermont.

It is essential to understand the meaning, relevance, and distinctions of the eight core competencies to appreciate their central place in practice and in the model. The brief descriptions listed here provide an initial step in this direction. Taken in their broadest and most generic meaning, each competence category is applicable to some extent to employees from the most subordinate to the most senior positions. The eight competency categories are listed in Box 25-1 along with some examples for each, on a continuum of simple to complex skills expected for diverse positions and circumstances.

1. *Assessment and Intervention Skills:* This competency includes all forms of assessment, data gathering, and monitoring and a range of technical, therapeutic, safety, managerial, or other intervention skills.
2. *Communication Skills:* This competency includes oral, written, and computer communication skills used to exchange information and to transmit messages with or about clients and others.
3. *Critical Thinking Skills:* This competency includes a broad array of skills along a continuum from simple problem solving and analysis to reflective judgment, scientific inquiry, and research-based knowledge development.
4. *Humanistic Caring Relationship Skills:* This competency includes skills related to promoting client-focused interests and concerns, interpersonal behaviors that demonstrate care for and with clients and significant others, sensitivity to diverse cultures and preferences, client advocacy, and social justice concerns.

5. *Teaching Skills:* This competency includes the transmission of information intended to instruct clients and others about topics essential to health care and well-being, from the simple telling and showing to the more advanced skills of formalized teaching episodes.

6. *Management Skills:* This competency pertains to such skills as managing time and resources, implementing activities to promote cooperation among relevant others, creating and implementing budgets, planning, delegating and supervising responsibilities of others, collaboration across disciplines, and related activities.

7. *Leadership Skills:* This competency includes activities that promote staff morale, cooperation, assertiveness, and risk-taking; creative planning for change and innovations; implementation of new policies or other protocols; and ongoing professional development of self and others.

8. *Knowledge Integration Skills:* This competency stretches along the continuum from using factual information, prior learning, and basic principles and procedures to supporting decisions and actions with relevant research-based evidence and integrating best practices from nursing and other health-related disciplines and the humanities, arts, and sciences disciplines.

BOX 25-1

LENBURG'S CONSTELLATION OF CORE PRACTICE COMPETENCIES: EXAMPLES FOR APPLICATION TO CASE MANAGEMENT

1. Assessment and intervention skills
   a. Promoting safety and protection: clients, families, personnel
   b. Assessing and monitoring: clients, personnel, practice protocols, audits, systems
   c. Managing therapeutic treatments and procedures: conventional, adaptive, innovative
   d. Promoting human–technology interaction and effectiveness
2. Communication skills
   a. Oral skills
      (1) Interacting, listening, processing, reflective feedback
      (2) Interviewing, history taking, data collection
      (3) Group discussion: interacting, leading, persuading
      (4) Giving directions, verifying, conflict resolution
      (5) Reporting, presenting
   b. Writing skills
      (1) Clinical reports, histories, clinical pathways, multidisciplinary action plans (MAPs), nursing care plans (NCPs), documentation
      (2) Agency documents: reports, forms, memos, letters
      (3) Manuscripts for publication, manuals, proposals
   c. Computing skills
      (1) Documentation related to/for clients, employers, authorities
      (2) Information search, investigation, discovery, synthesis, dissemination
3. Critical thinking skills
   a. Integrating, synthesizing pertinent data from multiple sources
   b. Problem solving, diagnostic reasoning, clinical decision making
   c. Outcomes and variance analysis, reflective judgment, ethical reasoning, prioritizing
   d. Scientific inquiry, investigation, research, evidence-based perspective
   e. Adaptation, creativity and innovation, quality improvements

Continued

| BOX 25-1 | LENBURG'S CONSTELLATION OF CORE PRACTICE COMPETENCIES: EXAMPLES FOR APPLICATION TO CASE MANAGEMENT—CONT'D |

4. Humanistic caring and relationship skills
    a. Moral, ethical, legal responsiveness and implementation for clients and others
    b. Cultural and individual respect, supportive interpersonal relationships
    c. Advocacy, sensitivity and compassion, social justice
5. Teaching skills
    a. Individuals and groups: clients, intradisciplinary and interdisciplinary staff development, others
    b. Health promotion, restoration, and maintenance, quality improvements
6. Management skills
    a. Administration and organization responsibilities; coordinate care and delivery systems
    b. Planning, delegation, supervision of others; maintain standards
    c. Interdisciplinary and intradisciplinary coordination, care conferences, discharge planning
    d. Human and material resource utilization, budgets, personnel, supplies, equipment
    e. Accountability and responsibility, performance appraisals, quality improvement
7. Leadership skills
    a. Intradisciplinary and interdisciplinary collaboration and negotiation, team building
    b. Creative vision to formulate alternatives, practice protocols, implement change
    c. Supportable assertiveness, persuasion, risk taking, persistence, flexibility
    d. Anticipatory planning, policy making, stimulating evidence-based decisions
    e. Ensure professional standards, adapt as needed, represent the profession to community leaders
    f. Continued professional development
8. Knowledge integration skills
    a. Use current knowledge pertaining to nursing and health-related disciplines and practice
    b. Incorporate humanities, arts, and sciences as well as business, economics, and politics into practice

It is important to note that the eight competencies listed in Box 25-1 are fixed; the examples of skills are just that—examples; the lists are not intended to be all-inclusive. Furthermore, some skills could be shifted to another competency category; to some extent, this depends on emphasis, preferences, and practice circumstances. These examples are listed to stimulate thought and discussion that ultimately could result in a revised draft with more specific skills for case managers in particular health care institutions or agencies. Nurses and case managers engage in many competencies simultaneously, and to some extent, their judgment and agency protocols will determine where specific skills should be listed (i.e., under which core competency).

The eight core practice competencies are very utilitarian and efficient; they can be used as follows:
- A template for writing outcome statements
- A comprehensive set for diverse practice levels
- A universal but flexible set for diverse settings and conditions
- A framework for specific skills and subskills
- A structure for ongoing quality improvement
- A guide for professional development (individual and groups)

Specific skills (and subskills) are listed under each competency category, consistent with the expectations for the particular level of practitioner; examples are listed later in the chapter. The targeted content and process for performance-based learning and assessment are based on the specific subskills listed under each competency category and their corresponding critical elements (Boyer, 2002; Luttrell et al., 1999;

Lenburg, 1999b). Critical elements are defined as the single, discrete, and observable behaviors that are mandatory for that skill and for the level of staff involved. They specify the baseline of acceptable performance and define "how good is good enough." The critical elements for any given skill, therefore, guide the content and processes for learning and evaluation.

Some basic descriptors of and criteria for writing critical elements are cited below. Additional descriptions and examples are found in references by Lenburg (1979, 1999, 1999b), Lenburg and Mitchell (1991), and Luttrell et al. (1999).

- The stated critical elements define competence, that is, how good is good enough? And how much is enough to validate competence in the specified skill?
- They are the essence of principles and required application of knowledge for competence; they are not conceived as steps in a procedure, even though they are arranged logically. They do not include everything known about the particular skill; that pertains to learning the content or skills.
- Critical elements are similar to written test questions in function, that is, evaluating essential ability, but by definition every critical element is mandatory. They comprise the standard to be met, the specific measures that define competence. In this criterion-referenced system, all critical elements (100%) are required to validate competence. Thus, deciding which critical elements truly are mandatory and how they are worded are extremely important in performance assessment because of the resulting consequences.

When writing critical elements

- Begin with one single verb that describes the highest level of expected skill performance.
- Use language that is clear, concise, precise, relevant, and unambiguous.
- Specify the range of acceptability for performance of that skill.
- Include specific methods or techniques as required.
- Include only behaviors that are mandatory for competence, not steps in the task.

It is important to understand the sequential and logical relationship among component parts of the model. First, write the competency outcome statements that determine broad practice abilities to be achieved (implemented); include all eight core competencies to some extent. Next, identify for each competency outcome the specific skills (and subskills where used) required for actual practice for the position. Then, for each skill listed, write the mandatory critical elements that will be assessed for that skill for the particular position, setting, and purpose. Finalize the process by writing the policies and procedures required for implementation.

The following guidelines are useful in making the transition to the competency-based practice

- Use the core competencies along with specific content to create competency outcome statements.
- Cluster specific skills under the competency categories.
- Write critical elements for specific skills based on criteria.
- Ensure internal consistency among all components.
- Implement program evaluation and use findings for improvements.
- Refine outcomes, assessment tools, and related materials for the next cycle.

APPLICATION TO CASE MANAGEMENT SYSTEMS

Literature related to nursing case management describes the variety of complex roles and abilities required for nurses in various settings. Tahan (1997) describes three role dimensions for the nurse case manager as the clinical role, the managerial role, and the financial/business role. While his overall categories differ from the COPA model, the competencies (skills) inherently have much in common. These competencies are elaborated further by Cohen and Cesta (1997). Taylor (1997) makes a valuable contribution in describing the competencies of nurse case managers regarding ethical issues. Lenburg chaired an Expert Panel of the American Academy of Nursing charged to explore cultural competence in education. Their work resulted in the monograph *Promoting Cultural Competence in Nursing Education*, which contains multiple recommendations related to expected outcomes and competencies for the many types of entities involved (Lenburg et al., 1995).

The predominant skills for nurse case managers include collaboration, negotiation, decision making, delegation, assessment, monitoring, planning, creating alternatives, applying specific interventions, teaching, supervision, and evaluating others. Using the COPA model, four major responsibilities could be extrapolated as competency outcomes and skills in terms for actual practice as listed below. Box 25-2 outlines the leading stem for these four examples followed by suggested related subskills, which in some circumstances also could be considered as their critical elements. Note that the statement of skills and critical elements should be edited depending on the needs, functions, and overall circumstances in the particular setting.

The stem is: The nurse case manager will

1. Coordinate patient care to maximize achievement of patient outcomes
2. Conduct utilization and resource management process
3. Implement discharge planning based on patient-related needs and established protocols
4. Promote the evolving definition of roles, functions, and practice competencies of the case manager and case management program (department)

An analysis of these competencies shows that the core competencies (as outlined in Box 25-1) potentially are included to some extent, although this is not obvious. Specific case management skills could be rewritten using the organizing framework of the eight core competencies to insure the required emphasis for the purpose at hand, as illustrated in Box 25-3. Using this organized approach, it becomes easier to determine whether all competencies are included and which are emphasized, overemphasized, or inadequately represented. This kind of competency analysis is fundamental for planning, revising, and evaluating orientation, instructional, and assessment programs; it makes inconsistency, redundancy, and omissions evident and identifies where corrective revisions need to be focused. It is a pragmatic, logical, and comprehensive process that promotes quality improvement and professional development. Either method could be used so long as an analysis confirms that all core categories are included to the extent required.

Figure 25-1 is a blank form designed as a worksheet on which case managers can list specific skills for each of the core competencies as they apply to the one or more primary roles of the position. The specific subskills vary by staff levels, practice settings, and types of case management system. For example, identify the following.

What *specific assessment* and *intervention skills* are performed by the nurse case manager?

What specific forms of written, oral, and computer *communication skills* are required from them?

What different forms of *critical thinking* apply to various levels of staff in the case management department?

The competency outcome categories facilitate the development of a comprehensive but specific framework to ensure that the learning, implementation, evaluation, and quality improvement processes are customized to the mission, environment, staffing patterns, and assigned staff roles of the agency or institution. The eight core competency categories also could be used as a framework for self-reflection and evaluation as part of an ongoing portfolio for professional development (Lenburg, 2000).

After the particular skills are listed under each of the eight core practice competencies required for the designated positions and settings, specific critical elements are written for each one. The set of critical elements define practice expectations required for the particular skill (e.g., for critical thinking, communication, or management). The process of identifying the precise behaviors expected in practice

Text continued on p.274

BOX 25-2	FOUR EXAMPLES OF CASE MANAGER COMPETENCIES (SKILLS) WITH SUGGESTED CRITICAL ELEMENTS

At the end of the designated period (orientation, annual review, etc.), the case manager will

1. Coordinate patient care to maximize achievement of patient outcomes
   a. Assess patient on admission to determine treatment based on best practice protocol
   b. Collaborate with members of care team to establish most effective plan of care based on patient-related data
   c. Engage patient and significant others in planning and implementing care
   d. Coordinate ongoing care according to standards of practice, guidelines (other criteria)
   e. Enforce privacy protection policy re patients and others
   f. Monitor care and variation in treatments and related costs by established categories
   g. Modify guidelines as needed, based on best practices, evidence, standards of care
   h. Recommend process and/or policy changes to improve patient outcomes and protocols
   i. Document patient care, responses, findings, and recommendations
2. Conduct utilization and resource management process (as determined: per unit, diagnosis, patient, etc.)
   a. Monitor care, treatment, progress according to standards of care, guidelines
   b. Promote implementation of established standards of care and other protocols
   c. Analyze identified deficiencies and variations in care, treatments, process
   d. Collaborate with others across care continuum to improve efficiency and effectiveness of care and use of resources
   e. Conduct managed care reviews on a timely (pre-established) basis using established protocols
   f. Negotiate lengths of stay and transitional plans with relevant others
   g. Write letters of appeal to reverse denials related to payment, length of stay, treatment, etc.
   h. Recommend process and/or policy changes to improve utilization of resources based on data
   i. Document research findings and policy recommendations with rationale for changes
3. Implement discharge planning based on patient-related needs and established protocols
   a. Outline patient's needs for ongoing health care, including outcomes to be achieved and accessible resources for each
   b. Engage patient and/or significant others in planning process
   c. Teach patient and/or significant others relevant aspects of care following discharge
   d. Make referrals to relevant providers or agencies to promote positive health outcomes
   e. Enforce privacy protection policy for patients and others
   f. Document discharge plan and interaction with patient and/or significant others
   g. Engage in actions to improve discharge planning guidelines and process
4. Promote the evolving definition of roles, function, and practice competencies of the case manager and case management program or department in diverse settings (local to national)
   a. Participate in activities designed to clarify case manager roles and competencies
   b. Conduct studies in local environment related to case managers, to determine such areas as the need for and responses to services, variations in roles and practice, and specific areas for clarification and improvement of practice competencies
   c. Make recommendations to improve policy, process, and practice of case managers, based on pertinent data, and evidence-based best practices
   d. Engage in team collaboration efforts to promote quality health care for consumers

BOX 25-3

SUGGESTED EXAMPLES OF SKILLS FOR CORE COMPETENCIES TO ASSESS PERFORMANCE OF THE NURSE CASE MANAGER

A. Core practice competence: Assessment and intervention
   Subskill: The case manager is able to
   1. Monitor effectiveness of clinical path protocols in achieving patient outcomes
   Critical elements:
   1. Obtain pertinent data to substantiate implementation of established protocols.
   2. Analyze obtained data in context of protocols to identify variances.
   3. Interpret findings to identify root cause factors associated with the variance.
   4. Recommend strategies to maximize implementation of protocols while promoting patient outcomes and satisfaction.

B. Core practice competence: Critical thinking
   Subskill: The case manager is able to
   1. Plan a study to investigate differences in variance for a designated protocol among patients with similar conditions or DRG classification.
   Critical elements:
   1. Write the specific question to be explored, with related components.
   2. Write the justification for investigating the specified problem.
   3. Describe methods to be used, including subjects, time-line, and methods of data collection and analysis.
   4. Develop a budget that is adequate and efficient for the purpose.
   5. Outline potential consequences of positive and negative findings.

C. Core practice competence: Teaching
   Subskill: The case manager is able to
   1. Teach a group of staff to implement changes in performance evaluation methods.
   Critical elements:
   1. Develop a plan for a staff workshop to include the following:
      a. Specific outcomes to be achieved
      b. Strategies to promote learning and support
      c. Methods to evaluate comprehension and agreement with new methods
   2. Interact with the group to determine perceptions of new methods described in material previously distributed.
   3. Implement persuasive strategies to maximize comprehension and support of new methods.
   4. Engage all members in discussion to maximize input of diverse examples, applications, and concerns.
   5. Evaluate comprehension and support of methods.

D. Core practice competence: Management
   Subskill: The case manager is able to
   1. Maintain practice standards by holding self and other providers accountable.
   Critical elements:
   1. Ensure that each staff member has completed orientation or education programs pertaining to specific standards.
   2. Implement specific methods by which staff will be oriented and evaluated.
   3. Evaluate staff performance of specific skills during designated periods using the preestablished standards.
   4. Use evaluation findings to assess the need for change to promote quality improvement in staff performance.
   5. Implement procedures designed to promote compliance with practice standards.
   6. Communicate with relevant agency authorities to report findings and recommendations.

| BOX 25-3 | SUGGESTED EXAMPLES OF SKILLS FOR CORE COMPETENCIES TO ASSESS PERFORMANCE OF THE NURSE CASE MANAGER—CONT'D |

E. Core practice competence: Leadership
 Subskill: The case manager is able to
 1. Collaborate with multidisciplinary team members to develop cost-effective protocols to achieve patient outcomes and patient and staff satisfaction.
 Critical elements:
 1. Collaborate with multidisciplinary team in ways that
   a. Contribute to achievement of outcomes from a nursing perspective.
   b. Show respect for differing perspectives and positions.
   c. Promote evidence-based decisions.
   d. Promote team-building and cooperation.
   e. Promote accuracy, clarity, precision, and relevance of findings, outcomes, interventions.
 2. Seek leadership opportunities to coordinate activities that promote achievement of outcomes.
 3. Use creative strategies to promote effectiveness and efficiency of care delivery protocols.

Name of Staff member:_____ **Position:**_____ **Date:**_____

List specific subskills for each competency category required for three to four primary roles for each particular position

Core Competencies	Role 1	Role 2	Role 3	Role 4
Assessment and intervention				
Communications				
Critical thinking				
Humanistic caring relationships				
Teaching				
Management				
Leadership				
Knowledge integration				

FIGURE **25-1** Individual skills identification worksheet.

is crucial to promoting competent practice and decreasing avoidable errors. The resulting document that includes the specific skills for each core competency with required critical elements provides the blueprint for instruction, orientation, and performance assessment; it also becomes one of the components for quality improvement planning. These components pertain to two of the four essential questions already described and provide the basis for the remaining questions. Specifying the core practice competencies with their related skills and critical elements provides clear direction for further development of both product and process to improve quality of care delivery.

Potential examples of subskills under several core competencies with related potential critical elements are outlined in Box 25-3. They pertain to the case manager but are general in nature to allow flexibility in development; specific skills, their wording, and the critical elements depend on many factors, as already noted, and can be written several different ways or to different levels of expectation. Both skills and critical elements will be more relevant if developed by the staff in the particular setting to comply with specific position descriptions. These examples, therefore, are suggestive and illustrate the concept; they are not intended to be complete, conclusive, or necessarily the most relevant for different settings. They are ideas to stimulate more precise development. Other examples are found in the references.

CPEs are developed from this beginning, as illustrated in Box 25-4. Space in this chapter does not permit description of all the components of this aspect of the COPA model (Lenburg, 1979, 1999b;

BOX 25-4 ▸ EXAMPLES OF COMPETENCY PERFORMANCE EXAMINATIONS (CPEs)*

CPE 1: Implement the nurse case manager role as manager of care for a group of assigned patients. At the designated time for assessment, the case manager will be able to

MET	NOT MET	COMPETENCIES AND CRITICAL ELEMENTS
_____	_____	1. Manage care delivered to assigned patients consistent with assessment of their needs
_____	_____	2. Delegate specific aspects of patient care to relevant staff according to qualifications
_____	_____	3. Prioritize patient care activities
_____	_____	4. Monitor patient care provided by assisting personnel
_____	_____	5. Ensure accurate administration of all therapeutic interventions assigned to patients
_____	_____	6. Manage time and resources consistent with patient needs and agency protocols
_____	_____	7. Incorporate universal competencies and related critical elements*:
_____	_____	a. Safety and protection
_____	_____	b. Standard precautions
_____	_____	c. Interpersonal communication
_____	_____	d. Critical thinking
_____	_____	e. Humanistic caring relationships
_____	_____	f. Professional responsibilities
_____	_____	g. Documentation
_____	_____	8. Integrate knowledge relevant to the roles of nurse manager

*Based on listing of critical elements for specific skills under competency outcome categories.

BOX 25-4	EXAMPLES OF COMPETENCY PERFORMANCE EXAMINATIONS (CPEs)—CONT'D

CPE 2: Implement the case manager leadership role on the designated unit(s). At the designated time for assessment, the case manager will be able to

MET	NOT MET	COMPETENCIES AND CRITICAL ELEMENTS
_____	_____	1. Coordinate care of a full caseload of patients with designated staff
_____	_____	a. Assign staff to patients consistent with patient needs, staff qualification, and unit needs
_____	_____	b. Delegate tasks to staff consistent with their qualifications and needs of the unit
_____	_____	c. Prioritize patient care activities
_____	_____	d. Monitor care for all patient care provided by assisting personnel
_____	_____	2. Manage time, human, and material resources consistent with patient needs and agency protocols
_____	_____	3. Communicate essential information during and at conclusion of shift to designated others
_____	_____	4. Collaborate with other health care providers to promote achievement of patient outcomes
_____	_____	5. Integrate knowledge relevant to the role of nurse manager
_____	_____	6. Monitor staff to ensure universal competencies are implemented (using critical elements)*
_____	_____	a. Safety and protection
_____	_____	b. Standard precautions
_____	_____	c. Interpersonal communication
_____	_____	d. Critical thinking
_____	_____	e. Humanistic caring relationships
_____	_____	f. Professional responsibilities
_____	_____	g. Documentation

Luttrell et al., 1999; Lenburg & Mitchell, 1991). Suffice it to say that the specified competencies and related critical elements form the basis for the assessment of competence of each employee at each level, based on the integration of the 10 psychometric concepts. Moreover, relevant policy statements and procedural directions must be developed, including, for example, exactly how the competency performance examination will be administered, by whom, when, and with what consequences. Holding staff accountable for competent practice is essential and the COPA model provides an innovative and comprehensive approach to this complex issue.

SUMMARY

The COPA model has the potential to increase the efficiency and effectiveness of case managers and case management departments as well as quality improvements in the care delivery organization. Some key characteristics that make the model attractive include its clarity and specificity of expected performance, potentially universal framework to guide both the learning and assessment of competence, flexibility, and adaptability to diverse staff levels and practice environmental settings. As designed, the eight core practice competency categories are useful as a guide for developing or revising statements pertaining to mission, practice-based outcomes, orientation programs, content and processes related to staff performance evaluation, and quality improvement strategies.

The creativity and commitment of the staff in a given setting will influence how the COPA model can be developed and implemented. The model is based on the belief in the need for a comprehensive, integrative, and organizing framework grounded in psychometric concepts that can be applied to complex practice environments to promote competent practice. Using all of its fundamental components, the model can be applied to diverse purposes, personnel, and settings. It presents a significant paradigm shift in perspective and approach in learning and the assessment of competence across the practice spectrum. In doing so, it promotes more efficient and effective quality improvement for patient care and employing agencies.

References

Bargagliotti, T., Luttrell, M., & Lenburg, C.B. (1999, Sept.). Reducing threats to the implementation of a competency-based performance assessment system. *Online Journal of Issues in Nursing*. Washington, D.C.: American Nurses Association.

Boyer, S. (2002). Vermont nurse internship project: A collaborative enterprise developed by nurse leaders from education, practice, and regulation. *Nursing Education Perspectives, 23*, 81-85. Available at www.springfieldhospital.org/vnip.html.

Cohen, E.L., & Cesta, T.G. (Eds.). (1997). *Nursing case management: From concept to evaluation* (pp. 153-160), 2nd edition. St. Louis: Mosby.

HIPAA. Available at www.hhs.gov/ocr/hippaa and at www.hipaa.org.

Lenburg, C.B. (2002, Oct.). Changes that challenge nursing education. *The Tennessee Nurse*. Available at www.tnaonline.org.

Lenburg, C.B. (2000, Jul./Aug.). Promoting competence through critical self-reflection and portfolio development: The inside evaluator and the outside context. *The Tennessee Nurse*. Available at www.tnaonline.org.

Lenburg, C.B. (1999a, Sept.). Redesigning expectations for initial and continuing competence for contemporary nursing practice. *Online Journal of Issues in Nursing*. Washington, D.C.: American Nurses Association.

Lenburg, C.B. (1999b, Sept.). The framework, concepts and methods of the competency outcomes and performance assessment (COPA) Model. *Online Journal of Issues in Nursing*. Washington, D.C.: American Nurses Association.

Lenburg, C.B. (1991). Assessing the goals of nursing education: Issues and approaches to evaluation of outcomes. In M. Garbin (Ed.), *Assessing educational outcomes*. New York: National League for Nursing.

Lenburg, C.B. (1979). *The clinical performance examination: Development and implementation*. New York: Appleton-Century-Crofts.

Lenburg, C.B., Lipson, J., Demi, A., Blaney, D., Stern, P., Schultz, P., & Gage, L. (1995). *Promoting cultural competence in nursing education*. Washington, D.C.: American Academy of Nursing.

Lenburg, C.B., & Mitchell, C.A. (1991). Assessment of outcomes: The design and use of real and simulation nursing performance examinations, *Nursing & Health Care, 12*, 68-74.

Luttrell, M., Lenburg, C.B., Scherubel, J.C., Jacob, S., & Koch, R. (1999). Competency outcome for learning and performance assessment: Redesigning a BSN curriculum. *Nursing and Health Care Perspectives, 20*, 134-141.

Redman, R., Lenburg, C.B. & Walker, P. (1999, Sept.). Competency assessment: Methods for development and implementation in nursing education and practice. *Online Journal of Issues in Nursing*. Washington, D.C.: American Nurses Association. Available at www.nursingworld.org/ojin/.

Tahan, H. (1997). The role of the nurse case manager. In E.L. Cohen & T.G. Cesta (Eds), *Nursing case management: From concept to evaluation* (pp. 197-209), 2nd edition. St. Louis: Mosby.

Taylor, C. (1997). Ethical issues in case management. In E.L. Cohen & T.G. Cesta (Eds), *Nursing case management: From concept to evaluation* (pp. 314-334), 2nd edition. St. Louis: Mosby.

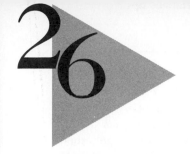

The Role of the Nurse Case Manager

Hussein A. Tahan

CHAPTER OVERVIEW

There is no standardization in the job description of the nurse case manager. Each institution implementing case management systems has established its own version of the roles and functions. This chapter, however, presents a thorough description of the role's, responsibilities, and functions of the case manager. It delineates the role's clinical, managerial, and financial aspects and discusses why nurses are, among all health care professionals, best fit to become case managers. In addition, it describes the skills and selection criteria required for the role. A special section of this chapter is designated for the various functions assumed by case managers while delivering patient care. Among these functions are change agent, clinician, consultant, coordinator and facilitator of care, educator, negotiator, manager, patient and family advocate, quality improvement coordinator, researcher, and risk manager.

Nurses have played a crucial role in the success of case management as a patient care delivery system since its inception. This is evidenced through the drastic changes such delivery systems have undergone. In the early 1980s, case management models were implemented by nursing executives as nursing efforts to meet the demands and challenges of the nursing shortage and the ever-changing health care system: cost containment and higher quality care. Today, however, these models are being implemented in a broader perspective as patient care delivery systems that are interdisciplinary, surpassing the boundaries of nursing care.

Despite the fact that for two decades case management models have been successful in improving quality of patient care, containing the incurred costs, and increasing patients' access to health care services, the literature regarding the nurse case manager's role description and functions is conflicting. Nurse case managers are introduced as integral members of interdisciplinary health care teams every time a health care institution implements a case management system for patient care delivery. The presence and achievements of case managers in such institutions are important for the success of the case management system. Regardless of the patient care setting in which these systems are implemented, the institutions rely heavily on the nurse case manager, who acts as the gatekeeper of the interdisciplinary health care team and as the coordinator, facilitator, and evaluator of care activities. The case manager in most institutions is a registered professional nurse who assumes an advanced practice nursing role.

There is no standardization in the role of the nurse case manager. The institutions that have implemented case management systems have created their own case manager's role in a way that correlates with their organizational chart and operations, policies and procedures, financial status, and the goals and aims of the case management system. Regardless of the type of health care institution, there is some common ground in the role of nurse case managers. A summary of these commonalities is based on the role dimensions defined by Tahan (1993) and revised in 1998 (Tahan, 1998a, 1998b), which are related to clinical/patient care, managerial/leadership, financial/business, information management/communication, and professional development/advancement.

THE NURSE CASE MANAGER'S ROLE DIMENSIONS

Case management is a compilation of functions and activities that a case manager performs within a particular care setting (i.e., acute care, home care, managed care organization), or provided by an independent practitioner such as the case in community nursing centers or private case management practices. Case management activities may also be provided to specific patient populations and communities such as the elderly, those with mental disorders, or residents of an underserved neighborhood (Goodwin, 1994).

Regardless of the care setting or the institution providing case management services, the following are some commonly used case management activities:

1. Patient outreach, screening, and risk assessment
2. Patient identification and intake
3. Assessment and problem identification
4. Development of the plan of care
5. Implementation of the plan
6. Care coordination, facilitation, expedition, and management
7. Transitional planning and referral to other health care providers (e.g., social worker) and brokerage of services (e.g., home care)
8. Ongoing assessment, reassessment, and follow-up
9. Patient/family education regarding health care needs and lifestyle changes
10. Monitoring and evaluation of care activities, patient responses to treatments, and outcomes
11. Patient/family advocacy
12. Quality assurance and improvement
13. Conducting research and research utilization
14. Cost control activities such as eliminating duplication and fragmentation, and expediting care provision
15. Writing reports and providing feedback to key stakeholders/personnel
16. Staff mentoring, coaching, and education (continuing education sessions)
17. Variance identification, analysis, and management
18. Managed care reviews, authorizations, and certifications
19. Consulting
20. Expert opinion
21. Public speaking
22. Writing for publication
23. Public health policy and politics
24. Data entry, analysis, and management
25. Documentation
26. Committee participation
27. Development and evaluation of case management plans

In acute care settings, for example, the nurse case manager is responsible for coordinating the care delivered to a group of patients (caseload/case mix) that begins at the time of admission and extends beyond discharge. This is carried out through the application of the nursing process (assessment, diagnosis, planning, implementation, and evaluation). . . . The nurse case manager ensures the delivery of cost-effective, outcome-oriented quality care, and access to health care. . . . The nurse case manager is accountable for applying nursing case management successfully to the daily activities of patient care (Tahan, 1993, pp. 55-56).

Nurse case managers can make sound decisions that reflect what is best for the patient and family, the interdisciplinary team, and the health care organization by applying Tahan's five role dimensions. Clarifying the nurse case manager's role and functions by applying these five dimensions provides a generic conceptual framework health care organizations can use as a guide to better design the case manager's job description, functions, and responsibilities (Table 26-1).

The Clinical/Patient Care Role Dimension

Nurse case managers are responsible for the assessment of patients and families every time a patient presents with a problem. They identify the existing or potential health problems by evaluating the patient's physical, functional, psychosocial, financial, cognitive, and spiritual condition. They then, in collaboration with other members of the interdisciplinary health care team, develop a plan of care that meets the patient's needs (Bower, 1989; Ethridge & Lamb, 1989; Giuliano & Poirier, 1991; Tahan, 1993, 1998a, 1998b; Zander, 1988a). The plan of care lists the key tasks, treatments, or events that must be

TABLE 26-1   THE NURSE CASE MANAGER'S ROLE DIMENSIONS AND ACTIVITIES

Role Dimension	Activities
Clinical/patient care	Patient outreach, identification, and intake Assessment and problem identification Development of the plan of care Implementation of the plan of care Ongoing assessment, reassessment, and follow-up Patient and family education
Managerial/leadership	Care coordination, facilitation, expedition, and management Transitional planning an referrals Monitoring and evaluation of care activities and outcomes Patient and family advocacy Quality assurance and improvement Staff mentoring, education, and coaching Committees participation Development of case management plans/clinical pathways
Financial/business	Cost control/reduction activities Variance identification, analysis, and management Managed care review, authorizations and certifications
Information management/communication	Data entry, analysis, and management Documentation Writing reports Providing feedback to key stakeholders/personnel
Professional development/advancement	Conducting research and research utilization Public/health policy and politics Writing for publication Public speaking

accomplished in handling patient problems and meeting the care goals, the patient and family teaching activities based on the identified health care needs, and the transitional plan that ensures a timely and appropriate patient discharge. The plan of care also includes prospectively determined/desired outcomes. The patient care activities and expected outcomes are presented with a specific time-line that delineates when an activity should be completed, and a particular outcome is expected to be achieved, denoting the patient's progress toward expected goals. Nurse case managers may use prospectively developed protocols/case management plans if any are available that meet patients' needs, diagnosis, and problems. If protocols are used, they are usually reviewed and revised to meet the individual patient's needs. Case managers use these protocols to direct, monitor, and evaluate patient treatments and nursing interventions, and to communicate the expected outcomes or responses to treatments (Cohen & Cesta, 1993; Tahan, 1993; Tahan and Cesta, 1995; Thompson et al., 1991; Zander 1988a).

When caring for patients, nurse case managers follow a holistic approach to care and spend a considerable amount of time discussing preventive services. They may or may not provide direct patient care activities. They assess the patient's and family's coping abilities, social support systems and networks, and financial/health insurance status. They intervene if a problem is identified. Case managers are also responsible for facilitating the patient's journey through the health care system, arranging for consultation with specialists or specialized services, and ensuring that transfers to more appropriate level of care areas are made when needed (Brockopp, Porter, Kinnard, & Silberman, 1992; Henderson & Collard, 1988; Leclair, 1991; Zander, 1988b).

As to case management plans, case managers play an active role in their development, revision, implementation, and evaluation. They participate in and collaborate with an interdisciplinary health care team for that purpose. When these plans are implemented to guide patient care, nurse case managers identify any variances from the standards and work with other team members to analyze and, when possible, resolve these variances (Cohen & Cesta, 1993; Ethridge & Lamb, 1989; O'Malley, 1988a; Tahan & Cesta, 1995).

The Managerial/Leadership Role Dimension

The managerial role dimension refers to the case manager's responsibility for facilitating, expediting, and coordinating the care of patients during the course of their illness (Cohen & Cesta, 1993; Ethridge & Lamb, 1989; Kruger, 1989; O'Malley, 1988a; Tahan, 1993, 1998a, 1998b; Zander, 1988a). Some examples of these functions are scheduling of and follow-up on tests, procedures, and treatments; patient and family teaching; transitional planning; negotiating and brokering community resources; monitoring patient care outcomes; and obtaining certification and authorizations from managed care organization (Cesta, Tahan, & Fink, 1998) for diagnostic and therapeutic services. The nurse case managers manage care by planning the treatment modalities and interventions necessary for meeting the needs of patients and families and the goals of the health care team. They determine, in collaboration with the interdisciplinary team, the goals of treatment, the projected length of stay of the episode of care, and the necessary treatments and services. This provides a clear time frame for accomplishing the care activities needed and their desired outcomes (Cesta, Tahan, & Fink, 1998; O'Malley, 1988b; Tahan, 1993).

Case managers also guide the patient care activities, nursing treatments, and interventions to be carried out by nurses and other health care professionals. They continuously evaluate the quality of care provided and the outcomes of treatments and services to prevent duplication, fragmentation, or misuse of resources (Ethridge & Lamb, 1989; Kruger, 1989; Loveridge, Cummings, & O'Malley, 1988; O'Malley, 1988b; Tahan, 1993; Zander, 1988a). In addition, they conduct retrospective and concurrent chart reviews for the purpose of utilization management, to evaluate the efficacy and efficiency of care, and to identify any quality improvement opportunities (Cohen & Cesta, 1993; Tahan, 1993).

Nurse case managers act as gatekeepers of the interdisciplinary care team. They facilitate communication among the various members and disciplines involved in the care of patients internally (e.g., medicine, nursing, rehabilitation, occupational therapy, social services, pharmacy, medical records, nutrition, and radiology) and externally (e.g., managed care organizations, home care agencies, nursing homes, and durable medical equipment companies). They are continuously involved, directly or indirectly, in the care of their caseload of patients. On one occasion, nurse case managers may be busy ensuring the timely implementation of necessary care activities. On another occasion, they are seen communicating certain outcomes of care to key health care providers such as physicians, or reassessing patients' conditions and updating managed care organizations of the latest developments so that they maintain appropriate reimbursement requirements/standards.

One informal responsibility of case managers is that of teacher and mentor. The case manager assesses staff development needs, especially among less experienced practitioners, and makes referrals to the appropriate person or resource (Brockopp et al., 1992; Cronin & Maklebust, 1989; Kruger, 1989; Leclair, 1991; Tahan, 1993). It is not uncommon to see nurse case managers conduct educational sessions related to the practice of case management for other health care providers, including physicians, nurses, therapists, and others. They may also function as preceptors for novice case managers, providing training on becoming successful case managers.

The Financial/Business Role Dimension

In collaboration with physicians and other health care team members, case managers initiate case management plans to ensure that patients do not receive inadequate care while trying to maintain appropriate resource allocation and length of stay and containing cost (Collard, Bergman, & Henderson, 1990; Tahan, 1993).

Case managers access information related to the prospective payment systems and reimbursement methods (e.g., diagnosis-related groups [DRGs]) and *Current Procedural Terminology* (CPT), the allocated cost for each diagnosis/procedure, the predetermined length of stay, and the treatments and procedures generally used for each diagnosis. They use this information to review resources and evaluate the efficiency of services related to the diagnosis. They exert a great influence over the quality and cost of care by determining, in a timely manner, the most important treatment for the patient. Case managers also assess variances (i.e., delays in care and services, and deviations from the norm) and act immediately to control these variances to contain costs and improve quality (Cohen & Cesta, 1993; Crawford, 1991; Tahan, 1993; Tahan & Cesta, 1995). They ensure consistency, continuity, facilitation, integration, and coordination of care activities to control any duplication or fragmentation in health care delivery, resulting in better allocation and consumption of resources and further cost containment (Henderson & Collard, 1988; O'Malley, 1988a).

To be effective, nurse case managers must access information on case mix indexes, cost and consumption of resources, and practice patterns. They must be familiar with the health care reimbursement methods including the prospective payment systems, current third party reimbursement procedures, and the operations of managed care organizations in today's health care environment of managed competition (Ethridge & Lamb, 1989; Kruger, 1989; Loveridge, Cummings, & O'Malley, 1988; McKenzie, Trokelson, & Holt, 1989; O'Malley, 1988b).

Case managers may work closely with utilization review nurses or may assume utilization management responsibilities, particularly in institutions that dissolved utilization review departments. They must identify long-stay patients, and control and prevent inappropriate hospital stays (Cohen & Cesta, 1993; McKenzie et al., 1989; Tahan, 1993) and access to emergency services. Moreover, they must ensure the use of necessary care activities, treatments, and procedures and that they are completed within acceptable and reimbursable time frames.

The Information Management/Communication Role Dimension

Information management and communication are integral functions of the nurse case manager. Without communication, information management, or feedback, nurse case managers cannot possibly succeed in their role. All their roles, responsibilities, and functions depend on information sharing. No matter what type of activity they may be involved in, some form of information is usually managed, transformed, discovered, or transmitted. Aspects of the nurse case manager's role that rely heavily on information are communication, negotiation, reporting, explanation, teaching, discussion, reinforcement, clarification, collaboration, coordination, facilitation, evaluation, monitoring, case-conferencing, certification, authorization, and feedback. Information included in these activities is always directed toward improving patient care processes, achieving clinical and organizational outcomes, or eliminating variances (i.e., delays, deviations, and omissions of services) of care.

Nurse case managers are involved in information management and communication in a variety of ways. The following are some examples:

1. Data collection, analysis, trending, and reporting (e.g., variances, data, quality assurance and improvement data, research data, or outcomes management data)
2. Report generation (e.g., logs of case managed patients, variances, cost analysis, cost-benefit analysis, cost-effectiveness analysis, denials and appeals, length of stay, admission and readmission rates, utilization management, and outcomes management)
3. Communicating and disseminating information (e.g., educational sessions, reports, case conferencing, grand rounds, patient and family education, managed care utilization reviews, authorizations/certifications)
4. Presentations/public speaking, storyboards, posters, and publishing
5. Providing feedback to case management plan development teams
6. Developing or revising policies and procedures
7. Sharing patient-related information with members of the interdisciplinary teams or external agencies such as managed care organizations
8. Documentation
9. Obtaining authorizations for services from managed care organizations and reporting findings of utilization review and management activities

The success of nurse case managers depends on how well they communicate with their patients and families, care providers, and payers. Special attention is paid to how influential they are with the customers and stakeholders of the health care organization and the case management system. Two types of stakeholders are highlighted here: internal (e.g., members of the interdisciplinary and administrative teams) and external (e.g., managed care organizations). In some situations, success is also a factor of computer literacy. As information networks in the field of case management have become highly dependent on and better facilitated by information technology (e.g., electronic communication and the use of Internet-based resources), computer literacy skills have gained increased attention in the role of the case manager.

The Professional Development/Advancement Role Dimension

Professional development and advancement are necessary for nurse case managers. Professional practice aids nurse case managers in gaining the respect and confidence of members of the interdisciplinary health care team. It is highly beneficial that nurse case managers maintain membership in related professional organizations, share their successes and innovations with others, and improve the conditions under which health care services are provided. Some of the advantages of maintaining memberships in related professional organizations such as the Case Management Society of America, the American Nurses Association, and other specialty organizations are as follows:

1. Networking with other case managers and case management societies
2. Exchanging information regarding the latest innovations in case management
3. Obtaining professional support from other case managers
4. Maintaining acceptable professional practice standards
5. Identifying common and national practice standards
6. Developing acceptable standards that promote ethics-based practice and help reduce ethical dilemmas or guide nurse case managers through the process of ethical decision making
7. Maintaining a political voice to advocate for the health of the population at large
8. Making the public policy agenda of case management practices known to other constituencies

There are two types of scholarly activities nurse case managers can involve themselves in to promote their professional development and advancement status: (1) activities that focus on improving the health care practice environment and (2) activities that focus on the nurse case manager's self-development and professional advancement. Examples of the activities that focus on improving the case management practice environment are the following:

- Conduction of research and utilization of research findings
- Promotion of evidence-based practice
- Outcomes management
- Patient and family advocacy
- Legislation and public policy
- Sharing of information at public forums (e.g., public speaking, poster presentation)
- Consulting and entrepreneurial activities

Examples of activities that focus on the nurse case manager's self-development are as follows:

- Pursuing higher education (e.g., graduate degrees in area of practice)
- Becoming certified in the area of specialty or in the practice of case management
- Writing for publication
- Training novice case managers
- Participating in continuing education forums
- Admitting to areas of deficit and seeking improvement in these areas
- Obtaining new skills that improve practice
- Remaining up-to-date with the latest health care practices and innovations

THE NURSE CASE MANAGER'S SKILLS

To be successful in their role, nurse case managers need to have certain skills that make them capable of carrying out their clinical, managerial, business, information management, and professional responsibilities. These skills and traits transcend the issues of where or by whom case managers are employed and are needed by case managers regardless of the care setting where they function or which professional to assume the role of the case manager. Table 26-2 presents a comprehensive list of the desired skills and personality traits of case managers. It is not mandatory that each case manager exhibits all the skills and traits. The list may be used by administrators of case management systems or supervisors of case managers to evaluate potential candidates for the case manager role and the actual performance of case managers.

As to their clinical skills, case managers need to be clinically astute and competent in all related diagnostic and therapeutic practices, tests and procedures, and national patient care management

TABLE 26-2	DESIRED SKILLS AND TRAITS FOR NURSE CASE MANAGERS	
Skills	**Traits**
CLINICAL/PATIENT CARE	
Direct/indirect care provision	Caring attitude
Expertise in clinical area	Tolerance
Patient and family teaching	Helpfulness
Transitional planning	Sensitivity
Coordination, facilitation, and expedition	Respect
of care activities/treatments	
Patient and family advocacy	Knowledge
Holistic and pastoral care	Resourcefulness
Crisis intervention and counseling	
Development and implementation of	
case management plans	
MANAGERIAL/LEADERSHIP	
Problem solving	Charisma
Conflict resolution	Emotional intelligence
Critical thinking and clinical judgment	Independence, autonomy
Project management	Vision
Conducting meetings	Confidence and self-esteem
Goal setting	Flexibility and adaptability
Management of change	Self-direction and motivation
Management of ethical and legal issues	Stress tolerance
Time management	Innovation and creativity
Priority setting	Commitment
Delegation	Advocacy
Negotiation	Cultural sensitivity
Cultural competence	
Consensus building	
Integration	
BUSINESS/FINANCIAL	
Resource allocation	Tolerance to numbers
Utilization review and management	Ability to compromise
Certification/authorization of care activities	Attention to details
Financial analysis	Open-mindedness
Cost-effectiveness analysis	Risk taking
Financial reimbursement procedures	Team player
Quality improvement	
Outcomes management	
Gatekeeping	
Claims and denials	
Health benefits and entitlements	
Variance analysis and management	

TABLE 26-2	DESIRED SKILLS AND TRAITS FOR NURSE CASE MANAGERS—CONT'D
Skills	**Traits**
INFORMATION MANAGEMENT/COMMUNICATION	
Customer relations	Presentation of self
Cultural sensitivity	Acceptance to criticism
Writing reports	Assertiveness
Information sharing	Motivated
Communication	Pleasant
Documentation	Practical
Brokerage	Teamwork
Dealing with challenging people	Diplomatic
Active listening	Realistic
Collaboration	
PROFESSIONAL DEVELOPMENT/ADVANCEMENT	
Membership in professional organizations	Success
Political and public policy issues	Excellence
Legislation	Willingness to learn
Specialty certification	Eager to gain new skills
Writing for publication	Admit to areas of deficit
Public speaking	Open to improvement
Research	
Advanced education	
Networking	
Consulting	

standards and clinical practice guidelines. They are considered role models and clinical experts for nursing and other staff. They should be skilled in coordinating patients' discharge and patient and family teaching activities and should be particularly knowledgeable in adult learning theory and the health belief model. Nurse case managers should also be able to function as mentors for less experienced staff.

Because they function as members of interdisciplinary health care teams, it is essential for nurse case managers to be highly skilled in communication, negotiation, contracting, teamwork, delegation, and conducting meetings. They also should be able to make sound decisions and resolve conflicts. To do all of this successfully, they should acquire critical thinking and problem solving skills. Because of their managerial responsibilities, case managers are required to write progress reports and quality improvement and length of stay reports, to speak publicly, and possibly to write for publication.

Looking at the business responsibilities embedded in the role of nurse case managers, one can see it is crucial that they have skills in financial analysis, contracting procedures of managed care organizations, financial reimbursement procedures, marketing, and customer relations. These skills are important, because nurse case managers are pressured to improve quality of care and reduce length of stay, hence containing cost.

SELECTION OF CASE MANAGERS

Health care administrators and policy makers have always struggled and still struggle with deciding who is best qualified to become the case manager. The question focuses on the following:

1. Should the case manager be a nurse-clinician or a paraprofessional staff member?
2. Are nurses the ideal candidates or are other professionals such as social workers and utilization reviewers equally effective in this role?
3. What is the financial implication of such a decision? Can the institution absorb the incurred cost?
4. Who best fits the institutional policies, procedures, and systems?

To respond to these issues, it is necessary to evaluate the case management system to be implemented and the proposed scope of practice and extent of responsibilities of case managers. Schwartz, Goldman, and Churgin (1982) argue that case managers should be clinicians because case management activities require substantial clinical knowledge and decision-making skills. Grau (1984) describes *case management* as a set of clinically based functions that require a clinician to obtain the optimum benefit for the client. This definition also stresses that the background of the case manager is important because it influences the kind of direct and indirect care activities to be provided and other aspects of care delivery and monitoring.

Cohen and Cesta (1993) and Mundinger (1984) support the argument that nurses are best fit for case management roles because they can provide most services that other professionals offer to clients. Professionals, other than nurses, are neither prepared for nor capable of providing the direct care activities for which nurses are responsible, which makes it more difficult for them to assume case management roles. Bower (1992) recommends nurses for case management roles because of their clinical abilities and skills that prepare them for better coordination of services to meet the total needs and concerns presented by patients and their families. Bower also argues that "nurses have skills and knowledge that extend beyond the biophysical and pathological aspects of care, bringing a holistic perspective and knowledge base to the care of case-managed clients" (p. 15). This strengthens the argument that nurses are the professional best prepared for this role.

According to Zander (1990a), nurses are born for the role of case managers because they are "the generalists; they are the detail people, and they excel in managing care. They are at the juncture of cost and quality, and they know the human implications of tradeoffs such as early discharge, patient education in groups, or the use of new technology" (p. 201). Case management responsibilities are an extension of the traditional role of nurses. These new functions advance the role, promote professionalism, and bring nursing to a higher level of professional standards among the other health care professions.

One might say that physicians are the case managers of their patients. This may not work well in case management systems, because physicians' care basically is centered on the medical management of the disease. The patients need professionals who can attend to all their other needs, however, not just the medical ones. Nurses can fill this need. They are prepared to address the total picture of patient care, the actual and potential problems (i.e., physical, psychological, social, spiritual) their patients may experience. Nurses in the case manager role act as facilitators and coordinators of care, a role that complements that of the physician. Because of their educational preparedness and clinical experience, nurses bring a wholeness approach to the total management of patient care. Such an approach complements the physician's role and the medical plan.

The literature is clear that nurses should be selected to assume the case manager role. But the question regarding the criteria that make the best nurse case manager remains to be answered. These criteria, as considered by most institutions implementing case management systems, are related to the educational preparation of nurses, communication skills, leadership skills, and clinical knowledge and experience. The personality traits of nurse case managers are important to their success as interdisciplinary team players, negotiators of care, and patient and family advocates.

Tahan, in 1993, examined the selection criteria for nurse case managers. In his study, 26 nursing administrators of case management systems were surveyed on their preferences and perceptions of the criteria that make a successful case manager. He found that:

- 40% of the nursing administrators recommended a BSN as the minimum requirement for the role
- 48% recommended 4 to 6 years of nursing experience, and 38% recommended 2 to 4 years
- 38% did not approve of the clinical ladder as a requirement for the role
- 61.9% did not have any preference for generalized versus specialized nursing experience; 28.6% preferred specialized practice
- Communication skills and certification in area of practice or specialty were recommended as prerequisites for the role

Most institutions employ registered nurses in the role of case manager. Some of them require a BSN degree as the minimum educational level; however, others use a combination of BSN and associate degree-prepared nurses. Bower (1992), in her book *Case Management by Nurses*, recommends a BSN degree as an entry level for nurse case managers. Loveridge et al. (1988) suggest that nurses with a BSN degree can assume case management responsibilities on a professional level, that is, no direct care activities. Loveridge and colleagues also recommend that those with associate degrees can act as case associates, that is, function on a technical level or be responsible for the provision of direct care activities.

Zander (1990b), on the other hand, suggests that other skills and experiences may be as important as the education level. These areas should be looked at when screening nurses for case management roles. Examples of such skills and experiences are (1) knowledge of the nursing process, (2) skills in collaborative practice and interdisciplinary teams, (3) managerial and leadership characteristics, and (4) communication skills.

Advanced educational degrees, graduate nursing degrees, or graduate degrees in a health care–related field are currently more commonly used as requirements for the nurse case manager's role, especially in academic medical centers. This shift has happened because administrators of case management programs view the case manager's role as an advanced practice role. Other reasons are the availability of more graduate degree programs in nursing case management today than ever existed during the past two decades and the awareness of the complex and progressive skills a master's prepared case manager brings to the role.

In a survey of acute care case managers regarding staff development activities and needs, baccalaureate prepared case managers identified clinical issues as most useful, compared with master's prepared case managers who identified systems-related issues as more important. This may indicate that master's prepared case managers have acquired a comfortable degree of clinical experience within their graduate degree preparation, making clinical issues of lesser need. In addition, graduate education may also have played a role in helping case managers become more attentive to systems-related issues (Nolan et al., 1998). After all, case managers spend a great deal of their time and efforts managing the system and resolving the systems-related problems.

CHARACTERISTICS OF THE ROLES OF NURSE CASE MANAGERS

Nurses who assume case management roles are given the opportunity to demonstrate effectiveness and efficiency in patient care. It is imperative that nurse case managers be able to ensure that the benefits of providing case-managed care exceed the incurred costs while maintaining or improving quality. The wide scope of functions, characteristics, and activities provided by nurse case managers illustrate many of the opportunities, challenges, and threats faced by nurses who are a part of any case management system. As a result, when delivering care, they tend to activate more than one role function or characteristic simultaneously. The nurse case manager's role characteristics and functions are best described in the following general categories.

Change Agent

Successful implementation of any case management system relies heavily on the change agents in the institution. Nurse case managers are integral to this change process (Cohen & Cesta, 1993). They are important in selling the new patient care delivery system to others in the institution, such as physicians, staff nurses, social workers, and personnel in the ancillary departments who are affected by the change. Nurse case managers act as resource persons, role models, and experts when promoting this change. They play a crucial role in teaching all health care personnel about case management systems and answer their questions and concerns. Nurse case managers act to spearhead change by encouraging health care personnel in their efforts to adapt to a new way of delivering care. In addition, they encourage patients in their attempts to quit smoking or to abstain from alcohol, or in other healthful lifestyle changes.

Implementation of case management systems is not an easy process. Some resistance (Cohen & Cesta, 1993; Tahan, 1993), mainly from those most affected by the change, may be encountered. Nurse case managers are prepared to meet this challenge before assuming their new role. They understand that resistance is one way some people might choose to deal with the change. But helping people go smoothly through the process is the case managers' number one challenge. They are well prepared in how to conquer resistance and are empowered by administration to use any approaches deemed appropriate for dealing with resistance and helping make the transition as easy and smooth as possible.

Clinician

Nurse case managers use their clinical expertise in assessing the patient's and family's current status and in identifying their actual and potential problems. They depend on their clinical knowledge and previous experiences when implementing the approaches to care that will help resolve these problems. Keeping abreast of the current advances in medical technology and the latest strategies in patient care is crucial to their meeting the client's needs across the health care continuum.

It is important for nurse case managers to be astute in the nursing (Bower, 1992) and case management processes. They must possess the necessary assessment skills that enable them to identify the patient's actual and potential health problems and be able to implement the interventions required to successfully resolve these problems and to evaluate the outcomes of care and responses to treatments.

The clinical skills enable nurse case managers to assess their clients as biopsychosocial beings and to plan the treatments to meet the clients' needs as a whole system and not just the disease. These skills allow them to establish more effective treatment goals and deliver better coordinated and timely care that helps the case-managed patients recover in a timely fashion.

Nurse case managers are also popular for their role modeling and clinical expert function. Because of their extensive clinical background, they act as a resource for less-experienced practitioners, some of whom may be from disciplines other than nursing.

Consultant

Nurse case managers guide the interdisciplinary team through the case management process of patient care. They act as consultants to physicians, house staff, fellow nurses, and other providers (Green & Malkemes, 1991; Meisler & Midyette, 1994). Because of their knowledge of institutional policies and procedures, operations, and systems, they provide the interdisciplinary team with a better understanding of the standards of care and practice and facilitate the coordination of tests and procedures, hence the provision of care. They play an important role in identifying the practices that best support efficient and effective care.

In addition, case managers act as consultants on clinical, ethical, legal, risk management, and administrative issues regarding the delivery of care. Nurse case managers coordinate the needs for consultants, especially for those patients with multiple, complicated needs, and ensure that consultations are obtained in a timely fashion. They are involved, as consultants, in comparing and evaluating medical products that provide the best patient outcomes in the most cost-effective manner (Meisler & Midyette, 1994).

Some nurse case managers may provide consultation services for patients and families via the telephone. This is best accomplished if case managers function in ambulatory and community-based care settings such as the emergency department, outpatient clinic, or home care or in the managed care organization setting when a client contacts the case manager for guidance or authorization regarding care.

Coordinator and Facilitator of Care

As patient care coordinators, nurse case managers collaborate with the interdisciplinary team members to meet the patient's needs and the goals of treatments. They are held responsible for coordinating and facilitating the provision of care on a day-to-day basis, the transitional plan, and the patient and family teaching efforts. They also coordinate the required tests and procedures as specified in the case management plan. These functions are essential to facilitate a timely delivery of care and patients' movement through the complex health care system, to reduce fragmentation or duplication of care activities, and to promote a collaborative practice atmosphere among the various care providers.

Nurse case managers consult and collaborate on an ongoing basis with other team members every time a problem regarding the provision of care arises or the patient's condition changes. This aspect of the role is important because it permits immediate intervention and change in the plan of care, timely communication with the appropriate personnel, and better decision making regarding patient care services. As coordinator and facilitator, the nurse case manager also prevents any delays in patients' discharge and helps control length of stay and resources and, hence, costs. This role responsibility makes nurse case managers important in the institution because they acquire the reputation of being "able to get things done." Health care providers then seek them out every time a problem arises or a certain care activity is not getting done.

It is easier for nurse case managers to assume responsibility for patient care coordination and facilitation because of their understanding of the operations of the institution, the existing systems, and the policies and procedures. However, nurse case managers are successful mainly because of the power, autonomy, accountability, and authority implicit in their role as granted to them by the organization's administration.

Educator

Patient and family education and staff development are other aspects of the nurse case manager's role (Cohen & Cesta, 1993; Meisler & Midyette, 1994; Smith, Danforth, & Owens, 1994; Tahan, 1993). Nurse case managers assess the patient's and family's educational needs at the time of admission to the hospital or during a health care encounter (e.g., clinic visit). They ensure that a teaching plan to meet these needs is put together to guide the nursing staff and other health care providers in the process of patient/family teaching. They may or may not be directly involved in conducting the actual teaching sessions. Case managers are responsible for making sure that patient and family teaching is completed, however, as indicated by the assessed needs. They also may act as members of institutional patient teaching committees responsible for developing patient and family teaching materials and overseeing the patient teaching process. Nurse case managers in most institutions play a significant role in ensuring compliance with the standards of regulatory and accreditation agencies associated with patient and family teaching and in promoting and enhancing compliance with the institutional policies and procedures.

Regarding staff development, nurse case managers help the clinical staff in professional growth and development by enhancing and disseminating new knowledge and skills. They assess the teaching needs of the nursing and support staff and plan educational sessions to meet these needs or make referrals to the training and development or continuing education departments. They also act as mentors and preceptors for junior and less experienced staff. In reference to case management systems, nurse case managers assume a crucial role in disseminating knowledge regarding case management models and resources, case management plans, and the role of case managers with all health care providers. This is done either formally through prescheduled classes or informally whenever the opportunity arises.

Manager

The manager aspect of the nurse case manager's role entails managing patient care and allocation of resources. As gatekeepers of care, nurse case managers ensure the completion of patient care activities in a timely fashion and the use of resources as appropriate and based on the needs of patients. As managers of care, they ensure that the plan of care or the case management plan reflects the patient's needs. They also direct and supervise the provision of care and optimize positive financial and clinical outcomes.

Nurse case managers conduct a review of current and past medical records to evaluate the cost of resources and quality of care. This review is important because it provides data regarding inefficient use of resources, medically unnecessary services, and the incurred costs. It also provides administrators with feedback regarding organizational performance and opportunities for improvement.

Negotiator

Nurse case managers assume a significant role in negotiating the plan of care of patients—the length of stay, the required services, and the time in which patient care activities should be completed—with members of the interdisciplinary team and, more important, with the patient and family and managed care organizations. They are popular for their negotiation skills in getting tests and procedures scheduled with ancillary departments in a timely manner and even in expediting reporting of results. Nurse case managers also play the role of gatekeeper of the interdisciplinary team, a role that requires a tremendous amount of negotiation. Using these skills, they improve the productivity of the team and ensure successful completion of its goals.

Nurse case managers are responsible for working closely with managed care organizations and insurance companies. They negotiate the approval (certification/authorization) of patient care services before the patient's hospitalization or the delivery of these services and the length of stay as determined by the patient's condition. This task is done before and on a regular basis during hospitalization. They exchange information with the representatives of the managed care organizations regarding patient care and the continued need of patients for medical attention.

Nurse case managers also negotiate the need for community services or nursing home placement with the physician and the patient and family. They then negotiate the approval of such services with appropriate managed care organizations and community resource agencies.

Patient and Family Advocate

Patient and family advocacy is an integral component of the case manager's role. This role is important in case management systems because nurse case managers are responsible for ensuring that the needs of patients and families are met. They always inform their clients of their treatment plans and options and of their progress and support them while they are struggling with decision making regarding the available options for care. They view these functions as important to ensure that the patients and their families make informed decisions regarding care choices. Nurse case managers may act as spokespersons for their patients with other health care team members or managed care organizations.

Nurse case managers convey the care options and diagnostic and therapeutic modalities to the patients, which may include the appropriate treatment plan, medications, tests and procedures, expected length of stay, and whether there is a need for any community services after discharge. They answer those questions raised by the patient or family that they can and seek answers to those they do not know. The role of nurse case managers as patient and family educators and facilitators of care are excellent examples of advocacy.

Quality Improvement Coordinator

Nurse case managers are responsible for ensuring that quality of patient care is maintained or improved at all times. With the current increased pressure on the health care system for cost containment, case managers are given the authority to ensure that quality of care is not compromised at the expense of reducing length of stay and costs. They act as quality improvement coordinators through their assigned responsibility for collecting and analyzing patient care–related data.

Case managers usually evaluate the provision of care by monitoring delays in patient care services and outcomes and deviations (variances) from the pre-established case management plans. They are proactive in improving patient care quality through developing, in collaboration with an interdisciplinary team of care providers, case management plans that reflect the ideal or best practices (e.g., nationally recognized practice guidelines and evidence-based treatment modalities). In these plans case managers delineate patient care activities and outcomes, including appropriate time frames for completion.

They also participate in continuous quality improvement teams as active members for monitoring patient care activities and outcomes, system problems, care quality, patient satisfaction, length of stay reduction, and so forth. They provide feedback on improvement efforts to all those involved in patient care on a unit level as well as on an administrative/organizational level. By virtue of their roles as case managers, they are always sought by health care providers, physicians and nonphysicians, to resolve delays in care processes and to investigate any patient care problems that arise.

Nurse case managers generate monthly variance reports that summarize patient care delays, omissions, and changes from the established case management plans. Such reports are an analysis and trending of the data collected. On the basis of these reports, case managers usually make recommendations for improving the organization's way of operating. They also suggest to the interdisciplinary teams any necessary revisions to be made in the case management plans to improve patient care delivery practices and outcomes and reduce delays or variances.

Researcher

In most institutions, research is considered an integral component of the role of nurse case managers. Case managers are encouraged to write grant and research proposals for studying patient care. They are active members of committees researching development, dissemination, and utilization of nursing knowledge and evidence-based practice. They evaluate patient care through research and make recommendations for changes in care standards, policies, and procedures on the basis of research results. They help bridge the gap between theory and practice by applying research in the clinical setting.

Nurse case managers are the best supporters of research related to product-line quality, health care issues, accessibility to care, professional issues, cost, system problems, and effectiveness of case management plans. Such research is important in the evaluation of the effectiveness of case management systems as patient care delivery models. Since they are at the forefront of patient care services, case managers are the best people for data collection in such research efforts.

Risk Manager

Risk management is scrutinized in all health care institutions. Nurse case managers play an important role in identifying patient care issues that present legal risk. As coordinators, facilitators, and managers of patient care, they pay close attention to patient care outcomes and ensure that these outcomes meet the preestablished patient care goals and that care is delivered in compliance with the following parameters:
- The institutional policies, procedures, and standards of care and practice
- The requirements and standards of managed care organizations
- The standards of regulatory and accreditation agencies on the state and federal level

It is important that there be a complete description of the case management system to be implemented and a clear definition of the nurse case manager's role. Most institutions expect case managers to
- Develop case management plans that presumably will improve quality of care
- Select the treatment option that is best for the patient and that is most cost-effective
- Manage the patient's total care to ensure optimum quality and outcomes

It is through these role functions that case managers reduce the medical liabilities an institution may face. They work closely with the legal or risk management departments to prevent any patient care problems from escalating into a medical liability. In their role as patient and family advocates and in their proactive approach to patient care, they are influential in preventing and reducing legal risk and potential law suits. Case managers may also minimize liability through the following activities:
- Immediate investigation and solving of patient care problems
- Constant review and revision of hospital policies and procedures and standards of care and practice
- Knowledge of managed care contracts and ensuring that care is precertified and provided in compliance with these contracts
- Supervision of appropriate allocation and utilization of resources
- Dissemination of information in a timely manner to key players and decision-makers

Transitional Planner

Nurse case managers play an important role in the delivery of cost-effective and efficient care services. They apply the concepts and principles of transitional planning in this aspect of their role. *Transitional planning* is simply defined as the act of moving patients from one level of care to another (i.e., from intensive/critical care, to intermediate, less acute, to stable) or from one care setting to another (i.e., acute to community or ambulatory) considered more appropriate and necessary based on the condition of the patient. It includes certain tasks, activities, and functions that focus on helping the patient transition to the predisease state or to an acceptable level of functioning as close to the patient's baseline as possible and one that is considered safe for the patient to return to a community setting.

Case managers use the discharge planning standards and guidelines of regulatory and accreditation agencies (federal and state) to ensure that appropriate services are provided to patients and their families and in the most appropriate and reimbursable care setting or level of care. They collaborate with other members of the interdisciplinary health care team to meet these requirements. In addition, case managers communicate with other providers on a daily and ongoing basis the findings of their assessment and evaluation regarding the patient's and family's health care needs and necessary community-based resources. Moreover, case managers communicate with external agents such as those who work for managed care organizations, home care agencies, and durable medical equipment companies to broker postdischarge services and resources and to ensure the patient's safe discharge back into the community.

The focus of nurse case managers on the continuum of care is essential for their success in transitional planning and case management. Their knowledge of the clinical, reimbursement, and eligibility guidelines for the provision of services in each of the varied settings of the continuum (preacute, acute, subacute, and postacute settings) ensure their compliance with the regulations and that the patients are transitioned safely and effectively from one level of care to another.

Utilization Manager

Nurse case managers cannot thoroughly meet their role expectations without a focus on utilization management. This role function is necessary for ensuring cost-effective care delivery and use of resources. Similar to transitional planning, nurse case managers focus on the continuum of care and the transition of patients from one level of care to another considered more appropriate as indicated by the patient's condition. They use preestablished criteria and guidelines such as those of Milliman and Robertson (Schibanoff, 1999) or InterQual (1998) to ensure the acceptable utilization management practices.

To ensure safe and appropriate use and allocation of health care resources, case managers match the patient's clinical condition and needed diagnostic and therapeutic interventions to the level of care being provided and in the necessary care setting. These activities enforce the efficient use of resources and the cost-effectiveness of care delivery practices.

Another aspect of utilization management case managers are involved in is obtaining certification and authorization for services from managed care organizations before they are delivered. This behooves case managers to examine the patient's condition, review the medical record and the treatment and transitional plans of care, and communicate the findings to the representatives of the managed care organizations. This type of communication may result in the managed care organization denying treatments or reimbursement for services provided. In this case, the nurse case managers engage in the denial and appeal process with the managed care organization to enhance or maximize reimbursement. Ultimately, the goals of utilization management are to ensure that patients receive the services they need and that the health care organization rendering the services receives appropriate reimbursement.

With the constant and rapid changes of health care delivery models, the role of nurse case managers has become more important than ever before. The popularity and success of case management systems have made these changes desirable. Nurse case managers have been empowered to function in advanced roles and to prove that their presence in such roles is crucial whenever any efforts are made to improve patient care quality and reduce cost and to help institutions maintain their financial stability, survival, and marketability.

References

Bower, K.A. (1989). Managed care: Controlling costs, guaranteeing outcomes. *Definition: The Center for Case Management, 3*(1), 3.

Bower, K.A. (1992). *Case management by nurses* (pp. 13-15), 2nd edition. Kansas City, Mo.: American Nurses Association.

Brockopp, D.Y., Porter, M., Kinnard, S., & Silberman, S. (1992). Fiscal and clinical evaluation of patient care: A case management model for the future. *Journal of Nursing Administration, 22*(9), 23-27.

Cesta, T., Tahan, H., & Fink, L. (1998). *The case manager's survival guide: Winning strategies for clinical practice.* St. Louis: Mosby, Inc.

Cohen, E.L., & Cesta. T.G. (1993). *Nursing case management: From concept to evaluation.* St. Louis: Mosby.

Collard, A.F., Bergman, A., & Henderson, M. (1990). Two approaches to measuring quality in medical case management programs. *Quality Review Bulletin, 16*(1), 3-8.

Crawford, J. (1991). Managed care consultation: The "house supervisor" alternative. *Nursing Management, 22*(5), 75-78.

Cronin, C..J., & Maklebust, J. (1989). Case-managed care: Capitalizing on the CNS. *Nursing Management, 20*(3), 38-47.

Ethridge, P., & Lamb, G. (1989). Professional nursing case management improves quality, access and costs. *Nursing Management, 20*(3), 30-35.

Goodwin, D. (1994). Nursing case management activities: How they differ between employment settings. *Journal of Nursing Administration, 24*(2), 29-34.

Grau, L. (1984). Case management and the nurse. *Geriatric Nursing, 5*(8), 372-375.

Green, S.L., & Malkemes, L.C. (1991). Concepts of designing new delivery models. *Journal of the Society for Health Systems, 2*(3), 14-24.

Giuliano, K.K., & Poirier, C.E. (1991). Nursing case management: Critical pathways to describe outcomes. *Nursing Management, 22*(3), 52-55.

Henderson, M.G., & Collard, A. (1988). Measuring quality in medical case management program. *Quality Review Bulletin, 14*(2), 33-39.

InterQual, Inc. (1998). *System administrator's guide.* Marlborough, Mass., InterQual.

Kruger, N.R. (1989). Case management: Is it a delivery model system for my organization? *Aspen's Advisor for Nurse Executives, 4*(10), 4-6.

Leclair, C. (1991). Introducing and accounting for RN case management. *Nursing Management, 22*(3), 44-49.

Loveridge, C.E., Cummings, S.H., & O'Malley, J. (1988). Developing case management in a primary nursing system. *Journal of Nursing Administration, 18*(10), 36-39.

McKenzie, C.B., Trokelson, N.G., & Holt, M.A. (1989). Nursing case management improves both. *Nursing Management, 20*(10), 30-34.

Meisler, N., & Midyette, P. (1994). CNS to case manager: Broadening the scope. *Nursing Management, 25*(11), 44-46.

Mundinger, M. (1984). Community-based care: Who will be the case managers? *Nursing Outlook, 323*(6), 294-295.

Nolan, M., Harris, A., Kufta, A., Opfer, N., & Turner, H. (1998). Preparing nurses for the acute care case manager role: Education needs identified by existing case managers. *The Journal of Continuing Education in Nursing, 29*(3), 130-136.

O'Malley, J. (1988a). Nursing case management. 1: Why look at a different model of nursing care delivery. *Aspen's Advisor for Nurse Executives, 3*(5), 5-6.

O'Malley, J. (1988b). Nursing case management. 2: Dimensions of the nurse case manager role. *Aspen's Advisor for Nurse Executives, 3*(6), 7.

Schibanoff, J.M. (Ed.) (1999). *Health care management guidelines.* New York: Milliman & Roberston.

Schwartz, S., Goldman, H., & Churgin, S. (1982). Case management for the chronic mentally ill: Models and dimensions. *Hospitals and Community Psychiatry, 33*(12), 1006-1009.

Smith, G.B., Danforth, D.A., & Owens, P.J. (1994). Role restructuring: Nurse, case manager, and educator. *Nursing Administration Quarterly, 19*(1), 21-32.

Tahan, H.A. (1998a). *The case manager's core competencies: Implications for education, training, and evaluation.* Contemporary Forum: Case Management Along the Continuum Conference. Chicago, March 16-18, 1998.

Tahan, H.A. (1998b). *Assuring success in the case manager's role: Skills, traits, and competencies.* Issues and Trends in Nursing Case Management Conference, Princeton, N.J., June 2, 1998.

Tahan, H.A. (1993). The nurse case manager in acute care settings: Job description and function. *Journal of Nursing Administration, 23*(10), 53-61.

Tahan, H.A., & Cesta, T.G. (1995). Evaluating the effectiveness of case management plans. *Journal of Nursing Administration, 25*(9), 58-63.

Thompson, K.S., Caddick, K., Mathie, J., Newlon, B., & Abrahams, T. (1991). Building a critical path for ventilator dependency. *American Journal of Nursing, 91*(7), 28-31.

Zander, K. (1988a). Nursing group practice: The "Cadillac" in continuity. *Definition: The Center for Case Management, 3*(2), 1-3.

Zander, K. (1988b). Why managed care works. *Definition: The Center for Nursing Case Management, 3*(4), 3.

Zander, K. (1990a). Case management: A golden opportunity for whom? In J.C. McCloskey & H.K. Grace (Eds.), *Current issues in nursing* (p. 301), 3rd edition. St. Louis: Mosby.

Zander, K. (1990b). Managed care and nursing case management. In G.G. Mayer, M.J. Madden, & E. Lawrenz (Eds.), *Patient care delivery models* (pp. 37-61). Rockville, Md.: Aspen Publications.

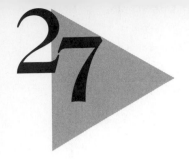

Credentialing for Case Management

Licensure, Certification, Certificate Programs, and Accreditation

Jeanne Boling
Marlys Severson

CHAPTER OVERVIEW

Licensure, certification, and certificate programs all play key roles in the assurance of a level of competence and quality for case management services provided by practitioners. Accreditation programs give the professional and public assurance of a level of competence and quality for case management organizations. This chapter describes the role of each type of credential and the benefits and concerns surrounding each. In addition, practical tips for evaluation are included to assist in navigating the expanding horizon of case management.

HISTORY OF CASE MANAGEMENT CREDENTIALING

In 1992 the National Case Management Task Force assembled representatives from 29 national stakeholder organizations in case management to discuss the need for standardization of case management services. The need was to protect the valuable services that case management professionals were providing to patients and their families from inexperienced, uneducated, and wrongly motivated individuals who called themselves "case managers." The result of this meeting was to appoint the Commission of Certification of Insurance Rehabilitation Specialists, now known as the Commission for Disability Management Specialists, to develop a certification for individual case managers using the criteria developed by the National Task Force. The resulting new credential became known as the certified case manager (CCM). This credential was conceived as a multidisciplinary entry level credential for the advanced practice of case management. The estimated 25,000 nationally certified case managers have demonstrated a basic professional licensure, a level of specific case management professional experience, and a knowledge level by obtaining a passing score on a research-based examination. The certification process, therefore, serves to distinguish a basic level of expertise to the vulnerable public.

Since the initial development of the CCM examination, the number of additional certifications for case managers has grown with the specific interests of case managers as the field has developed. Once case management was recognized as a successful strategy in the management of health care quality, efficiency, and cost, it began to be practiced in every conceivable setting: hospitals, home care, subacute care, behavioral health care, all forms of managed care organizations, rehabilitation facilities, insurance and reinsurance carriers, independent case management organizations, elder care, long-term care, military, all clinical specialties, Medicare, Medicaid, Champus/Tricare, occupational health, and Workers' Compensation settings. It became obvious that individual case managers could be practicing at the highest level but could be severely impeded by the system in which they practiced. Thus came the need for evaluation of the system used by the organization supporting the individual case manager. This then called for the accreditation process. In the same manner that a valid certification process ensures the public of a level of individual competence, an accreditation process ensures purchasers of case management services (employers, health plans, insurers) of the competence of the case management organization's structure and system. Initiated in 1997 and 1998, both the Commission on Accreditation of Rehabilitation Facilities (CARF) and the American Accreditation HealthCare Commission/URAC have developed accreditation programs for case management organizations.

What Questions Does Credentialing Answer?

Case management professionals provide a service to a medically less knowledgeable and vulnerable public. At the time of their greatest need and lowest ability to evaluate, they are asked to trust a case manager to assist them in making highly complex decisions and accessing necessary resources. How can they be ensured that the case manager with whom they are working has the level of knowledge and expertise to guide them through this process? How do they know it is safe to trust the case manager with whom they are working? A hospital human resources department needs to hire for case management positions. How will they evaluate the skill level of the individuals interviewed? A manufacturer buys health care coverage for employees. Three health plans respond to an employer's request for proposal. All have case management. How can the company do a comparative analysis for the quality of the case management services marketed? The answers to these questions rest in the credentialing provided by state licensure, certification, and accreditation bodies charged with protecting the public. We will look at the messages sent to the public by licensure, certification, certificate programs, and accreditation in case management.

LICENSURE

Licensure by individual states ensures the public that the individual health care professional has completed the basic education for the profession, has passed a knowledge-based examination, and has not committed any criminal acts (Box 27-1). Licensure conveys to the public a minimal level of competency to practice. Each profession defines the parameters of the basic entry practice.

Case management, as outlined in the Case Management Society of America's (CMSA) *Standards of Practice*, is recognized as a multidisciplinary function and requires that the case manager will "strive to achieve and maintain current professional licensure, national certification, and/or higher education in

BOX 27-1 ▶ LICENSURE
A license or permit to practice medicine or a health profession within a defined scope issued by any state of the United States. Examples include RN, MD, LCSW, and RPT.

case management or in a health and human services profession directly related to the individual's case management practice" (Case Management Society of America, 2002).

Because case management is not yet recognized as an independent professional discipline, the licensure of case managers is critical to the evaluation of the practice of case management.

CERTIFICATION

When practice requires experience, expertise, or knowledge beyond the basic level of practice, disciplines have addressed advanced practice with additional requirements for education, demonstrated competency, or experience (Box 27-2). Certification is the process of validating that knowledge and expertise. It is typically based on standards that are the result of input from industry experts and publications as well of ongoing industry research. Most certification bodies require an active health care license and varying educational achievements and amounts of professional experience in the field of case management to be able to sit for the examination. Once the certification test is passed, the individual is certified for an initial period, which is typically between 3 to 5 years. Recertification is based on continued acceptable employment and continuing education requirements or retaking the examination. The individuals who achieve certification status are given a specific designation to use when signing their name that goes behind their professional licensure such as RN, CM. Most of the certification bodies have qualifying examinations at least annually and some are semiannually. The choice of which certification to obtain is a very individual decision based on the person's discipline, specialty, geographical location, and practice area.

INDIVIDUAL CONSIDERATIONS FOR SELECTION OF A CREDENTIAL

In addition, consideration must be given to the following:

- Do you practice case management throughout the continuum of care, or is it limited to a part of that continuum?
- Does your case management practice encompass the entire process of case management as described in the CMSA *Standards of Practice for Case Management* (Box 27-3), or does your job entail completing a part of the process of case management?
- Does the state in which you practice mandate any particular certificate in the practice arena in which you function?
- How does the certification relate to your discipline?
- What is the value of the certification compared with the costs of obtaining and maintaining the certificate?

BOX 27-2	CERTIFICATION

An adjunctive credential available to an individual who meets eligibility criteria of a particular examination and subsequently achieves a passing score on the examination. This certification can be granted by a national certifying body, signifying that an individual has met the qualifications for case management practice established by that certifying body.
Examples include CCM, CRRN, CDMS, A-CCC, COHN, CMC, C-MAC, and CPHQ.

BOX 27-3	CASE MANAGEMENT PROCESS

Common to performance of case management functions is the process used, including assessment, problem identification, outcome identification, planning, monitoring, evaluating, and outcome reporting.

- Do you have the educational background and work experience necessary to qualify for certification?
- How will the certificate benefit you in your present position and fit into your career path?

Once all of these questions have been answered, a review of the available certifications must be made. Care must be taken to review the employment situation and to match it with the eligibility criteria of whatever certification is thought to be most appropriate. Without a match between eligibility criteria of the examination and the present job description of the individual, the process cannot continue.

Evaluating Certification Programs for Validity

The certification program must also be examined for validity. Questions to ask are as follows:
- Is it a not-for-profit agency with a program that is national in scope?
- Is it administratively and financially independent of the parent association and free from conflict of interest?
- Is the certifying agency separate and independent from any associated educational body?
- Is the examination free of bias and nondiscriminatory with published demographic data?
- What is the program for periodic recertification to ensure continued competence?
- How are pass/fail cutoff scores established? Has anyone been granted the credential without achieving a passing score?
- Is there a code of conduct and a formal disciplinary policy designed to protect the public?
- Are the eligibility criteria logically appropriate to relevant job requirements?
- Does at least one public member serve as a member of the governing board?
- Are reliability statistics produced after each administration of the examination?
- Has the validity of the examination been established by conducting ongoing national job analysis surveys?
- Is the certification process research based?

This choice of a credential is a highly individual and personal choice that must be weighed carefully. As the practice of case management matures, there will continue to be more certifications available. It is not surprising that there is a great deal of confusion among the credentials. They may be related to particular disciplines, a particular practice arena, or particular disease entities. The various certifying bodies are able to forward eligibility criteria and information regarding the certification. Carefully review this information and contact them for clarification if necessary. Finding the best match is the priority. Carefully weigh the choices and choose the certification that is most appropriate. Table 27-1 illustrates a representative sample of the certifications available.

There are a number of perceived benefits of case management certification for the individual case manager, the case manager employer, the public client/patient, and their families (Box 27-4).

Likewise, time and effort go into the offering and obtaining of any credential. This time is equivalent to value. Concerns about the relative value of the credential compared with the cost of obtaining it are the primary issues in case management as well as other professional disciplines (Box 27-5).

Text continued on p.304

TABLE 27-1 CASE MANAGEMENT CERTIFICATIONS

Certification	Acronym	Primary Focus	Organization Provided by	Contact Information
American Board of Disability Analyst	ABDA	Rehabilitation medicine, case management	American Board of Disability Analysts	ABDA Central Office Park Plaza Medical Bldg. 345 24th Avenue N, Suite 200 Nashville, TN 37203 Telephone: 615-327-2984
American Board of Quality Assurance and Utilization Review Physicians	ABQAURP	Utilization management physicians and allied health physicians	American Board of Quality Assurance and Utilization Review Physicians	American Board of Quality Assurance and Utilization Review Physicians 2120 Range Road Clearwater, FL 33765 Telephone: 727-298-8777 www.abqaurp.org
Case manager, certified	CMC	All health care professionals	The American Institute of Outcomes Case Management	The American Institute of Outcomes Case Management 12519 Lambert Road Whittier, CA 90606 Telephone: 562-945-9990 www.aiocm.com
Certification in continuity of care, advanced	A-CCC	Multidisciplinary discharge planners/ case managers	National Board for Certification in Continuity of Care	National Board for Certification in Continuity of Care 1350 Broadway, Suite 1705 New York, NY 10018 Telephone: 212-356-0691 www.nbccc.org
Certified case manager	CCM	Multidisciplinary, multiple-practice setting case managers	Commission for Case Management Certification	Commission for Case Manager Certification 1835 Rohlwing Road, Suite D Rolling Meadows, IL 60008 Telephone: 847-818-0292 www.ccmcertification.org

Certification	Abbreviation	Target group	Organization	Contact
Certified disability management specialist	CDMS	Disability managers, insurance-based rehabilitation specialists, vocational counselors	Certified Disability Management Specialists Commission	Certified Disability Management Specialist Commission 1835 Rohlwing Road, Suite D Rolling Meadows, IL 60008 Telephone: 847-818-0292 www.cdms.org
Case management administrator certification	CMAC	Case management administration	The Center for Case Management	The Center for Case Management 6 Pleasant Street South Natick, MA 01760 Telephone: 508-651-2600 www.cfcm.com
Care manager, certified	CMC	Gerontology, counseling care management	National Academy of Certified Care Managers	National Academy of Certified Care Managers 244 Upton Road PO Box 669 Colchester, CT 06415 Telephone: 800-962-2260 www.ngccm.net
Certified managed care nurse	CMCN	Nurses in managed care	American Board of Managed Care Nursing	American Board of Managed Care Nursing 4435 Waterfront Drive, Suite 101, Glen Allen, VA 23060 Telephone: 804-527-1905 www.abmcn.org
Certified life care planner	CLCP	Multidisciplinary case manager, vocational counselor life care planners	University of Florida/MediPro	The Commission on Health Care Certification 13801 Village Mill Drive Suite 204 Midlothian, VA 23114 Telephone: 804-378-7273 www.mediproseminars.com

Continued

TABLE 27-1   CASE MANAGEMENT CERTIFICATIONS—CONT'D

Certification	Acronym	Primary Focus	Organization Provided by	Contact Information
Certified nurse life care planning	CNLCP	Nurse life care planners	American Association of Nurse Life Care Planners	American Association of Nurse Life Care Planners Certification Board 498 E. Golden Pheasant Drive Draper, UT 84020 Telephone: 888-575-4047 www.aanlcp.org
Certified occupational health nurse–case manager	COHN-CM COHN-S/ CM	Occupational health case management	American Board of Occupational Health Nursing–Case Manager	American Board of Occupational Health Nurses 201 E. Ogden Avenue, Suite 114 Hinsdale, IL 60521 Telephone: 630-789-5799 www.abohn.org
Certified professional disability management	CPDM	Disability Managers	Insurance Education Association	Insurance Education Association 1201 Dove Street Newport Beach, CA 92660 Telephone: 800-655-4432 Ext 1 www.iea.to
Certified professional in health care quality	CPHQ	Quality managers, utilization managers, risk managers	Healthcare Quality Certification Board of the National Association HealthCare Quality	HealthCare Quality Certification Board of the National Association HealthCare Quality PO Box 19604 Lenexa, KS 66285 Telephone: 913-599-4173 www.cphq.org

Certification	Abbreviation	Who	Organization	Contact
Certified professional utilization review/utilization management	CPUR/CPUM	Utilization managers, case managers	McKesson HBOC/Interqual	McKesson HBOC,Inc./InterQual Products Group 293 Boston Post Road West, Suite 180 Marlborough, MA 01752 Telephone: 508-651-2600 www.interqual.com
Certified rehabilitation registered nurse Certified rehabilitation nurse–advanced	CRRN CRRN-A	Rehabilitation nurses	Rehabilitation Nursing Certification Board	Association of Rehabilitation Nurses Certification Board 4700 W. Lake Avenue Glenview, IL 60025 Telephone: 800-229-7530 www.rehabnurse.org
Certified social work case manager Certified social work case manager–advanced	CSWCM CASWCM	Social work case managers	National Association of Social Workers	National Association of Social Workers Credentialing Center 750 First Street NE, Suite 700 Washington, DC 20002 Telephone: 202-408-8600 www.socialworkers.org
Certified nursing case manager	RN, CM	Nurse case manager	American Nurses Credentialing Center	American Nurses Credentialing Center 600 Maryland Avenue SW, Suite 100 West Washington, DC 20024 Telephone: 800-284-2378 www.nursingworld.org/ancc/cert.html

---

BOX 27-4 ▶ PERCEIVED BENEFITS OF A CASE MANAGEMENT CERTIFICATION

- Provides a benchmark of knowledge and assurance to employers of case managers.
- Contributes to the ethical standards of the practice of case management.
- Most experts agree that having a certification indicates that a case manager is attempting to broaden his/her base of knowledge and stay current with trends in quality and patient care.
- Provides assurance to the public that the case manager has attained a specific level of knowledge.

BOX 27-5 ▶ CONCERNS RELATED TO CASE MANAGEMENT CERTIFICATION

- Some case managers feel pressured by an increasingly competitive job market to take advantage of the recent proliferation in case management credentials (Case Management Society of America, 1995).
- Some experts are critical of the trend toward raising the educational requirements for the top case management certifications. An issue is whether the bachelor of science in nursing should be regarded as a minimum standard for the practice of case management, since a baccalaureate degree is required in allied health professions (Case Management Society of America, 1995).
- Credentialed case managers command higher salaries. Some case management employers do not wish to pay more.

BOX 27-6 ▶ CERTIFICATE

The award of a paper certifying completion of a given educational program.

Certificate Programs

A growing number of programs provide continuing education certificates. Some certificate programs are based with for-profit continuing education entities, some are academically based, and some are based with not-for-profit organizations (Box 27-6).

These programs may or may not screen applicants for experience or professional licensure. They may or may not test the individuals to demonstrate a knowledge level attained. They do offer an educational program for a fee, at the conclusion of which is offered a certificate. Because there is considerable variation in the quality of these programs, care must be taken to evaluate the value of the certificate. Some certificate programs, although funded by a for-profit entity, not only offer the certificate but also grant the individual completing the class a designation to use after their name. This suggests to the untrained public, employer, or professional that the program is ensuring the public of a level of expertise and therefore protection. However, such is not the case unless the program offers a research-based examination and generally follows the criteria set forth by the National Association for Certifying Agencies (NACA), a division of the National Organization for Competency Assurance (NOCA) based in Washington, D.C. It is important to distinguish a certificate program from a national research–based and recognized certification credential.

These certificate programs may be useful in obtaining an entry level of knowledge before entering the field of case management. Also, some certificate programs provide an overview of case management to prepare the participant for a case management certification examination.

Accreditation

Certification establishes a benchmark only for individual practice. However, with certification only, the health care industry still faces the problem of qualified individuals practicing within a system that may not understand or support the role of the case manager. Accreditation of case management organizations helps to shape the system and thereby assists individual case managers in reaching the full extent of their practice capability. Accreditation also serves as a measure of quality of a case management program to the public and to purchasers of case management services. Accreditation is difficult in the case management arena due to the variety of definitions, organizations, and programs practicing case management. These organizations must adhere to varying legalities and governing bodies. For accreditation to be valuable, the standards must be broad enough to allow for the diversity and yet encompass the general principles surrounding organization excellence. Steps to such organizational accountability include the following:

- Defining the operational parameters of case management, including business and clinical goals
- Encouraging the standardization of definitions and various case management practices, but without inappropriately restricting innovation and customization
- Implementing written policies & procedures to promote operational integrity
- Pursuing quality improvement and quality assurance programs
- Benchmarking best practices and promoting outcomes measurement (*Case Manager's Desk Reference,* 2001)

Two organizations, CARF and the American Accreditation HealthCare Commission/URAC, offer accreditation programs for case management departments. Both became available in 1999. The CARF standards are geared more toward medical rehabilitation case management, whereas the Commission/URAC standards apply more to payer-based programs. Other accrediting bodies incorporate the case management process and case management principles in their standards, but they do not specifically accredit case management programs or organizations, as do CARF and URAC.

Commission on Accreditation of Rehabilitation Facilities

CARF has multiple case management accreditation programs that depend on the practice arena. These include the following

- Medical Rehabilitation Case Management
  It occurs in a variety of settings that include, but are not limited to, a health care environment, a private practice, or the payer community. Key areas include the following:
  - Initial and ongoing assessments
  - Knowledge and awareness of care options and linkages
  - Effective and efficient use of resources
  - Individualized plans based on the needs of the persons served
  - Predicted outcomes
  - Regulatory, legislative, and financial implications
- Employment and community services programs: Case Management/Service Coordination and Behavioral Health Standards–Case Management/Service Coordination

These two programs provide goal-oriented and individualized supports focusing on improved self-sufficiency for the persons served. They may be separate, freestanding programs; an independent program within a large organization; or a specifically identified activity within a system of care. Key areas include the following:

- Assessment
- Planning
- Linkage
- Advocacy
- Coordination
- Monitoring activities
- Occasional supportive counseling
- Crisis intervention services

The following sections comprise the CARF Case Management Accreditation Standards.

LEADERSHIP

The leadership section addresses who is responsible for managing and directing medical rehabilitation case management. It also outlines who in leadership would be responsible for various areas of case management activity, such as fiscal management, ethics, strategy, health, safety, and transportation.

INFORMATION AND OUTCOMES MANAGEMENT

This section addresses how information is gathered at the level of the individual and the level of the program to determine the outcomes of interventions completed by case managers. It also discusses public disclosure of information gathered.

REHABILITATION PROCESS FOR PERSONS SERVED

The rehabilitation section addresses the rights of the client and how case managers interact with the client and the rehabilitation team, as follows:

- Full participation of the case manager in decision making related to the services, equipment, and supplies provided to the persons served, community resources used, and efficient movement of the client through the continuum of care
- The role of the case manager in the continuum of care and use of the continuum of care
- Coordination with all stakeholders
- Advocacy for clients

American Accreditation HealthCare Commission/URAC

URAC has developed a modular approach to accreditation. They have developed CORE Standards that all accredited organizations must meet as a foundation for accreditation. There are 43 CORE standards, which cover the following areas:

- Organizational structure
- Policies and procedures
- Interdepartmental coordination
- Information management
- Business relationships
- Oversight of delegated/subcontracted functions
- Staff qualifications
- Staff management
- Clinical oversight
- Regulatory compliance

- Quality management program
- Quality management committee
- Quality management documentation
- Quality improvement projects
- Financial incentives
- Communications
- Satisfaction
- Access to services
- Complaints and appeals

In addition to the CORE standards, URAC has multiple modules to address many of the specialty functions of health care. The Case Management Accreditation module is one of those specialty accreditations. It encompasses 24 standards that cover the following areas:

- Policies and procedure
- Staff structure and qualifications
- Staff management and development
- Information management
- Organizational ethics
- Case management process
- On-site case management
- Complaints

Where Do the URAC Standards Apply?

The standards apply to "case management organizations," which are defined as organizations and/or programs that provide telephone and/or on-site case management services in conjunction with a private or publicly funded benefits program. Such services may be provided by a stand-alone case management organization or by an organization that conducts case management in conjunction with a range of managed care services such as utilization management or disease management (AAHC/URAC, 1999).

Accreditation Process

Unlike licensure and certification, accreditation is not granted as the result of receiving a passing score on a content specific test. Rather, accreditation is the cumulative evaluation of the structure and processes that are in place within a case management organization. It not only reviews the documentation of policies and procedures but also looks at how well the organization implements the policies and procedures that exist.

The accrediting body develops a set of guidelines that become the basis of the evaluative process. These guidelines are usually established using input from experts in the field, may be based on the standards that exist for the industry being accredited, and, in most accrediting organizations, are opened for public comment.

The accreditation process usually encompasses a review of documentation and on-site interviews. The organization then makes a determination of the type and length of the accreditation being provided. The review of documentation is an overview of policies, procedures, and processes of the organization. It is a cursory review to determine if the organization meets a basic level of compliance with the standards. For instance, does the organization have the necessary policies and procedures in place to meet the accreditation standards? During this review, the examiner may desire additional information from the organization or pose specific questions to be reviewed. This review may occur before or during the on-site assessment.

The review process culminates in an on-site evaluation. During this phase of the process, reviewers engaged by the accrediting organization schedule an on-site assessment of the organization to evaluate if indeed the organization is functioning in a manner consistent with the guidelines established. The team usually conducts interviews of key staff members and may review additional internal documents for evidence of compliance (e.g., patient charts or minutes of meetings). If the organization displays a level of operation in keeping with the standards outlined, they are granted a particular accreditation status depending on their compliance with the standards for a specified period of time.

As one might imagine, any process that requires time and establishes a level of accountability is debated as to the relative value to society. Boxes 27-7 and 27-8 list the benefits and concerns of accreditation.

The following areas must be addressed by accrediting entities requiring outcomes data so criteria can be refined.

1. Case load size
2. Case management qualifications
3. Evaluation of quality in case management programs
4. Collection and analysis of data
   - Cost
   - Confidentiality
   - Access
5. Outcomes studies

How Does Case Management Program Accreditation Affect Individual Case Managers?

Accreditation will help to standardize case management practices by measuring case management programs against consistent benchmarks. It is hoped that some of the results will be (1) increased organizational focus on quality, (2) clearer operational policies and procedures governing case management, and (3) sufficient organizational support for case management services. Accreditation can also make customers and clients more confident in the case management services they receive.

As the development of case management continues, the need for research-based continuing quality improvement will become critical. It is the hope of the industry that professional organizations can work jointly with certification and accrediting bodies to collect data, identify best practices, and advise practicing case managers concerning which case management strategies are most effective.

As can be seen, licensure, certification, certificate programs, and accreditation all play a role in ensuring the public and those purchasing case management services of a level of professional care (Box 27-9). The reader is strongly encouraged to evaluate and reach for the most appropriate credential.

BOX 27-7   BENEFITS OF ACCREDITATION

- Encourages sufficient organizational support for case management
- Clarifies operational procedures and policies governing case management
- Encourages increasing organizational focus on quality management
- Promotes organizational accountability
- Ensures that case managers can practice in a manner consistent with the profession's standards (D'Andrea & Hamill, 1999)
- Once the accreditation is established and recognized by state legislatures, it may substitute for organization licensure. This can save significant time and money for multistate organizations (Key to Quality Healthcare)

BOX 27-8 ▶ CONCERNS RELATED TO ACCREDITATION DEVELOPMENT

- Some case management employers are concerned that the cost of preparation for accreditation will add to the cost of case management and ultimately drive up the cost of health care (American Health Consultants, 1998).
- Small case management firms and individual case managers are concerned over the developmental costs of the accreditation and their continued survival in the marketplace.
- There is concern that state legislatures may require accreditation to conduct business within the state.

BOX 27-9 ▶ ACCREDITATION BODIES

Accreditation Association for Ambulatory Health Care (AAAHC)
3201 Old Glenview Road, Suite 300
Wilmette, IL 60091-2992
Telephone: 847-853-6060
Fax: 847-853-9028
www.aaahc.org

Accreditation Commission for Health Care, Inc. (ACHC)
5816 Creedmore Road, Suite 201
Raleigh, NC 27612
Telephone: 919-785-1214
Fax: 919-785-3011
www.achc.org

American Association HealthCare Commission/URAC
1220 L Street, NW, Suite 400
Washington, DC 20005
Telephone: 202-216-9010
Fax: 202-216-9006
www.urac.org

Commission on Accreditation of Rehabilitation Facilities (CARF)
4891 E. Grant Road
Tucson, AZ 85712
Telephone: 520-325-1044
Fax: 520-318-1129
www.carf.org

Joint Commission on Accreditation of Healthcare Organizations (JCAHO)
One Renaissance Boulevard
Oakbrook Terrace, IL 606181
Telephone: 603-792-5000
Fax: 603-792-5005
www.jcaho.org

Continued

BOX 27-9	ACCREDITATION BODIES—CONT'D

National Committee for Quality Assurance (NCQA)
2000 L Street NW, Suite 500
Washington, DC 20036
Telephone: 888-275-7585
Fax: 202-955-5615
www.ncqa.org

References

2003 CARF Program Descriptions.

Accreditation programs: Key to quality healthcare. Available at http://www.urac.org/Key-to-quality.htm.

American Accreditation HealthCare Commission/URAC Case Management Accreditation Standards. 1999.

American Health Consultants (1998, Dec.). *Hospital case management.*

American Nurses Credentialing Center (1998). *Nursing Case Management Catalog.*

Case Management Society of America. (2002). *Standards of practice for case management* (pp. 14-18).

Commission for Case Management Certification (1997). *CCM Certification Guide,* Certified Case Manager.

Commission on Accreditation of Rehabilitation Facilities (1999). *1999 Medical rehabilitation standards manual,* Medical Rehabilitation Case Management Program.

D'Andrea, G., & Hamill, C.T. (1999). Case management organization accreditation under way. *The Case Manager, 10*(1), 53-61.

Gilpin, S. (2003). The Commission for Case Manager Certification's 10th anniversary. *The Case Manager,* 14(3).

Mullahy, C.M. (1998). *The case manager's handbook* (pp. 154-157, 435-441), 2nd edition. Gaithersburg: Aspen Publications.

Powell, S.K. (1996). *Nursing case management* (pp. 49-51). Philadelphia: Lippincott-Raven.

Powell, S.K., & Ignatavicius, D. (2001). *Core curriculum for case management* (pp. 99-111). Philadelphia: Lippincott Williams & Wilkins.

Snowden, F. (2001). *Case manager's desk reference, second edition.* (pp. 49-53, 240-246). Gaithersburg: Aspen Publications.

URAC Case Management Standards, Version 2.0.

URAC Core Standards 2002.

28

Facilitating Educational and Career Mobility

Online Case Management

Gayle Preheim

CHAPTER OVERVIEW

Today's competitive and chaotic managed care environment provides the impetus for acquiring or updating knowledge and skills to meet the demand for employment opportunities and expanded roles in nursing, including managing care across a continuum of services and settings. This chapter describes the challenges and opportunities for developing case management competencies through innovative strategies that support educational mobility and career advancement through online courses delivered via the Internet.

Current trends in education have redefined the who, what, where, and how of teaching and learning. The World Wide Web and interactive educational technology allow for the creation of virtual classrooms with increased relevancy and availability and without the rigid constraints of time, place, or pace. Best practices in education using interactive technology emphasize creating an active learning environment to promote discovery, critical thinking, and collaboration. Student and faculty roles are changed in a Web-based environment, and the responsibilities for learning and teaching are shared. Experiences with online case management courses provide insights into the advantages and potential pitfalls. The value and need for opportunities to facilitate educational and career mobility guide the design, delivery, and evaluation of Web-based educational programs. Registered nurses seeking to enhance their professional nursing careers develop case management competencies in an online RN-BS degree completion program at the University of Colorado Health Sciences Center School of Nursing.

TRENDS IN EDUCATION

Roles and concepts of teaching and learning are being restructured (Sherry & Wilson, 1997). The expanding World Wide Web and emerging virtual communities provide professional nurses with previously unimagined access to multiple databases and a rich national and international community for collaborative practice. A focus of education is to rapidly respond to the learning needs of registered nurses by designing and delivering quality and accessible educational programs. The Colorado Nursing Articulation Model (Colorado Council of Nursing Education, 2000) provides a pathway for registered nurses to build on previous education and experience and earn a baccalaureate degree. Innovative strategies integrate educational technology into teaching and learning to provide nurses with additional tools to achieve goals of personal growth and professional advancement.

Relationship of Case Management and Online Learning in Promoting Educational and Career Mobility

The study and practice of case management are well suited to online learning and resources. Professional nurses recognize the need and benefit of updated knowledge and skills to manage complex health care needs. Current knowledge is needed to be able to affect the coordination of care and influence the organization for improved cost and quality outcomes in the delivery of health care. Self-directedness, flexibility, collaboration, effective communication skills, and commitment to inquiry and discovery for problem solving and decision making are skills necessary for both effective care coordination and successful Web-based learning.

Proficiency in using technology is a commonly required competency in the workforce today (Twigg & Oblinger, 1996). The amount and type of information professionals must process and communicate are changing. As the use of computer technology and information increases, individuals who have not developed adequate computer skills are at a disadvantage. Professional nurses must be skilled in the use of computers to access, manage, and communicate information (Robin, 1998). They must be able to access and use the rapidly changing and increasing volume of database resources, consumer information, clinical guideline and practice standards, and accrediting and regulatory information available on the Web.

"In a world of accelerated change, learning must be a lifelong process" (Knowles, 1980, p. 19). Professionals are expected to build new skills on past knowledge, apply theory in practice, and become increasingly self-directed problem solvers and decision makers (Mast & Van Atta, 1986). The American Association of Colleges of Nursing (2000) declared the baccalaureate degree in nursing as minimal preparation for professional practice, citing the need for educational preparation to be commensurate with the diversified responsibilities associated with expanding clinical knowledge and the complexities of health care. Specifically, the movement of health care delivery from hospitals to the community and the focus on prevention, as well as inpatient care, prompts the need for practice competencies to include clinical decision making, case management, and cost-effective coordinated care.

Practicing nurses eager to update their competencies to adapt to the changing health care environment view educational mobility as the vehicle to gain new knowledge and skills. The American Association of Colleges of Nursing (1998) recommended distance learning technologies be implemented to increase access and flexibility in curriculum design and methods to accommodate students with varied educational and experiential backgrounds, citing the imperative of continuous, life-long learning in the nursing profession. Furthermore, the American Association of Colleges of Nursing White Paper, "Distance Technology in Nursing Education" (1999), recognized the significant impact of technological advances on access to quality nursing education for adult, working students who represent the majority of the undergraduate nursing population.

Nurses whose educational program integrates the essential competencies of case management with skill building in network telecommunications have greater potential to do the following:

- Be knowledgeable about health care issues and changes occurring locally, and nationally through the Internet and World Wide Web.
- Be knowledgeable about economic trends, local needs and resources, and alternative problem-solving and decision-making strategies through health care information systems.
- Develop skills in using clinical information systems for the practice of nursing case management and the delivery of nursing care.
- Develop skills to evaluate and manage programs and projects through the use of clinical knowledge, knowledge of health policy, knowledge of clinical and cost data management, and manipulation, analysis, and interpretation of data.
- Develop skills in using computerized information systems in health care to support clinical and administrative decision making.

- Develop information management skills to functionally collect, aggregate, organize, move, and present information in effective and economical ways useful to others.
- Improve communication, understanding, and management of information for care delivery and coordination.
- Maximize the accuracy, timeliness, and usefulness of information for improved health care planning, delivery, and monitoring.
- Transform data or information from one form to another to increase meaningfulness and usefulness.
- Provide insight into structures of information for processing and using appropriate transformations, including algorithms and rules of thumb useful in the practice of nursing case management.
- Work together across boundaries of time, multiple roles and responsibilities, and urban and rural geographies.
- Discover a vision of the future that includes technology and information systems in health care.

Shifts in Expectations and Approaches in Education

Four elements of teaching and learning, relevant to the professional development of case managers, are shifting (Boettcher, 1998) and will be outlined here.

WHO IS LEARNING?

Today's view of education is nontraditional. As pragmatists who face the realities of the workplace daily, case managers view education for its use value rather than enrichment. Nurses are returning to school for retooling, an additional degree, or certification for professional advancement. Learner demographics show shifts from full time to part time, from younger to more mature, from inexperienced with computer technology to skilled in the use of computers and the Internet. Online teaching and learning strategies are appropriate for case managers who may be distant from campus, hold positions of employment, or have workloads that require the readily available course materials and opportunities for faculty and peer interaction at a flexible pace and convenient place. According to Fulkerth (1998), education is evaluated according to the expectations of a consumer-oriented culture: "What do I get? How much will it cost? How convenient is it? How will it be delivered? What is the warranty?"

WHO IS TEACHING?

A collaborative movement between the teacher and student is shifting the teacher's role from controlling the course content and delivery to creating an environment for learning. The teacher as teller with the sole authority and single answer is drifting as an appreciation for the complexity of real world problems and diversity of possible responses is growing (Sherry & Wilson, 1997). As a facilitator, guide, and mentor, the teacher creates the learning environment with learning tools. Students are accountable for their own learning and share the responsibility for teaching each other (Fulkerth, 1998). In an innovatively designed Web-based environment, interaction and collaboration are promoted by providing access to unlimited numbers of case management experts in the field, clinical and educational resources, and knowledge bases.

WHAT IS IMPORTANT TO LEARN?

Expectations are changing about what students need to learn, as well as the delivery mechanism and technology available to serve the need. A shift is occurring from teaching content to enabling students to develop lifelong learning skills. Clinical practice disciplines are becoming more complex and more interdisciplinary. In addition to mastering the nursing discipline's knowledge base, case managers must know how to access, analyze, and use rapidly changing information such as clinical guidelines, health policy, and accrediting and regulatory criteria (Collins, 1996; Fulkerth, 1998). The focus is on the learner and authentic problems (Sherry & Wilson, 1997). The capacity for learning how to learn is essential. Facts are less important than processes, relationships, and interactions. Essential competencies in preparation for a successful career and a useful life are the ability to think critically, communicate effectively, and collaborate with others (Twigg, 1994).

WHERE IS LEARNING OCCURRING?

Accessibility to innovatively designed educational programs using technology is increasing to meet the nurse's changing learning needs and expectations. Online courses are leading the development of new learning environments (Campbell, 1997). The World Wide Web represents a new way of looking at teaching and learning. Used in combination with Internet communication tools such as email, the Web can be used for material delivery or as an environment for interactive learning. Distributed learning allows faculty, case managers, and educational materials to be placed at independent locations so that teaching and learning can occur at any time, in any place, and at any pace (Boettcher, 1998).

The Impact of Educational Technology

Distance learning programs counter the nursing workforce shortage by providing convenient access to nurses who seek education and career mobility but have lack of access to traditional, campus-based education due to family, work, and economic considerations. Internet delivered courses and student supports are designed using a variety of tools, including CD-ROMs, video conferencing, asynchronous discussions, or synchronous chat to provide interactive learning and develop a sense of connection (Cillay, 2003). Students continue to serve their patients in their own communities while they complete degrees via technology (American Association of Colleges of Nursing, 2000). Educational technology provides a new arena for relationship building and the learning milieu for social and behavioral skill development needed for a humanistic, practice-oriented discipline. Web-based courses are designed to address different learning styles, illuminate difficult concepts, accelerate knowledge acquisition, and prepare students for a lifetime of learning. According to Sherry and Wilson (1997), educational technology impacts learning in the following ways:

- Enhancing the quality of education through active learning and teaching strategies
- Guiding educational redesign from instructing to facilitating learning
- Creating relevant and accessible learning environments for learners with differing learning styles and constraints of time and location
- Promoting shared responsibility between the faculty and the learner for the quality of the learning process
- Advancing active learning strategies that motivate and satisfy learners because of the improved quality of learning

INNOVATIVE ONLINE TEACHING AND LEARNING STRATEGIES

A Web-based learning environment can be attractive to both traditional and nontraditional nursing students who seek a rigorous learning experience yet require flexibility. Communications technology allows asynchronous learning experiences, providing continuous access to the course. Increasingly, learners use networks to interact with peers, their instructors, professional experts, and other information resources available on the World Wide Web (Twigg & Oblinger, 1996).

Assessing Readiness for Online Learning

A self-assessment of learning readiness and goals is necessary before investing time and energy in online learning. Consider motivations, ability to be self-directed and self-disciplined, the degree of direction and structure preferred, and skills for working in a virtual environment, including willingness to use a computer as a medium for interacting with people. The following questions will help determine if an online course is the learning alternative of choice:

- Why do I want or need to take this course?
- What are my available options, who else offers them, at what cost, with what schedule, and for what benefit?
- Is this the right time for me to take the course, given my workload, organizational support, family support, financial capability, availability of tuition reimbursement, and motivation?
- How will this course meet my needs in terms of content, schedule, outcomes, application, technical support, mentoring, and collegiality with other learners?
- Do the educational technology and delivery methods suit my learning style, and do I have access to the appropriate hardware, software, and computer skills?
- What skills do I have to contribute to promoting a community on line? (Billings, 1996)

Recommendations for Selecting an Online Offering

An online course should have comprehensive requisites to support learning, including a resource team for ensuring quality in design, delivery, and technical support. Essential factors to consider include the following:

- Evidence of design team (expert content faculty, Web developer, instructional designer/graphic designer, technical assistance) collaboration and commitment to excellence in the use of educational technology with a valued place in the school
- Evidence of a well-organized educational offering that includes planning, course materials, specific computer hardware and software requirements, access instructions, timelines, computer literacy expectations for students, enrollment procedures, and a plan for obtaining necessary help/support
- Faculty reputation as skilled facilitator, group mediator, communicator, and proven demonstrations of attentiveness, empathy, patience, flexibility, humor, and ability to establish trust in the faculty–learner relationship
- Evidence of student involvement and feedback integrated in the course offering, and reflection of student evaluation data from previous offering integrated into the current offering
- User-friendly enrollment procedures, advising, and access to text, course materials, and library resources that ensure careful and prompt attention to student needs, including those of distant learners
- Availability of technical assistance at the educational institution and clear protocol for accessing as needed
- Appropriate opportunities for orientation to the technology before the course begins and socialization to the roles of the learner (self-directed learning, independent learning, collaborative learning) and faculty and as a member of an online learning community
- Availability of help for students to learn how to learn online via learning guides, presentation handouts, or introductory training modules
- Peer support; success of online learning depends on shared commitment and enthusiasm of learners
- Opportunities for formative and summative evaluation by the students of the course/delivery so recommendations for improvements can be integrated in an ongoing manner

- Access to information systems support at the workplace if Internet access is expected during work hours
- Administrative or employer support for your enrollment, including opportunities to integrate course learning activities with workplace issues or initiatives (Billings, 1996)

Innovative Strategies to Promote Learning Outcomes

The Internet as a delivery method has potential advantages relevant to access, convenience, and flexibility. However, the teaching and learning strategies used to facilitate the mastery of higher order learning are more important than the delivery method (Campbell, 1997). The course design, whether unstructured or highly structured, should increase the learner's competency through purposeful interaction. Instruction includes the elements of motivating the learner, explaining what is to be learned, linking new information with previous knowledge, providing instructional material, and testing comprehension (Ritchie & Hoffman, 1998). Online strategies may include a wide variety of tools and techniques, such as distributed lectures and instructional materials, interactive media textbooks, one-to-one communication using email, access to library resources, asynchronous group communications for posting messages and submitting assignments, synchronous group discussions or chat areas for same-time, different-place meetings, simulation exercises, and online assessment and evaluation (Billings, 1996).

Instruction, however, is not learning. Learning requires initiative, interest, interaction, innovation, and involvement. In 1987 the American Association of Higher Education recognized that networked communication systems and information technologies were becoming major resources for teaching and learning. The "Seven Principles of Best Practice in Education" (Chickering & Ehrmann, 1996) describe appropriate ways to maximize the use of educational technology, as follows:

1. Encourage contacts between students and faculty. Interacting encourages students to think about their own experiences and learning goals and is a most important factor in student motivation.
2. Develop reciprocity and cooperation among students. Learning is a social process. Thinking is improved and understanding is deepened when student–student interaction and collaboration are promoted.
3. Use active learning techniques. Learning involves thinking, speaking or writing reflectively, relating to experience, and applying to daily lives.
4. Give prompt feedback. Knowing what you know and what you don't know focuses learning. Frequent opportunities to perform and receive feedback on performance should be provided. Students can learn to self-assess their learning needs.
5. Emphasize time on task. Allocating realistic amounts of time and energy promotes learning.
6. Communicate high expectations. Expecting the student to perform well becomes a self-fulfilling prophecy. Peer evaluation and learning teams can encourage investment in learning.
7. Respect diverse talents and ways of learning. Different students bring different strengths and styles of learning. Self-direction, self-discovery, and self-discipline are worthwhile learning tasks.

A "constructivist" learning environment to promote active learning outcomes is appropriate for the World Wide Web. This environment creates opportunity for involvement and the generation of self-directed learning. Generative learning is based on the ability to reflect on existing knowledge and integrate alternative points of view. "Students must work with information, manipulate it, change it, relate it to existing knowledge structures, and use it to support problem solving. Students learn how to use or apply information they learn. Generative learning activities require students to take static information and generate fluid, flexible, usable knowledge" (Kommers, Grabinger, & Dunlap, 1996, p. 273).

A learning environment should be created that includes activities such as collaboration, autonomy in learning, critical reflection, and authentic interactions with real-world problems. Students should participate in activities that promote high-level thinking processes, including problem solving, experimentation, original creating, and discussion and examination of topics from multiple perspectives (Bostock, 1997). However, to become capable problem solvers, students must know how to learn and be willing and able to take responsibility for identifying learning deficits, setting learning goals, managing the learning process, and monitoring the learning strategies they use (Grabinger & Dunlap, 1996).

Role Expectations and Shared Responsibilities

In a Web-based environment, teaching and learning come together as a partnership. Faculty provide the framework and manage the learning process. The learner actively participates and collaborates with other learners and resources to enhance comprehension, understanding, and knowledge (Doherty, 1998). Students become investigators and problem solvers. Teachers become facilitators and coaches rather than presenters of knowledge (Knowles, 1980).

The goals of online learning are consistent with the principles of adult and active learning, whereby nurses tend to be self-directed and accept responsibility for their own learning. Adult learners have developed individualized learning styles, depending on what works best for them. Some learn most effectively through action, interaction, or participation; others through reading and reflection. A Web-based environment blends these approaches. Online learning provides the opportunity and expectation that individuals will select learning materials that they perceive have immediate applicability to life tasks. The focus of learning is on problem solving and generating products of value. It emphasizes self-determination, self-assessment, and the involvement of the whole person in the learning process (Kinzie & Sullivan, 1989; Lawless & Brown, 1997). Learner control is enhanced in online learning because the case manager can direct his or her own learning experiences, including the path and pace. Depending on learning style and needs, the depth of study, range of content and type of media, and time spent are tailored by the individual. The learner's perceptions of competence, self-determination, and intrinsic interest may increase (Lawless & Brown, 1997).

The faculty role in online learning has often been described as the "guide on the side" rather than the "sage on the stage." As facilitators, faculty should be resources for self-directed learners rather than imparters of a body of knowledge. Designing a framework for constructive discourse and negotiation of meaning among students is a primary responsibility. Learning guides and content resources may be provided. Learners' participation and activities are monitored, and social support for the learning community is provided through encouragement, feedback, and mentoring.

As important as the concepts of self-directed learning and active involvement are for the student, and facilitation and guidance are for the faculty, the critical element for successful online learning is the development of a community of learners. Through the dynamic community, peers and experts in the field develop and share toolkits with useful application for professional development and personal growth. The new model for education is a learning network: a community of learners who work together in an online environment. The American Association for Higher Education (1998) outlined "Learning Principles and Collaborative Action," as follows:

1. Learning is fundamentally about making and maintaining connections.
2. Learning is enhanced by taking place in the context of compelling situations.
3. Learning is an active search for meaning by the learner, constructing knowledge rather than receiving it, and shaping it as well as being shaped by experiences.
4. Learning is a developmental and cumulative process.
5. Learning is by individuals who are intrinsically tied to others as social beings.
6. Learning is strongly affected by the educational climate.
7. Learning requires frequent feedback if it is to be sustained.
8. Learning takes place informally and incidentally.

9. Learning is grounded in particular contexts and individual experiences.
10. Learning involves the ability of individuals to monitor their own learning.

"Network learning enables anyone, anywhere, at anytime to be a learner or a teacher. It enhances the link between theory and practice, and the classroom and the real world" (Kersley, 1993, p. 70). A community of learners has come together when learners gather to provide mutual support and scaffolding for learning and performance. Indicators of an effective learner support environment are as follows (Sherry & Wilson, 1997):

- Learners solve their own problems and share solutions.
- Effective learning resources are located or developed and made available to the entire learning community.
- Learners are encouraged and rewarded for taking initiative.
- Learners' areas of expertise are valued.
- Technical support and guidance are made available to each other through online resources and a buddy system.
- The informal culture encourages risk-taking and innovation.

EVALUATION OF ONLINE LEARNING EXPERIENCES

The Web is effective in providing quality and accessible educational opportunities, promoting interaction among learners across geographical boundaries, and guiding application to practice. However, offerings must be carefully designed and strategies cautiously implemented to achieve the desired outcomes of content mastery and competency development. What engages, motivates, and reinforces student learning? What student/faculty preparation is needed and how can barriers be managed? Which methods are most useful for redesigning roles, structuring learning experiences, assessing competencies, and facilitating learners' ability to perform in the practice setting?

Many models, instruments, and methodologies exist to evaluate the use of educational technology and the value of the virtual classroom. The Flashlight Evaluation Project (Ehrmann & Zungia, 1997) uses a conceptual model for evaluating the impact of informational technology on teaching and learning. Changes in learning outcomes, access, and cost are measured. Examples of key learner-focused educational issues include active and collaborative learning strategies, using time productively, high expectations for all students regardless of learning style, rich and rapid feedback, engagement in learning, faculty and student interaction, cognitive and creative outcomes, accessibility, respect for diversity, and application to work (Ehrmann & Zungia, 1997).

Courses designed to provide opportunities for collaboration, problem- or project-based experiences, and focus on high-level activities, such as integration and critique, are most effective in promoting learning (Billings, 1996).

Learners' Perceptions of the Benefits of Online Learning

Satisfaction is directly related to the availability of learner support for using the technology and changes in approaches to teaching and learning. Russell (1999) reviewed 255 studies conducted from 1928 to 1997 and found no significant differences in the competencies of students taught by traditional classroom methods versus distance education methods. In comparisons of online courses with real-time courses offered on campus, students' responses to online courses were positive (Billings, 1996; Forsyth, 1996; Twigg & Oblinger, 1996). Themes related to online learning included the benefits of accessibility, convenience, and flexibility. Students believed they spent more time with the course material because learning was more meaningful to them. They generally felt connected, interacted more with faculty and peers, learned to use classmates as resources, and reflected more on their interactions with the course content (Carlton, Ryan, & Siktberg, 1998). The ability to share examples, discuss works in progress, and critique each other's work was valuable. The need to take more responsibility for their learning was acknowledged, as was the high technology learning curve. The consensus was that course and personal learning goals were accomplished.

Lessons Learned by Exploring, Experimenting, and Evaluating

An existing didactic case management course offered at the University of Colorado School of Nursing was redesigned for Internet delivery to maximize access to current Web-based resources and stimulate the use of technology in the practice of case management. Ongoing modification occurs with each subsequent offering. A design team consisting of content experts, instructional designer, and Webmaster developed and operationalized the course using WebCT (2002), an authoring software program. The conceptual framework for the content includes the Case Management Society of America Standards of Practice and the Commission for Case Manager Certification Essential Activities and Core Areas of Case Management. The course features six content modules with competency outcomes, interactive learning activities and resources, a conference center for asynchronous discussion, and individual and group assignments with critical elements for competency evaluation. A teaching and learning environment emphasizes a caring educative pedagogy and reinforces the "Seven Principles of Best Practices in Education" (Chickering & Gamson, 1987).

The process of transforming a course for internet delivery includes *exploring* a variety of traditional and innovative strategies for consistency with the goals of competency-based education within an educative caring pedagogy; *experimenting* with multiple learning strategies to determine usefulness and effectiveness in content mastery and competency development, including problem-based learning projects, presentations, peer review, quizzes, reflection papers, group work, and research using Internet resources; and *evaluating* the efficacy of methods from student and faculty viewpoints. Formative and summative evaluation methods are used to assess the impact of learning strategies and competency assessment methodologies. Consistent themes include agreement that the course design supported learning, confidence in ability to learn difficult and complex material was enhanced, meaningful communication was encouraged, and application of learning to the real world was emphasized. Students agreed they would enroll in another Internet course and recommend the course to others. Responses were used in an ongoing manner to improve content, teaching strategies, and level of presentation. Recommendations for design and evaluation strategies have guided subsequent Web-based offerings and facilitated the evaluation of curriculum concepts and organizing frameworks.

DEVELOPING CASE MANAGEMENT COMPETENCIES

Design-Develop-Deliver-Decide Model

Partnerships among educational institutions and clinical agencies are evolving for the purpose of achieving shared goals of quality education and care delivery with limited resources. Nursing case managers play critical roles in satisfying the need for quality health services in a cost-effective environment and require updated knowledge and skills. Nursing administrators recognize the immediate need for quality educational programs and professional development to support the evolving role of nursing case manager and to positively impact clinical and cost outcomes. Nursing educators are committed to promote the fusion of learning and work and to design and deliver educational programs using interactive learning strategies and technology to increase accessibility and relevance. The result was the faculty-developed *"Design-Develop-Deliver-Decide"* model to create, market, implement, and evaluate a case management Web-based course offered by the University of Colorado School of Nursing. Practicing registered nurses from a variety of tertiary care and health maintenance organizations have successfully completed the course within the RN-BS program of study or for professional development.

In *design*, the educational setting, strategies, and players are redefined. The employing organization demonstrates to its members a commitment to learning, the expectation and support for competency development, and continuous improvement. The educator–employer partnership is established to assist in achieving the goals. A needs analysis identifies the employer's performance expectations of the practicing nurse. Competency outcomes are determined collaboratively. The return on investment must be determined: Will the educational program result in increased knowledge, evidenced by improvement in the performance of essential skills at a reasonable cost?

Collaborative planning in the *develop* phase ensures course structure and process to enhance competency development. A design operationalizes the course, which features interactive strategies selected to promote self-directed learning, content mastery, and application to practice. Responsibility is shared among the employer and the course development team to ensure a learner-centered Web environment.

In traditional educational settings the student–teacher relationship starts and ends with the *delivery* or offering of the course. In a collaborative partnership the relationship with the employer has preceded the learner–facilitator relationship and may be extended beyond the duration of the current course offering. After expectations are mutually clarified, protocols are established for participant identification, tuition reimbursement, assessment of basic computer skills and Internet access, and time frames. Recognition, encouragement, and reward by the employer are important, as the responsibility for the quality of the process is shared among educator, employer, and learner.

Throughout the course, learners, employers, and educators must *decide* whether the anticipated outcomes are achieved. Evaluation data provide a quantitative and qualitative picture of the strengths and areas of improvement. Recommendations from formative data collected at the end of each module are incorporated to continually shape the educational experience to meet learning needs and expectations. Key learning, continued learning needs, and one-word journals clarify students' perspective of competency achievement. Summative course evaluation data provide a comprehensive review of the Web-based learning environment and evidence of learning. Finally, evidence of learning relevant to practice, including functional, interpersonal, and critical thinking competencies, are summarized and presented in educator-employer conferences. Employer feedback is solicited, providing an opportunity to assess their perspective of the success of the project, strategize about future possibilities, and forge partnerships that enhance both service and education.

Implications for Enhancing Educational and Career Mobility

Practicing nurses, employers, and educators promote professional development and achievement of shared goals to improve care coordination, quality, and cost outcomes. When flexible teaching and learning strategies are planned and implemented in a Web-based environment to advance case management competencies, nurses have an opportunity to demonstrate initiative in self-directed learning to achieve cognitive, attitude, and skill outcomes. As the nurse is guided by the structured modular activities and resources, continuing learning needs are identified and new learning is reinforced by online interaction. Involvement is maximized as convenience and accessibility are increased by altering time and space constraints through networked educational technologies. Professional working relationships, networking, and mentoring opportunities are enhanced when nontraditional learners are provided convenient and accessible educational programs.

Learning as an integral part of life and work is reinforced as the educational experiences integrate current practice roles and responsibilities with education throughout professional nursing careers. Online courses for case management competency development align goals, strategies, and resources with eager learners for advancing their education and career options throughout their professional nursing practice.

References

American Association of Colleges of Nursing (1998). *Educational Mobility.* Washington, D.C.: American Nurses Publishing. Available at http://www.aacn.nche.edu/Publications/positions/edmobil.htm.

American Association of Colleges of Nursing (1999). *AACN White Paper: Distance Technology in Nursing Education.* Washington, D.C.: American Nurses Publishing. Available at http://www.aacn.nche.edu/Publications/positions/whitepaper.htm.

American Association of Colleges of Nursing (2000). *Issues bulletin: Distance learning is changing and challenging nursing education.* Washington, D.C.: American Nurses Publishing. Available at http://www.aacn.nche.edu/Publications/issues/jan2000.htm.

American Association of Colleges of Nursing (2000). *The baccalaureate degree in nursing as minimal preparation for professional practice.* Washington, D.C.: American Nurses Publishing. Available at http://www.aacn.nche.edu/Publications/positions/baccmin.htm.

American Association for Higher Education, American College Personnel Association, National Association of Student Personnel Administrators: Joint Task Force on Student Learning Final Report (1998). *Powerful partnerships: A shared responsibility for learning.* Available at http://www.aahe.org/assessment/joint.htm.

Billings, D. (1996). Distance education in nursing: Adapting courses for distance education. *Computers in Nursing 14*(5), 262-263, 266.

Boettcher, J. (1998). The turtle is moving. *Syllabus Magazine, 12*(2).

Bostock, S. (1997). Designing Web-based instruction for active learning. In B.H. Kahn (Ed.), *Web-based instruction,* Englewood Cliffs, N.J.: Educational Technology Publications.

Campbell, J. (1997). Evaluating ALN: What works, who's learning? *ALN Magazine 1*(2). Available at http://www.aln.org/publications/magazine/v1n2/campbell_alntalk.asp.

Carlton, K, Ryan, M., & Siktberg, L. (1998). Designing courses for the internet: A conceptual approach. *Nurse Educator, 23*(3), 45-50.

Collins, B. (1996). *Tele-learning in a digital world.* London: Thomson Computer Press. Colorado Council on Nursing Education (2000). *Colorado Nursing Articulation Model 2000-2005.* Denver, Colo.: Colorado Trust.

Chickering, A., & Ehrmann, S. (1996). *Implementing the seven principles: Technology as lever.* Washington, D.C.: American Association for Higher Education. Available at http://www.tltgroup.org/programs/seven.html.

Chickering, A., & Gamson, Z. (1997). Principles for good practice in undergraduate education. *American Higher Education Bulletin,* March.

Cillay, D. (2003). Multi-model deliver and diverse interaction in an instructional design course. The Technology Source. Available at http://ts.mivu.org/default.asp?show = article&id = 1000.

Doherty, P. (1998). Learner control in asynchronous learning environments, *ALN Magazine, 2*(2). Available at http://www.aln.org/publications/magazine/v2n2/doherty.asp.

Ehrmann, S., & Zungia, R. (1997). *The flashlight evaluation handbook.* Washington, D.C.: Teaching, Learning and Technology Group, American Association on Higher Education.

Forsyth, I. (1996). *Teaching and learning materials and the Internet,* London: Kogan Page.

Fulkerth, B. (1998). A bridge for distance education: planning for the information-age student. *Syllabus Magazine, 12*(4).

Grabinger, S., & Dunlap, J. (1996). *Make learning meaningful.* In P. Kommers, S. Grabinger, & J. Dunla (Eds.), *Hypermedia and multimedia learning environment: instructional design and integration.* Mahwah, N.J.: Erlbaum Associates.

Kersley, G. (1993). Speaking personal with Linda Harasim. *The American Journal of Distance Education, 7*(3):70-73.

Kinzie, M., & Sullivan, H. (1989). Continuing motivation, learner control and CAI. *Educational Technology Research and Development, 37*(2):5-14.

Knowles, M. (1980). *The modern practice of adult education,* Chicago: Follet Publishing.

Kommers, P., Grabinger, S., & Dunlap J. (1996). *Hypermedia and multimedia learning environment: instructional design and integration.* Mahwah, N.J.: Erlbaum Associates.

Lawless, K., & Brown, S. (1997). Multimedia learning environments: Issues of learner control and navigation, *Instructional Science*, 25.

Mast, M., & Van Atta, J. (1968). Applying adult learning principles in instructional module design, *Nurse Educator*, *11*(1), 35-39, 1986.

Ritchie, D., & Hoffman, B. (1998). Instructional design principles in the World Wide Web, NAU/Web.com, Flagstaff, Ariz.

Robin, M. (1998). Models of online courses. *ALN Magazine 2*(2). Available at http://www.aln.org/publications/magazine/v2n2/mason.asp.

Banks, L. Graebner, C., & McConnell, D. (Eds.), *Networked lifelong learning: innovative approaches to education and training through the Internet*, conference proceedings, University of Sheffield.

Russell, T. (1999). *The no significant difference phenomenon.* Raleigh, N.C.: North Carolina State University.

Sherry, L., & Wilson, B. (1997). Transformative communication as a stimulus to Web innovations. In B.H. Kahn (Ed.), *Web-based instruction*, Englewood Cliffs, N.J.: Educational Technology Publications.

Twigg, C. (1994). The need for a national learning infrastructure, *Educom Review 29*(4,5,6,). Available at http://www.educause.edu/nlii/keydocs/monograph.html.

Twigg, C., & Oblinger, D. (1996). *The virtual university: a report from a Joint Educom/IBM Roundtable.* Washington, D.C. Available at http://www.educause.edu/nlii/VU.html.

WebCT (2002). *Leveraging technology to transform the educational experience.* Available at http://www.Webct.com/service/ViewContent?contentID=4464759.

VII

IMPLEMENTATION

Taking a Systems Process Approach

Building on Unit VI, Unit VII takes the reader on a journey through all the key steps in the implementation process. Of particular interest is the application of the case management design to a variety of clinical settings. In addition, an understanding of today's case management planning tools, including multidisciplinary action plans, and case management documentation tools is included in this section. Today's case managers deal with a myriad of ethical issues, which are explored here. A discussion of the information technology arena and of compliance and regulatory issues completes this very eclectic section.

29

The Cast of Characters

CHAPTER OVERVIEW

Primary nursing models no longer meet the changing needs of either the health care environment or the patients. In this chapter, the multidisciplinary approach is discussed in terms of its relative value to the case management model. Both this approach and case management in general are presented in response to an increasingly complex health care environment. How to form teams and how to gain the support and trust of colleagues are two of the topics discussed.

GETTING OUT OF THE PARALLEL PLAY SYNDROME

Those who began their nursing careers in the 1970s were trained and educated to function as independent professional nurses. With the advent of the primary nursing model, *professional* meant doing everything oneself (Bakke, 1974). The team spirit and sense of esprit de corps were lost in the fight to prove nursing a worthy profession. In the attempt to show just how important nursing was to the patient, other disciplines, which also provided unique and necessary services, were neglected.

Perhaps nursing had to go through this process. Perhaps it was necessary as part of the profession's evolutionary growth. Because nurses were so used to nursing being viewed as a second-class profession, they were riding high on the conviction that they could do it all and do it all well.

Out of this generation of parallel play came terms such as *burnout, fatigue syndrome,* and *fragmented care.* Under the primary nursing model, it was expected that the nurse would meet all the patient's needs, from the bed bath to the discharge plan. With the nursing shortage that began in 1985 and the prospective payment system that resulted in shortened lengths of stay, nurses found it almost impossible to function under the primary nursing system.

Increased complexity and technology required that registered nurses become experts in a narrower range of tasks, which meant that other tasks had to be relinquished or returned to the other disciplines. Nursing care had to become more specialized as it responded to changing patient needs both in the hospital and after discharge.

Because the hospital stay was shortened in response to the prospective payment system, the phrase "discharge them quicker, but sicker" was being quoted by both health care practitioners and patients. Members of the public were losing confidence in the health care system because they felt rushed through the process by the insurers as well as the health care providers, who now had to keep the hospital stay as short as possible.

Flexible time (flex time) measures, which were designed to attract more people to the profession and to retain those already in the workforce, contributed to fragmented nursing care. Fragmentation was chiefly an outcome of these measures, which resulted in the advent of 10- and 12-hour shifts. Flex time was very attractive to employees because it allowed them to have long blocks of time off to spend with their families and to continue their education. Unfortunately, these long blocks of time created a tremendous gap in patient care. Trying to be all things to the patient for 12 hours and then not being present for 3 days was meeting the worker's needs at the patient's expense. The accelerated hospital stay compounded the situation. It was conceivable that patients might see a different nurse during each day of an average 4-day hospital stay. Patients complained that no one knew them or their needs, and they were unable to develop professional relationships with any of their nurses. These patients felt that no one practitioner was responsible for their care. Nursing appeared to have failed because accountability for patient care had been lost.

Although nursing departments across the country tried to keep functioning in primary nursing systems, the new environment made it impossible to do so. Primary nursing had been founded on the notion that the registered professional nurse would be responsible for all aspects of the patient's care from admission to discharge. This became unattainable with the introduction of the flex time system. Although theoretically nurses were responsible, extended absences from the unit prevented a true continuation of their relationship with the patient or the other members of the health care team.

In addition, patient assignments continued, in many instances, to remain geographic, with each nurse on the shift assigned a particular geographic part of the nursing unit. If the patient was moved to some other area of the unit, it was likely that the primary nurse would no longer be caring for that patient. Such changes meant care had become extremely fragmented.

At the same time, the role of the head nurse or nurse manager was moving away from the bedside. More and more administrative responsibility was given to these middle managers as upper management positions were eliminated. In the past the nurse manager had been able to clinically monitor all the patients on the floor and still carry out managerial responsibilities. As the administrative duties increased, this became more difficult to accomplish. In addition, the average length of stay was dramatically shortened, so that patients were admitted and discharged from the unit faster than they could be followed up by a busy manager with other responsibilities.

THE EFFECTS OF A CHANGING ENVIRONMENT

During the 1970s, nurses and other health care providers first began to complain of stress-related problems such as chronic fatigue and burnout. In 1974 a psychologist named Freudenberger coined the clinical term *burnout*. Burnout was described as the degeneration of a once highly productive individual into a negative, exhausted one. It was seen as a direct response to work stress when the worker no longer had the resources available to deal with other people's emotional, psychological, and physical problems.

Burnout follows a particular pattern that generally begins with feelings of emotional exhaustion. Such exhaustion results from being emotionally overextended and exhausted by one's work with others (Maslach, 1976, 1978, 1982). This exhaustion is followed by feelings of depersonalization, which have been described as negative, unfeeling, and impersonal responses toward the recipients of one's care. As the syndrome becomes more severe, the worker may describe feelings of reduced personal accomplishment. Personal accomplishment is characterized by feelings of competence and successful achievement in one's work with people (Maslach, 1976, 1978, 1982). By placing registered nurses in a position that required them to be all things to the patient, the nurses experienced an incredible amount of on-the-job stress.

Role overload was yet another outcome of work stress that was identified in some nurses (Cesta, 1989). Role overload is characterized by the worker's subjective feelings of being unable to complete the work because of inadequate personal or environmental resources (French & Caplan, 1972; Hardy, 1976; Ritzer, 1977). These feelings have been reported to be particularly high in nurses who are in their first 2 years of employment (Cesta, 1989; Das, 1981; Maslach, 1982).

When role overload combined with feelings of burnout, the nurse's ability to deal with work began to change and gradually diminished (Cesta, 1989).

Nurses began to adjust the primary nursing system in an attempt to address changes in the health care arena. This new system eventually became known as *modified primary* and retained the theory that the nurse was accountable for all aspects of care. This did not mean, however, that the nurse retained responsibility for the patient from admission to discharge. Primary nursing responsibilities were applicable only to the day the nurse worked.

Once these modifications were made in the primary model, the stage was set for the development of a more appropriate model that addressed all the foregoing issues (Loveridge, Cummings, & O'Malley, 1988). The alternative model combined elements of team and primary nursing (Zander, 1985). There was really nothing new or revolutionary about the case management model for nursing care delivery. The basic premise of the model was a team or collaborative approach that allowed the case manager to function as the evaluator and coordinator of care or facilitator of the team. This new role was similar to that of the primary nurse, except that the case manager was now removed from direct patient care responsibility.

With the addition of this role, nursing moved away from attempting to be all things to the patient. Members of the profession began to admit that they could not do all things equally well and that other members of the team were needed to provide their particular areas of expertise. Nursing was finally getting out of the parallel play syndrome and was moving toward a more dynamic and interactive modality.

FORMATION OF THE COLLABORATIVE PRACTICE GROUPS

It is perhaps easier now for nurses to reintroduce themselves to the team approach. Although social workers and physicians had functioned that way for years, nurses had been struggling to achieve independence and autonomy. Nurses felt more confident and ready to join the team after gaining prestige among other health care providers (Farley & Stoner, 1989).

Institutions implementing case management models for the first time must explain to team members why nurses are returning to the team approach. At first, this reintroduction of the team approach may be observed with some suspicion and doubt. Without making the intentions of the team clear, it will be impossible to institute collaborative practice groups.

Physicians and other health care providers may have preconceived ideas about case management, some of which stem from their familiarity with the managed care systems introduced in health maintenance organizations (HMOs). Generally, many health care providers see these managed care systems as negative or as one more way for their practices to be regulated and controlled and their services to be rationed (Knight, 1998; Schwartz & Mendelson, 1992).

Collaborative practice groups cannot be formed until all members adopt the model as their own and see its benefit for both themselves and the patient. It should be emphasized that case management is not just a nursing care model but a way for all the disciplines to form plans of care that avoid duplication of effort, unnecessary tests and procedures, or misuse of resources.

Each discipline involved in patient care activities develops a plan that meets the objectives for that discipline as they relate to the patient. Case management provides, for the first time, the opportunity for all the disciplines to come together in an effort to use each other's expertise for maximum benefit to the patient.

Cast of Characters

Who then comprises the cast of characters, and how do they come together as a group? Formation of these interdisciplinary groups is one of the first steps for implementation, and it must take place before any real clinical changes can occur.

In a unit-based case management approach, who is in the group depends on the types of case management plans being developed. At the least, each group should consist of members from the following disciplines: nursing, medicine, social work, discharge planning, and nutrition. People from these areas make up the core of any group, and each one provides input related to the clinical objectives of that member's discipline. Of course, the central figures in any such team are the patient and family.

Other members are added as they relate to the particular diagnosis or procedure planned. Other disciplines that might be included are physical therapy, occupational therapy, respiratory therapy, and nutrition.

In some cases the groups may have already been formed as part of the implementation of a non–unit-based case management approach. In this approach, groups are formed around a particular diagnosis, and all members of the team are experts in that clinical area. For example, a team might be formed to manage diabetic patients throughout the hospital. A diabetes case management team is often headed by a diabetologist and a nurse case manager who together provide the leadership to direct the other members of the team. A cardiac case management team might be headed by a cardiologist and a cardiac nurse case manager. The members of a case management team follow the patients' cases regardless of where they might be within the hospital. Therefore the team remains constant while the patients and their locations change.

Because the case management team is developed before the arrival of the patient, these non–unit-based groups have already determined protocols and care methods for their specific types of patients. It is not necessary for the case manager to identify the members of the team at the time of the patient's admission to the hospital because the team is already in place. In the unit-based case management model, however, the members of the team are determined by the patient problem. These teams are fluid and constantly changing.

After the patient's admission the attending physician, case manager, social worker, nutritionist, and others are identified and the specific plan of care for the patient is formalized. The use of internal techniques and relationships should not be underestimated in the formation of the multidisciplinary groups. If a nonthreatening, informal relationship has been developed first, it will be much easier to obtain the cooperation of some professionals. Inviting key players to lunch, meeting in the library, or just chatting on the unit can do much to gain trust and respect.

There may be occasions when a member of another discipline who is in a position of authority may be needed to intervene on the part of the case manager to obtain concurrence for collaborative practice. For example, some physicians admit large numbers of patients to the hospital every year and are therefore considered to have a great deal of power and independence in their everyday practice within the hospital. These individuals may not immediately see the advantage of joining a multidisciplinary team effort because it may not appear to benefit them, or they may view the effort to form teams as an attempt to control their practices. In a case like this, it may be necessary to have a physician administrator intervene on the behalf of the case management team. Usually, once the benefits are presented to the physicians, they give their support. Also, they may need to get their superiors' consent to participate.

Another technique to gain the support of some of the more resistant professionals is to begin working first with those who have already agreed to the model. It is sometimes more effective to begin with these individuals than to try to convert the resisters right away. Perhaps when success is proved with those who have been immediately receptive, the others will give their support. Once again, support may depend on people's perceptions of what the model can do for them. There will always be a certain percentage of players who will sit on the fence, waiting to see if implementation succeeds or fails. Once success is evident, they will cross over to the case manager's side.

In both the unit- and non–unit-based case management approach, the team becomes the focal point for care delivery, with each member lending information from a specific area of expertise. Most institutions rely on the case manager to be responsible for smooth operation and communication among team members. In some instances, however, social workers or physicians have been used to coordinate communication. Nurses function well in this role because they are educated to take a holistic approach to care delivery and because they are the ones who become involved in all aspects of the patient's care.

For example, it is less likely that a social worker will have the clinical skills of a registered nurse, but most registered nurses have the basic skills required to provide discharge planning and referral services to patients after discharge. Case managers should be able to identify patients at high risk and to refer such patients to the appropriate discipline. Patients with high-risk discharge planning needs can be referred to the discharge planner or social worker, as appropriate to the organization. At the very least, the case manager should be able to work the system to the patient's advantage, knowing the appropriate members to call as needs arise. An advanced understanding of the patient's medical and nursing needs helps to make this assessment complete. The case manager can then refer the problem to the appropriate practitioner.

In the unit-based approach, it may be difficult or impossible for the complete team to meet at one time. Once again, case managers fill this gap. They provide the thread that holds all the members together. In this sense the case managers must have excellent communication skills. The information they translate between team members and to patients and families must be accurate and concise or the thread is broken and the team falls apart.

The team should be assembled as a group whenever possible. Dialogue and opinion can thus be shared on a face-to-face basis. It is often during meetings of this type that difficult patient problems are resolved.

The case manager may spend a good deal of time during the beginning of implementation trying to ensure that the team becomes a reality and remains on target to provide the best possible care for the patient.

The case manager role consists of the following three dimensions (Tahan, 1993, Chapter 17). The first dimension is the *clinical role*, which requires collaboration with the interdisciplinary team and involves the development of protocols that list the key tasks or events that must be accomplished for handling patient problems. Case managers use these protocols to direct, monitor, and evaluate patient treatment and the outcomes or responses to treatment (Thompson et al., 1991; Zander, 1988). Case managers identify variances from the standard protocols and work with other health care team members to analyze and deal with these variances of care (Cesta, Tahan, & Fink, 1998; Ethridge & Lamb, 1989; O'Malley, 1988b).

The second dimension is that of the *managerial role*, which refers to the case manager's responsibility for coordinating the care of patients during the course of hospitalization (Ethridge & Lamb, 1989; Kruger, 1989; O'Malley, 1988a; Zander, 1988). The case manager manages care by planning the nursing treatment modalities and interventions necessary for meeting the needs of the patient and the family. Goals of treatment are set at admission, and length of stay is determined as it relates to the diagnosis-related group (DRG). The discharge plan is formed as early in the hospital stay as possible (O'Malley, 1988b).

Case managers also guide the activities, nursing treatments, and interventions of other nursing staff members (Ethridge & Lamb, 1989; Kruger, 1989). They continuously evaluate the quality of care provided and outcomes of treatments and services to prevent misuse of resources (O'Malley, 1988a).

One of the informal responsibilities of the case manager is that of teacher and mentor (Cronin & Maklebust, 1989; Kruger, 1989). The case manager assesses staff development needs, especially among the less-experienced practitioners, and refers them to the appropriate person or resource (Leclair, 1991).

As part of the teaching responsibilities of the role, case managers conduct patient and family teaching sessions during the hospitalization period (Cronin & Maklebust, 1989; Zander, 1988).

The third dimension of the case manager role involves *financial aspects.* In collaboration with the physician and other health care members, case managers activate a caregiving process for each patient and use a case management plan, which is a generic tool for managing care and keeping it consistent with the predetermined financial outcomes for a defined case type (Adams & Biggerstaff, 1995; O'Malley, 1988b; Zander, 1988). The use of such clinical treatment standards helps ensure that patients do not receive inadequate care because of cost containment measures (Collard, Bergman, & Henderson, 1990; Mass & Johnson, 1998).

Case managers access information related to DRGs and case types, the cost of each diagnosis, the allocated length of stay, and the treatments and procedures generally used for each diagnosis. They use this information to review resources and evaluate the efficiency of care related to the diagnosis (Cronin & Maklebust, 1989). The case manager has a great influence on the quality and price of care by helping to determine in a timely manner the most pertinent treatment for the patient (Henderson & Collard, 1988). Case managers also assess variances for each case type and act immediately to control these variances to contain costs (Cesta & Tahan, 2002; Crawford, 1991). They assure consistency, continuity, and coordination of care to control for duplication and fragmentation in health care delivery, which results in better resource allocation and further cost containment (Henderson & Collard, 1988; O'Malley, 1988a).

To be effective, case managers must access information on case mix index, cost of resources, and consumption and must be familiar with the prospective payment system and current third-party reimbursement procedures, including managed care and capitation (Ethridge & Lamb, 1989; O'Malley, 1988b).

Case managers work closely with the utilization review department in identifying long-stay patients and planning with that department to control and prevent inappropriate hospital stays (Cronin & Maklebust, 1989). In other cases the case manager assumes the functions of utilization review/management. These functions generally include reviewing cases for medical necessity and resource utilization and providing this information to third party payers, particularly managed care organizations (MCOs). When these functions are integrated into the role of the case manager, work with third-party payers becomes less fragmented and better coordinated. Communication and cooperation with the MCO is enhanced.

References

Adams, C.E., & Biggerstaff, N. (1995). Reduced resource utilization through standardized outcomes-focused care plans. *Journal of Nursing Administration, 25*(10), 43-49.

Bakke, K. (1974). Primary nursing: Perceptions of a staff nurse. *American Journal of Nursing, 74*(8), 1432-1434.

Cesta, T.G. (1989). *The relationship of role overload and burnout to coping process in registered professional staff nurses newly employed in a hospital setting.* Doctoral dissertation. University Microfilms, Inc., Publication No. 9016399.

Cesta, T.G., & Tahan, H.A. (2002). *The case manager's survival guide: Winning strategies for clinical practice.* St. Louis: Mosby.

Collard, A.F., Bergman, A., & Henderson, M. (1990). Two approaches to measuring quality in medical case management programs. *Quality Review Bulletin*, 3-8.

Crawford, J. (1991). Managed care consultant: The "house supervisor" alternative. *Nursing Management, 22*(5), 75-78.

Cronin, C.J., & Maklebust, J. (1989). Case-managed care: Capitalizing on the CNS. *Nursing Management, 20*(3), 38-47.

Das, E.B.L. (1981). Contributing factors to burnout in the nursing environment. Doctoral dissertation, Texas Woman's University. *Dissertation Abstracts International, 42*, 04B.

Ethridge, P., & Lamb, G. (1989). Professional nursing case management improves quality, access and costs. *Nursing Management, 20*(3), 30-35.

Farley, M.J., & Stoner, M.H. (1989). The nurse executive and interdisciplinary team building. *Nursing Administration Quarterly*, 24-29.

French, J.R.P., & Caplan, R.D. (1972). Organizational stress and individual strain. In A.J. Morrow (Ed.), *The failure of success* (pp. 30-66). New York: AMACOM.

Freudenberger, H.J. (1974). Staff burn-out. *Journal of Social Issues, 30,* 159-165.

Hardy, M.E. (1976, Aug.). Role problems, role strain, job satisfaction, and nursing care. Paper presented at the annual meeting of the American Sociological Association, New York.

Henderson, M.G., & Collard, A. (1988). Measuring quality in medical case management programs. *Quality Review Bulletin,* 33-39.

Knight, W. (1998). *Managed care: What it is and how it works.* Gaithersburg, Md.: Aspen Publications.

Kruger, N.R. (1989). Case management: Is it a delivery system for my organization? *Aspen's Advisor for Nurse Executives, 4*(10), 4-6.

Leclair, C. (1991). Introducing and accounting for RN case management. *Nursing Management, 22*(3), 44-49.

Loveridge, C.E., Cummings, S.H., & O'Malley, J. (1988). Developing case management in a primary nursing system. *Journal of Nursing Administration, 18*(10), 36-39.

Maslach, C. (1976). Burned-out. *Human Behavior, 5,* 17-21.

Maslach, C. (1978). Job burn-out: How people cope. *Public Welfare, 36,* 56-58.

Maslach, C. (1982). *Burnout. The cost of caring.* Englewood Cliffs, N.J.: Prentice-Hall.

Mass, S., & Johnson, B. (1998, Nov.). Case management and clinical guidelines. *The Journal of Care Management.* Special Edition.

O'Malley, J. (1988a). Nursing case management. I: Why look at a different model for nursing care delivery? *Aspen's Advisor for Nurse Executives, 3*(5), 5-6.

O'Malley, J. (1988b). Nursing case management, part II: Dimensions of the nurse case manager role. *Aspen's Advisor for Nurse Executives, 3*(6), 7.

Ritzer, G. (1977). *Working.* Englewood Cliffs, N.J.: Prentice-Hall.

Schwartz, W., & Mendelson, D. (1992 Summer). Why managed care cannot contain hospital cost without. *Health Affairs* 100-107.

Tahan, H.T. (1993). The nurse case manager in acute care settings: Job description and function. *Journal of Nursing Administration, 23*(10), 53-61.

Thompson, K.S., Caddick, K., Mathie, J., Newlon, B., & Abraham, T. (1991). Building a critical path for ventilator dependency. *American Journal of Nursing,* 28-31.

Zander, K. (1992 Fall). Quantifying, managing, and improving quality: III. Using variance concurrently. *The New Definition, 7*(4), 1-4.

Zander, K. (1985). Second generation primary nursing: A new agenda. *Journal of Nursing Administration, 15*(3), 18-24.

Zander, K. (1988). Managed care within acute care settings: Design and implementation via nursing case management. *Health Care Supervisor, 6*(2), 27-43.

Variations Within Clinical Settings

CHAPTER OVERVIEW

Case management models provide an opportunity for health care institutions to provide quality, cost-effective services regardless of the type of setting or financial resources. The model is flexible and can be adapted to meet the needs of both clinical and institutional settings.

    This chapter describes how the case management model can be adapted to a variety of clinical settings, including medicine, surgery, critical care, nursing homes, clinics, and other ambulatory care settings. The way in which a case management model is used depends on the goals of the organization using it. The chapter also discusses the challenge facing case management in linking the inpatient and outpatient settings.

FLEXIBILITY OF CASE MANAGEMENT

One thing that makes case management models particularly appealing is that the structure is extremely flexible. A case management design can be modified to fit the needs and budgets of any clinical setting. Because the primary goals of case management are to reduce costs while maintaining quality, the model can, in many circumstances, be implemented for a minimal cost (Ethridge & Lamb, 1989).

    There are probably as many variations on the case management theme as there are nursing units in the United States. There is no right or wrong way to design a case management system. The design is not as important as the roles and functions of the system's members. Each person's functions are what make the model unique, not the number of workers involved. Today's health care environment calls for flexibility and creativity, and the institutions that display these features will probably be the most successful ones over the next 10 years (Armstrong & Stetler, 1991).

    For an institution implementing case management for the first time, the exact design structure for the units will be based on an array of factors. Choosing the first units to participate is an important decision. If the first units are successful, the institution will be more likely to support continued implementation. On the other hand, if the first units are less than successful, the leaders of the organization may not be willing to allow the implementation process to continue. Therefore the first units should be chosen carefully.

    The units selected for initial implementation should have the following characteristics:

- Homogeneous patient population
- High-volume case types
- Potential for improvement in length of stay

- Committed nurse manager
- Receptive physician group
- Interested nursing staff
- Open full-time equivalent (FTE) position (if possible)

Of course, it may not be possible to obtain each of these elements on every nursing unit. Finding a unit with as many of these factors as possible will help ensure a positive transition to a case management model.

A homogeneous patient population is beneficial because it may mean a smaller number of professionals involved in patient care on the unit. A homogeneous population also reduces the number of case management plans that need to be written. Most units that specialize in certain diseases or surgical procedures will have a smaller physician group with which to interact. A smaller group will allow for a more rapid transition to the model and will be more helpful in formulating the case management plans because the group will probably be more likely to agree on plans of care.

A large percentage of high-volume case types will also help when generating case management plans that will cover a wider number of patients on the unit. In general, if a unit admits more than 50% of its patients to five or fewer diagnosis-related (DRG) categories, the unit may be a good candidate for conversion to case management.

However, it is important to analyze these high-volume case types for their potential in reducing length of stay. High volume does not necessarily mean a reduction in length of stay. For example, some patient problems are on protocols that are already as brief as possible; chemotherapy is one example. Reductions might not be attainable around the diagnosis, but other elements of hospitalization, such as preadmission blood work or prehydration therapy, may allow for reductions.

The transition to a case management system will require total commitment from those on the unit. One of the most important people in the change process is the nurse manager. The nurse manager has 24-hour responsibility and accountability and has the primary administrative responsibility for the smooth functioning of the unit. Most of the other professionals enter and exit the unit because their responsibilities take them to other areas of the hospital. The nurse manager's sole responsibility is the nursing unit. It is vital that nurse managers have a working knowledge of case management so that they can function both formally and informally as advocates for change. Nurse managers can be instrumental in obtaining the cooperation of physicians with whom they have long-standing relationships.

Most of the activities on a nursing unit revolve around nurse managers who have administrative authority for their units. Their responsibilities may include staffing, budgeting, maintaining supplies, and caring for patients. No changes in these responsibilities should be made without the nurse managers' input and support.

When selecting units for conversion to case management, at least a majority of physicians affiliated with the unit should support the change. This, of course, may not always be possible. Obtaining the support of some physicians can be enough for making a positive transition.

It is important that the chief medical officer be supportive of the conversion to case management. Chairpersons of individual clinical areas should also be engaged in the change process as early as possible and should be supportive of case management.

When a case management model is implemented, it is helpful but not crucial to begin with a nursing staff that volunteered to be among the first units in the institution to convert. Often such enthusiasm came from the unit's nurse manager and filtered down to the other nurses on the unit. Again, this may be a factor that is not immediately obtainable.

Most institutions converting to a unit-based model try to do so at minimal cost to the organization. This may mean using an already existing FTE position or a budgeted position that has never been filled. It is not wise to eliminate an employee to make room for a case manager. The open FTE position should be acquired through attrition whenever possible because elimination of an employee can cause ill will, resentment, and insecurity among other staff nurses on the unit.

Some organizations have had to use other creative approaches to obtaining case management positions. Some have converted existing departments or positions, such as utilization managers, discharge planners, social workers, or nurse managers. No position should be eliminated unless others in the organization are able to absorb the workload of the eliminated position(s). During this time, job descriptions should be reviewed and, if necessary, role functions reallocated. Examples might include the development of discharge planning criteria for patients that slot them into either high- or low-risk categories. Lower-risk patients might remain the responsibility of the staff nurse or case manager, whereas high-risk patients are referred to the discharge planner or social worker. Retaining these additional FTE positions raises the cost of the overall design of the model. As organizational resources continue to dwindle, these types of designs will become increasingly less possible. During the initial design phase, it is always preferable for the organization to look for opportunities to integrate these functions under the role of the case manager. This provides for the most efficient, least expensive design.

It is often possible to create additional positions once some success has been shown. For these reasons it is again imperative that the initial units selected indicate a great potential for successful transition.

MEDICAL UNIT

Medical units may be among those with the most case management patient needs. Medical patients are often elderly and have more complex discharge plans. These patients are often the least likely to be advocates for themselves and can fall through the cracks during an extended and complicated hospital stay. They are among the most costly to hospitals and are often resource intensive.

Medical patients are also among the most difficult to plan for because their hospital course can be unpredictable. Ironically, these are also reasons that a case manager can be a great asset to a medical unit. The medical patient whose hospital course changes daily needs someone to ensure that everything is happening as planned and that nothing is missed.

There are usually more case managers on a medical unit than on any other type of unit in the hospital. Because of the increased complexity and severity of the cases, the organization should aim to have every medical patient under the authority of a case manager. The number of case managers should be based on an average caseload of about 20 to 25 patients. If every patient on the medical unit cannot be followed by the case manager, then criteria must be developed for selecting those patients who will benefit the most by being followed. In general, the case load of the case manager on the medical unit must be somewhat smaller than what would be seen on either a specialty unit or a surgical unit because these patients tend to need more resources and the number of interventions per patient will probably be greater.

Criteria for selecting patients on a general medical floor must be individually determined through a retrospective audit of those patients who seem to represent patterns of increased resource use. However, this is not the only factor to be evaluated. Other patients who might benefit from a case manager include those with the following characteristics:

- Advanced age (older than 70 years)
- Noncompliance with treatment
- Potential for falls
- Potential for skin breakdown
- Discharge placement problems/complicated plan
- Complicated medical plan
- Home care needs
- Complicated teaching needs

SURGICAL UNIT

Surgical cases can be as complicated as medical cases. In general, however, the hospital course of a surgical patient is somewhat more predictable and amenable to a predetermined plan. Many surgeons practice with protocols, which manage the patient's postoperative course in the same way that the case management plan does. Although there are exceptions to every rule, the expected course can be planned around an anticipated length of stay. Surgical patients are often elective admissions, which means that there may be less potential for in-hospital complications.

For these reasons, a surgical case manager may be able to carry a larger patient caseload than a case manager on a medical unit. A caseload of about 25 patients is probably manageable on most surgical units. One complication to this equation is the extremely short lengths of stay on surgical units that will translate to rapid turnover for the surgical case manager. Although the patients may be less complex clinically, this accelerated turnover may mean a workload for the surgical case manager that is comparable to that of the medical case manager. The rapidity of turnover should be factored in when determining an appropriate caseload for the surgical case manager.

It may not be necessary to have every surgical patient under the direction of a case manager. Criteria for selecting patients should include patient need and complexity or severity of condition. Patients who are admitted for emergency surgery and who require medical clearance before surgery also might need the attention of the case manager. Patients who develop postoperative complications, which may result in a prolonged length of stay, should also be considered.

CRITICAL CARE UNIT

The critical care unit may be the last area of the hospital to convert to case management. Because this area has a lower nurse/patient ratio and a more responsive health care team, these patients are already receiving a form of case management.

Critical care can be viewed as one episode in the course of hospitalization. Case management in critical care can help with clinical management issues such as admission and discharge criteria. These criteria can support patient throughput.

The case manager and case management plans may be the only elements missing from these areas. Most intensive care units have a 2:1 or a 1:1 nurse/patient ratio. In these situations, it may be possible to use the nurses, in their current positions, to function in a case management role. Thus all registered nurses working in the unit would be case managers and would carry out the functions and responsibilities of the case manager as well as provide direct patient care.

Case management plans can be developed around particular clinical problems, such as ventilator weaning, which would support and assist the staff nurses acting as case managers. Protocols for withdrawing patients from care as they improve could be incorporated into critical care case management plans.

There are problems with this system, but solutions do exist. The first problem is that continuity of care is still an issue if the unit is on flextime. Also, it may be difficult for nurses working with critically ill patients to take on the added responsibilities associated with the case manager role. They may not have the time needed to create managed care plans or to be involved in team formation. They may simply be absent from the unit too much to care for patients and function as case managers.

One option for staffing critical care areas with case managers is to cohort the acute unit with the critical care unit. For example, the surgical case manager would also be responsible for patients transitioning in or out of the surgical intensive care unit. The cardiology case manager might also be responsible for the critical care unit, and so on. This type of design provides continuity for the patients and does not require a case manager dedicated to those areas.

The emergency department lends itself to the development of case management plans. Plans can be developed for the efficient treatment of specific disease entities such as asthma or for the clinical management of patient treatments such as conscious sedation. Case management plans can also be developed for beginning the "ruling-out" process, as in the treatment of abdominal pain, and the identification of tuberculosis or human immunodeficiency virus (HIV) infection. Emergency department case managers can perform a number of important functions, including the following:

- Management of treat-and-release patients, including standardization of the treatment processes
- Referrals of "soft admissions," who might be discharges from the emergency department instead of admitted. Referrals to primary care physicians, clinics, home care, or subacute care are possible referral options
- Expeditious treatment and admission of patients admitted to the hospital, including beginning the appropriate treatment (e.g., antibiotics) in the emergency department

NURSING SKILLED NURSING FACILITY

The skilled nursing facility (SNF) is an example of a non–acute care facility that can financially benefit from a case management system. A case management model can ensure a higher quality of patient care with fewer resources. As the population ages and life expectancy increases, the needs of extended-care facilities will rise proportionally. As do most other health care institutions, nursing homes struggle with increased regulations and decreased resources (Smith, 1991).

In the nursing home setting, a case manager can ensure patient outcomes. This can reduce the use of registered nurses and increase the use of ancillary personnel.

SNFs are required to provide plans of care and goals for their patients. In general, personnel other than registered nurses can carry out these plans. Regulation requires that a registered nurse be present in most instances, but this nurse could be better used as a facilitator, an educator, or a coordinator of services to the patient. This approach can enhance quality of life and slow deterioration of functional ability.

SUBACUTE CARE FACILITY

Another area of consideration for case management are subacute units. *Subacute care* is defined as follows:

- A level of care that blends acute and long-term care skills and philosophies
- Care that bridges long-term and acute care
- One of the fastest growing segments on the continuum of health care

Subacute care is less invasive than acute care and less diagnostically oriented. Patient care is more intense but of shorter duration than that given in an SNF. Care usually occurs immediately following hospitalization, but in some cases it may be used instead of hospitalization. For appropriate case management in a subacute setting, patients must be in stable condition, but well enough to go home. Subacute program models include the following:

- Short-term medically complex
- Short-term rehabilitative
- Long-term or chronic (20% of all subacute cases)

Short-term medically complex patients are usually postsurgical patients or those with complex medical conditions who are medically stable but still require intensive medical/nursing management and/or ancillary services. Examples include the following:

Wound care
Respiratory management
Total parenteral nutrition
Dialysis
Intravenous therapy
Postsurgical recovery
Oncology
Acquired immune deficiency syndrome (AIDS) care
Complications due to prematurity
Terminal care

Short-term rehabilitative patients are those who have a potential for functional improvement who also have significant medical and nursing needs and are too ill or unable to tolerate the intensity of acute rehabilitation. Short-term rehabilitative therapies include physical, occupational, and speech therapy. Typical diagnoses would include stroke, amputation, total hip or knee replacement, and brain injury.

Long-term or chronic care patients have an extended acute care stay (e.g., longer than 25 days) but can be discharged earlier to a subacute setting if an appropriate one is available. They may be medically stable, but have high nursing/ancillary care needs.

Long-term patients may include those requiring preventative maintenance or needing maintenance of functional level, those in a coma, patients who are ventilator dependent, and those with head injuries.

Subacute case managers may function in free-standing SNFs, in hospital-based SNFs, in acute care hospital rehabilitation units, in long-term care hospitals, or in specialty hospitals or units.

A team approach with the nurse manager as a case manager can be cost effective and ensure improved quality of care. Many institutions have attempted to use the nurse manager in this facilitator role. As in the acute care setting, this dual role has become increasingly difficult in the nursing home setting. By using a case manager in addition to a nurse manager, greater quality and more efficient clinical outcomes can be achieved.

AMBULATORY/OUTPATIENT SETTING

Case management crosses all boundaries of the health care spectrum. The patient's quality of life may depend on the kind of clinical management this person receives in the primary care setting. The approach used in most ambulatory settings is a form of case management. Continuity of caregivers is often attempted for a patient's return visits. For many patients without a private family physician, these clinic visits provide their only links to the health care system. Use of the team approach to manage patients enhances quality of care. To this end, the American Academy of Ambulatory Care Nursing (AAACN) included case management skills in their competencies for professional practice (AAACN, 1997).

With the implementation of prospective payment for hospital-based clinics, emergency departments and ambulatory surgery in 2000, the need for case management in, and across these settings, has become even more vital. Limited resources and reimbursement requires aggressive case management strategies to reduce fragmentation, duplication, and redundancy. By applying case management interventions in the ambulatory settings, patients will receive more coordinated, cost-effective care. In addition, the disconnect that often occurs between inpatient and outpatient settings, the loss of continuity, and poor communication are reduced or eliminated when case management systems are applied across the continuum of care.

The future challenge for case management models will be to link the inpatient and outpatient settings in a way that promotes a smooth transition for the patient and ensures continuity of care once the patient returns to the community.

Development of case management plans can be based on expected outcomes for each patient visit. Such an approach can control the resources applied and the goals of care for each visit. This approach can also be used for home care visits or for clinic visits. If care is guided by the expected outcomes, progress can be tracked and monitored and appropriate interventions made in response to the patient's reaction to treatment.

Documentation of the patient's level of compliance after discharge from the hospital can provide valuable data as to the effect hospitalization had on the patient's quality of life. In addition, a case manager's unique relationship with the patient, as well as follow-up visits and telephone calls, can ensure patient compliance with postdischarge health care follow-up.

References

American Association of Colleges of Nursing (1997). *Nursing in ambulatory care: The future is here.* Monograph. Washington, DC: American Nurses Publishing.

Armstrong, D.M., & Stetler, C.B. (1991). Strategic considerations in developing a delivery model. *Nursing Economics, 9*(2), 112-115.

Ethridge, P., & Lamb, G. (1989). Professional nursing case management improves quality, access, and costs. *Nursing Management, 20*(3), 30-35.

Smith, J. (1991). Changing traditional nursing home roles to nursing case management. *Journal of Gerontological Nursing, 17*(5), 32-39.

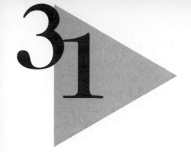

Brainstorming

Development of the Multidisciplinary Action Plan

CHAPTER OVERVIEW

The case management plan is the documentation that drives the case management system. Institutions implementing case management models need to determine the content of the documentation format they wish to adopt.

This chapter reviews the evolution of case management plans and the step-by-step process of development. This chapter also discusses the links between the prospective payment system, diagnosis-related groups (DRGs), and the case management plan.

Health care organizations must go beyond what the DRG suggests when designing these plans. The principal procedure or diagnosis should be used with the DRG as the underlying guide for determining the extent of the plan.

EVOLUTION OF THE CASE MANAGEMENT PLAN

Just as there are many ways to adapt case management models to fit the needs of a particular organization, there are multiple ways to develop a case management documentation system. Since the inception of case management, most hospitals have been using the *critical path* label on their case management plans. When introduced in 1985 by the New England Medical Center in Boston, the critical path was the first system that attempted to incorporate expected outcomes within specified time frames. The term *critical path* means that the plan defines the critical or key events expected to happen each day of a patient's hospitalization (Giuliano & Poirier, 1991; Zander, 1991, 1992).

Since 1985 critical paths have been adapted to meet the needs of organizations implementing case management models. The paths remain an extremely flexible method of planning and documenting. In addition to *critical path* and *clinical pathway*, other labels, such as *multidisciplinary plan, multidisciplinary action plan (MAP)*, and *action plan*, have been attached to these case management plans. All these terms are the same in theory. Each of the plans attempts to outline the expected outcomes of care for each discipline during each day of hospitalization. Some of these care plans place greater emphasis on the nursing plan, while some emphasize the medical plan of care. Some others, such as the MAP discussed here, incorporate all disciplines.

Some case management organizations use case management plans as one-page guides. Essentially, these one-page plans are multidisciplinary protocols for the problem or diagnosis. The details of the plan depend on the goals of the organization in which the plan is being used. In some cases, nursing documentation can be recorded directly onto the form. This format is also easily adapted to a hospital computer system. Computerization of the plan allows the case manager the flexibility of changing the plan as the patient's needs change. For those organizations without a computer system, the case management plan is still an easy, flexible tool to use.

The case management plan can also be used in place of the traditional nursing care plan. Nursing care plans have been criticized by some as useless exercises in writing. The plans are written to meet the needs of regulatory agencies but are often not used by nurses to guide or plan their day-to-day care. Once written, the plans are often never looked at again. These plans are not even written to provide a plan of care that correlates with the expected length of stay. For this reason, these plans are not the preferred form for planning care in case management models.

It is no accident that the critical path or MAP format came into existence. These MAPs are the driving forces behind case management models because they help determine the plan of care and arrange that plan around the expected length of stay. Unlike the nursing care plan, MAPs are multidisciplinary and take into account the unique contributions of each discipline. MAPs also link case management with the prospective payment system by using the DRG for determining the appropriate length for the plan. The most current reimbursements are consulted when any plan is started.

When developing the MAP, keep in mind that the state reimbursable length of stay may be longer or shorter than the federal length of stay. Also, it would be impractical to develop standard plans for patients with varying types of insurance coverage. Instead, these variations in reimbursable length of stay can be averaged. Another technique is to determine the length of stay the physician expects and measure it against the reimbursable length of stay. It may turn out that the stay the physician hoped for is shorter than the reimbursable length of stay. In a case like this, the physician's preference would determine the length of stay outlined in the MAP.

Milliman and Roberston's *Health care management guidelines* (1997) should also be used as a benchmark reference. Guidelines such as these provide not only length of stay expectations but also alternative settings and options for managing the length of stay. They are used by many managed care organizations during the review process for determining reimbursable hospital days.

If the length of stay the physician expects is longer than the reimbursable length of stay, a compromise must be reached. The federal and state rates should be reviewed with the physician in relation to the physician's plan. Areas for reduction should be discussed to reduce the length of stay so that it matches or comes below the reimbursable length of stay. A general guideline is to design the plan so that it is shorter than the reimbursable length of stay. This allows for some margin of error in case the patient requires an additional day of hospitalization.

The case manager can control the length of stay by overseeing the movement of the patient through the system. It is difficult to implement MAPs that will be effective without the position of case manager in place. Instituting plans without a professional to drive the process is not a likely way to achieve the desired results. The staff nurse and the case manager are responsible for ensuring that the expected outcomes, as outlined on the MAP, are carried out. If the expected outcomes cannot be achieved, the case manager analyzes the patient's situation and documents the outcome that cannot be accomplished. This outcome is then documented as a variance, which is anything that does not happen when it is supposed to happen.

The DRG must be used as a guide for projecting the length of stay indicated on the MAP. Because the DRG categories are designed for determining hospital reimbursement rates, they are too heterogeneous to assess the effectiveness of the clinical plan at the bedside. For example, if an MAP is written to plan the care of a lumbar laminectomy patient, the discharge diagnosis of lumbar laminectomy might fall under a wide variety of DRGs, such as "medical back procedure" or "spinal procedure." Therefore, if someone wanted to look at the length of stay of all laminectomy patients within a case management system in the hospital, asking for length of stay records for one DRG would not include the majority of laminectomy patients, who might have been classified under other DRG categories.

Other DRGs are heterogeneous in another way. For example, the DRG for chemotherapy, DRG 410, includes any and all chemotherapy protocols, whether they are for 1 or 5 days. The Centers for Medicare and Medicaid Services (CMS) reimbursement rate for chemotherapy is 2.6 days, regardless of the type of chemotherapy being given. Once again, the DRG system will not be a suitable tool for analyzing whether the MAP decreases the length of stay, reduces resource use, or provides the most effective quality care for that problem.

If an organization wants to determine the true effectiveness of case management plans used among a specific patient group, the DRG cannot be used. Clinicians must dig deeper, using a microanalysis approach. Patients' reviews should be based on their principal procedure or diagnosis at the time of discharge. This way the plan's effectiveness can be determined. After all, there is no MAP called "medical back problem," and there cannot be one called "chemotherapy" because these would be too general. It follows, therefore, that analysis must be as specific as the level of the diagnosis. Once again, it should be emphasized that other data sets, such as the Milliman and Roberston guidelines, should be referenced when making care planning decisions.

The case management plan for chemotherapy would be specific to the type of chemotherapy being administered and the specific protocol being followed. In the interest of cost-effectiveness, several chemotherapy protocols can be combined on one MAP. At the time of admission the patient's specific protocol is identified from a menu of several possible choices on the MAP. All these plans would fall under the same DRG, even though they would be different.

The process for developing the case management plan must be based on several specific elements. The organization must first decide on the form that the plans will take. Factors that affect the form include degree of complexity, extent to which the plan will include other disciplines, and whether the form will include nursing documentation. These factors help determine the plan's design and content. Each factor must be decided before the content is developed.

Once the format has been decided and approved, the organization must decide which diagnoses or procedures are to be planned first. It is obvious that every plan cannot be developed simultaneously. Some general guidelines can be useful in making these decisions. If the model being implemented is a case management, diagnosis-specific approach, then these decisions have probably already been made. Many organizations begin with a few specific diagnoses that are easily planned. Some examples of commonly used diagnoses include "fractured hip," "open heart surgery," and "transurethral prostatectomy" (TURP). These are easily written and followed because these types of procedures are already the subjects of many protocols. It is generally easier to get the cooperation of surgeons who are managing these cases because they are already managing their patients in a protocol-oriented way. It is also easier to reduce length of stay because the chance of complication or comorbidity is slightly lower in these patient populations than in some others.

If the organization is adopting a unit-based case management model, then deciding which diagnosis to begin with is slightly more complicated, although technically it is the same as for the non–unit-based approach. One of the first factors to consider is the number of patients to include in the implementation of one plan. This involves examining the high-volume case types for the organization. Once this is done, an attempt should be made to match these high-volume case types to the units being converted to a case management model. These two factors point to the types of patient problems that should be considered first. After these determinations, a match is then made to physicians who work with these patients and who are willing to help develop and adopt case management plans.

Only after all these steps have been taken can the actual process of writing begin. There will be several parts to each plan. In general, the longest of these are the nursing and medical plans. Plans for medical problems are developed from chart review, consultation with experts in the field, and literature review, all to create the "best possible plan" or ideal plan for that patient problem. To make the most of each person's time, individual brainstorming sessions between the case manager and a representative from each discipline are most effective. The case manager can make some preparation to begin the shell of the plan before meeting with anyone. The case manager can determine the approximate length of the plan, based on state and federal reimbursements, and then can begin to plan out the nursing portion of the plan, indicating the expected nursing outcomes for each day of hospitalization.

Once these pieces are complete, the case manager arranges to meet with members of the other disciplines. The most logical person to begin with is the physician. Plans need to be physician specific, but this means that several physicians agree as a group to the same plan. Under no circumstances should a completed plan be presented to a physician until it is first made clear that the individual preferences and practice patterns of that practitioner will be taken into consideration. Plans should be individualized as much as possible.

Another technique to use is a team approach in which the members of the team physically meet as a group at specific, assigned times. The team can begin the process by developing a tool to review patient records. The tool should include demographic and clinically specific information. Clinical issues that "appear" to be affecting length of stay should be highlighted. Examples of these include progressive ambulation, timing of removal of tubes or drains, switches from intravenous to oral medications, and response time for consults. The clinical issue being studied will drive this list. Once the tool is developed, the team can begin reviewing charts. A representative number of charts should be selected randomly. For most diagnoses at least 30 charts should be reviewed. Validating the issues that "appear" to be affecting length of stay will help drive the clinical content of the plan (Adler, Bryk, Cesta, & McEachen, 1995).

Most physicians have a clear sense of their expectations or of what they would routinely order for the average patient with a particular problem. Of course, not every patient can or will fit exactly into this projected plan. Each plan must be tailored to the patient after admission. The physician should remember that the projected plan is designed for the average patient with a particular problem. This plan could be considered an aggregate of all patients the physician has treated, discounting unusual or aberrant conditions or circumstances.

On average, the plan development process can be completed in less than 1 hour. This hour is a small contribution compared with the amount of time it would take for the physician to individually inform all the health care providers of the care plan. Development of an MAP not only saves the physician time but also eliminates the second guessing that sometimes occurs.

One approach for developing an MAP is to simply ask the physician what would routinely be ordered for each day of hospitalization. Systematically running through each day ensures that nothing is neglected. Once all disciplines have completed this process, each should be afforded the opportunity to review the plan one last time. If a group of physicians is involved, each physician should have the chance to provide input. This content should be checked against the data collected on chart review.

The decision as to which disciplines will be represented in the plan depends on the diagnosis or procedure being planned. For some, physical therapy will be important. For others, respiratory therapy may be necessary. In most institutions, social work is a separate component but an integral part of the patient's plan, so this department should be given its own section on every plan. In other institutions some specialties such as skin care nurse may always be included. The disciplines involved will vary from institution to institution, but in general, nursing, medicine, and social work should be on every plan (Tahan, 1998).

Once each representative has participated in the plan development process, it would be beneficial to have as many of these people as possible sit down together to review the plan. This form of brainstorming may expose redundant treatments or procedures. This is another way of significantly reducing resource utilization while providing the best possible quality of care.

MAP TIME-LINES

MAPs can be time-lined in hours, days, weeks, or months, depending on the clinical area. Emergency department treatment might be mapped out in terms of hours or parts of an hour. Typical diagnoses, including common medical problems or surgeries, usually fall within a day's time frame. Weeks might be used for those diagnoses that have a longer length of stay, such as those that might be found in a neonatal intensive care unit, where the length of stay is 3 or 4 months. Month time frames might be relevant in long-term care facilities, such as those for patients with chronic mental disorders, where clinical progress is extremely slow and lengths of stay are measured in years. Nursing home patients provide another example of patient goals that might be evaluated in terms of months.

Once these time frames are determined, variance time frames must be decided. In other words, when does something become a variance? In what time period should every outcome listed for a particular day be achieved? A *variance* is anything that does not happen when it is supposed to happen. The hospital must decide what kind of leeway will be allowed for achieving these outcomes. Day 1 will seldom begin at 6 AM on the day of admission, because most patients are admitted later in the day. For example, emergency admissions may arrive on the unit in the late afternoon or night shift. It is clear that the beginning and end of any one day in the hospital is a loose concept. Institutions should be generous when deciding on variance time frames. If not, it is possible to set up a situation where almost everything becomes a variance. A plan lasting at least 5 days might not place something into the variance category unless it is not completed within 24 hours. The expected time frame should drive the time frames for variances. For example, if the plan is developed around 15-minute intervals, anything beyond that time period becomes a variance.

Documentation of Variances

An area designated for documenting variances should be on the plan. Each variance can be identified and categorized, if desirable. Typical variance categories include the following:

Operational

Health care provider

Patient

Unmet clinical indicators

An example of operational variances is the breakdown of a piece of equipment, which prevents the completion of a test. Another example is the inability to discharge a patient because no long-term care facilities in the area have an available bed. These are examples of operational variances that go beyond the confines of the hospital. More examples are presented in the Boxes 31-1 and 31-2.

BOX 31-1 ▸ OPERATIONAL VARIANCE EXAMPLES

Broken equipment
Lost requisition slips, causing delays
Departmental delays due to staffing or other causes
Interdepartmental delays
Larger system delays affecting discharge, such as home care services, equipment, or insurance availability

BOX 31-2	HEALTH CARE PROVIDER VARIANCE EXAMPLES

Deviation from plan because physician varied the practice pattern
Change related to health care provider's practice patterns, level of expertise, or experience

BOX 31-3	PATIENT VARIANCE EXAMPLES

Refusal
Change in status
Emotionally or physically unable

Health care provider variances include any situations in which a health care provider is the cause of the delay in achieving an expected outcome. Discretion must be used when documenting these variances because some may involve a risk management issue. For example, if the resident is paged several times during the night because a patient has pulled out the nasogastric tube and the resident does not respond for several hours, the patient misses several doses of medication. Other variances in this category may be associated with the physician's alteration or adjustment of the traditional plan of care.

Patient variances include any patient-related delays (Box 31-3). The patient delay may be caused by complications of the patient's medical condition, which require a delay in completion of a test or procedure. For example, the patient may have spiked a fever and may be unable to leave the floor for magnetic resonance imaging (MRI). In other circumstances, the delay may be because the patient refused to allow the test or procedure; noncompliance frequently causes patient delays. When a patient refuses a test or procedure, the absolute need for the test or procedure should be questioned and evaluated. This sort of stringent review and follow-up is an example of how a checks-and-balances system in case management can help reduce unnecessary resource use. Tests and procedures cost the institution money not only in terms of the expense of the supplies and equipment but also in terms of the human resources needed to administer the test and evaluate the results. More timely completion of appropriate tests means a reduction in the length of stay for all patients.

Another type of patient variance is called *patient variance on admission*. This variance type is also known as a *preexisting condition* or *comorbidity*. Case management plans are simple guidelines or expected plans for particular diagnoses or procedures. Regulatory agencies require individualization of any predetermined plans of care during patient admission. This process should be a routine part of putting any patient on a case management plan. The patient's case should be reviewed in relation to the prewritten plan. Anything different or unusual about the patient's case should yield a change in the plan to make it specific to the patient; one plan is not going to be appropriate for every patient. This process ensures that the plan meets the needs of the patient in question. For example, if the plan calls for a specific medication and the patient is allergic to that medication, the plan should be altered to adjust to that particular patient's clinical condition.

The fourth type of variance is unmet clinical quality indicators (Box 31-4). Clinical quality indicators are developed in conjunction with the MAP. They are created by the physicians to benchmark clinical outcomes that reflect quality of care rendered. These clinical outcomes can be either intermediate or discharge patient outcomes (Morrison & Beckworth, 1998). The box contains examples of clinical quality indicators that would be developed for asthma team patients.

| BOX 31-4 | UNMET CLINICAL QUALITY INDICATORS: ASTHMA |

INTERMEDIATE OUTCOMES
Patient off intravenous Solu-Medrol when peak flow >200

DISCHARGE OUTCOMES
Peak flow measurement >250 L/s
Patient out of bed without shortness of breath
Patient able to return demonstration of the use of metered-dose inhaler with spacer

Variance data are abstracted from the patient's medical record and MAP. The analysis of these data is invaluable in determining why an expected patient outcome or clinical quality indicator has not been met. In addition, these data allow for trending of patient outcomes, length of stay, and evaluation of the quality of patient care.

Appendix 7-1 is an example of an MAP developed and used at the St. Vincent's Catholic Medical Centers of New York. This MAP is clinically specific, not DRG specific. The format illustrated is a preprinted, bound booklet that outlines the expected outcomes for care for each day of hospitalization for each discipline involved. Medicine, nursing, social work, and discharge planning are automatically included on every plan. Other departments are included as needed. Each department is given a standard place on the form, and content is filled in by members of the discipline during formation of the plan.

The length of the booklet is guided by the reimbursement for the DRGs usually associated with the diagnosis or problem. This information is correlated with what the physician expects the length of stay to be. Generally the physician will adapt to the reimbursement length of stay if this information is supplied in a positive way. If more than one DRG is involved, which is usually the case, then some judgment must be used in determining the shortest possible plan that takes into account the possibly varying reimbursable lengths of stay. In other words, it may be necessary to look at the most commonly used DRGs and follow an average or usual length of stay. Clearly, these expected lengths are "guesstimates" and will not be completely accurate every time. Each plan may be lengthened or shortened, depending on patient-related variations, but some professional judgment must be used. If a plan is 7 days in length and the patient is ready to go home on the sixth day, an earlier discharge would be completed, and the documentation would be written to reflect the reasons why. A delayed discharge must be documented in the same way with variances that caused the delay being documented and explained.

During the early phases of DRG use in case management systems, the finer points of the DRG were not always synchronous with the system itself. As the system evolved into more of a financial one, clinical applications of the system needed to remain flexible, and the limitations of such uses needed to be clarified for those clinicians using the system.

Space for nursing documentation has been incorporated into the form of some MAPs. In this space the registered nurse documents whether expected outcomes for the day were achieved and any appropriate responses of the patient. Progress notes are included only when a more elaborate or detailed form of documentation is needed, and narrative nurses' notes are eliminated unless an exception arises. This detailed list of outcomes provides the nurse with an action plan that is specific for that day and keeps the patient on track toward discharge.

For the novice nurse who is less able to project patient needs because of a lack of experience, the MAP provides a plan that is outcome oriented and guides the new nurse through that particular day of hospitalization. Rather than correcting problems after they have happened, the MAP provides an advanced, detailed plan with tasks that can be carried out in a timely fashion.

The case manager is the driving force behind the success of the managed care plan. It is generally the case manager who checks on variances related to both cause and remedy and who is accountable for the patient's continued success in moving through the system. Using the plan as a guide, the case manager directs all other health care providers toward achieving the expected daily outcome of care.

Another responsibility of the case manager is to provide patient teaching when necessary and to find out why a test or procedure has not been done. The case manager also reviews the care plan with the physician and ensures timely outcomes. Finally, the case manager coordinates with the social worker, discharge planner, family, and patient to ensure that the best possible discharge plan has been made and that it is ready when the patient goes home. This entire process is communicated to other members of the team through the MAP format and through the case manager's documentation. All in all, the case manager views the whole picture and ensures proper and accurate progress of the patient through the hospital system.

Staff nurses work in collaboration with the case manager and other members of the health care team to ensure that the outcomes of care are achieved within the time frames specified on the MAP. The patient's outcomes are documented by the staff nurse and relate the clinical story of the patient's progress during hospitalization. Appendix 31-1 contains a sample critical path that has been adapted to the needs of a particular institution; Appendix 7-1 provides an additional example.

PATIENT PATHWAYS

The case management plan can be adapted for use by patients and families. The existing plans rewritten in language understandable to patients and their families can be an effective tool. It is not necessary for these adapted plans to contain as much in-depth information as the case management plans used by the health care providers. Rather, only specific information relevant to the patient's needs can be summarized from the more-detailed plan.

An issue to consider in the selection of the content is the inclusion of a discussion in patient-friendly language of the general course of events patients can expect during their hospital stay. Care should be taken not to be too specific clinically because as changes are made to the medical plan, patients may become concerned that there is something wrong or that their clinical progression toward discharge is not going as planned.

Benchmarks should be outlined in the patient's version of the case management plan. These benchmarks should include milestones during the course of the hospital stay as well as discharge indicators. For example, asthmatic patients might be told that their intravenous medication will be stopped when their peak flow reading is 200 L/s. In this way the patient will clearly understand the goal of care as well as why their intravenous medication was switched to an oral medication. Other benchmarks should relate to the patient's clinical condition and should reflect the benchmarks or indicators outlined in the clinician's case management plan.

Another useful technique is to give the patient and family a patient version of the critical pathway. Such a document presents the discharge indicators or the factors that indicate when a particular case type is safe and ready for discharge. Again, these pathways should be written in language that is understandable to lay people and given to the patient soon after admission to the hospital. In this way the patient once again knows the indications for safe discharge and can work with the health care team toward these goals. In addition, the patient also sees that a decision to discharge is based on predetermined criteria and is not arbitrary in any way.

References

Adler, S.L., Bryk, E., Cesta, T.G., & McEachen, I. (1995). Collaboration: The solution to multidisciplinary care planning. *Orthopaedic Nursing, 14*(2), 21-29.

Doyle, R.L., & Schibanoff, J.M. (1997). *Health care management guidelines*, New York: Milliman & Roberston.

Giuliano, K.K., & Poirier, C.E. (1991). Nursing case management: Critical pathways to desirable outcomes. *Nursing Management, 22*(3), 52-55.

Morrison, R.S., & Beckworth, V. (1998). Outcomes for patients with congestive heart failure in a nursing case management model. *Nursing Case Management, 3*(3), 108-114.

Tahan, H.A. (1998). The multidisciplinary mandate of clinical pathways enhancement. *Nursing Case Management, 3*(1), 46-51.

Zander, K. (1991). Care MAPs: The core of cost/quality care. *The New Definition, 6*(3), 1-3.

Zander, K. (1992). Physicians, care MAPs, and collaboration. *The New Definition, 7*(1), 1-4.

Appendix 31-1

St. Michael Hospital, Milwaukee, Wisconsin

Uncomplicated MI Critical Path

DRG: _____

HCFA LOS: _____ Exp. LOS: _____

Physician: _____

Date Reviewed by Physician/RN: _____

Day/Date					
Floor	**DAY 1** ED	**DAY 1** CCU	**DAY 2**	**DAY 3** TRANSFER TO MCU	**DAY 4**
Consults			Cardiac Rehab PT and OT – – – – Definition	– – – →	

Tests	CBC
	ECG
	Electrolytes
	Glucose
	BUN
	Creatinine
	CXR
	Cardiac enzymes
		CCU Standing
		  Orders – – – →
		ECG – – – – –
		Assess Need:
		CPK
		Isoenzymes × 3 (total)
		  per protocol
		Chem profile &
		  electrolytes
			ECG – – – – – –
			
			Electrolytes
			in AM
				ECG – – – – – – –
				Stress test/cath ordered
				  Day 7 or 8
					ECG

Activity	Bed rest – – – –	– – – – – – →	Bed rest with commode PRN	Up in chair & progress – – – – – – – → Progression of self-care ADL – – – – – →	
Treatments	IV D5W Ko – – → Cardiovascular Assessment & VS q 10-15 min & PRN – – – → Monitor – – – –	Daily weights I & O – – – – – – – VS q 4° & PRN – – – – – – – – – – – –	Heplock VI –	– VS q 8° & PRN – – – – – – – – – – – – – – –	– – – – – – – – – – – – – → – – – – – – – – – – – – – –
Medications	Nitrates – – – – O₂ 2-4 PNC – – – Analgesics – – – Lidocaine	– → – – – – – – – → – – – – – → Stool softener Beta blockers Calcium channel blockers	O₂ PRN – →		

UNCOMPLICATED MI CRITICAL PATH—CONT'D					
Floor	**DAY 1** ED	**DAY 1** CCU	**DAY 2**	**DAY 3** TRANSFER TO MCU	**DAY 4**
Diet		Low cholesterol			
Discharge planning	Complete ED data base	Complete data base. Assessment of home situation	Mutual goal setting – – – – → *Multidisciplinary Staffing (T or F) Assessment of IP & OP plans of care. (*Inpatient Cardiac Rehab only)		Assess D/C needs & date Contact SW/ HC PRN
Key nursing diagnosis/interventions	Orientation to ED, staff & equipment. *Assess & monitor:* -Head-to-toe assessment – × 1 -Hemodynamic & cardiovascular stability (4) *Instruct:* -Pain scale 1-10 (1) -Preparation for admission to CCU(2) [ ]brochure given [ ] family/sig. other notified -Offer emotional support	-Orientation to CCU routine, equipment, CCTV, & care delivery system -Assess pain q 30" until under control (1) -Reinforce use of pain scale (1) Position for comfort q 2° or prn (1) *Assess & Monitor:* -Head-to-toe assessment q 4° or prn -Activity restriction (3) -Hemodynamic & cardiovascular stability (4) -Arrhythmatic disturbances (4)	Position for comfort q 2° or prn (1) -Parent booklet given (2) -Orient to CCTV, channels 3 & 11 (2) Review basic medication instruction with administration of routine doses (2) *Instruct:* -ID risk factors specific with patient (2) -Diet modification (2) -Gradual progression of activity (3) – – – – – –	Assess patient readiness to learn, observe verbal/non-verbal cues, patient's condition (2) *Instruct:* Stress Reduction (2) -Stress management relaxation techniques – – – – – – – – -Time management -ID support systems & resources – – – – – – – – – – – – – – → – – – – – – – – → – – – – – – – – →	– – – – – – → – – – – – – → – – – – – – → – – – – – – → – – – – – – → – – – – – – → – – – – – – →
Key patient activities/ outcomes	-Patient &/or significant other verbalizes fears & anxiety -Patient rates pain & intensity on 1-10 scale (1) – – → -Patient &/or significant other verbalizes reason for hospitalization (2)	-Patient demonstrates use of call light – → – – – – – – – – → – – – – – – – – → -Patient's behavior indicates pain reduction or elimination (1) -Patient verbalizes that pain is decreased, alleviated, or under control (1)	-Patient verbalizes understanding of diagnosis (2) -Patient voices specific concerns related to coping with illness (2) -Patient watches CCTV (2)	-Patient behavior shows progress toward acceptance of illness (2) – – – – – – – – -Patient able to identify own learning needs (2) – – – – – – – – -Patient demonstrates readiness to learn (2) – – – – – – – – -Patient verbalizes own risk factors (2)	– – – – – – → – – – – – – → – – – – – – → Behavior shows signs of: -Stress management (2) Relaxation techniques (2)

Continued

UNCOMPLICATED MI CRITICAL PATH—CONT'D				
Floor	**DAY 1** ED	**DAY 1** CCU	**DAY 2**	**DAY 3** TRANSFER TO MCU	**DAY 4**
				-Patient demonstrates gradual progression of energy using energy-conservation techniques (3 & 4)	-Patient verbalizes time management skills (2 & 4) -Patient verbalizes support system & resources (2)

Day/Date

Floor	**DAY 5** TRANSFER TO 2N WITH TELEMETRY	**DAY 6**	**DAY 7-8**	
Consults		Assess need OP cardiac rehab		
Tests			Stress test/Cath	
Activity	Ambulate bid	Up ad lib		
Treatments	CS q 8° & PRN I & O	VS bid or q shift D/C I & O	D/C Heplock	
Medications				
Diet	Low Cholesterol →			
Discharge Planning		D/C orders D/C meds Follow-up MD appointment		
Key nursing diagnosis/interventions	Review previous learning (2)	Review home program (2) -Post-MI status -Diet -Meds a) Schedule b) Indications/side effects c) Med sheet given -Follow-up with MD -Program given by patient	OP cardiac rehab Post list	Possible nursing diagnoses 1. Pain 2. Knowledge deficit (learning needs with diagnosis of MI) 3. Activity intolerance 4. Decreased cardiac output * Nursing care guide available

UNCOMPLICATED MI CRITICAL PATH—CONT'D				
Floor	**DAY 5** Transfer to 2N with telemetry	**DAY 6**	**DAY 7-8**	
Key patient activities/ outcomes	Patient verbalizes understanding of cardiac disease and/or MI (2)	Patient plans activity progression and after D/C (home, work, sexuality, social) using energy conservation/work simplification techniques (2,3,4)	Patient describes home med schedule with indications/side effects (reference med sheet) (2) Patient verbalizes follow-up MD, early warning signs, and emergency plan (2)	WIPRO Criteria → All Met and Documented before Discharge 72 hours before D/C No evidence of ECG changes. 48 hours before D/C. No change in type/dosage of antiarrhythmic drug(s). Chest pain controlled with anti-anginal drugs. Vital signs WNL for patient 24 hours before D/C. Lab values WNL for patient (electrolytes, BUN, enzymes) Oral temp <99° without antipyretic. Invasive monitoring devices removed. Activity/mobility/ambulation documented as improved/stabilized. Improved clinical status (e.g., chest clear, rales & wheezing, absence of friction rub & S, gallop). If DC'd to self-care, document completion of patient education. D/C plan documented. **If hospital stay <3 days for rule out MI, no evidence of ECG changes or enzyme rise.**

DEFINITIONS

Decreased cardiac output: A state in which the blood pumped by the individual's heart is sufficiently reduced that it is inadequate to meet the needs of the body's tissues.

Pain: A state in which an individual experiences and reports the presence of severe discomfort or an uncomfortable sensation.

Activity intolerance: A state in which an individual has insufficient physiological or psychological energy to endure or complete required or desired daily activities.

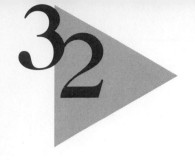

Interdisciplinary Care Planning and Documentation Using Nursing Interventions Classification and Nursing Outcomes Classifications

Kathleen Smith
Vivienne Smith

CHAPTER OVERVIEW

Current focus on the preservation of patient safety requires that health care information be documented in ways that maximize interdisciplinary communication, improve clarity, and make data accessible to those directly involved in the patient's care. Three primary elements are necessary to develop such a comprehensive, interdisciplinary record of patient care.

First, basic system design should reflect dynamic, collaborative care planning, which is evident in a well-constructed, integrated clinical documentation system. Second, a standard language system is essential to clearly describe, examine, and evaluate the work of health care providers and relate this in a way that is easily understood by others. Third, a computer information system is necessary for organization and display of patient information, as well as providing support for outcome data collection.

Ultimately, the goal is to link the interdisciplinary care plan, clinical charting, and the documentation of outcomes. This chapter reviews these three elements and the efforts of one hospital to accomplish the goal.

INTRODUCTION

In recent years, renewed emphasis has been placed on health care quality and safety issues. One trend has been to implement cohesive team care planning that meets the needs of the patient by maximizing communication and capitalizing on the unique contribution of each team member. Typically, however, hospitals struggle to demonstrate evidence of such collaborative effort, especially when it comes to care planning. Review of documentation still reveals fragmentation and duplication of effort, a situation that inevitably leads to lack of information sharing between disciplines. An effective documentation system can be the key to communicating the care plan as well as providing a tool to support the integrated team approach.

Although the concept sounds simple, the task can seem overwhelming because historically health care disciplines have documented independently on paper systems designed to support the individual approach. Efforts to actualize the concept have been bolstered by external regulatory forces. The Joint

Commission on Accreditation of Healthcare Organizations (JCAHO) and the National Committee for Quality Assurance (NCQA) are just two of the organizations that have placed their focus on safety during the delivery of patient care (O'Leary, 2001). The successful integration of interdisciplinary care plans, standardized documentation, and information technology applications can help organizations meet the goal of safe, high-quality patient care.

INTERDISCIPLINARY CARE PLANNING AND DOCUMENTATION

Patient care plans have been around in one form or another since the 1930s. They have been developed to greater or lesser degrees by individual disciplines, with some representing a dynamic, useful tool driving patient care activities. Others are more static documents, making them less useful on a day-to-day basis. It has become clear that these discipline-specific care plan documents must somehow be merged and should include expected goals and outcomes. At the same time, there must be enough flexibility to allow all care providers to identify additional problems and appropriate interventions for individual patients.

Most health care disciplines rely on their own version of the patient care plan. The kardex is generally the tool that is used by nurses. A critical first step is to replace the system that supports multiple care plans, including the kardex, with one comprehensive and fluid document that is used by all or most members of the care team. After identification of patient problems, individual goals must be set forth along with specific interventions that are necessary to meet those goals. All disciplines should participate in development and constant revision of the plan so that it becomes a meaningful plan of action. In this way, patient assessments performed by all disciplines can be incorporated into one, main plan of care.

A second step must be to link the plan to documentation so it is clear how that plan was carried out. This step can transform the care plan into a living document. Charting should be driven by elements contained within the plan so that patient care process is clearly purposeful. In addition, outcomes must be documented to show evidence that interventions are both appropriate and effective. Lack of desired progress should naturally prompt care plan revisions.

If this type of interdisciplinary model is to be successful, it must be designed with the ability to capture the minimum data elements for each discipline. In addition, the framework for documentation should be standardized so the information is easily understood by others. And all of this must be accomplished without losing the unique contribution of each type of care provider!

THE CONTRIBUTION OF STANDARDIZED LANGUAGE

Structured vocabularies are necessary to clearly describe, examine, and evaluate the work of health care providers. Because staff may use multiple terms to describe the same phenomenon, it becomes impossible to collect the data necessary for comparing similarities or differences in the care and outcomes of particular patient populations (McCloskey & Bulechek, 1996). Standardized language systems of care elements have been developed to address these problems. The benefits of incorporating standardized data into clinical documentation are that they enable us to explicitly describe the patient care process, thereby increasing the visibility of the contributions of each discipline. They also improve communication between the health care team enhancing the continuity of care for patients. In addition, computerization of clinical documentation, if it is to provide useful outcome data, is possible only through the use of standard, codified language systems.

Background

Werley and Lang (1988) first recognized the need for nursing to develop a standard set of data elements that could be collected by nursing to measures outcomes. This data set, called the Nursing Minimum Data Set (NMDS), is a minimum set of items of information with uniform definitions and categories concerning the specific dimension of professional nursing that meet the information needs of multiple data users in the health care system. (Werley & Lang, 1988).

The elements of the NMDS are divided into three categories (Table 32-1). Items in the first two categories are collected by existing standardized data sets, for example, the Uniform Hospital Discharge Data Set. However, the third category of elements including nursing diagnoses, interventions, outcomes, and care intensity has historically not been collected due to lack of standardization of the terms. On the other hand, the medical community has developed several classification systems to describe medical care. Examples are the *International Classification of Diseases (ICD), Current Procedural Terminology (CPT)*, and the diagnosis-related group (DRG) coding systems. Major work has been undertaken in recent years and remains ongoing to develop nursing standard language and classification systems for inclusion in national health care databases.

Role of the American Nurses Association in Nursing Language Development

A Steering Committee on Databases to Support Clinical Nursing Practice was established in 1989 by the American Nurses Association (ANA) to oversee the development of nursing languages within the framework of the NMDS. In 1998, this committee was renamed the Committee for Nursing Practice Information Infrastructure (CNPII) to reflect a broader context for its oversight of nursing terminology systems and to ensure that nursing has a role in the development of health care policy. The CNPII recently updated previous criteria for evaluation of nursing data sets, classifications, taxonomies, and nomenclatures (Coenen et al., 2001). The ANA uses these new criteria to evaluate language systems.

The ANA currently recognizes two data sets: the Nursing Minimum Data Set (NMDS) and the Nursing Management Minimum Data Set (NMMDS). In addition, they have endorsed two nomenclatures: the International Classification for Nursing Practice (ICNP) and the Systemized Nomenclature of Medicine Reference Terminology (SNOMED RT), as well as eight nursing classification systems: North American Nursing Diagnosis Association (NANDA) Taxonomy II, The Omaha System, Nursing Intervention

TABLE 32-1	NURSING MINIMUM DATA SHEET	
Demographic Elements	**Service Elements**	**Nursing Care Elements**
Personal identification	Facility or service agency number	Nursing diagnosis
Date of birth	Health record number of client	Nursing intervention
Sex	Number of principal registered nurse	Nursing outcomes
Race and ethnicity	Providers	Intensity of nursing care
Residence	Episode admission or encounter date	
	Discharge or termination date	
	Disposition of client	
	Expected payer of bill	

Classification (NIC), Home Health Care Classification (HHCC), Nursing Outcomes Classification (NOC), Patient Care Data Set, Perioperative Nursing Data Set, and the Complete Complementary Alternative Medicine Billing and Coding Reference (Coenen et al., 2001).

Two of these systems contain terms used by a variety of health care disciplines. They are SNOMED RT, which is a reference terminology originally developed for medicine, and The Complete Complementary Alternative Medicine Billing and Coding Reference, which is a coding system used for reimbursement of alternative medicine services. This indicates the necessity for integration of nursing terminologies into the broader health care arena. Because it has been recognized that no single language and classification system can meet the needs of nurses in a variety of settings in all countries, a project spearheaded by the International Council of Nurses is under way to provide a unifying framework for all nursing language systems throughout the world. They are currently developing the ICNP, which is a terminology system that provides the language for nursing phenomena, nursing actions, and nursing outcomes and enables existing vocabularies and classifications to be cross-mapped to allow comparison of nursing data generated from a variety of sources (Coenen, 2003).

Nursing Classification Systems

The ANA currently recognizes four classification systems that focus on particular clinical areas. The Omaha System (Martin & Scheet, 1992) and the Home Health Care Classification (Saba, 2002) both focus on nursing practice in community health settings. The Patient Care Data Set was created to capture clinical data in the acute care setting (Ozbolt, 1996). The Perioperative Nursing Data Set provides the data elements that define and describe nursing practice in the perioperative setting (Beyea, 2000).

The ANA also recognizes NANDA, NIC, and NOC, which are more comprehensive taxonomies, containing terms for patient problems, interventions, and outcomes. These are the most frequently used and can be applied by clinicians in a variety of settings.

Nursing diagnosis was originally introduced in the early 1970s (Gebbie & Lavin, 1975). Since then, the NANDA has continued the work of classifying nursing diagnoses. A nursing diagnosis is defined as a "clinical judgement about individual, family, or community responses to actual or potential health problems/life processes" (NANDA, 2003, p. 263). The definition contains a label with defining characteristics and related factors. The most current version is the NANDA Taxonomy II, containing 167 approved diagnoses classified into 46 classes and 13 domains.

NIC is a comprehensive taxonomy of 514 interventions that describe treatments that nurses perform. These treatments include all specialties in all types of settings (Dochterman & Bulechek, 2004). An *intervention* is the label given to a set of specific activities that nurses carry out to assist patients as they move toward an outcome. Interventions can be both nurse initiated and physician initiated. The classification is organized into a three-level taxonomy of 7 domains, 30 classes, and the 514 interventions. Each intervention has a label name with a definition and is coded with a unique four-digit number. There is list of suggested activities for each intervention, and they can be modified to individualize the care of the patient.

NOC provides the language for the evaluation step of the nursing process and outcome element of the NMDS (Moorhead, Johnson, & Maas, 2004). It includes a set of 330 outcome labels sensitive to nursing care. A nursing-sensitive outcome is defined as a patient or family caregiver state, behavior, or perception that is measurable along a continuum and responsive to a nursing intervention. The taxonomy is organized into seven domains. Each domain contains classes or groups of related outcomes. The outcomes each have a definition, label name, and a list of indicators with a five-point scale for use in rating the status of the outcome. Each outcome is coded to designate domain, class, outcome, indicator, rating scale, and the 1-to-5 evaluation score. NOC enables the examination of links between diagnoses, interventions, and outcomes. It allows the measurement of patient status at different points along the care continuum.

Efforts are under way to create a common structure for NANDA, NIC, and NOC to enable clinicians to more easily integrate and link the three elements when planning and documenting patient care (Dochterman & Jones, 2003). In the proposed taxonomy diagnoses, interventions and outcomes would be organized under the same domains and classes, thereby facilitating the incorporation of the languages in information system databases.

DESIGN AND IMPLEMENTATION

Critical evaluation of the documentation system at our hospital prompted the patient care leadership group to appoint a small task force to brainstorm and develop a plan for improvement. The group eventually expanded to include administrative leaders, quality management staff, and direct patient care providers. From the beginning it was clear that without a standardized framework, the task of organizing and capturing the minimum data elements would be almost impossible. The NIC and NOC systems were selected because they provide a comprehensive, patient-focused framework that crosses multiple clinical settings, while still allowing individualization of the care plan.

The next step was to develop an electronic care planning tool using the McKesson Horizon Clinical suite of software, primarily utilizing the Care Manager application. This software had already been purchased at our site, and the order entry component was in use on a house-wide basis. However, it did not include an effective care planning module, so a creative solution had to be developed by combining features of the order entry and clinical guidelines applications. Care plans were constructed using a basic set of "core" NICs, interventions essential for the care of all patients regardless of problem or diagnosis. One example of a core NIC is Pain Management. Because all patients must be routinely assessed for pain, this intervention is always applicable.

Care plans were created with the expectation that all care providers would assess individual patients and customize the plan as needed. However, once a plan has been developed, it is essential to apply it to the patient care process and subsequently link it to documentation. This ensures that the care plan determines which charting elements are necessary, giving more meaning to all documentation. In our system, NIC charting screens can be accessed only by selecting corresponding elements from the plan. If a screen is not available for documentation, it is usually a trigger that an additional NIC should be added to the care plan.

Computerized documentation screens were developed by multidisciplinary workgroups to take advantage of the perspective and knowledge of many clinical experts. Each discipline first developed their own unique admission assessment screen to capture required data elements. In this way, all providers have the opportunity to add interventions or patient-specific goals to the care plan based on their discipline-specific assessment. NIC charting screens were then developed according to evidence-based standards and protocols in use at our facility. In some cases, specialized patient care activities were added to accommodate more in-depth charting needs. For example, detailed activities were added to the NIC Discharge Planning screen to enable case manager documentation of patient care conferences and patient placement activities.

Working together with the multidisciplinary group proved to be a critical step because it engaged clinical specialists from several nonnursing disciplines and provided an opportunity to review just how comprehensive the NIC system can be. As these clinical specialists worked alongside the core nursing group it became apparent that there were sufficient commonalties to allow many types of providers to share intervention labels and related activities.

The use of NOC also proved to be acceptable to all disciplines. Patient goals are formulated for patients and placed on the care plan. For example, the goal for the intervention of "Teaching: Prescribed

Medication" for our transplant patients is that they will have substantial knowledge of their immuno-suppressive medications on discharge. Thus the NOC "Knowledge: Medication" is measured daily and charted against using a five-point Likert scale that ranges from none (0) to extensive, with 4 indicating substantial. The use of NOC facilitates the ability to capture outcomes data to be used in monitoring the quality of our patient care.

The final design uses the computer to manage and display problem-based care plans that consist of NICs and patient-specific goals. NIC charting screens are accessed by selecting an NIC from the care plan and linking to the appropriate charting screen. Outcomes are documented on these screens using NOCs appropriate for the intervention. The computer displays all this patient data in real time and integrates input from multiple types of care providers so a comprehensive review of patient progress is always available. The electronic medium allows the entire record of care to be accessed online, making it possible for multiple disciplines to participate. Table 32-2 provides an example of an interdisciplinary care plan using NANDA, NIC and NOC.

TABLE 32-2	INTERDISCIPLINARY CARE PLAN USING NANDA, NIC, AND NOC FOR POST-OPERATIVE RENAL TRANSPLANT PATIENT	

Nursing Diagnosis/ Patient Problems	NANDA
	  Risk for fluid volume deficit
	  Risk for infection
	  Pain
	  Risk for altered nutrition
	  Impaired physical mobility
	  Knowledge deficit: medications	

Nursing Treatments/ Intervention	NIC: Fluid Monitoring
	NIC: IV Therapy
	NIC: Urinary Elimination Management
		NOC: Fluid Balance
		  BP in expected range
		  Body weight stable
		  24 hr I & O balanced
		  CVP in expected range
		  Serum electrolytes in expected range

	NIC: Wound Care	NOC: Wound Healing: Primary Intention
		  Skin approximation
		  Resolution of drainage

	NIC: Pain Management	NOC: Pain Level Reported pain

	NIC: Teaching: Prescribed Meds	NOC: Knowledge Medication
		  Description of actions of medication
		  Description of correct administration of medication

	NIC: Self-Care Assistance	NOC: Self-Care: ADL Hygiene Toileting

Continued

TABLE 32-2	**INTERDISCIPLINARY CARE PLAN USING NANDA, NIC, AND NOC FOR POST-OPERATIVE RENAL TRANSPLANT PATIENT—CONT'D**	
	NIC: Skin Surveillance	NOC: Tissue Integrity, Skin and Mucous Membranes Skin intactness
	NIC: Surveillance Safety NIC: Emotional Support NIC: Nutrition Management NIC: Medication Management NIC: Bowel Management	
Nutrition Services	NIC: Nutrition Therapy	NOC: Nutritional Status Food and fluid intake Biochemical measures
Rehabilitation Services	NIC: Exercise Therapy: Ambulation	NOC: Mobility Level Ambulation: walking
Respiratory Therapy	NIC: Oxygen Therapy NIC: Cough Enhancement	NOC: Respiratory Status Oxygen saturation within normal limits
Case Management	NIC: Discharge Planning	NOC: Knowledge Health Resources Description of plan for follow-up care Description of community resources available for assistance

AUTOMATING THE PROCESS

Clinical information systems (CISs) are an essential part of any plan to develop a documentation system that seeks to describe and standardize patient care. They can provide the framework for organizing patient care. Most systems already provide features that support input, display, and reporting of patient information. However, not all systems have kept pace with the rapidly changing needs of the industry. It is essential that in addition to a framework for nurses to use at the bedside, the CISs have the ability to codify data that can later be retrieved and analyzed. The system should support data collection that can be used to determine best practices for desired outcomes, variability in practice, and the most effective utilization of resources.

At this time, one of the greatest challenges is in trying to find ways to make current CISs support the vision of a problem-oriented, interdisciplinary care plan. Such plans represent major practice changes for care providers, so the CIS must facilitate and support this. Merely replicating what exists today on paper will not accomplish the goal of linking documentation to care plans.

One of the most difficult aspects of health care informatics is to articulate the patient care process for software vendors. When entering into discussions about technical feasibility, it is imperative to bring clinical perspective to the table, shifting the paradigm away from traditional charting systems. Patient care is a process with great complexity and many components. Although these components are often addressed well in individual software modules, they are typically not integrated in a way that supports continuity of patient care. The result is that managing a caseload of patients over the continuum can seem cumbersome and inefficient. It is incumbent on health care informatics specialists to articulate this to vendors so they can understand the vision of a CIS that not only collects and retrieves data but also supports workflow. Programming changes take time, however, so in the meantime it is wise to explore creative ways to use existing products while continuing to communicate needs to vendors.

SUMMARY

Computerized documentation systems must be designed in such a way as to demonstrate an interdisciplinary care plan, implementation of that plan, and evaluation of outcomes for patients. Designing and implementing a system that blends input and perspective from multiple disciplines can be challenging. Add to that the introduction of a standardized language and the time needed for adoption is even greater. Because the computer is often introduced as the tool for managing this type of integrated system, it is frequently regarded as the object of blame when the change process becomes tough.

The authors of *Clinical Information Systems, A Framework for Reaching the Vision* point out that continued learning and growth are needed for health care providers to accept innovation. They state, "In the clinical systems arena, if not in other areas, there is an acute need for serious soul searching and self-examination around our openness to giving up old models and behaviors, old frameworks of reality, and to embrace learning new methodologies and skills" (Androwich et al., 2003).

As we move forward with greater emphasis on patient safety, systems must be developed that promote interdisciplinary communication, care planning, and documentation. Use of standardized language within a CIS that supports workflow can bring us closer to this goal. Significant paradigm shift is needed on the part of clinicians as well as software vendors if this goal is to be realized. Meanwhile, beginning steps have been taken as we begin the journey.

References

Androwich, I. et al. (2003). *Clinical information systems: A framework for reaching the vision.* Washington, D.C.: American Nurses Publishing.

Beyea, S.C. (2000) *Perioperative nursing data set: The perioperative nursing vocabulary.* Denver: AORN.

Coenen, A., et al. (2001). Toward comparable nursing data: American Nurses Association criteria for datasets, classification systems, and nomenclatures. *Computers in Nursing, 19*(6), 240-246.

Coenen, A. (2003, Apr. 3). Nursing Classifications "The International Classification for Nursing Practice (ICNP) Programme: Advancing a Unifying Framework for Nursing" *Online Journal of Issues in Nursing.* Available at nursing world.org/ojin/tpc7/tpc7_8.htm. Accessed May 22, 2003.

Dochterman, J., & Bulechek, G. (Eds) (2004). *Nursing Intervention Classification (NIC)*, 4th ed. St. Louis: Mosby–Year Book.

Dochterman, J.M., & Jones, D.A. (2003). *Unifying nursing languages: The harmonization of NANDA, NIC, and NOC.* Washington, D.C.: NursesBooks.org.

Gebbie, K.M., & Lavin, M.A. (1975). Classification of nursing diagnosis: Proceedings of the first national conference. St. Louis: Mosby.

Johnson, M. (2002). Criteria for standardized nursing languages. *Outcomes Management, 6*(1), 1-3.

Martin, K., & Scheet, N. (1992). *The Omaha system: Applications for community health nursing.* Philadelphia: W.B. Saunders.

McCloskey, J.C., & Bulechek, G.M. (Eds.) (2000). Iowa Intervention Project. In *Nursing intervention classification (NIC)*, 3rd ed., St. Louis: Mosby.

Moorhead, S., Johnson, M., & Maas, M. (Eds.) (2004). *Nursing outcomes classification (NOC)*, 3rd ed., St. Louis: Mosby.

North American Nursing Diagnosis Association (2003). *Nursing diagnoses: Definitions & classification 2003-2004.* Philadelphia: NANDA International.

O'Leary, D. (2001). *Statement of the Joint Commission on Accreditation of Health care Organizations before the U. S. Senate and the Subcommittee of Labor, Health and Human Services and Education of the Senate Committee on Appropriations, February 22, 2001.* Joint Commission on Accreditation of Health Care Operations. Available at http://www.jcaho.org/. Accessed May 17, 2003.

Ozbolt, J.G. (1996). From minimum data to maximum impact: Using clinical data to strengthen patient care. *Advanced Practice Nursing Quarterly, 1*(4), 62-69.

Saba, V.K. (2002). *Home Health Care Classification system (HHCC): An overview.* Available at nursingworld.org/ojin/tpc7/tpc7_7.htm. Access May 22, 2003.

Werley, H., & Lang, N. (1988). *Identification of the Nursing Minimum Data set.* New York: Springer.

Ethical Issues in Case Management

Sister Carol Taylor

CHAPTER OVERVIEW

This chapter explores the ethical issues related to case management. The essential elements of ethical competence are described, and strategies for developing and evaluating ethical competence are offered. The nurse case manager's potential for influencing the well-being of patients is highlighted with a discussion of advocacy. The principle- and care-based theoretical and practical approaches to clinical ethics are presented with a discussion of the nurse case manager's role in clinical ethics. The chapter concludes with a discussion of moral integrity and with an examination of the six recurrent issues confronting nurse case managers.

Nurse case managers literally hold human well-being in their hands. Repetitious execution of the multiple administrative and clinical tasks that make up the workday of each nurse case manager often blinds us to the truth of this statement. Renewed attention to what we do, and reflection on *why* we do what we do will quickly remind us that the "cases" we "manage" are actually people with unique life histories and needs. Moreover, we will readily see the links between who we are and how we conduct ourselves professionally and the well-being of those society entrusts to our professional care. This concluding chapter examines why ethical competence is essential for nurse case managers, explores the role of the nurse case manager in clinical ethics, and examines specific challenges to the professional and personal integrity of nurse case managers.

ETHICAL COMPETENCE AND THE NURSE CASE MANAGER

Ethical Competence as a Core Competence

Is ethical competence a core or an elective competence? Is it like knowing the general principles of asepsis or like knowing how to run a neonatal intensive care unit? Although some nurses continue to think about ethical competence as a specialized expertise that nurses can choose to develop, in 1991 the American Nurses Association (ANA) published standards of professional performance that hold all nurses accountable for ethical practice. Boxes 33-1 and 33-2 present the ANA Code of Ethics and Standards of Professional Performance. Today nurses are legally liable if their practice is ethically deficient.

> **BOX 33-1** ▸ THE AMERICAN NURSES ASSOCIATION'S CODE OF ETHICS FOR NURSES
>
> 1. The nurse, in all professional relationships, practices with compassion and respect for the inherent dignity, worth, and uniqueness of every individual, unrestricted by considerations of social or economic status, personal attributes, or the nature of health problems.
> 2. The nurse's primary commitment is to the patient, whether an individual, family, group, or community.
> 3. The nurse promotes, advocates for, and strives to protect the health, safety, and rights of the patient.
> 4. The nurse is responsible and accountable for individual nursing practice and determines the appropriate delegation of tasks consistent with the nurse's obligation to provide optimum patient care.
> 5. The nurse owes the same duties to self as to others, including the responsibility to preserve integrity and safety, to maintain competence, and to continue personal and professional growth.
> 6. The nurse participates in establishing, maintaining, and improving health care environments and conditions of employment conducive to the provision of quality health care and consistent with the values of the profession through individual and collective action.
> 7. The nurse participates in the advancement of the profession through contributions to practice, education, administration, and knowledge development.
> 8. The nurse collaborates with other health professionals and the public in promoting community, national, and international efforts to meet health needs.
> 9. The profession of nursing, as represented by associations and their members, is responsible for articulating nursing values, for maintaining the integrity of the profession and its practice, and for shaping social policy.
>
> Reprinted with permission from American Nurses Association, *Code of Ethics for Nurses with Interpretive Statements*, © 2001 Nursebooks.org, Washington, D.C.: American Nurses Association.

Elements of Ethical Competence

Part of the difficulty in holding ourselves and one another accountable for ethical competence lies in the failure to define exactly what it is that constitutes ethical competence. When hiring a new nurse case manager, we generally have a clear idea of the intellectual, clinical, and administrative competencies essential to the successful execution of the role. Rarely, however, are the requisite ethical competencies clear in our mind, and we thus fail to evaluate candidates in this arena. Listed below are some basic characteristics of the ethically competent nurse case manager. Following the list are reasons why these characteristics are important and ways they can be evaluated in a prospective employee interview. Ethically competent nurse case managers are able to do the following:

- Be trusted to act in ways that advance the best interests of the patients entrusted to their care
- Hold themselves and their colleagues accountable for their practice
- Act as effective patient advocates
- Mediate ethical conflict among the patient, significant others, the health care team, and other interested parties
- Recognize the ethical dimensions of practice and identify and respond to ethical problems
- Critique new health care technologies and changes in the way we define, administer, deliver, and finance health care in light of their potential to influence human well-being

BOX 33-2	THE AMERICAN NURSES ASSOCIATION'S STANDARDS OF PROFESSIONAL PERFORMANCE

STANDARD 12. ETHICS

Measurement Criteria
The registered nurse:
Uses the *Code of Ethics for Nurses with Interpretive Statements* (ANA, 2001) to guide practice.
Delivers care in a manner that preserves and protects patient autonomy, dignity, and rights.
Maintains patient confidentiality within legal and regulatory parameters.
Serves as a patient advocate, assisting patients in developing skills for self-advocacy.
Maintains a therapeutic and professional patient-nurse relationship with appropriate professional role boundaries.
Demonstrates a commitment to practicing self-care, managing stress, and connecting with self and others.
Contributes to resolving ethical issues of patients, colleagues, or systems as evidenced in such activities as participating on ethics committees.
Reports illegal, incompetent, or impaired practices.

Additional Measurement Criteria for the Advanced Practice Registered Nurse
The advanced practice registered nurse:
Informs the patient of the risks, benefits, and outcomes of health care regimens.
Participates in interdisciplinary teams that address ethical risks, benefits, and outcomes.

Additional Measurement Criteria for the Nursing Role Specialty
The registered nurse in a nursing role specialty:
Participates on multidisciplinary and interdisciplinary teams that address ethical risks, benefits, and outcomes.
Informs administrators or others of the risk, benefits, and outcomes of programs and decisions that affect health care delivery.

Reprinted with permission from American Nurses Association, *Nursing: Scope and Standards of Practice*, © 2004 Nursebooks.org. Washington, D.C.: American Nurses Association.

COMMITMENT TO PATIENT WELL-BEING

Commitment to patient well-being as an element of ethical competence would seem to be self-evident, because all those in helping professions in general and in health care professions in particular have as their reason for being commitment to human well-being. Unfortunately the health care system is changing in ways that make it increasingly difficult to assume this orientation. The nurse case manager's first challenge and core responsibility is to keep the entire system of care and the caregiving team focused on meeting the needs of the patients it purports to serve. One nurse case manager voiced frustration when she was unable to find a bed on the unit a patient with acquired immunodeficiency syndrome (AIDS) requested when he was being readmitted for new complications. She was told that worrying about which unit had a bed was not "her job." She quickly responded to her colleague that if this was important to the patient, then it was important to her because she did not know who else was going to worry about it.

EXAMPLE. Nurses working in an oncology unit are discovering that patients enrolled in certain managed care companies have had their access to mental health services severely restricted. Their options are to accept the restricted services as a given or to begin to gather the data that will demonstrate that these restrictions are dramatically influencing the health and well-being of the patients being served. If commitment to the health and well-being of patients is their primary commitment, they will not allow this change in the system to go unchallenged.

RESPONSIBILITY AND ACCOUNTABILITY

As systems for delivering health care continue to fragment, it is not unusual for patient health problems to go undiagnosed or, when diagnosed, to be ignored or inadequately addressed. The diffusion of power and authority in complex caregiving teams makes it easy to assume that "someone else" is responsibly monitoring the problem. By virtue of the coordinating role they play in the caregiving team, nurse case managers are well positioned to monitor the effectiveness of the plan of care and to call to accountability those whose efforts remain uncommitted: *If I hold myself accountable for the well-being of those committed to my care, I need more than a task orientation to each day's work. It isn't enough for me to be "busy" doing professional activities. These activities must be contributing to the well-being of those I serve. My workday is complete when I am confident that everything necessary is being done for those entrusted to my care.* This critical distinction is often overlooked in practice today.

EXAMPLE. Nurses on your unit are pleased that the newly implemented critical pathway for women undergoing a modified radical mastectomy seems to be streamlining care and ensuring a better quality of care for all. Each staff nurse has been encouraged to keep women "on the path" postoperatively so that discharge outcomes can be met within specified time intervals. One nurse voices a concern that one patient seems to need more time and that she is afraid that nurses are impatient with her lack of outcome achievement. The nurse case manager who assumes responsibility for patient well-being is able to counsel staff nurses about the importance of respecting individual patient needs and about their need to assume responsibility for advocating that patients receive the time they need to meet critical outcomes. At issue is our ability to remember that we are first accountable to the patient and then to a new system of care.

EXAMPLE. Although everyone in your hospital knows something about advance directives and some are even enthusiastic about their potential for eliminating or reducing conflict over end-of-life decision-making, the hospital has not identified who is responsible for actually helping patients to specify their preferences in a meaningful way. Each patient receives literature on advance directives in the admitting office, but after that is at the mercy of any health care professional who elects to pursue this conversation. More often than not, no one pursues this concern. You can elect to raise this issue and attempt to change the system to ensure that this need is being addressed or you can accept the status quo.

ABILITY TO ACT AS AN EFFECTIVE ADVOCATE

Most of us have heard stories from friends or acquaintances about someone's terrifying hospitalization. "I don't know how people in hospitals survive without a family member in constant attendance to make sure the patient gets the ordered care and to prevent mix-ups!" Although numerous variables influence the amount and type of advocacy required by different patients, it is generally true that someone must act as advocate for the patient on multiple levels and in particular for the patient whose self-advocacy is impaired. Again the nurse case manager is in the ideal position to "work the system" both within and outside the hospital to ensure that the patient's needs are met. In the current climate of financial "bottom-line" decision-making, the need for strong patient advocacy is even more pronounced.

EXAMPLE. A managed care company decides to reimburse hospitals for only the first 12 to 24 hours after delivery, and nurses begin to find that women need a longer hospital stay after delivering to realize valued maternal-infant outcomes. The nurse case manager must choose whether to advocate for these women. A nurse case manager can decide to accept that some outcomes simply cannot be realized in this short time frame or can work to change the system to ensure that these needs are met either in the hospital or at home. An effective advocate will work with individual patients on a case-by-case basis as well as try to marshal forces to change the system.

ABILITY TO MEDIATE ETHICAL CONFLICT
Ethical conflict is inherent in health care practice today. Among the forces contributing to this conflict are the following:
- The multiple therapeutic options available for most health problems and the lack of consensus about their medical effectiveness, benefit, and burdens
- The raging debate about who should get how much of our scarce health care resources and the increasing tendency to dismiss certain patients as "poor investment risks" or as simply "unworthy" of indicated medical care
- The condition of moral pluralism; the fact that we seem to grow more heterogeneous daily in our religious and cultural beliefs and values

Ethically competent nurse case managers need to be skilled in identifying patients, families, and caregiving teams that are at risk for ethical conflict and in addressing the factors contributing to this conflict. When nurse case managers can effectively mediate problematic situations or invite ethics consult teams to perform this service, the conflict does not escalate and the alienation that sometimes results between patient and families and caregiving individuals, team, or institution can be avoided. A chief objective is to identify the sources of common problems and to change the system to prevent their recurrence.

EXAMPLE. The wife of one of the patients on your unit comes to you and tells you that a gastrointestinal consultant has just informed her that they need to take her husband back to surgery because he has developed a mesenteric infarct. She tearfully tells you that she knows her husband would refuse this surgery if he were able to speak but that no one seems to be listening to her. He did not do well after surgery to remove a recurrent meningioma. She said that he only reluctantly consented to repeat surgery after much pleading from his adult children. You can side with the medical team who seems to be of the mind that this is a reversible problem that must be addressed or you can try to find out more about the wife's reluctance to consent and get the caregiving team to sit down with the wife and family to decide what actually is in the patient's best interests. The nurse case manager must choose whether to ignore the conflict (or hope that someone else assumes responsibility for its resolution) or to intervene to mediate the conflict.

ABILITY TO RECOGNIZE ETHICAL DIMENSIONS OF PRACTICE
The ethical dimensions of practice range from sensitivity to threats to human dignity in the caregiving environment to concerns about limited access to basic health care services. The nurse case manager who recognizes the ethical dimensions of practice and who knows how and when to intervene can provide effective leadership in this domain.

EXAMPLE. Nurses in a medical intensive care unit are voicing frustration with the unevenness with which ethical dimensions of care are addressed in the unit, depending on which attending physician is leading the resident team that month. Two of the four attending physicians who make rounds with the residents are supportive of and encourage discussion of ethical questions, whereas the other two seem to believe that these discussions distract attention from the "critical," that is, medical, aspects of the case. At issue is how comfortable the nurses and medical residents are in addressing the topic of do-not-resuscitate (DNR) orders and in initiating advance planning for critical end-of-life decisions. While one case manager allows the attending physician to determine what can be discussed in morning rounds, another invites all four attending physicians to a meeting in which nurses present a plan to make ethical concerns a priority item in the discussion of each patient during rounds. The time gained with patients for whom there are no current ethical questions will allow for a timely discussion of issues when they do come up.

ABILITY TO CRITIQUE POTENTIAL TO INFLUENCE HUMAN WELL-BEING

A final critical element of ethical competence for the nurse case manager is the ability to critique new health care technologies and changes in the way we define, administer, deliver, and finance health care in light of their potential to influence human well-being. The nurse skilled in this ability remains sufficiently distant from and critical of all aspects of caregiving to evaluate them in terms of their human consequences. Examples of successful intervention in this regard occur in both beginning and end-of-life care. In the not so distant past physicians always interjected the latest medical technology into the processes of childbearing and dying. Although this type of care continues to meet the needs of some high-risk patients, we fortunately now have the options of natural childbirth and hospice care for patients who elect to go a different route. These alternative types of care were made available after reflective health care professionals challenged the need for the latest medical treatment for all beginning and end-of-life care.

EXAMPLE. A critical care nurse comments there is almost no need to spend time in the patient's room any more because sophisticated monitoring equipment allows everyone at the nurses' station to know more than they ever wanted to know about each patient at any moment in time. A nurse case manager listening to this comment begins to wonder how beneficial this equipment is, in its totality, to the patient. How much of it is merely a convenience to the nurses and physicians? What benefits are gained for the patient, and at what cost in terms of burden and discomfort? He decides to study this concern and involves other interested nurses. As a result of the data they collect and especially because of what they learn from patient interviews, one type of monitor is "retired" and another is used only for patients with special monitoring needs. When they share their findings with the company who manufactures many of the products they use, they discover that the company is interested in the topic of humanizing technology and seeks their collaboration in a research project.

Evaluating Ethical Competence

To evaluate ethical competence in prospective nurse case managers, it is helpful to present case scenarios common to the practice setting and elicit their response (Box 33-3). Responses should demonstrate their ease and competence in recognizing and addressing ethical concerns. Box 33-3 offers sample scenarios for evaluating ethical competence and highlights the specific competencies they test. These scenarios could also be used in an informal or a formal staff meeting to spark conversation about ethical competence and to encourage reasoning about how case managers identify and meet ethical obligations to individual patients and to society. After several hypothetical scenarios are explored, staff can be invited

BOX 33-3	EVALUATING ETHICAL COMPETENCE

Sample Case Scenarios for Interviewing Prospective Employees

INTERVIEWER: "Among the competencies we find to be essential for our nurse case managers is ethical competence. I'd like to get a sense of your competence and confidence in responding to some hypothetical situations. I'll describe a situation and invite you to tell me how you would respond if you were the responsible case manager."

SCENARIO 1

The wife of a patient with end-stage cancer seeks you out and tells you that she is afraid that her husband is "losing hope" and "giving up." She tells you that she has just learned that one of the patients on the unit was evaluated for inclusion in a clinical trial that offers some promise of arresting the disease if the patient receives the experimental drug. She wants you to get her husband in this trial and to do whatever you can to ensure that he receives the experimental drug. You are not familiar with the criteria for inclusion in this trial and think that it would probably be futile for her husband given his condition. You have to be at an administrative meeting in 20 minutes. What do you say to her?

Evaluate Response for:
Commitment to patient well-being
Sense of responsibility and accountability
Ability to be an effective patient advocate

SCENARIO 2

One of the staff nurses on your unit complains that the medical staff is treating patients differently and that it is making a lot of the nurses "mad." The unit has both wealthy, well-insured patients and a large number of minority, Medicaid, and Medicare patients. She reports that a number of the attending physicians seem to bend over backward to ensure that the preferences of the wealthy patients are known and met while doing the bare minimum for other patients. You suspect that she is probably right but also know that this system is well entrenched.

Evaluate Response for:
Commitment to patient well-being
Sense of responsibility and accountability
Ability to be an effective patient advocate
Ability to recognize ethical dimensions of practice

SCENARIO 3

A woman who has just delivered her first baby and who appears utterly fatigued after a lengthy labor and overwhelmed by the new demands of parenting confides to you that she needs to stay in the hospital for a couple of days until she feels comfortable caring for her newborn. You are concerned about her level of stress but also know that her health maintenance organization will only fund the first 24 hours of care after delivery and that this couple has limited financial resources.

Evaluate Response for:
Commitment to patient well-being
Sense of responsibility and accountability
Ability to be an effective patient advocate
Ability to critique system's potential to influence human well-being

Continued

BOX 33-3   Evaluating Ethical Competence—cont'd

Sample Case Scenarios for Interviewing Prospective Employees—cont'd

Scenario 4

Marita, a 16-year-old high school junior with congenital heart defects and a long history of hospitalizations, surgical and pharmacological interventions, and chronic illness, now needs a heart transplant or she will die. She adamantly refuses the transplant and says she prefers death to the ordeal of the transplant. Her mother cannot accept this decision and refuses to even discuss this with her daughter. The staff is split as to whether to side with the patient or her mother and differ in their assessments of the probability of the transplant's ultimately benefiting her. You sense the team's growing frustration and know that if the transplant option is pursued, the sooner it is done, the better will be the prognosis.

Evaluate Response for:
Commitment to patient well-being
Ability to be an effective patient advocate
Ability to mediate ethical conflict

Scenario 5

While making rounds, you encounter an 82-year-old patient who was admitted from the local prison with complications secondary to his emphysema. You recognize him from previous admissions and in talking with him listen to his descriptions of how horrible the conditions are in the prison for the aging convicts like himself. Listening to his story you recall other elderly prisoners who have been on your unit during the last 3 or 4 years who have shown some signs of neglect. He tells you that he will do anything to get admitted to the hospital and that most of the other elderly prisoners would, too. "Not even a dog should have to live the way we do." You sense that he is probably being honest and that he does not seem to be manipulative or playing on your sympathies.

Evaluate Response for:
Commitment to patient well-being
Sense of responsibility and accountability

Scenario 6

An 11-year-old Native American boy in the pediatric oncology unit tells you to make sure that "Ellen never takes care of me again." When you question him, he tells you how "mean" she is and that she never treats him nicely like the other nurses do. You respect Ellen's clinical competence and know that this patient has a reputation for being a problem.

Evaluate Response for:
Commitment to patient well-being
Sense of responsibility and accountability
Ability to be an effective patient advocate

---

to present situations they have experienced so that the team can talk together about different ways of responding. When these discussions are regularly scheduled, they communicate the expectation that ethical competence is critical to the performance of the nurse case manager's roles and that it needs to be consciously developed and updated in the same way that clinical and administrative competencies are approached.

Theoretical and Practical Approaches to Clinical Ethics

Ethics, broadly defined, concerns itself with right and wrong moral conduct, with how we ought to live (and die) and why. *Clinical ethics*, a relatively new branch of ethics, addresses ethical issues and problems that arise in the context of caring for actual patients in varied clinical settings, in the hospital, residential facility, clinic, and home. The ethically competent nurse case manager will be familiar with at least two common approaches to clinical ethics: the principle-based approach and the care-based approach. Brief descriptions of these follow, and references are cited for those wishing to learn more about these methods.

PRINCIPLE-BASED APPROACH

One of the leading theories of bioethics and clinical ethics has been termed the *four-principle approach*. Popularized by Beauchamp and Childress (1994), this approach identifies four ethical principles derived from common moral beliefs and uses them to identify, discuss, and analyze the moral features of particular situations. The four principles include *autonomy* (self-determination), *beneficence* (benefiting or helping), *nonmaleficence* (avoiding harm), and *justice* (treating fairly). Other theorists list as key principles veracity (truth telling), confidentiality (respecting privileged information), fidelity (keeping promises), and avoiding killing. All of these are held to obligate health care professionals in a prima facie manner; that is, all things being equal, *I am obligated to respect patients, benefit them, cause them no harm, treat all fairly, be truthful, and so on. A moral dilemma results when I am unable to simultaneously execute two prima facie obligations.* For example, a woman with AIDS begs you not to inform her sexual partner and the father of her child that she has AIDS because she is afraid that he will leave her. While you have an obligation to respect her privacy and to keep privileged information confidential, you also have an obligation to prevent harm to identifiable third parties. Seemingly you cannot do both. Unfortunately there is no agreed-on hierarchy of principles that specifies which principles supersede others. Clouser and Gert (1994) offer a strong critique of this method, which they term *principlism*. Many nurses have been critical of this methodology because popularized versions seem to promote a type of quandary ethics of the to-pull-the-plug-or-not variety, which has not been sensitive to the everyday ethical concerns of practicing nurses.

CARE-BASED APPROACH

Dissatisfaction with the principle-based approach to nursing ethics combined with attentiveness to Gilligan's (1982) ground-breaking work in moral development led some nurse theorists to begin to articulate an ethic of care (Benner & Wrubel, 1989; Fry, 1989; Watson, 1985). Central to this perspective is the nature of the nurse-patient relationship and attention to the particulars of individual patients viewed within the context of their lives. Operating within this methodology, nurses pay attention to the human needs and interests that underlie ethical conflict with the intent of restoring and strengthening bonds between professionals, patients, and families. Characteristics of the care perspective include the following:

- Centrality of the caring relationship
- Promotion of the dignity of and respect for patients as people
- Acceptance of particular patients and health care professional variables (beliefs, values, relationships) as morally relevant factors in ethical decision-making
- Norms of responsiveness and responsibility
- Redefinition of fundamental moral skills (Taylor, 1993)

ETHICALLY RELEVANT CONSIDERATIONS

Whichever ethical approach the nurse case manager uses, the following list of ethically relevant considerations is helpful in the analysis of ethically problematic cases and in the discussion of these cases with others. Fletcher, Miller, and Spencer (1995, pp. 11-13) suggest that the following eight considerations offer a bridge between ethical principles, an ethics of caring, and the clinical situation:

1. Balancing benefits and harms in the care of patients
2. Disclosure, informed consent, and shared decision-making
3. Norms of family life
4. Relationships between clinicians and patients
5. Professional integrity of clinicians
6. Cost-effectiveness and allocation
7. Issues of cultural and religious variation
8. Considerations of power

Resources for Ethics for the Nurse Case Manager

Because clinical ethicists in general and nurse ethicists more specifically are still something of a rarity and infrequently are employed by health care agencies and institutions, nurse case managers who are interested in developing ethical competence may need to look outside their institutions for resources. Many professional nursing organizations such as the American Nurses Association (and individual states' associations) and the Association of Critical Care Nurses have task forces and committees that deal exclusively with ethical matters. These organizations and others frequently host conferences and seminars that address ethical issues and can refer nurses to the educational resources most likely to address their needs. Box 33-4 highlights some of the better known ethics resources. Some geographical areas are served by regional networks of ethics centers or by university-based ethics centers.

Advocacy and the Nurse Case Manager

Nurse ethicist Sally Gadow defines advocacy as the moral commitment to enhance patients' autonomy. "Among all of the professionals surrounding a patient, nurses often are the most capable of fostering patient self-determination. The practice of advocacy in nursing thus involves development of the nurse-patient relationship as the medium for expression of patients' values" (1989, p. 535). To function effectively as a patient advocate, nurse case managers must understand the basic dynamics in health care decision-making.

Basically there are three models of health care decision-making that are "alive and well" in most clinical settings (Table 33-1). In paternalism or maternalism, the clinician is "boss" and makes decisions to benefit patients, who are viewed as generally lacking sufficient knowledge to make right decisions. When this model works well, patients are spared the anguish of making tough decisions, and competent and compassionate clinicians make good decisions in the patient's best interests. When this model does not work well, patients receive unwanted care and live with the consequences long after the clinician exits the scene. The patient sovereignty model evolved to correct the problem of patients receiving unwanted care. Championing the patient as "boss" and the principle of autonomy, this model claims that no one knows what is best for the patient better than the patient himself or herself. In this model, patients receive the care they desire or demand, and the chief drawback is that there is often no one to protect patients from their poor or ill-advised choices.

In the early 1980s the President's Commission for the Study of Ethical Problems in Medicine and Biomedical and Behavioral Research rejected both of these models and recommended a model of shared decision-making. This model is also based on autonomy but respects the fact that both the patient and clinicians bring something of importance to the process of decision-making and calls for both to participate in the decision. The objective in this model is not simply that patients choose but that patients make the choice that is right for them, that is, a choice consistent with their values, moral identity, and decisional history. In this model clinicians are obligated to provide the support patients need to make

---

BOX 33-4 ▸ RESOURCES FOR ETHICS

American Nurses Association Center for Ethics and Human Rights
600 Maryland Avenue, SW
Suite 100 West
Washington, DC 20024-2571
(202) 651-7055
www.nursingworld.org/ethics/
Publishes the *Ethics and Human Rights Communiqué*, which provides an ongoing vehicle of communication for nurses facing ethical and human rights dilemmas in practice. *Communiqué* informs readers about important upcoming events and resources of interest such as bibliographies, surveys, grants, ANA conferences, ethical continuing education offerings, and new ANA publications.

National Reference Center for Bioethics Literature
Kennedy Institute of Ethics
Georgetown University
Box 571212
Washington, DC 20057
1-888-BIO-ETHX
www.georgetown.edu/research/nrcbl/nrc
A specialized collection of library resources concerned with contemporary biomedical issues in the fields of ethics, philosophy, medicine, nursing, science, law, religion, and the social sciences. Call for bioethics information, BIOETHICSLINE searches (computerized database), search strategies, reference help, and publication orders.

The Hastings Center
21 Malcolm Gordon Road
Garrison, NY 10524
(845) 424-4040
www.thehastingscenter.org
A nonprofit, nonpartisan organization that carries out educational and research programs on ethical issues in medicine, the life sciences, and the professions. Publishes *The Hastings Center Report*.

---

good decisions. It is in this respect that the decision-making model differs from the patient sovereignty model, which is a model of noninterference.

Even this brief introduction of models will make clear why the advocacy role of the nurse is problematic. Although most ethicists agree with the President's Commission and recommend a model of shared decision-making, clinicians may be found who subscribe to each of the three models. Not surprisingly these clinicians differ in their estimate of whether patients and families need advocates and in their acceptance of the differing responsibilities of advocates.

CLINICAL ETHICS AND THE NURSE CASE MANAGER

Promoting Autonomy

Among our most prized human abilities is the freedom to make choices in light of what we value or deem good. Individuals are autonomous to the extent that they are self-determining. Much of the bioethics debate in the United States has focused on how we can safeguard the right of patients to be

TABLE 33-1 MODELS OF HEALTH CARE DECISION-MAKING

Model	Description	Principle	Justification	Dangers
Paternalism	Physician is the boss.	Beneficence	Patients often do not understand enough about medicine to make the "right" decision.	Patients may receive care they do not want and must live with the consequences.
Patient sovereignty	Patient is the boss.	Autonomy (self-determination)	No one knows better than the patient what is in his or her overall "best interests"; right to be self-determining ought always to take precedence.	No one protects patients from a "poor" or "ill-advised" choice; "easy-out" for health care practitioners.
Shared decision-making	Patient and health care team work together.	Authentic autonomy	Patient may need support in being authentically autonomous.	Can easily slide into paternalism.

autonomous. Nurse case managers by virtue of their position and authority in the health care system can play a critical role in safeguarding patient autonomy.

Individuals with an intact decision-making capacity have the right to consent to and to refuse all medically indicated therapy. Because judgments about decision-making capacity ideally are made by those who know patients best, nurse case managers ought to participate in efforts to determine and document capacity. Criteria for decision-making capacity include the following:

1. Ability to comprehend information relevant to the decision at hand
2. Ability to deliberate in accord with a relatively consistent set of values and goals
3. Ability to communicate preferences

Nurse case managers who are effective advocates will help patients with decision-making capacity to anticipate the types of health care decisions they may need to make in the future and to explore their treatment options. It is important that patient preferences be documented and that nurses be familiar with state law about advance directives. Nurse case managers can play a leading role in making sure that the agency or institution they are affiliated with has a policy that identifies the parties responsible for obtaining and documenting patient preferences.

It is important that case managers working with patients with complex needs support authentically autonomous decision-making, that is, ensure that decisions reflect the identity, decisional history, and moral norms of the patient. This frequently will mean walking patients through the various treatment options to see what each will mean for this patient in terms of real-life benefits and burdens. When institutional, caregiver, or family interests interfere with the autonomy of the patient, nurse advocates will support the patient and ensure that his or her interests are protected.

Lack of decision-making capacity does not of itself negate the right to be self-determining. Known preferences of the incapacitated individual are to be respected. Advance directives—a living will or durable power of attorney for health care—legally protect an individual's preferences concerning health care. Case managers advocate for incapacitated patients by supporting their surrogate decision makers. The surrogate decision maker is the voice for a patient who can no longer speak for himself or herself. Surrogates should use their knowledge of the patient and the patient's values to make the choice the patient himself or herself would make if he or she were able to do so.

Valid moral surrogates have intact decision-making capacity, understand the information pertinent to the decision at hand, know the patient's preferences to the extent it is possible, have no undue conflict of interest, and are not experiencing severe emotional problems. Legally valid surrogates who are financially or emotionally dependent on a patient may make treatment decisions based on their own needs rather than on the interests of the patient. Nurse advocates can teach such surrogates that they are the voice for a now incapacitated patient and that they should decide as the patient would decide. If surrogates persist in making decisions that run counter to the patient's previously expressed wishes, health care professionals may need to explore legal means to challenge the surrogate's decision-making authority.

Promoting Patient Well-Being

The first task of the nurse advocate is to work with the patient, family, and health care team to clarify and communicate the appropriate goal of therapy: cure and restoration, stabilization of functioning, or preparation for a comfortable, dignified death. Although this would seem to be a given, often confusion makes it difficult to ensure that all interventions are consistent with the goal. Obviously, treatment goals may need revision when a patient makes unexpected progress or fails to progress. In one tertiary medical center, a decision was made to terminate aggressive treatment for a man with an advanced stage IV glioblastoma. He was transferred out of the neurology step-down unit to a general floor. Unfortunately the transfer was made on a weekend evening when communication was poor, so when the patient had spiked high temperatures, an aggressive workup was done and therapy for sepsis was initiated. If the intent of the therapy was comfort and the therapy was consistent with preparing him for a dignified death, the intervention was appropriate. However, if it was merely a knee-jerk response to a life-threatening complication and was aimed at restoration and cure, it was inappropriate for this patient. The family of an incapacitated, frail, debilitated patient may need great support in determining what is in the best interest of the patient and in deciding when to treat a condition aggressively and when to let nature take its course. Unfortunately there is no clear line between promoting life and needlessly prolonging dying.

Pellegrino (1989) recommends analysis of therapy along two lines: effectiveness and benefit/burden ratio. A treatment is effective when it reverses or ameliorates the natural progression of the disease. Surgical repair has a high probability of being effective treatment for a mesenteric infarct. This is an objective medical determination—to the degree that medicine as a science can be objective. Whether the benefits of that surgery would advance the overall best interests of the patient described earlier who had had a recurrent meningioma and outweigh the burdens of the surgery is, however, a subjective determination that can be made only by the patient or by those who know the patient best. Nurses may need to remind physicians that more is at stake in treatment decisions than whether the proposed therapy is "medically indicated." Nurses' knowledge is also critical in the determination of the probability that a particular intervention will contribute to or compromise a goal such as comfort.

Nurses advocating for the patient's interests will also ensure that the patient's priority needs are addressed (biologic, psychosocial, and spiritual needs). As health care reform increasingly fragments services, the likelihood decreases that patients will be cared for by health care professionals, including nurses, familiar with them. Nurse managers must critique nursing systems of care in which no one nurse is responsible for the overall care plan and for identifying and resolving concerns important to patients and families. Often the only patient problems receiving attention today are physical problems. It is nursing's charge to ensure that holistic, individualized, prioritized care is a reality, especially for today's elders.

Preventing and Resolving Ethical Conflict

Nurse case managers who wish to prevent ethical conflict will work in care settings where it is established that preventing and resolving ethical conflict fall within the authority of each health care professional engaged in patient care. This conviction will facilitate early recognition of problematic situations and timely communication among all those involved in decision-making. When communication among the patient, family, and caregiving team fails to resolve the problem, an ethics consult or meeting of the institutional ethics committee may be indicated. Sensitivity to and the ability to communicate about the factors contributing to ethical conflict are essential to successful mediation of these conflicts. When mediation is not attempted, conflicts tend to escalate, and it is not unusual for patients and families to develop hostile adversarial relationships that all too frequently end in litigation or at the very least in alienation and a distrust of health care professionals that colors future interactions with caregivers. Nurse case managers should be aware of the ethics resources available in their institutions and professional community and use them when needed (see Box 33-4). Mastery of ethical decision-making to simplify conflict resolution is also important, as shown in Box 33-5. Box 33-6 summarizes critical elements of the advocacy role of the nurse case manager.

█ MORAL INTEGRITY AND THE NURSE CASE MANAGER

Mark Siegler (1984), a physician ethicist, describes three stages in the evolution of medicine and notes how medicine's focus has changed from one stage to the next. In the first stage, the *age of paternalism*, physicians focused on the good of the patient as defined by the physician. In the second stage, the *age of autonomy*, the focus remained the good of the patient but as defined by the patient himself or herself. In the third stage of medicine, which Siegler termed *the age of bureaucratic parsimony*, the good of the patient is weighed against the good of society. Today we can add a fourth stage of medicine to Siegler's list, which might be termed *the age of for-profit medicine*, in which health care professionals (or other decision makers) weigh the good of the patient against the good of stockholders. These are profound paradigmatic changes that have the potential to dramatically influence the practice of professional nursing. Nurse case managers who wish to preserve their moral integrity in today's changing health care milieu face multiple challenges. Six of these challenges are explored on the following pages.

Challenge 1: Fidelity to the Unique Needs of Individual Patients

When asked to list descriptors of quality care, many nurses use words like *holistic, individualized, prioritized,* and *continuous.* It is interesting to reflect on the reality that underlies these descriptors and to ask if we are still able to practice nursing in a way that makes this type of care anything more than interesting rhetoric. Are the type of nurse-patient relationships that make holistic, individualized, and prioritized care possible a reality today, or are they mere relics of a bygone past when nurses had the time to really get to know their patients? For example, nurses in a medical center were discussing the care received by a patient who had recently died from end-stage breast cancer. Apparently the patient was concerned about seeing her two children, ages 17 and 20 years, who had stopped coming to visit because they were overwhelmed by the degree of her illness, especially since their father had died of a brain tumor 2 years earlier. What the staff realized after the patient died was that no one had picked up on her requests to see her children and had not arranged a visit, so the patient died without ever seeing her children again. Horrified that this had been allowed to happen, the nurses realized that not one of them had seen this request as his or her responsibility in their attempts to provide highly technical rescue medicine that was responsive to each medical complication and crisis. One nurse caught herself saying, "I am familiar with 'the case' but didn't really know this woman."

BOX 33-5 ▶ **A PROCESS OF ETHICAL DECISION-MAKING**

ASSESSMENT
Gather and document pertinent medical and nonmedical facts:
- *Who:* persons who have the authority for decision-making and the responsibility for its consequences and the effect on them personally of the decision needing to be made
- *What:* patient's medical condition, prognosis, and therapeutic options and probable consequences of treatment and nontreatment; patient's beliefs, values, interests; related family, caregiver, and institution beliefs, values, and interests; pertinent legal and administrative considerations
- *When:* time parameters
- *Where:* setting
- *Why:* variables creating or fueling conflict

DIAGNOSIS
Identify the ethical issue(s) as clearly as possible. Distinguish ethical problems from communication or general patient care management problems.

Planning
1. Identify the objective of doing the ethics workup.
2. List and explore courses of action likely to achieve this goal. Think through the short- and long-term consequences of each.
3. Think of the ethical justification for each course of action and defend it against competing options:
   a. Compatibility with aims of nursing and demands of nurse-patient relationship
   b. Approaches to ethical inquiry: ethical principles, care perspective, virtue theory, communitarianism
   c. Grounding and source of ethics: philosophical (based in reason), theological (based in religion), sociocultural (based in custom)
4. Clearly identify what you believe to be the moral obligations of the nurse.
5. Select the course of action you are best able to defend against counter arguments.
6. Seek assistance if unable to work through the above steps independently.

IMPLEMENTATION
Implement the selected course of action and assess consequences.

EVALUATION
Critique your decision, incorporating feedback from involved participants if possible. Decide how you would respond to a similar case in the future. Determine whether you need to do something now to optimize future responses. Interventions may be personal (e.g., learn more about advance directives) or institutional (e.g., clarify the hospital's DNR policy and reeducate caregivers about the policy).

From Taylor, C. (1997). Ethical perspectives. In M.M. Burke & M.B. Walsh (Eds), *Gerontologic nursing: Care of the elderly,* 2nd ed. St. Louis: Mosby.

Clinical practice guidelines based on aggregate data, critical pathways, and algorithms all seem to draw attention away from individual patients to population aggregates. Each of these standardizing methodologies has the potential to improve patient outcomes by keeping achievable target outcomes consciously before patients and the caregiving team. Whether these methodologies are used to improve care for individual patients or to force individuals to jump through predetermined hoops that may or

---

BOX 33-6 ▶ ADVOCACY COMPETENCIES

SUPPORTING AUTONOMY
1. Determining and documenting the patient's decision-making capacity; ensuring that agency or institution policies specify how this is to be done, and identify responsible parties
2. Protecting the right of patients with decision-making capacity to be self-determining
   a. Facilitate communication and documentation of the patient's preferences
   b. Anticipate the types of treatment decisions that likely will need to be made
   c. Assist in the preparation of advance directives
3. Promoting authentic autonomy; authentic decisions reflect the individual's identity, decisional history, and moral norms
4. Identifying the morally as well as legally valid surrogate decision maker for patients who lack decision-making capacity
5. Supporting the surrogate decision maker, clarifying the surrogate decision maker's role
6. Identifying limits to patient or surrogate autonomy and limits to caregiver autonomy
7. Developing agency or institution policies that identify the caregivers responsible for and the procedures to be used to identify and support the appropriate decision makers

PROMOTING PATIENT WELL-BEING
Clarifying the goal of therapy: cure and restoration, stabilization of functioning, preparation for a comfortable, dignified death
1. Determining the medical effectiveness of therapy
2. Weighing the benefits and burdens of therapy
3. Ensuring that all interventions are consistent with the overall goal of therapy
4. Ensuring that the patient's priority needs are addressed (biologic, psychosocial, and spiritual needs)
5. Ensuring continuity of care as patient is transferred among services and within and without the institution
6. Weighing the moral relevance of third-party interests (family, caregiver, institution, society)
7. Identifying and addressing forces within society and the health care system that compromise patient well-being

PREVENTING AND RESOLVING ETHICAL CONFLICT
1. Establishing that preventing and resolving ethical conflict falls within the authority of all health care professionals engaged in the care of a patient
2. Developing awareness of and sensitivity to the conscious and unconscious sources of conflict
3. Facilitating timely communication among those involved in decision-making: one-on-one meetings and periodic meetings of the patient, family, and interdisciplinary team to clarify goals and plan of care
4. Documenting pertinent information on the patient record
5. Referring unresolved ethical issues to the ethics consult team or the institutional ethics committee
6. Identifying and addressing system variables that contribute to recurrent ethical problems

From Taylor, C. (1997). Ethical perspectives. In M.M. Burke & M.B. Walsh (Eds), *Gerontologic nursing: Care of the elderly*, 2nd ed. St. Louis: Mosby.

may not contribute to their well-being may in large part be determined by the stance adopted by nurse case managers. Never before have patients been so in need of nurse advocates who know the system well enough to ensure that it is responsive to the unique needs of individual patients and their families. In the past our lack of skill in "working the system" limited our power to effectively serve as advocates for patients. Today the nurse case manager has the authority to pull together and to coordinate the services each individual patient needs and to modify systems that are unresponsive to patient need. How this authority will be used remains to be seen.

Challenge 2: Competing Loyalties

The nurse case manager's ability to modify the system to meet individual patient needs depends on his or her loyalties. When asked to whom are you accountable, nurse case managers may reply, "to the patient," "to the hospital," "to my boss," "to myself," or "to the caregiving team." *If I see myself as primarily accountable to an employing institution who pays my salary and who is driven by a financial bottom line, I may be reluctant to advocate for a patient who needs additional time to achieve target outcomes before discharge.* It is helpful to consciously reflect on one's loyalties and to identify potential conflicts. Once again, the rhetoric of nursing reminds us that our primary concern is the patient. Unfortunately, today it is not uncommon for nursing practice to reflect concern for anything but this reality.

Challenge 3: Resolving Role Conflict

Among other things, the nurse case manager is a service coordinator, an advocate, a counselor, and a gatekeeper. Obviously, where one works, the needs of the patients served, and the mix of professionals on the caregiving team will all influence the roles played by the nurse case manager and the amount of time spent in each role. It can be helpful to use a pie chart to record the portion of time you spend in each role, on average, on any given day and to compare your chart with those of others in comparable positions. Reflection and discussion should yield greater insight into whether your personal mix of roles is adequately serving your patients and your employing institution. An important question to ask is, "What determines which of your roles takes precedence when role conflict exists?"

> The needs of your employer: "Utilization review says she has to be out of here by noon tomorrow at the latest."
>
> The needs of your patient: "We just have to get her pain under better control before she goes home, and this might take another day or two; they just changed her medicine this evening."
>
> Your unique talents: "I don't know how utilization review does it. . . . I could never talk with an already overburdened family about the need to take their mom or dad home before they think they are ready."

Our moral integrity makes it imperative for us never to allow our priorities to be dictated solely by our employing agency or institution. As the health care system changes, we need to reflect more carefully on what may be termed the "nonnegotiables" of our practice. What are those elements of professional nursing care that we cannot surrender without ceasing to be nurses?

Challenge 4: Owning Responsibilities to Underserved Populations

Nurses have both individual and corporate responsibilities to underserved populations. Nurse case managers are uniquely situated to gather the type of data that can be used to demonstrate to policy makers that the needs of select groups of patients are not being adequately addressed. Recurrent admissions of patients whose problems could have been more successfully addressed had the patients been seen earlier should be a signal that health needs are not being adequately met. Whether the patients are homeless men and women; a large population of abused children, spouses, or the elderly; incarcerated individuals;

those with psychiatric or mental health problems; or simply those with inadequate insurance, nurse case managers can, if they choose, lead caregiving teams in gathering the type of data that will convince policy makers of the need for system reform.

Challenge 5: Identifying Personal Biases

In the interests of providing care that is just and oriented to giving each person his or her due, it is essential that nurse case managers attempt to identify personal sources of bias or discrimination. Reflection usually reveals the presence of some factors that positively or negatively predispose us to patients. An air of helplessness in a patient may elicit one nurse's mothering instinct and disgust in another. Similarly, age, gender, body size, occupation, skin color, nationality, culture, religion, financial status, and lifestyle factors can all influence the way we perceive and relate to patients. One nurse case manager who had worked in an AIDS unit for several years confided that she slowly realized after reflecting on her work that she treated patients differently on the basis of how they had acquired AIDS. "I'm much more patient and giving of myself to those who acquired it through sexual transmission rather than by sharing needles." This brief vignette illustrates the importance of identifying our personal biases. We need to be as conscious as we can of what inclines (or disinclines) us to "go to bat" for a patient whose needs are not being met.

Challenge 6: Balancing Care for Others with Appropriate Self-Care

A final word of caution. The tremendous potential nurse case managers have for influencing the delivery of health care in the United States may result in some nurses literally sacrificing themselves on the altar of quality care for those entrusted to their practice. While responsibility and accountability are essential elements of ethical competence, in excess they can fan the flames of burnout and quickly reduce a competent, caring professional to a lifeless mannequin. When deficient, nurses poorly serve their patients and colleagues, who quickly learn not to trust nurses who consistently place their needs and well-being over and above the needs of those they work for and with. The ethically competent nurse knows how to balance competing responsibilities to self, family, and work and is able to skillfully meet both professional and personal obligations. This dimension of moral integrity merits ongoing reflection and may be aided by discussion with colleagues. Because no two nurse case managers will view their responsibilities to patients, the caregiving team, and themselves in exactly the same way, discussions about what constitutes acceptable boundaries of responsibility and accountability can be helpful.

These are exciting times. More individuals than ever before are claiming as an achievable goal quality affordable care for all. Unfortunately, some of the means being used to achieve this goal are already suspect. Nurse case managers are on the front lines of the revolution in health care. Never before have the everyday choices of practicing nurses had greater potential to set standards of excellence that will serve us all. Ethical competence is not an option for nurse case managers. The health and well-being of all those we serve literally depend on their ethical competence.

References

American Hospital Association (1991). *Put it in writing: A guide to promoting advance directives.* Chicago: American Hospital Association.

American Nurses Association (2004). *Nursing: Scope and standards of practice*, 2nd ed. Washington, D.C.: American Nurses Publishing.

American Nurses Association (2001). *Code of ethics for nurses with interpretive statements.* Washington, D.C.: American Nurses Publishing.

Beauchamp, T.L., & Childress, J.F. (1994). *Principles of biomedical ethics*, 4th ed. New York: Oxford University Press.

Benner, P., & Wrubel, J. (1989). *The primacy of caring.* Menlo Park, Calif: Addison-Wesley Publishing Co.

Clouser, K.D., & Gert, B. (1994). Morality vs. principlism. In R. Gillon, (Ed.), *Principles of health care ethics.* New York: John Wiley & Sons.

Concern for Dying (1991). *Advance directive protocols and the patient self-determination act: A resource manual for the development of institutional protocols.* New York: Concern for Dying.

Fletcher, J.C., Miller, F.G., & Spencer, E.M. (1995). Clinical ethics: History, content and resources. In J.C. Fletcher, C.A. Hite, P.A. Lombardo, & M.F. Marshall (Eds.), *Introduction to clinical ethics* (pp. 3-17). Frederick, Md.: University Publishing Group.

Fry, S. (1989). The role of caring in a theory of nursing ethics. *Hypatia, 4,* 88-103.

Gadow, S. (1989). Clinical subjectivity: Advocacy with silent patients. *Nursing Clinics of North America, 24*(2), 535-541.

Gadow, S. (1980). Existential advocacy: Philosophical foundations of nursing. In S.F. Spicker & S. Gadow (Eds), *Nursing: Images and ideals: Opening dialogue with the humanities* (pp. 79-101). New York: Springer.

Gilligan, C. (1982). *In a different voice: Psychological theory and women's development.* Cambridge, Mass.: Harvard University Press.

The Hastings Center. (1987). *Guidelines on the termination of life-sustaining treatment and the care of the dying.* Bloomington and Indianapolis: Indiana University Press.

Jameton, A. (1993). Dilemmas of moral distress: Moral responsibility and nursing practice. *AWHONN's Clinical Issues in Perinatal and Women's Health Nursing, 4*(4), 542-551.

Patient Self-Determination Act of 1990, in OBRA 1990 (P.L. 101-508, H.R. 5835). Pellegrino, E.D. (1989). Withholding and withdrawing treatments: Ethics at the bedside. *Clinical Neurosurgery, 35,* 164-184.

Pellegrino, E.D. (1989). Withholding and withdrawing of treatments: Ethics at the bedside. *Clinical Neurosurgery, 35,* 164-184.

President's Commission for the Study of Ethical Problems in Medicine and Biomedical and Behavioral Research (1982). *Making health care decisions* (Vols. 1-3). Washington, DC: U.S. Government Printing Office.

President's Commission for the Study of Ethical Problems in Medicine and Biomedical and Behavioral Research (1983). *Deciding to forego life-sustaining treatment: Ethical, medical, and legal issues in treatment decisions.* Washington, DC: U.S. Government Printing Office.

Siegler, M. (1984). Should age be a criterion in health care? *Hastings Center Report, 14*(5), 24-27.

Taylor, C. (1993). Nursing ethics: The role of caring. *AWHONN'S Clinical Issues in Perinatal and Women's Health Nursing, 4*(4), 552-560.

Taylor, C. (1995). Rethinking nursing's basic competencies. *Journal of Nursing Care Quality, 9*(4), 1-13.

Watson, J. (1985). *Nursing: The philosophy and science of caring.* Boulder, Colo.: Colorado Associated University Press. Content adapted from Taylor, C. (1997). *The morality internal to the practice of nursing.* Unpublished doctoral dissertation, Georgetown University, Washington, D.C.

Case Management and Information Technology

Roy L. Simpson

CHAPTER OVERVIEW

Information technology is pivotal to the future success of case management because of its potential to help professional nurse case managers perform their jobs more effectively and efficiently. This is especially true for those who are involved in beyond-the-walls case management, which still depends heavily on paper-based processes. Because of its pervasiveness, information technology's greatest opportunity for case managed care lies in the development of a national information network that links nursing information systems with patients in their own homes via computers. Such a network would allow nursing professionals to satisfy the patient's need for confidentiality and 24-hour access to information support while meeting nursing's need to reach ever-growing patient populations.

Among innovative efforts already under way that successfully offer case-managed care via computer networks to patients with diseases such as acquired immunodeficiency syndrome (AIDS) and Alzheimers is ComputerLink, a special computer network designed to help nurses support home-based care. The computer's capacity to offer daily follow-up contact, to serve as a medium for asking and answering questions, to provide voice reminders or alarms to signal anything from medications to checkups, and to contain costs are characteristics that will contribute to the success of networks that both case management professional and patient alike can access. The acceptance of a universal nursing minimum data set to codify nursing knowledge will also be crucial to this process.

Despite advances in information technology, case management in the mid-1990s continues to be a largely manual, labor-intensive process. Yet information technology, like no other tool available to professional nurse case managers, promises to make case management more viable, effective, and powerful. To be sure, technologically sophisticated hospitals using within-the-walls case management protocols likely are already benefiting greatly from existing clinical information systems and patient tracking systems. In these institutions, automation primarily is used for documentation assistance and managing patient follow-up schedules.

When it comes to beyond-the-walls case management, however, few institutions have the information technology tools needed to liberate professional nurse case managers from intensive paper-based processes. Yet it is precisely in this area—in case management beyond the walls of the institution—that information technology holds the greatest promise.

The real opportunity for case-managed care lies in the direction in which technology is currently and rapidly moving—toward the advent of *pervasive* technology or *pervasive* health care information networks or infrastructures.

A pervasive technology is one that is more noticeable by its absence than its presence, in the same way that automobiles, televisions, and telephones are today. In other words, a hotel room—or even a hospital room—today without a phone or television would be an unpleasant surprise. Yet it is likely that within 10 years, a hotel room or a hospital room without a *computer as well* will also be an oddity. The wild excitement over the Internet and the World Wide Web is only a hint at how powerfully the information superhighway is beginning to permeate the consciousness of American society.

This is particularly true of younger generations who are as comfortable with computers as toddlers of previous generations were with telephones. With this in mind, it is important to remember that only people born before a technology becomes pervasive think of it as "technology"; all others think of it as part of the environment. Thus today's schoolchildren do not think of television and telephones as technology; they simply cannot imagine life without them. They are part of the landscape of modern existence. Tomorrow's children—and tomorrow's nurses—will feel the same way about computers.

In this march toward pervasiveness, technology historically passes through the following four predictable stages:

1. Development as experimental curiosities as individuals try to solve a particular problem in laboratories or—in the case of computers—in their garages or basements
2. Use by a small number of specialists to solve a specific problem
3. Mass development as it becomes easily manufactured and commonplace (although still used primarily by a small fraction of the population who have specialized training)
4. Total pervasiveness and accessibility by the average citizen, as exemplified by telephones, televisions, and radios.

Although health care technology will never move beyond the third stage (after all, it will always require individuals with specialized training to operate), the *network* in which information is shared will indeed become pervasive. One need only look at the explosion of current interest in the Internet and the World Wide Web to get a glimpse of how information networks will pervade American society. Indeed the technology to deliver multimedia services over telephone wires via the television has existed since the early 1990s. Cable television companies and telephone operating companies are fighting it out to determine who will "own" the ability to deliver information technology services to the home. In other words, this convergence of technology means that the television—the current focus of entertainment in most American homes—will also be the focus for computer interaction (i.e., the television will also *be* the computer—it will be possible to go from watching a television show to attaching a keyboard to the set and to instantly begin "surfing" information networks or communicating with caregivers via bulletin boards).

The development of a pervasive national information network has tremendous ramifications for the nurse case manager. A national network will link nursing information systems and, as a result, nurse case managers, to patients in their own homes via computers (or multimedia centers—the television as computer or vice versa). It is even imaginable that within 10 years all homes will come equipped with a television, just as they come equipped with ovens. Prognosticators also predict that there will be a computer company or information company, similar to the telephone company, that individuals will call to get their computer turned on and linked into the network (just as one calls the power company to get the power turned on). Taken to its logical conclusion, this prediction sees an information utility company just like the telephone or electrical utility. This information utility will likely be run like any other utility, with some sort of public service commission in charge and with hefty governmental laws that regulate distribution of services.

NETWORK LINKAGE AND HOME CARE

With network linkage connecting patients with each other and with nurses through a computer network, the nursing professional can satisfy the patient's need for confidentiality and 24-hour access to informational support. Network linkage also supports nursing's need to reach out to an ever-expanding patient population. Today nurses are already experimenting with case-managed care via computer networks for such diseases as acquired immunodeficiency syndrome (AIDS) and Alzheimer's with immensely positive results.

Consider the work of Patricia Brennan, associate professor of nursing and systems engineering at the Frances Payne Bolton School of Nursing at Case Western Reserve University, who used computer networks to link AIDS and Alzheimer's disease patients' family caregivers to nurses and with each respective subgroup. Participants in the study were provided with terminals and modems and given access to ComputerLink, a special computer network designed to help nurses support home-based care. Users were free to access the network any time of the day or night at no cost. Each participant was provided with 1.5 hours of free training and ongoing assistance in using the system.

The ComputerLink network offered the following three primary modules:

1. Communications module, which included a bulletin board area for "conversing" with others in the same predicament and a question-and-answer section for anonymous postings to nurses
2. Decision support model, which helped participants make self-care choices using a structured decision analysis method
3. Information module, a database filled with encyclopedic data about the disease

A project nurse was assigned as chief moderator, responsible for reading all public "conversations" and notations (and therefore for assessing information gaps in the participating populations), maintaining the currency of the electronic encyclopedia, troubleshooting for all participants, and acting as clinical expert in all capabilities.

The results were positive. The typical user got on the system 125 times, or an average of four to five times a week. According to Brennan, "testimonial evidence of perceived support abounded in both groups of participants. Postings on the public forum contained messages of encouragement, ideas for self-care and for managing with the formal health system, and counsel to peers" (Simpson, 1994).

There were also many nursing benefits. Case managers were able to disseminate information to patients more easily and quickly. Nurses could also control misinformation by ensuring that outdated information was not accessible to users. Privacy over the network ensured that all users could learn from an interaction, not just one patient at one time.

Brennan's research project proved that "continuity of care in home care can be achieved through both traditional and non-traditional means—sending nurses out to the homes or through novel use of existing technology such as computer terminals" (Simpson, 1994).

NETWORK LINKAGE AND CASE MANAGEMENT

Having a network that can be accessed by case management professionals and patients alike will be key to the success of case management in the future. If computers do indeed become as ubiquitous as telephones and televisions in people's homes, case management beyond the walls becomes a viable reality. Without ever leaving the hospital, nurses could have daily contact with patients for follow-ups, questions about medications, patient follow-through, and so on.

With voice or sound computer-generated reminders or alarms, nurses could remind patients or family members about everything from taking insulin shots, to changing their dressings, to coming in for a check-up. Via the same network, patients could report to the caregiver unusual symptoms or concerns about their care. Although such communications could never replace the personal contact and personal care that is so important to the professional practice of nursing, they would certainly alleviate the strain on nurses who must manage the details involved in community-based health care delivery.

In addition, using networked computers would support the institution's desire to contain costs. If day-to-day communications and educational issues are addressed via computer, resources could be allocated more cost effectively, ensuring that nursing professionals spend their face-to-face time with more critical situations.

Once a nationwide network of health care information is in place, it can be surmised that "back office" linkage will be an important part of the network. And it will likely be expected that the case manager will manage the various critical pathways and treatment protocols outlined by different payers. In this way the case manager truly becomes an advocate for the patient and an intermediary for the institution, ensuring not only that the patient receives the best care but also that the institution follows prescribed protocols to obtain reimbursement.

Insurance companies and third-party payers are already playing a big part in the development of the health care information network so that benefit and financial information can be managed quickly and efficiently on the patient's behalf. Payers and institutions alike will likely be the focus for collecting all the data related to patient care, performing variance analyses and indicating benchmark outcomes in an ongoing attempt to determine the best protocols while containing costs. The debate as to who will set critical pathways and treatment protocols continues to rage: the payers or the providers? To have a strong voice in this process, nursing must be able to identify and codify nursing services and outline its contributions to the patient's outcomes.

The result of establishing benchmarks and of being held to standards of care will be profound. For example, if 3 of 10 patients with a cholecystectomy develop a nonsocomial infection after surgery and the benchmark is 1 of 10, the competence of the nursing care will be closely scrutinized. Nurse managers and case managers must be prepared for this eventuality.

Clearly a pervasive network of this kind will empower nurses, particularly case managers, at the same time that it makes them more accountable for their actions. The case manager of the future needs to be an expert not only in clinical care but also in critical analysis of enormous amounts of data on which decisions will be based.

PREPARING FOR THE FUTURE

A common health care network would not, and could not, replace nursing contact. However, it would serve as a powerful support tool in the evolution of case management. It may be 10 years or more before a pervasive network is in place whereby nursing would have both the informational infrastructure and the ability to contact and communicate with patients electronically. The advent or acceptance of a universally accepted nursing minimum data set is critical to this process. Nursing must be able to codify its knowledge in order to be able to properly use computer networks and share nursing information and outcomes with other medical and nonmedical caregivers.

Nursing has always been able to adapt to technological advances. Fifty years ago, there was no such thing as an intensive care unit (ICU). Today, nurses are critical to the success of ICUs. In the same way we must prepare for a future that will be dramatically different—a future of vast computer connections that can link patients with caregivers, caregivers with each other, and more. The promise of case management will be achieved by using information technology to share information and communicate with patients and caregivers beyond the walls of the institution. It is up to nurses *today* to prepare themselves for such a future.

Reference

Simpson, R.L. (1994, Winter). Computer networks show great promise in supporting AIDS patients. *Nursing Administration Quarterly, 18*(2), 92-95.

35 Telehealth Applications for Case Management

Diane J. Skiba
Lena Sorensen
Mary B. McCarthy
Vicki J. Brownrigg

CHAPTER OVERVIEW

The purposes of this chapter are to introduce the concept of telehealth; provide examples of telehealth use in women's health, chronic disease management and mental health; summarize the evidence to support telehealth; and identify existing issues and challenges. This chapter ends with a case scenario that illustrates how the case manager of the future will incorporate telehealth tools into her practice.

Imagine a world where no matter who you are or where you are, you can get the health care you need when you need it.

Office for Advancement of Telehealth, 2001

INTRODUCTION

Telehealth opportunities using emerging technologies have the capacity to shape and transform the delivery of health care and how case managers interact with their clients. These telehealth tools will allow case managers to interact with their clients and other health care professionals without concerns for geographic or time boundaries. Telehealth tools allow case managers to augment their practice, extend their reach into communities, and collaboratively interact with patients and other health care professionals.

DEFINITIONS AND HISTORY

The concept of telehealth evolved over the last century. Providing health care at a distance is not a new phenomenon. Telemedicine efforts can be traced to the introduction of the telephone. Its first documented use in the journal *The Lancet* was in 1897, when it was used to diagnosis a child with croup (Darkens & Cary, 2000). Pion, Altman, Hyatt, & Linden (1999) give the following two other early examples. First, in 1879, subscribers to the telephone were assigned telephone numbers because of a measles epidemic (before the epidemic, there were no assigned numbers). A Massachusetts physician recommended the numeric coding. Second, in 1870s, a telephone exchange was set up between 20 physicians and a local drugstore in Hartford, Connecticut. Most health care professionals attribute the start of telemedicine in the late 1950s with initial efforts focused on providing health care consultation to rural or remote environments (Bloch, 1999). An early example was the use of a closed-circuit television system to provide education and clinical consultation between the Nebraska Psychiatric Institute and a remote state mental facility. A project in Boston connecting Logan International Airport with Massachusetts General Hospital demonstrated the use of real-time consultations using the state-of-the-art technology of 1973, black and white television cameras and monitors. These are only a few of the historic examples of using technology to support and provide health care.

Maheu, Whitten, and Allen (2001) reported that Willemain and Mark (1971) were the first to coin the term *telemedicine*, and it simply meant the provision of health services, clinical information, and education over a distance using some form of telecommunications. The definition of *telemedicine* varies, but there are common elements found across all definitions. It has been simply defined by Wootton (1995) as "health care carried out at a distance." The Institute of Medicine (1996) broadly defined *telemedicine* as "the use of electronic information and communication technologies to provide and support health care when distance separates the participants."

In nursing, the American Nurses Association (ANA, 1997) wanted a more inclusive term and proceeded to define *telehealth* as "delivery of health care services or activities with time and distance barriers removed and using technologies such as telephones, computers, interactive video transmissions." Thus, *telehealth* is an umbrella term that encompasses *telemedicine, telenursing, teleradiology*, and *telepsychiatry*. Accordingly, telenursing is considered a form of telehealth where nursing practice is delivered via telecommunications.

According to the Office for the Advancement of Telehealth (2001),

> Telehealth is the use of electronic information and telecommunications technologies to support long-distance clinical health care, patient and professional health-related education, public health and health administration.

Additional terms were added to our vocabulary as new technologies emerged and as the use of the Internet by patients increased. Two such terms are *e-health* and *e-disease* management. *E-health* is used to refer to all types of electronic health care delivered over the Internet (McLendon, 2000). Health care broadly encompasses direct care, informational, educational, and commercial services as well as computer applications (Savas, Parekh, & Fisher, 1999). Many view e-health as being different from telehealth in that it is consumer centric. Eysenbach (2001) best summarizes it as follows:

> "e-Health is an emerging field in the intersection of medical informatics, public health and business, referring to health services and information delivered or enhanced through the Internet and related technologies. In a broader sense, the term characterizes not only a technical development, but also a state-of-mind, a way of thinking, an attitude, and a commitment for networked, global thinking, to improve health care locally, regionally, and worldwide by using information and communication technology." (p. e 20)

According to LeGrow and Metzger (November, 2001), e-disease management is defined as "any application of web-based technologies to organize disease management" (p. 6). e-Disease management includes tools that facilitate patient self-management, support for clinicians, and collaborative support between patients and their clinicians. In their report, LeGrow and Metzger (November, 2001) outlined that *e-disease* management tools can support the following components:
- Patient risk screening
- Population screening
- Guidelines and protocols
- Decision support at point-of-care
- Patient empowerment
- Outreach care management

- Cross-continuum coordination
- Team-based care
- Alternate encounters
- Performance feedback

TELEHEALTH APPLICATIONS

With this introduction and review of definitions, we can explore examples of telehealth tools used by nurses to manage their clients. These examples represent a fraction of the activity in nursing and health care and illustrate the unique telehealth tools that can augment a case manager's practice. Many examples have contributed to the growing evidence to support the use of telehealth. First is a look at telehealth applications in women's health care. Nurses, highly involved in the management of women's health care, used several telehealth tools to augment their practice. Another set of examples illustrates the use of telehealth tools in the ever-burgeoning area referred to as *e-disease management.* The final area to explore is the use of telehealth applications to address mental health issues. One of the early uses of telecommunications was video conferencing to extend psychiatric services to rural areas. It is not surprising that behavioral change management strategies now include the use of information and communication technologies.

WOMEN'S HEALTH

Although still nascent, tools used in the management of women's health care continue to develop as information and telecommunications technologies evolve, enabling case managers to expand their roles and extend their reach in providing efficient, cost-effective, high-quality standards of individualized care for this vast population. Attesting to the cost-effectiveness (as well as increased favorable outcomes) of telehealth are the results of a 3-year study of 100 women, within health maintenance organizations, diagnosed with preterm labor (PTL) in single-gestation pregnancies. The patients were divided into: *Group 1* (telehealth group), comprised of 60 women who received telehealth services (home uterine activity monitoring [HUAM] with daily telephonic nursing contact); and *group 2* (control group), consisting of 40 women who received standard care without the HUAM outpatient service. Group 1 averaged later gestational age and higher average birth weight at time of delivery, fewer average total nursery days, and fewer neonatal intensive care admissions than did Group 2 (6.7% versus 40%). The average total per pregnancy cost in group 1 was $7,225, as opposed to $21,684 for group 2, a savings of $14,459 (Morrison, Bergauer, Jacques, Coleman, & Stanziano, 2001).

Introduced by nurses in the late 1800s, telephone triage remains the most widely used and recognized element of telephone nursing. Routinely included in this invaluable service are the dispensing of advice, exchange of information, appointment scheduling, referrals, symptom and disease management, and demand management (Greenberg, 2000), such as ordering of patient medications, supplies, and equipment. For example, nurse case managers and clinical pharmacist support for patients are available from Matria Healthcare, Inc., telephonically toll-free 24 hours a day, 7 days per week (B. Doyle, personal communication, May 9, 2003). Thus, PTL patients with activity restrictions can obtain tocolytic medications for their subcutaneous infusion pumps, diabetics can obtain insulin, and obstetric patients on anticoagulant therapy can obtain heparin when timely administration of these medications is critical.

The importance of any tool that supports the case management functions of assessment, planning, implementation, and evaluation (Greenberg, 2000), or those that further enhance their roles as coordinators, facilitators, and advocates (Redford & Parkins, 1997), cannot be overemphasized. There are still a significant number of people for whom health care through the use of computers, or other electronic devices, is not feasible because of a lack of training or access or when communication by computer is not possible because of personal incapacity. For these patients, the telephone is an especially vital case management tool.

Largely because of its unique TRAX system, which offers a broad array of secure and Health Insurance Portability and Accountability Act (HIPAA)-compliant features, Matria Healthcare has become the technology leader in evidence-based disease and case management services. It has attained this position by consistently adhering to practices of administration and delivery of criteria-based assessments, education, interventions, and outcomes reporting commensurate with nationally recognized critical and high-quality standards for the entire population it manages. Patients are managed 24 hours a day, 7 days a week, and data updates are transmitted using state-of-the-art information technology equipment. As patient outcomes are tracked and graphed, their authorized providers or case managers throughout the continuum of care can access real-time data. (B. Doyle, personal communication, May 9, 2003). Matria has been in the vanguard of case management since 1984 and is exemplar in offering a wide variety of services to help manage women's health patients, among others. The types of case management services include patients with PTL, pregnancy-induced hypertension (PIH), diabetes in pregnancy (through their *Care* Link program), preterm premature rupture of membranes (pPROM), management of multiple gestation pregnancies, coagulation disorders, and intravenous hydration (to include management of patients with hyperemesis gravidarum), and nutrition services. The TRAX system also aids in the management of non–pregnancy-related cancer, cardiac disease, asthma, chronic pain, diabetes, and depression (B. Doyle, personal communication, May 9, 2003).

In further support of the needs of these patients and their case managers, Matria's secure and HIPAA-compliant TRAX system offers case note and decision support capabilities, user to-do lists, demographic data, individualized patient care plans, real-time access to management and outcomes reports, and online summaries of condition-specific assessment reports to authorized users. This case management system also restratifies after each assessment (B. Doyle, personal communication, May 9, 2003), keeping the patient's status updated while including the patient as an active partner in the health care process, rather than an object in it, thereby strengthening the patient-provider relationship.

Matria's peripheral devices, which allow daily and PRN home monitoring of all patients, such as uterine activity monitoring of patients at risk for preterm delivery; the blood pressure, weight, fetal movement, and proteinuria of pregnancy induced hypertension (PIH) patients (with their OB-1 device); and the vital signs and blood glucose readings of diabetic patients, can all be transmitted electronically and immediately downloaded into computers while alerting nurse case managers in red when thresholds are exceeded. Monitoring results are also immediately recorded into the computer's outcomes reports section (B. Doyle, personal communication, May 9, 2003).

Videoconferencing, or interactive televideo, is another means by which women's health care may be enhanced because it allows for spontaneous meetings, reaching near or remote areas, particularly when travel may be difficult or ill advised. For example, a woman with a multiple gestation pregnancy in rural Montana may easily be included in the patient care conference being held on her behalf, along with her case manager, nurses, physicians, and social worker. The flexibility of this technology encourages collaboration between all members of the health care team while maintaining a provider-patient partnership, enhancing patient empowerment while accelerating the decision-making process and allowing team members to obtain expert advice from distant sites. In addition, it may allow a nurse case manager caring for a patient with a history of postpartum depression to assess her patient's affect and thereby perhaps contribute significantly to improved patient care outcomes.

E-DISEASE MANAGEMENT

It is within the telehealth application of monitoring and tracking of patient status that the majority of telehealth studies are reported. Most are investigating the application of telehealth technology in chronic illnesses such as diabetes mellitus (Ahring, Joyce, Ahring, & Nadir, 1992; Marrero et al., 1995; Whitlock, Brown, Moore, & Pavliscsak, 2000), cardiovascular disease (Ades et al., 1999; Cartwright, Dalton, Swindells, Rushant, & Mooney, 1992; Friedman et al., 1996), and asthma (Finkelstein, Hripcsak, & Cabrera, 1998).

In the diabetes studies, Whitlock et al. (2000) found significantly lower hemoglobin A1c (Hb_{A1c}) and greater weight loss in an experimental group of type 2 diabetic patients after 3 months of weekly audio/videoconferencing with telehealth nurses and monthly conferencing with primary care physicians. In diabetes studies with similar designs using modem transmission of blood glucose data over the telephone, Ahring et al. (1992) reported a significant lower Hb_{A1c} in their study of 42 adults with type 1 diabetes, whereas Marrero et al. (1995) failed to find significance in 106 children with diabetes. The two studies reported similar methodology with the exceptions of the frequency of transmission of data and the age of the subjects. The Ahring study transmitted the glucose information weekly, whereas the Marrero study transmitted the information every 2 weeks.

In a randomized controlled study of 267 patients aged 60 or above receiving telehealth cardiovascular monitoring and counseling, Friedman et al. (1996) found significant changes in adherence to antihypertensive medications, systolic blood pressure, and diastolic blood pressure. Ades et al. (2000) found no significant differences in peak aerobic capacity and quality of life domains between patients undergoing cardiac rehabilitation in their homes using electrocardiographic and voice transtelephonic monitoring and patients undergoing traditional, on-site cardiac rehabilitation. In a study of hypertensive obstetric patients, Cartwright et al. (1992) found no difference in anxiety levels between those undergoing home blood pressure monitoring and those being monitored in the hospital. A majority of those enrolled in the study voiced a preference for home monitoring.

In a randomized clinical trial of 121 adults with essential hypertension, Rogers, Small, Buchan, Butch, Stewart, Krenzer, and Husovsky (2001) reported a lower mean arterial pressure for patients in the home monitoring group. Patients in the experimental group transmitted their blood pressure recording over the telephone. Each day, patients were required to take their blood pressure with their monitoring device that automatically dialed into a service. The service converted that data into a meaningful report that was transmitted to their physician. Daily monitoring provided necessary data for physicians to make more frequent changes in the type and dose of antihypertensive medications.

Baer, DiSalvo, Cail, Noyes, and Kvedar (1999) tested the feasibility of electronic home monitoring of congestive health failure patients. The Partners Health Care System used a Vital Signs System (VSS) monitoring device that measured weight, blood pressure, and heart rate of congestive heart failure (CHF) patients. A total of 22 CHF patients participated in a study to assess reliability of the measures, feasibility of using this device in the home, and acceptability by patients. Of the 22 CHF patients, a total of 18 managed to stay enrolled in the study over a 5-month period. This feasibility study demonstrated that the VSS measures were reliable (differences between electronic and manual measures were within an acceptable range), accepted by both nurses and patients and deemed appropriate to monitor CHF patients at home.

In a study involving asthma, Finkelstein, Hripcsak, and Cabrera (1998) describe the use of the Home Asthma Telemonitoring (HAT) system. The system consists of a palmtop computer connected to an electronic flowmeter. Patients report their symptoms, medication use, and other data using the palmtop computer while their peak expiratory flow is measured by the electronic flowmeter. Results are submitted to a central clinical information system, and there is an ongoing communication link between providers and patients. Finkelstein et al. (1998) found subjects with little previous computer experience were able to use a home-based asthma telemonitoring system without difficulty, and there was an overall high level of acceptance by adult asthma patients from a lower-income, inner-city population.

The Veterans Administration (VA) health care system is currently testing the effectiveness of five different e-health technologies with different VA populations. The first experiment uses videophone "reassurance visits" for patients with chronic disease conditions and mental health difficulties, mainly posttraumatic stress syndrome, schizophrenia, and clinical depression. Initial results are promising, with a reduction in the average number of prescription drugs and with patient satisfaction well above 90% (Kleyman, 2001). In a second experiment, patients with complex chronic conditions received a telemonitor unit that check heart rate, glucose, and other health indicators. Perhaps the most interesting experiment is the use of Health Buddy, a simple appliance that is connected to a standard telephone. The Health Buddy unit is an in-home messaging device that beeps each morning and prompts the patient to answer anywhere from 6 to 10 questions. The patient responds to each question by pressing one of four buttons to correspond to their answers. The care coordinator then sees a light flashing at her or his office in one of three colors: green ("okay"), yellow ("change in health status"), or red ("call patient now").

The Congestive Health Active Management Program (CHAMP) had their case managers use the Health Buddy device with 200 patients and monitored their responses using the Health Hers Web page. The patients with the Health Buddy device answered daily questions sent by the case managers compared with the other 200 patients who were in the usual care group. The study (as cited in LeGrow & Metzger, 2001) found that using case managers and the Health Buddy device has a significant impact on health outcomes, such as reduced emergency department visits, reduced hospitalizations, and a direct variable costs saving of $7,885 per patient per year. The Health Buddy group decreased their hospitalization and emergency department visits by 73%.

MENTAL HEALTH SERVICES

VideoLink of St. Peter's (Helena, MT) began operation in January 1995 (funded by the U.S. Office of Rural Health Policy) encompassing a 12-county, 28,509-square-mile area with a population of 190,000. This telemental health service provides video connections to 26 Montana communities, connecting a variety of mental health providers including psychologists, psychiatrists, psychiatric nurse practitioners, social workers, and case managers. This telemental health network provides medication consultation, psychological testing, discharge and follow-up planning, forensic evaluations, and family therapy. The state hospitals are able to do preadmission screening, discharge planning, and family visitation throughout the state. The patient and case manager are present at one end and the consulting provider at the other. This video teleconferencing (VTC) has proved to be especially helpful for family therapy for families separated with patient living at an institution (Stamm, 1998).

Hunkeler, Meresman, Hargraves, et al. (2000) conducted a randomized clinical trial that compared three different treatments for a total of 302 patients starting antidepressant drug therapy. The three treatment methods were usual care, telehealth care, and telehealth care with peer support. The telehealth care consisted of emotional support and focused behavioral interventions in ten 6-minute phone calls over 4 months. The third method consisted of the same telephone calls as well as in-person visits by trained health plan members who had recovered from depression. The telehealth methods allowed patients with or without peer support to improve by 50% on the Hamilton Depression Rating Scale. This was in comparison to 37% improvement in the usual-care group. The telehealth groups also improved significantly more than the usual-care group in the Beck Depression Inventory at the end of 6 months. Other results included reported less symptoms on the Hamilton scale at 6 months, improved mental functions, and treatment functioning at 6 weeks for the telehealth groups. It was concluded that telehealth in the form of telephone support improved clinical outcomes of antidepressant drug therapy for adult patients in managed care clinics.

One of the barriers to quality treatment for mental illness is the lack of access to quality treatment systems and providers. The new communication technologies have the capability for providing quality services through case management and improving the quality of life for people living with mental illness (Hunkeler et al., 2000; Jerome et al., 2000). *Behavioral eHealth* refers to the variety of psychological services offered via the Internet. These services can range from psychoeducational information, consultation, and supervision to psychotherapy. Behavioral eHealth will not replace traditional mental health clinical activities but will expand providers and patients access to health care services and information (Nicholson, 1998; Rabasca, 2000a, 2000; Stamm, 1998). Increasingly, psychologists and mental health providers are using telehealth to deliver services; Medicare now covers some telehealth psychotherapy services (Ballie, 2001; Puskin, 2001; Rabasca, 2000a). With this increased use, there is increased attention as to its effects and appropriateness.

EVIDENCE-BASED STUDIES TO SUPPORT TELEHEALTH

In the area of telehealth, there have been several systematic reviews published in the literature. The first review (Balas, Jaffrey, Kuperman, Boren et al., 1997) evaluates the evidence related to the efficacy of communication technologies in health care. These studies focus on electronic communication using either a telephone or a computer. Studies included clinical trials for telephone follow-up and counseling, computerized communications, telephone reminders, interactive telephone systems, telephone access, and telephone screening. The two main conclusions were that (1) electronic communications enable greater continuity of care by improved access and facilitation of care coordination and (2) this communication is not limited just to physicians with clients.

A second review by Balas and Iakovidis (1999) examined the use of home monitoring devices. This review, not a traditional systematic review, stated "electronic monitoring of home promises cost effective health care, more active involvement of patients in their health care and a new sense of realism in making a diagnosis" (Balas & Iakovidis, 1999). Home monitoring equipment discussed in this article included such devices as glucometers, fetal monitoring, and blood pressure measures.

A third systematic review (Mair & Whitten, 2000) examined patient satisfaction with telemedicine. In this review, video-based clinical consultations were the focus. It turns out there were relatively few studies to assess and therefore there was limited generalizability of patient's satisfaction with video consultations.

Another review conducted by Currell, Urquhart, Wainwright, and Lewis (2001) examined telemedicine versus face-to-face patient care and the effects on professional practice and health care. The original study, completed several years earlier, was recently updated. This study used the Cochrane criteria for systematic reviews. They concluded that it is feasible to establish telemedicine studies but there is variable and inconclusive evidence to support outcomes of these studies. This is particularly true for cost effectiveness. The review highlighted the need for further research.

Whitten and colleagues (2002) conducted a systematic review of cost-effectiveness studies for telemedicine applications. Their analysis that yielded 55 cost studies of 612 articles; only 24 met the criteria for inclusion in the review. Of these studies, only 20 had collected any cost data. Most collected simple cost comparisons without any sensitivity analyses and none conducted a cost utility analysis. Thus, they concluded there is no good evidence that telemedicine is a cost-effective means of delivering health care (Whitten et al., 2002).

Two additional evidence-based practice studies were conducted at the Oregon Health Sciences Center, and they examine the effectiveness of telemedicine with Medicare populations. The first report, Telemedicine for the Medicare Population (2001), examined the use of telemedicine in three different categories: store and forward, self-monitoring/testing, and clinician interactive services. The review examined efficacy, safety, and cost-effectiveness variables. In general, they found that the top six uses of telemedicine were (1) consultations or second opinions, (2) diagnostic interpretations, (3) chronic disease management, (4) postdischarge follow-up, (5) emergency department triage, and (6) specialist visits. In terms of evidence, there is a growing body of literature to demonstrate that the technology can work and that there are clinical and economic benefits. Unfortunately, methodological issues such as small sample sizes preclude a definitive evidence of its efficacy. A supplemental report that specifically examines pediatric, obstetric, and clinician-indirect home interventions found similar results.

There is emerging evidence to support the use of telehealth applications in health care. Although each of the systematic reviews point to this growing evidence, it is apparent that more research that is targeted at clinical trials that examine both clinical outcomes and costs are urgently needed.

ISSUES AND CHALLENGES

Several issues and challenges remain as barriers to the implementation of telehealth applications in nursing practice. The first, *privacy and confidentiality*, is an ever-present issue with any technology. This is of particular concern to patients as their care enters the world of cyberspace. A second area of concern is *standards of practice* and ensuring that a nurse's practice within his or her scope of practice and in accord with any regulatory statues. There also is a fear by nurses that without standards of practice for telehealth, patients will receive less-than-optimal care and that technology will replace nurses. Practice guidelines were designed to ensure quality care and to attest to the use of telehealth applications to augment, not replace a nurse's, practice. A final area of concern focuses on licensure and reimbursement.

Maintaining a patient's right to privacy has always been a concern of health care providers and institutions, but the increasing use of information technology and technology networks in all health care systems has complicated and extended the scope of this concern. Federal and state governments have enacted a number of laws in attempts to create standards for ensuring the right to privacy and confidentiality of personal information while still creating electronic systems that will enhance and improve all levels of health care systems. Individual institutions have developed policies and security systems that ensure these rights within their own system, but once any information is transmitted across various forms of media networks, the mechanisms for ensuring this privacy become extremely complex.

The federal government has created a number of ways to regulate these rights. HIPAA, which took effect in April 2003, is considered by many to be among the most significant pieces of health care legislation in the history of the U.S. health system. The purpose of this legislation is to improve the efficiency and effectiveness of information systems and to establish a common set of standards and requirements for performing and securing electronic information exchanges. The Privacy Rule defines how patient information may be used or disclosed, and the Security Rule sets baseline standards for the confidentiality, availability, and integrity of patient information (Kumekawa, 2001).

During the Clinton administration, a Joint Working Group on Telehealth was established and charged with coordinating all federally funded telemedicine studies and projects as well as to examine and recommend standards related to patient safety, the efficacy and quality of services provided, and the legal and economic issues related to telehealth (http://telehealth.hrsa.gov/jwgt/jwgt.htm; http://telehealth.hrsa.gov/jwgt/certdraft.htm). The Office for the Advancement of Telehealth (OAT) part of the DHHS, Health Resources and Services

Administration found that many of the privacy concerns unique to telehealth were associated with issues of licensure regulations and reimbursement (Kumekawa, 2001; Wachter, 2000).

The ANA published "Core Principles on Telehealth" (1998), "Competencies for Telehealth Technologies in Nursing" (1999), and "Developing Telehealth Protocols: A Blueprint for Success" (Hutcherson, 2001). The American Telehealth Association (ATA) has produced a guide for health care professionals and patients using eHealth services (http://www.atmeda.org/ehealth/guide.htm), and the Internet Healthcare Coalition has published the eHealth code of ethics "to ensure that people worldwide can confidently and with full understanding of known risks realize the potential of the Internet in managing their own health and the health of those in their care" (http://www.ihealthcoalition.org/ethics/ehealthcode0524.html). The Health Internet Ethics Coalition, which includes a commitment to adopt a privacy policy, enhanced privacy protection for personal health information, and safeguarding consumer privacy and disclosing ownership and sponsorship information (http://www.hiethics.org).

Currently state laws regulate who can practice medicine and nursing, and they define the practice parameters for each. But as health care delivery and consultations cross geographic boundaries via telehealth, these standards of regulations do not work. There has been much discussion about how we can ensure quality standards of all providers in telehealth. A number of models have been suggested for how to deal with this (http://telehealth.hrsa.gov/pubs/licenstxt.htm; http://telehealth.hrsa.gov/pubs/licens.htm).

As health care practice crosses many state and national boundaries in telehealth, issues of licensure and jurisdiction become increasingly complex. Historically, state-based boards have regulated practice. How should issues of ensuring standards across state boundaries of the people who are providing, consulting, or developing health information electronically be handled? Recognizing the changing regulatory issues related to telehealth/eHealth, The Pew Health Professions Commission has shifted from state-based health care work force regulations to a national one (Gaffney, 1999). Nursing has responded to this shift by proposing national standardized competencies and regulations. *Telenursing* is defined as the practice of nursing over distance using telecommunications technology (National Council of State Boards of Nursing). In 1997, the National Council of State Boards of Nursing (NCSBN) proposed an interstate licensing model, the Interstate Nurse Licensure Compact (http://www.ncsbn.org), to ensure the quality of all nurse providers in telehealth (Gaffney, 1999). This compact was passed into law in 2000. To date, 15 states have enacted the interstate compact, with legislation being considered in additional states.

Along with the concern about interstate licensure, there have also been questions about a need for certification or additional credentialing. The compact covers the practice of registered nurses and licensed practical nurses but not advanced practice nurses (APNs) (Gaffney, 1999). In 2002, the NCSBN approved the adoption of model language for a licensure compact for APNs so states that had passed the Nurse Licensure Compact could implement a compact for APNs (http://www.ncsbn.org/public/nurselicensurecompact/aprncompact.htm). The consensus has been that the current licensure authorizes professional practice and that no additional credentialing is necessary.

There has also been an international effort made among the G8 countries on setting baseline recommendations for teleconsultation. The Subproject 4 Group (SP4 Group) of the Global Health Care Applications Project set forth teleconsultation practice guidelines. They define *teleconsultation* as "consultation, when necessary, between distant health care professionals concerning a patient's diagnosis and treatment, using telecommunication and information technology to bridge the spatial and functional distance between the participants" (Nerlich et al., 2002, p. 412). The SP4 panel gave specific recommendations for provider, institution, and organization and suggested a set of guidelines for conducting teleconsultation. (Nerlich et al., 2002).

How will these services be reimbursed? In the past, individual organizations and insurance agencies managed the individual contacts and contracts. However, until the 1990s, private and public payers generally did not have explicit policies that covered telehealth services. In 1999, Congress required the

Healthcare Financing Administration to pay for telemedicine consultation services under the Balanced Budget Act of 1997. A *telehealth visit* is defined as "one occurring between an originating site, that is the site where the patient is located at the time the service is provided by a telecommunications system, and a distant site, the site where the practitioner providing the professional service is located at the time the service is provided via a telecommunications system" (Pushkin, 2001). These reimbursement requirements were restricted to patients in rural Health Professional Shortage Areas requiring care from consulting specialists and had a fee-sharing requirement. In December 2000, Congress passed the Medicare, Medicaid, and SCHIP Benefits Improvement and Protection Act of 2000, which expanded the coverage of telehealth services to include to all "non-metropolitan statistical areas and any entity that participated in a Federal telemedicine demonstration project... as of December 31, 2000" (Pushkin). It now covers professional consultations (by Medicare billing practitioners), office or other outpatient visits, individual psychotherapy, medication management, and any other services specified by the Secretary of Health and Human Services (Ballie, 2001; Puskin, 2001). The fee-sharing requirement was also eliminated.

Home health, which is largely the practice domain of nurses, is not yet eligible for reimbursement as a telehomecare visit, although the expanded act does state that home health agencies "may adopt telehealth technology that it believes promotes efficiencies or improves quality of care" and record it with other Medicare-covered services (use prospective payment dollars) to cover its use (Puskin, 2001). Twenty states currently have developed reimbursement systems through Medicaid for telehealth (http://cms.hhs.gov/states/telelist.asp). There remains a long way to go before an adequate system has been established that provides for fair and appropriate reimbursement systems in telehealth.

FUTURE CASE SCENARIO

As a final challenge, take a look at a future case scenario of how a case manager might interact with a client in the community.

Mrs. Young is a 76-year-old diabetic woman who lives by herself at home. In addition to her diabetes, she has a heart condition and arthritis. Her case manager visits with Mrs. Young once a week through a videophone. During her weekly visit, Mrs. Young's heart condition is monitored with a digital Heart-Shaped brooch. Her other vital signs are monitored through a combination of digital devices such as her intelligent bathroom scale, which graphs her weight gain/loss on the bathroom mirror, and wearable sensors like her smart socks, whose sensate liner technology can warn of potential skin breakdown. Her daily glucose readings are electronically transmitted through her wireless personal digital assistant (PDA) cellphone. The case manager talks with Mrs. Young about her general mood and well-being while she is observing her environment through the various scanned images of Mrs. Young captured on the embedded cameras in the kitchen and living room. Mrs. Young's data are compared with her clinical pathway and adjusted according to the latest evidence available from the case manager's knowledge repository. Mrs. Young's videophone and digital tools are housed in a remote controlled robotic device that also contains her talking pill dispenser. This talking dispenser repeats the name and reason for taking the pill, and it records the date and time. Mrs. Young's videophone and her wireless PDA cellphone are connected to the Internet so she can retrieve her daily emails and check into her electronic support group. Because her eyesight has been failing, she uses voice-activated commands and her smart agent, Audrey, assists her with electronic interactions. Her daily e-mails consist of messages from her case manager and daily talking graphs of her vital signs and glucose readings. This graph provides continual feedback to Mrs. Young about her progress and connects her with customized Web pages to talk about her diabetes and its myriad of complications. She belongs to an electronic support group that helps her in managing her diabetes. Her smart agent helps Mrs. Young with the interpretation of her results and records her questions for the case manager's smart agent, Florence. Telehealth allows Mrs. Young to receive care and the necessary supports to live at home.

SUMMARY

Case managers have a great opportunity to examine the potential of telehealth applications in their practice (Skiba & Cohen, 2000). Extending one's reach in the community and providing access to a multitude of resources to support patients are benefits that can be easily derived from telehealth applications. It is time for case managers to seize the opportunity and develop telehealth applications that can best serve their client population. The growth of telehealth applications, particularly in e-disease management, is increasing every year. As more health care delivery systems recognize the benefits of telehealth, there will be more institutions that implement systems. It is incumbent on the care manager to investigate these opportunities and ensure that cost-effective and quality care is provided to all clients.

References

Ades, P., Pashkow, F., Fletcher, G., Pina, I., Zohman, L., & Nestor, J. (2000). A controlled trial of cardiac rehabilitation in the home setting using electrocardiographic and voice transtelephonic monitoring. *American Heart Journal, 139*(3), 543-548.

Ahring, K., Joyce, C., Ahring, J., & Farid, N. (1992). Telephone modem access improves diabetes control in those with insulin-requiring diabetes. *Diabetes Care, 15*(8), 971-975.

American Nurses Association (Mar. 25, 1998). *Core principles on telehealth.* Washington, D.C.: American Nurses Publishing.

American Nurses Association (Mar. 19, 1999). *Competencies for telehealth technologies in nursing.* Washington, D.C.: American Nurses Publishing.

American Nurses Association (1997). Telehealth—Issues for nursing. Policy Series No. 96-PRA-03. Available at www.ana.org/readroom/tele2.htm. Accessed December 5, 2003.

Baer, C., DiSlavo, T., Cail, M., Noyes, D., & Kvedar, J. (1999). Electronic home monitoring of congestive heart failure patients: Design and feasibility. *Congestive Health Failure, 5*(3), 105-113.

Balas, E., Jaffrey, F., Kuperman, G., Boren, S., Brown, G., Pineiroli, F., & Mitchell, J. (1997). Electronic communication with patients: Evaluation of distance medicine technology. *JAMA, 278*(2), 152-159.

Balas, E., & Iakovidis, I (1999). Distance technologies for patient monitoring. *British Medical Journal, 319,* 1309-1311.

Ballie, R. (2001). Medicare will now cover some telehealth psychotherapy services. (Electronic version) *APA Monitor, 32*(10). Available at www.apa.org/monitor/nov01/telehealth.html. Accessed December 5, 2003.

Bloch, C. (1999). *Federal Telemedicine Activities and Internet Sites.* Potomac, Md.: Bloch Consulting Group.

Cartwright, W., Dalton, K., Swindells, H., Rushant, S., & Rooney, P. (1992). Objective measurement of anxiety in hypertensive pregnant women managed in hospital and in the community. *British Journal of Obstetrics and Gynecology, 99,* 182-185.

Currell, R. Urquhart, C., Wainwright, P., & Lewis, R. (2001). Telemedicine versus face to face patient care: effects on professional practice and health care outcomes (Cochrane Review). In: *The Cochrane Library, Issue 3,* 2001. Oxford: Update Software.

Darkens, A., & Cary, M.A. (2000). *Telemedicine and Telehealth: Principles, policies, performance, and pitfalls.* New York: Springer.

Eysenbach, G. (2001) What is e-Health? [editorial]. *Journal of Medical Internet Research 3*(2): e20. Available at www.jmir.org/2001/2/e20/. Accessed December 5, 2003.

Finkelstein, J., Hripcsak, G., & Cabrera, M. (1998). Patients' acceptance of Internet-based home asthma telemonitoring. In C. Chute (Ed.), *AMIA '98 Annual Symposium Proceedings* (pp. 346-340). Philadelphia: Hanley & Belfus.

Friedman, R., Kazis, L., Jette, A., Smith, M., Stollerman, J., Torgerson, J., & Carey, K. (1996). A telecommunications systems for monitoring and counseling patients with hypertension. *American Journal of Hypertension, 9,* 285-292.

Gaffney, T. (May 31, 1999). The regulatory dilemma surrounding interstate practice. *Online Journal of Issues in Nursing.* Available at www.nursingworld.org/ojin/topic9/topic9_1.htm. Accessed December 5, 2003.

Greenberg, M.E. (2000). The domain of telenursing: Issues and prospects. *Nursing Economics 18*(4), 220. [Electronic version].

Hunkeler, E.M., Mersesman, J.F., Hargreaves, W.A., Fireman, B., Berman, W.H., Kirsch, A.J., et al. (2000). Efficacy of nurse telehealth care and peer support in augmenting treatment of depression in primary care. *Archives of Family Medicine, 9,* 700-708.

Hutcherson, C.M. (2001). Legal considerations for nurses practicing in a telehealth setting. *Online Journal of Issues in Nursing, 6*(3). Available at www.nursingworld.org/ojin/topic16/tpc16_3.htm. Accessed December 5, 2003.

Institute of Medicine (1996). *Telemedicine, A Guide to Assessing Tele-communications in Health Care.* Washington, D.C., National Academy Press.

Jerome, L.W., DeLeon, P.H., James, L.C., Folen, R., Earles, J. & Gedney, J.J. (2000). The coming of age of telecommunications in psychological research and practice. *American Psychologist, 55*(4),407-421.

Kleyman, P. (November-December, 2001) VA sunshine network tests five technologies. American Association of Aging. Aging Today [Electronic version]. Retrieved December 2, 2003 from: http://www.asaging.org/at/at-226/infocus_vasunshine.html.

Kumekawa, J.K. (2001). Health information privacy protection: Crisis or common sense? *Online Journal of Issues in Nursing, 6*(3). Manuscript 2. Available at www.nursingworld.org/ojin/topic16/tpc16_2.htm. Accessed December 2, 2003.

LeGrow, G., & Metzger, J. (2001). E-disease management. *California Healthcare Foundation.* Available at www.chcf.org/topics/view.cfm?itemID = 12864. Accessed December 2, 2003.

Mair, F., & Whitten, P. (2000). Systematic review of studies of patient satisfaction with telemedicine. *British Medical Journal, 320,* 1517-1520.

Maheu, M., Whitten, P., & Allen, A. (2001). *E-Health, telehealth, and telemedicine: A guide to start-up and success.* San Francisco: Jossey-Bass.

Marrero, D., Vandagriff, J., Kronz, K., Fineberg, N., Golden, M., Gray, D., Orr, D., Wright, J., & Johnson, N. (1995). Using telecommunication technology to manage children with diabetes: The Computer-Linked Outpatient Clinic (CLOC) study. *The Diabetes Educator, 21*(4), 313-319.

McLendon, K. (2000). E-commerce and HIM: Ready or not, here it comes. *Journal of the American Health Information Management Association, 71*(1), 22-23.

Morrison, J.C., Bergauer, N.K., Jacques, D., Coleman, S.K., & Stanziano, G.J. (Nov. 2001). Telemedicine: Cost-effective management of high-risk pregnancy. *Managed Care.* Available at www.managedcaremag.com/archives/0111/0111.peer_highrisk.html. Accessed December 2, 2003.

Nerlich, M., Balas, A., Schall, T., Stieglitz, S-P., Filzmaier, R., Asbach, P., et al. (2002). Teleconsultation practice guidelines: Report from G8 Global Health Applications Subproject 4. *Telemedicine Journal and e-Health, 8*(4), 411-418.

Nickelson, D. (2003). Telehealth and Internet resources for psychologists and consumers. American Psychological Association. Available at www.apa.org/practice/telehealth.html.

Nickelson, D.W. (1998). Telehealth and the evolving health care system: Strategic opportunities for professional psychology. *Professional Psychology: Research and Practice, 29,* 527-535.

Office for the Advancement of Telehealth (2001). Welcome. Available at www.telehealth.hrsa.gov/welcome.htm. Accessed December 1, 2003.

Pion, R., Altman, S., Hyatt, L., & Linden, R. (1999). *Home health telecommunications: Technology to improve revenues.* New York: McGraw-Hill.

Puskin, D.S. (2001). Telemedicine: Follow the money. *Online Journal of Issues in Nursing, 6*(3). Available at www.nursingworld.org/ojin/topic16/tpc16_1.htm. Accessed December 2, 2003.

Rabasca, L. (2000a). Taking telehealth to the next step. [Electronic version] *APA Monitor, 31*(4). Available at www.apa.org/monitor/apr00/telehealth.html. Accessed December 2, 2003.

Rabasca, L. (2000b). Taking time and space out of service delivery. (Electronic version) *APA Monitor, 31*(4). Available at www.apa.org/monitor/apr00/teledelivery.html. Accessed December 5, 2003.

Redford, L.J., & Parkins, L.G. (1997). Interactive televideo in rural case management. *Journal of Case Management* 6(4), 151-157.

Reed, G., McLaughlin, C., & Milholland, K. (2000). Ten interdisciplinary principles for professional practice in telehealth: Implications for Psychology. *Professional Psychology: Research & Practice, 31*(2), 170-178.

Rogers, M., Small, D., Buchan, D., Butch, C., Stewart, C., Krenzer, B., & Husovsky, H. (2001). Home monitoring service improves mean aterial pressure in patients with essential hypertension. *Annals of Internal Medicine, 134*, 1024-1032.

Savas, S., Parekh, M., & Fisher, L. (1999, November 11). Health e-opportunities in e-health? *Goldman Sachs Investment Research*, p. 3.

Skiba, D.J., & Cohen, E. (2000). Case management and technology: A necessary fit for the future. *Nursing Administration Quarterly, 25*(1), 132-141.

Stamm, B.H. (1998). Clinical applications of telehealth in mental health care. *Professional Psychology: Research and Practice, 29*(6), 536-542.

Telemedicine for the Medicare Population. File Inventory, Evidence Report/Technology Assessment Number 24. AHRQ Publication No. 01-E012, July 2001. Agency for Healthcare Research and Quality, Rockville, Md. Available at www.ahcpr.gov/clinic/epcsums/telemedsum.htm. Accessed December 5, 2003.

Telemedicine for the Medicare Population: Pediatric, Obstetric, and Clinician-Indirect Home Interventions. File Inventory, Evidence Report/Technology Assessment Number 24, Supplement. AHRQ Publication No. 01-E060, August 2001. Agency for Healthcare Research and Quality, Rockville, Md. Available at www.ahrq.gov/clinic/epc-sums/telmedsup.htm#Availability. Accessed December 5, 2003.

Wachter, G. (April 4, 2000). HIPAA's Privacy Rule Summarized: What does it mean for Telemedicine? Available at www.tie.telemed.org/legal/privacy/privacy00.asp. Accessed December 5, 2003.

Whitlock, W., Brown, A., Moore, K., Pavliscsak, H., Dingbaum, A., Lacefield, D., Buker, K., & Xenakis, S. (2000). Telemedicine improved diabetic management. *Military Medicine, 165*, 579-584.

Whitten, P., Mair, F., Haycox, A., May, C., Williams, T., & Hellmich, S. (2002). Systematic review of cost effectiveness studies of telemedicine interventions. *British Medical Journal, 324*(1), 1434-1437.

Willemain, T.R., & Mark, R.G. (1971). Models of remote health systems. *Biomedical Sciences Instrumentation, 8*, 9-17.

Wootton, R. (1995). Telemedicine fad or future? *Lancet, 345*, 73-74.

Compliance and Regulation

Rebecca F. Cady

CHAPTER OVERVIEW

Because of developments during the past 10 years in state and federal law and law enforcement, case management has become inextricably intertwined with the legal issues of compliance and regulation. Nursing case managers must be aware of the key issues in compliance and regulation as they pertain to the nursing case manager's professional activities to avoid both personal and corporate liability.

INTRODUCTION

Compliance and regulation have become, in recent years, issues about which all health care providers must be aware. Unfortunately for most of us, the laws and the regulations developed to enforce the laws are among the most confusing ever created. Entire volumes have been devoted to explaining the intricacies of these two issues. To understand these issues as they relate to case management, it is necessary to first review the applicable government health care programs and the laws that govern them.

Overview of Governmental Health Care Programs

Case managers deal with many patients who are insured by Medicare and Medicaid. Medicare, enacted in 1965, is a federally funded health insurance program contained in Title 18 of the Social Security Act (42 USC Sections 1395 et. seq.). In general, it is designed to provide health insurance benefits to Social Security recipients over age 65 years and to those who are permanently disabled as defined under the Social Security Act. Medicare is entirely a federal program and pays only for services that are "reasonable and necessary for the diagnosis or treatment of illness or injury or to improve the functioning of a malformed body member" [42 USC Section 1395y(a)(1)(A)]. Participating providers are required to ensure that any services rendered to Medicare recipients are supported by sufficient evidence of medical necessity [42 USC Section 1320c-5(a)(1)]. Under the statutes that govern Medicare, the Secretary of Health and Human Services regulates the administration of the program via the Centers for Medicare and Medicaid Services (CMS) with regulations totaling over 1600 pages. Medicaid, also enacted in 1965, is jointly financed by the federal and state governments and is administered by the states. Medicaid provisions are contained in Title 19 of the Social Security Act (42 USC Sections 1396 et. seq.). Medicaid authorizes federal grants to states for medical assistance to low-income persons who are age 65 years or over, blind, disabled, or members of families with dependent children or qualified pregnant women or children (42 CFR Section 430.0).

The Secretary of Health and Human Services is primarily responsible for the administration of the government's various health care programs established under the Social Security Act. In 1978 the Office of the Inspector General (OIG) was created by Congress to detect and prevent fraud and abuse in the Medicare and Medicaid programs [5 USC App. Section 2(2)]. State Medicaid Fraud Control Units are authorized by the Medicare-Medicaid Anti-fraud and Abuse Amendments to the Social Security Act. The purpose of these state units is to conduct a statewide program for the investigation and prosecution of violations of all applicable state laws regarding all aspects of fraud in connection with any aspect of the provision of medical assistance and the activities of providers of such assistance under the federal Medicaid program [42 USC Section 1396b(q)(3)]. To obtain Medicaid funding, a state must have a plan for medical assistance, which must contain procedures relating to payment for services sufficient to ensure that payments are consistent with quality of care [42 USC Section 1396 a(a)(30)(A)]. Each state must have a fraud detection program, and the state plan must provide for exclusion of persons who have committed fraud or abuse. The federal statute defines abuse as "provider practices that are inconsistent with sound fiscal, business, or medical practices, and result in an unnecessary cost to the Medicaid program, or in reimbursement for services that are not medically necessary or that fail to meet professionally recognized standards for health care" (42 C.F.R. 455.2).

TRICARE is the federal health insurance program for Department of Defense employees. Like Medicare, TRICARE pays only for medically necessary services and supplies [32 CFR Section 199.4(a)(1)(i)].

Nursing Case Management

To understand how nursing case management activities are affected by laws regarding compliance and regulations, the role and duties of the nursing case manager must be reviewed. Nursing case management is noted to be a model of care delivery that focuses on achieving optimal patient outcomes in expected time frames while containing costs, which meets the standards of regulatory agencies and is in line with health care reform activities at the federal level (Elizondo, 1994). The goals of nursing case management are (1) achieve expected patient outcomes within specific time frames; (2) improve quality of care; (3) deliver multidisciplinary care throughout hospitalization; (4) contain costs; (5) ensure appropriate length of stay; and (6) improve patient, family, and caregiver satisfaction (Elizondo, 1994). Bower (1995, p. 166) defines case management as follows:

A clinical system that focuses on the accountability of an identified individual or group for coordinating a patient's care (or group of patients), across an episode or continuum of care; negotiating, procuring, and coordinating services and resources needed by patients/families with complex issues; ensuring and facilitating the achievement of quality, clinical, and cost outcomes; intervening at key points for individual patients; addressing and resolving patterns of issues that have a negative quality-cost impact; and creating opportunities and systems to enhance outcomes.

Nursing case management activities must meet compliance requirements as well as conform to many federal and state regulations. This chapter identifies the critical issues that nursing case managers must be aware of, outline rules to follow, and illustrate the consequences of not following these rules by discussing the penalties and punishments that may ensue.

Historical Background: Compliance and Regulation

In May 1995 the Department of Health and Human Services (DHHS) began a 2-year demonstration project entitled Operation Restore Trust (ORT). The purpose of this project was to test several new approaches to fighting fraud and abuse in the Medicare and Medicaid programs. This program initially targeted five states: California, Florida, Illinois, New York, and Texas. These states were chosen because collectively these states' residents included more than one third of all Medicare and Medicaid beneficiaries. The goal of ORT was to increase enforcement in health care programs where the government believed that fraud and abuse were prevalent. The project also focused on high-growth program areas, which included home health agencies, nursing homes, hospice care, and durable medical equipment suppliers.

In 1996 the OIG's fiscal year medical and audit review indicated that 30% of all claims reviewed did not comply with Medicare laws and regulations. This report estimated that the dollar value of improper Medicare benefit payments made during fiscal year 1996 was $23.2 billion, or approximately 14% of the $168.6 billion in processed fee-for-service payments reported by the CMS. This report also estimated that improper home care claims accounted for $3.6 billion, or 15.74% of the improper payments (Gibbs-Brown, 1997). This report identified the four leading causes of improper Medicare payments as (1) insufficient or no documentation (46%), (2) lack of medical necessity (36.78%), (3) incorrect coding (8.53%), and (4) not covered or allowed services (5.26%).

The OIG's fiscal year 1997 medical and audit review revealed that only 11% of the total Medicare outlays constituted payment of improper claims, a 3% reduction from the previous years' statistics (Schorr, 1998). This suggested to the OIG that overall claims accuracy was improving. It was also found that claims submitted without documentation had decreased as well, from more than $3 billion in erroneous payments during fiscal year 1996 to only $850 million in fiscal year 1997 (Schorr, 1998). As a result of the initial success of this program, HHS decided to expand it through 2000 to include all 50 states.

The Health Insurance Portability and Accountability Act of 1996 (HIPAA) established a national Health Care Fraud and Abuse Control Program (HCFAC), under the joint direction of the Attorney General and the Secretary of Health and Human Services, acting through the Department's Inspector General (HHS/OIG). This program was designed to coordinate federal, state, and local law enforcement activities to identify and prosecute health care fraud, to prevent future fraud and abuse, and to protect program beneficiaries. In 2001, federal prosecutors filed 445 criminal indictments in health care fraud cases, and 465 defendants were convicted for health care fraud related crimes (HHS/Department of Justice [DOJ], 2002). In 2002, there were 517 criminal convictions (OIG, 2002).

THE REAL COST OF HEALTH CARE FRAUD

Judgments and settlements in health care fraud cases exceeded $1.2 billion in 2001 and over $858 million in 2002 (McCallum, 2002). The HHS/OIG indicates that improper payments under Medicare's fee for service system totaled an estimated $11.9 billion during 2000, the lowest estimate to date (HHS/DOJ, 2002).

Fraud is also a problem in the private sector. A survey done by the Health Insurance Association of America revealed that 9 of 10 private insurers has launched antifraud programs since 1995. The savings from these private insurers' antifraud programs totaled a staggering $260 million, an average $2.3 million per insurer, which constituted a savings of $7.50 for each dollar spent on fraud detection (White, 1998). According to Greg Anderson, director of corporate finance investigations for Blue Cross/Blue Shield of Michigan, billing for services not rendered and upcoding fraud* constitute 100% of the provider fraud in fee-for-service plans (White, 1998, p. 32).

In 1998 a review by the DHHS OIG found that portable chest radiographs performed in long-term care facilities cost up to nine times more than nonportable chest radiographs. The OIG also found, after

---

*Upcoding is a term used to describe the practice in which a different billing code is used to maximize reimbursement for a service or procedure done instead of using the specific code designated for that service or procedure.

reviewing medical records in California, New York, Florida, Texas, and Illinois, that there was "no indication in more than 50% of the beneficiaries' medical records that they would be unable to be transported outside of the nursing home for medical services." As a result, the OIG recommended that the CMS enforce the Medicare requirement that a physician must justify the need for portable services. According to CMS, the result of such enforcement would be a savings of as much as $63.7 million per year and $371.9 million over 5 years (Schwartz, 1998). In 1998 Cambridge Information Services, a Massachusetts-based health care information research company, used data obtained from CMS to determine that U.S. hospitals may have overbilled Medicare for as much as $482 million for laboratory tests performed between 1990 and 1997. As a result, they estimated that the DOJ could potentially recover at least $750 million in overbillings and penalties (Medicare Report, 1998). During the first half of 1999, Medicare erroneously paid approximately $48.5 million for medically unnecessary, undocumented, and inadequately documented therapy (HHS/DOJ 2002).

Ultimately, the cost of this fraud is passed on to consumers and their health care providers in the form of lower payments for services rendered, higher co-pays, and higher costs of health insurance.

FALSE CLAIMS

The False Claims Act

The federal False Claims Act (31 USC Section 3729) prohibits presenting any false claim for reimbursement to the United States if the provider knows the claim is false or where there is deliberate ignorance or reckless disregard of the claim's falsity. This law also prohibits submitting or causing to submit a false claim, conspiring to obtain a false claim, and making or using false records to obtain a payment. This means that employers may be liable for the acts of employees as well as contractors who submit claims that are false. In the health care setting the False Claims Act can be used to prosecute the institution, entity, or individual provider for a variety of actions, including the following (Kleiman, 1999):
1. Billing for goods and services not provided
2. Billing for unnecessary goods and services
3. Submitting false cost reports
4. Billing for substandard care
5. Acceptance or giving of kickbacks
6. Unbundling of services or supplies that should be grouped together

It is important for clinicians to realize that the False Claims Act allows for actions against individual clinicians. Therefore false claims are not merely a problem for the health care corporation. Nursing case managers must exercise caution when billing for their services to avoid the submission of potentially false claims.

Whistleblowers

The whistleblower, or "Qui Tam," provisions of the False Claim Act allow individuals, known as "relators," to file suit on behalf of the United States against those who have falsely or fraudulently claimed federal funds. Kleiman (1999) reminds us that fraud in any program depending on federal funding* may be prosecuted under this act. The whistleblower can be a current or former employee, a patient, a competitor,

---

*This includes Medicare, Medicaid, the Veterans Administration, TRICARE, and private health insurance purchased for federal employees, as well as federal support for medical or nursing education or biomedical research.

or any other individual who obtains knowledge of fraudulent and or abusive behavior. Generally, the knowledge must be firsthand, that is, it cannot come from a public source. Persons who file Qui Tam suits can recover from 15% to 25% of any settlement or judgment reached in a case if the United States intervenes in the action, or up to 30% if they pursue it on their own [31 USC Section 3730(d)(1)]. Given the stiff penalties that apply in fraud and abuse cases, the whistleblower can receive a great deal of money if the government prevails in such a case. As a result, the number of these lawsuits, known as "Qui Tam" cases, has increased dramatically since 1993, with 131 cases filed in 1993 and 530 cases filed in 1997 (DOJ, 1997). According to figures from the DOJ, over 50% of the Qui Tam cases filed in 1997 were home health care related (DOJ, 1997). Recoveries in Qui Tam cases as of October 1997 were $625 million (DOJ 1997). As of 2002, almost 70% of the Attorney General's fraud division cases consisted of cases filed on behalf of the federal government by private citizens (McCallum, 2002).

In fiscal year 2001, the federal government intervened in 61 Qui Tam cases; in 2002, it was just over 34 cases (McCallum, 2002).

Under the False Claims Act, an employee who is fired, demoted, or otherwise discriminated against for furthering an investigation into false claims is entitled to double back pay with interest, litigation costs, attorney's fees, general damages, and reinstatement [31 USC Section 3730(h)]. This reflects the fact that whistleblowers are protected by law against retaliatory actions for investigating or reporting fraud. Both federal and state laws protect whistleblowing employees. In addition, the U.S. Supreme Court has ruled that federal civil rights law protects employees who are fired to deter them from testifying in a federal trial against their employers (*Haddle v. Garrison*, 119 S.Ct. 489, 1998). Kleiman (1999) notes that since all False Claim Act suits must be filed under seal, the defendant may not know about the suit for months or even years, with the result that the whistleblower may remain anonymous and may continue working in the industry during most of the time the suit is in process.

Dealing with Whistleblowers

When the case manager must deal with a subordinate employee who is a whistleblower, great caution must be exercised. The case of *Neal v. Honeywell* (826 F. Supp 266, 7th Cir. 1994) is instructive in how not to deal with a whistleblower. In this case a human resources department psychologist reported fraud to the company hotline. She immediately experienced retaliation, despite promises of anonymity. After she was forced to quit, she sued her employer under the False Claims Act for the retaliation. In this case, the plant manager, who had been involved with the fraud, was promoted with a salary increase. The whistleblower, Dr. Neal, was given a 1-month paid leave when she was subjected to death threats and was denied a routine promotion. Dr. Neal was eventually awarded $294,000. Her employer was also required to pay nearly $1 million of Dr. Neals' attorney's fees. Even though she did not file a false claims case, this whistleblower was able to use the False Claims Act to receive compensation for the retaliatory actions of her employer.

Kleiman (1999) notes that retaliation does not always mean firing the employee. Courts may also consider actions such as breaking promises of confidentiality, reducing the responsibilities of employees who come forward with problems, or subtly punishing them in other ways to be retaliation. This means that when faced with the need to take action regarding an employee who has reported fraud and or abuse, it would be prudent to discuss the matter with your institution's risk manager or in-house attorney before acting.

Qui Tam Case Studies

In April 2003, Poudre Valley Health Care, Inc. settled a False Claims Act case for $2.9 million; the relator, a former employee, received $565,500 as his share of the proceeds of the settlement (DOJ, 2003). In June 2003, HCA (formerly known as Columbia/HCA and HCA–The Healthcare Company) agreed to pay the United States $631 million in civil penalties and damages arising from false claims. This amount, together with previous fines paid in criminal cases of $840 million, and an administrative settlement with the CMS of $250 million resulted in this case becoming the largest recovery ($1.7 billion) ever reached by the government in a health care fraud investigation (DOJ, Mar. 6, 2003). The settlement resolved fraud allegations against HCA and HCA hospitals in nine false claims act Qui Tam cases pending in federal court in the District of Columbia. The whistleblowers received a combined share of $151,591,500, the highest qui tam award ever paid out by the government (DOJ, Mar. 6, 2003). In March 2003, the San Diego Hospital Association and one of its facilities, Sharp Memorial Hospital, settled a false claims act Qui Tam case for $6.2 million for fraudulently misstating organ acquisition costs (DOJ, Mar. 6, 2003). The whistleblower, a heart transplant coordinator at Sharp, received $1.2 million (DOJ, Mar. 6, 2003).

CORPORATE COMPLIANCE: MANAGING THE RISK

The nursing case manager must be aware of the requirements regarding compliance plans for several reasons. First, if the nursing case manager is involved in developing or administering the compliance program, it is imperative to be familiar with the standards against which the program will be judged. Second, each nursing case manager must be familiar with his or her own employer's compliance plan and program, and being aware of the standards will provide a background of understanding why the plan was developed as it was.

The Compliance Program and Plan

If an agency or institution finds itself in question of having violated legal prohibitions against fraud and abuse, one of the most beneficial defenses it will have is a well-developed corporate compliance program. The Federal Sentencing Guidelines (2002) provide for decreased monetary fines and other penalties if the defendant entity had in place at the time of the alleged fraud and abuse a corporate compliance program that was developed and carried out in accordance with these guidelines. Stahl (1998) notes that while adopting and implementing a compliance program is voluntary, the OIG believes that such programs prevent fraud, abuse, and waste and at the same time further providers' fundamental mission to provide quality care.

There are two aspects to corporate compliance described by Cantone (1999): the corporate compliance program, which is the total of a corporation's efforts to comply with the various laws and regulations, and the corporate compliance plan, which is a detailed document specifically addressing those areas identified as presenting the corporation with significant liability.

Cantone (1999) identifies several benefits to a corporate compliance plan for healthcare organizations, including the following:

1. Potential reduction of civil or criminal wrongdoing
2. Potential reduction of administrative or civil penalties if a violation occurs
3. Provision of a more accurate view of employees' behaviors
4. Identification and elimination of criminal and unethical conduct
5. Provision of a means for efficient dissemination of information relating to changes in government requirements
6. Establishment of a structure that encourages employees to deal with concerns internally, which reduces the potential for Qui Tam actions and governmental investigations

Stahl (1998) identifies additional benefits of a compliance program, cited by the OIG in its guidelines for compliance, which were released on February 11, 1998:

1. Ensures that accurate claims will be submitted to government and private payers
2. Enables the hospital/facility to fulfill its caregiving mission
3. Assists hospital/facility in identifying any weaknesses in internal systems and management
4. Demonstrates a strong commitment to honest, responsible provider and corporate conduct
5. Improves quality of care
6. Develops a procedure that allows for prompt, thorough investigation of alleged misconduct by corporate officers, managers, employees, independent contractors, physicians, other health care professionals, and consultants
7. Initiates immediate and appropriate corrective action
8. Minimizes the loss to the government from false claims, and thereby reduces the hospital's/facility's exposure to civil damages and penalties, criminal sanctions, and administrative remedies

Developing a Compliance Plan

When developing a corporate compliance plan, the Federal Sentencing Guidelines must be referred to carefully. To meet the Federal Sentencing Guidelines, a compliance plan must include the following (Cantone, 1999; Federal Sentencing Guidelines, 2002):
1. Compliance standards and procedures
2. Overall compliance program oversight by high-level personnel
3. Due care delegating authority
4. Employee education and training
5. Monitoring, auditing, and reporting systems
6. Consistent enforcement and discipline
7. Response and corrective action

In developing a compliance plan, the first step is to perform a baseline risk assessment to determine responsibilities and existing processes for compliance, focusing on the most common types of compliance problems (Cantone, 1999). Part of this risk assessment should include auditing clinical charts, financial operations, policies and procedures, contracts, and billing processes to search for miscoding, double billing, and credit balances (Cantone, 1999). Common areas of risk can include the following:
1. Billing for services not provided
2. Plan of care documents not signed by the physician
3. Falsification of physician signatures
4. Backdating physician signatures
5. Physician consultation and administrative fees
6. Kickbacks
7. Cost report fraud

The second step is to establish a code of conduct, which will apply across the board in the organization. A code of conduct should include the following:
1. Ethical principles
2. Explanation of laws
3. Schedule for amending the code
4. Vehicle to report potential compliance issues
5. Nonretaliation policy for whistleblowers
6. Description of disciplinary measures

Third, oversight for the compliance program must be assigned to a high-level person in the organization. In some institutions a corporate compliance officer (CCO) is solely responsible for compliance. In others the functions of the CCO are assigned to a high-level corporate officer such as the chief financial officer or the executive director. Some organizations also appoint a compliance committee that provides oversight to all compliance activities.

It is crucial to remember that to meet federal guidelines, the compliance plan must be more than just artfully written documents. The plan must truly function in accordance with the guidelines provided by the Federal Sentencing Guidelines (2002), as follows:

1. The organization must have established compliance standards and procedures to be followed by its employees and other agents that are reasonably capable of reducing the prospect of criminal conduct.
2. Specific individuals within high-level personnel of the organization must have been assigned overall responsibility to oversee compliance with the standards and procedures.
3. The organization must have used due care not to delegate substantial discretionary authority to individuals whom the organization knew, or should have known through the exercise of due diligence, had a propensity to engage in illegal activities.
4. The organization must have taken steps to communicate effectively its standards and procedures to all employees and agents.
5. The organization must have taken reasonable steps to achieve compliance with its standards.
6. The standards must have been consistently enforced through appropriate disciplinary mechanisms, including as appropriate, discipline of individuals for failure to detect an offense. Adequate discipline of individuals responsible for an offense is a necessary component of enforcement; however, the form of discipline that will be appropriate will be case specific.
7. After an offense has been detected, the organization must have taken all reasonable steps to respond appropriately to the offense and to prevent further similar offenses, including any necessary modifications to its program to prevent and detect violations of law.

Documentation

Good documentation can be an important way to defend against charges of fraud and abuse. Stahl (1998) suggests that policies and procedures related to the processing and submitting of claims should do the following:

1. Provide for proper and timely documentation of all physician and other health care professional services that substantiate billed services.
2. Specify the documentation requirements in the patient's medical records, which, at a minimum should include the length of time spent in providing the service, who provided the service, why the service was provided, and the clinical outcomes. This documentation is essential to justify reasonableness and medical necessity.

It is imperative, however, that documentation never be falsified. The Federal False Entry Statute (18 USC Section 1001) provides that

> . . . [W]hoever, in any matter within the jurisdiction of the executive, legislative, or judicial branch of the Government of the United States knowingly and willfully:
>
> 1. falsifies, conceals, or covers up by any trick, scheme, or device a material fact;
> 2. makes any materially false, fictitious, or fraudulent statement or representation; or
> 3. makes or uses any false writing or document knowing the same to contain any materially false, fictitious or fraudulent statement or entry; shall be fined under this title or imprisoned not more than five years, or both.

Providers have an obligation to ensure that their Medicare-funded services are "supported by evidence of medical necessity . . . as may reasonably be required by a reviewing peer review organization." [42 USC Section 1320c-5(a)(3)].

Duty to Report

If an institution receives an overpayment from Medicare, whether this arises from simple negligence or from the presentation of false claims, it must report this overpayment to the CMS. Stahl (1998) notes that when violations of the compliance program are identified, the matter must be reported to the appropriate governmental authority within a reasonable time frame but no later than 60 days after the violation is identified. If administrators are aware of overpayments and fail to report them, they could be liable for concealment of a felony. U.S. Code Title 18, Section 4 states:

> "Whoever, having knowledge of the actual commission of a felony cognizable by a court of the United States, conceals and does not as soon as possible make known the same to some judge or other person in civil or military authority under the United States, shall be fined under this title or imprisoned not more than three years, or both."

To date, no health care professionals have been prosecuted under this law; however, personnel who fail to report knowledge of false claims do so at risk of their entire professional and personal lives.

POTENTIAL PENALTIES FOR LACK OF COMPLIANCE

Penalties for fraud and abuse can literally ruin a health care provider's personal and professional life. Cantone (1999) notes that the potential consequences for failing to comply include the following:
1. Probation and a court-imposed, government-designed program
2. Fines set at an amount sufficient to divest the organization of all of its net assets
3. Exclusion from the Medicare and Medicaid programs
4. Management liability
5. Stockholder lawsuits
6. Qui Tam lawsuits

Exclusion

Section 1320a-7 of Title 42 provides that individuals can be excluded from participation in Medicare and state health care programs under certain circumstances, including (1) conviction relating to fraud, (2) conviction relating to obstruction of an investigation of Medicare fraud, (3) claims for fraud or excess charges, and (4) furnishing patient services of a quality that fails to meet professionally recognized standards of health care [42 USC 1320a-7(b)]. A minimum 5-year exclusion from participation in Medicare and/or any state health care program is mandatory for any individual or entity that (1) has been convicted for Medicare-related crimes, (2) has been convicted of a criminal offense relating to neglect or abuse of patients, or (3) has been convicted of a criminal offense related to the delivery of an item or service under Medicare, Medicaid, or any state health care program [42 USC Section 1320a-7(a) and 1320a-7(c)(3)(B)]. In general, when a provider is going to be excluded, that provider is provided with a notice indicating that within 60 days of the notice, they can request a hearing before an administrative law judge to challenge whether they were in fact convicted, whether their convictions were related to the delivery of an item or service, and the length of their exclusion from the program. In 2001, the DHHS excluded 3756 individuals and entities from participating in federally sponsored health care programs, a record number [42 USC Section 1320a-7(a) and 1320a-7(c)(3)(B)]. In 2002, there were 3448 individuals and entities excluded (OIG, 2002).

Suspension of Payments

A state Medicaid agency is also allowed to suspend provider payments "upon receipt of reliable evidence that the circumstances giving rise to the need for a withholding of payments involve fraud or willful misrepresentation under the Medicaid program" [42 CFR Section 455.23 (a)]. The regulation provides that payments may be suspended "without first notifying the provider" but requires that notice be given within 5 days of taking such action and specifies that the provider may request and must be granted administrative review where state law so requires [42 CFR Section 455.23(a)].

Financial Penalties

The False Claims Act allows potentially enormous financial penalties for individuals or facilities found liable under the act, including treble damages and straight fines of up to $10,000 for *each* false claim submitted.

License Revocation

The individual state in which a practitioner convicted of fraud against a government program is licensed can also take action against that practitioner, including revocation of professional licenses and imposition of fines in addition to those imposed by the federal government. For example, in Louisiana the statutory maximum penalty for Medicaid fraud is 5 years with or without hard labor and/or a fine of not more than $10,000 (Louisiana Statutes Annotated, R.S. 14:70.1). Many states have adopted the Federal Sentencing Guidelines as mandatory in dealing with Medicaid fraud cases on a state basis. In the New York case of *Harshad v. DeBuono* (1997), the New York appeals court upheld the decision of the State Board for Professional Medical Conduct to revoke the medical license of a physician who was convicted on his plea of guilty to a felony charge of insurance fraud.

FALSE CLAIMS ISSUES RELATED TO NURSING CASE MANAGEMENT

False Claims Resulting from Substandard Care

The most potentially devastating type of false claims case to a case manager is a case involving false claims as a result of substandard care. There have been several important cases alleging fraud in substandard care. The first case occurred in the Eastern District of Pennsylvania in February 1996. At this time, the U.S. Attorney's office filed a civil complaint against the owner and former manager of Tucker House, a 180-bed nursing facility located in Philadelphia. This lawsuit alleged that three former residents had been subjected to substandard care, in that inadequate nutrition was maintained, as evidenced by the development of multiple stage III and IV pressure ulcers, secondary infections in the ulcers, precipitous and severe weight loss, and other symptoms of malnutrition, as well as improper wound care. The government also found that the staff failed to recognize the malnutrition or intervene early enough to prevent further decline of the patients' health.

   The suit was based on both the False Claims Act and the Nursing Home Reform Act (NHRA, 42 USCA Section 1396 r et. seq.). The government's contention was that the defendants had violated th · False Claims Act by submitting claims for services provided to these residents when the residents had not been provided with adequate care. The government's argument was that noncompliance with quality of care standards applicable to nursing facilities under both federal and state law was the same as intentional noncompliance with the required Medicare and Medicaid provider certification agreement between the government and the facility. This is because, under the certification agreement, all providers are charged with knowing all federal and state laws that apply to them and to the services they provide; the government has interpreted the knowledge requirement to be a compliance requirement as well. Because submitting claims for services to the government is a certification that all such services were provided in compliance with all quality of care laws and regulations, submitting such claims while not complying with the quality of care standards was false certification actionable under the False Claims Act.

The NHRA requires nursing facilities participating in Medicare and Medicaid to ensure that their residents are cared for adequately and appropriately. The regulations under the NHRA specifically require that facilities identify when a resident's nutritional status falls below what is considered acceptable for that patient's age and health status and must correct, if possible, whatever is causing the nutritional problem [42 CFR Section 483.25(i)]. This act also requires comprehensive assessment and treatment of pressure ulcers [42 CFR Section 483.25(c)]. In this case, state laws in Pennsylvania also required that facilities meet daily nutritional requirements of patients (28 PA Code Section 211.6a) and that the director of nursing services ensures that all prescribed health services for patients are properly implemented (28 PA Code Section 211.12e).

One of the important facts of this case was that the medical records of these patients indicated that the facility's staff had or should have had some knowledge that the nutritional intake of the residents was not sufficient. Even worse, the nursing staff's treatment notes were not entirely consistent with the severe problems obviously present in these patients. The fact that the facility failed to determine what the patients' true conditions were before submitting the claims constituted, in the government's eye, reckless disregard for the truth. The case was settled for $500,000 and consent orders imposing rigorous quality of care standards on the facility (Kleiman, 1999; Kurlander, 1997).

Two years later, in January 1998, the same U.S. attorney filed a similar action against three additional nursing homes. This case also settled for $500,000 and an agreement to implement the same kinds of quality of care standards as in the Tucker House case (Kleiman, 1999). In August 1998, the U.S. attorney's office in Baltimore filed suit against Greenbelt Nursing and Rehabilitation Center. The suit was settled only 1 month after it was filed. In a detailed court order agreed to by both parties, Greenbelt's owner agreed to strict standards for staffing, staff training, quality assurance, medical and nursing care, nutritional needs, psychiatric services, wound care, and resident safety. Greenbelt was also required to hire a monitor and an interim manager to be approved by the government. Most important, Greenbelt agreed that the U.S. government could interview its staff outside the presence of supervisors and without company lawyers present (Kleiman, 1999). In 2001, the principal operator and co-owner of two nursing homes and other health care businesses in Pennsylvania agreed to a 5-year exclusion for his role in providing substandard care to residents of those homes, representing the first time HHS/OIG excluded the owner of a health care facility based on the owner's responsibility for poor care at the facility (HHS/DOJ, 2002). In 2001, Manor Care, Inc. settled a civil false claims act case arising from inadequate care to Medicare patients at one it its skilled nursing facilities and paid a $90,000 fine to the government as well as agreeing to retain an independent consultant to monitor quality of care at the facility (HHS/DOJ, 2002).

The Problem of the Dually Eligible Client

Compliance presents a potentially very complicated problem for all health care providers, but most especially for nursing case managers. Often the case manager is forced to juggle the regulations and rules of both Medicare and Medicaid simultaneously when dealing with a single patient. Mitchell (1997) notes that Medicare and Medicaid overlap significantly, especially where persons with chronic conditions are concerned. Saucier (1995) noted that nearly all elderly Medicaid beneficiaries and up to a third of Medicaid beneficiaries with disabilities also qualify for Medicare. When patients are dually eligible, the federal government (through Medicare) is responsible for primary, acute, and a growing amount of chronic care and the state (through Medicaid) is responsible for long-term care and wraparound coverage (Mitchell, 1997). Although the two funding sources complement each other in that Medicaid covers gaps in Medicare coverage for the dually eligible, the existence of two payers does not, by itself, ensure coordination of care. Mitchell (1997) suggests that this is due to the fact that the systems remain bifurcated, which potentially undercuts the benefits of managed care for those dually eligible patients, as the current system creates obstacles to providing good and cost-effective care. What this means for the nursing case manager is that extra care must be taken when dealing with dually eligible clients to avoid potential compliance issues.

Management and Evaluation of Medicare Patients

Under the Medicare management and evaluation regulations, which were published in 1989, nurses can provide reimbursable case management services for home health patients with chronic problems to prevent rehospitalization of those patients. This regulation was significant because it was the first time Medicare rules did the following:

1. Recognized and reimbursed nurses as case managers in the home
2. Reimbursed for prevention and health promotion in the home
3. Acknowledged and reimbursed chronic rather than exclusively acute care (Allen, 1994; Knollmeuller, 1993; National Association for Home Care, 1992).

Management and evaluation (MAE) is defined as providing case management for patients with chronic illnesses and multiple skilled or nonskilled disciplines involved, where rehospitalization or nonadherence to the care plan is likely (Allen, 1994; HCFA, 1989). Allen (1994) notes that the regulation provides for the continued care of persons at high risk for rehospitalization who can benefit from a registered nurse ensuring that the care plan developed with the patient and family is maintained.

The rules regarding MAE resulted from a lawsuit brought in 1987, which asserted that fiscal intermediaries of CMS had randomly and without permission narrowed the definition of eligible Medicare home services and denied reimbursement of home care agencies and that CMS had failed in its oversight of these intermediaries. The suit also challenged CMS's 1986 modification of the definition of eligible care regarding part-time/intermittent care, as well as its narrow definition of "medically necessary" and arbitrary reimbursement decisions based on the semantics of the claim rather than on medical need (Allen, 1994). The courts agreed with the claimants and ordered CMS to rewrite the eligibility rules and broaden the definition of allowable Medicare-reimbursed services provided in the home. As a part of these rule changes, MAE of the patient's care plan was introduced as a reimbursable skilled service under Medicare (Allen, 1994); MAE services have the following three goals:

1. To allow registered nurses to monitor the delivery of skilled and unskilled care provided in the patient's home
2. To coordinate services with an appreciation for the interrelationship of the caregiving services given the potential for adverse consequences
3. To provide a reimbursement avenue to respond to care plan complications

Allen (1994) notes that MAE is a skilled service and thus may be provided as a stand-alone service to Medicare recipients. Criteria for identifying patients who could benefit from MAE services include various physical, environmental, psychosocial, and health-related behaviors and conditions. The physical criteria include potential for deterioration and complex, multiple care needs. Environmental criteria include an unhealthy or unsafe environment and actual or potential safety issues. Psychosocial criteria include unorganized or fragmented informal caregivers, lack of or inconsistent support system, and limited financial, mental, or intellectual resources. Health-related behavior criteria include multiple health care providers and/or community services, unstable or inconsistent self-care, need for coordination and teaching of formal or informal unskilled care, and high turnover of caregivers, with a need for continuity and instruction of unskilled providers (Allen, 1994). To avoid potential trouble with false claims arising from MAE services, the case manager must document the criteria in nursing notes, must evaluate the criteria at regular intervals to ensure that they are current problems, and must document interventions (Allen, 1994). Documentation is critical in this area because although the regulations do not limit the visit frequency or duration, the documentation must reflect that the patient continues to need the skilled service.

Allen (1994) notes that there are three potential problems with use of MAE. First, MAE cannot be used only to continue a home health aide, as MAE is not meant to provide long-term homemaker or activities of daily living assistance only. Second, MAE is not appropriate for continued management of an unstable situation. Third, MAE requires an updated working care plan that reflects the skilled and unskilled care that is being provided. Nursing case managers performing MAE must be careful to avoid these problems and to document thoroughly.

OTHER RELEVANT FEDERAL AND STATE LAWS PERTAINING TO COMPLIANCE AND REGULATION OF NURSING CASE MANAGEMENT

In addition to charges under the False Claims Act, providers may be charged with mail fraud in violation of 18 USC Section 1341 if they have used the U.S. mails in furtherance of their fraudulent behavior, and they may be charged with wire fraud in violation of 18 USC Section 1343 if they have engaged in telephone conversations or used wire transmissions in furtherance of their fraudulent behavior.

The Medicare anti-kickback statute [42 USC Sections 1320a-7b(b)] represents a culmination of several years of congressional effort to combat fraud and abuse in the Medicare and Medicaid programs. Congress first enacted these laws in 1972. The law made it a misdemeanor to solicit, offer, or receive any "kickback or bribe in connection with" furnishing covered services or referring a patient to a provider of those services (Social Security Amendments, 1972).

In 1977 Congress expanded on the 1972 statute, making violations of the statute a felony and additionally proscribing the solicitation or receipt of any "remuneration," including any kickback, bribe, or rebate, in return for referring a patient to a provider of covered services, regardless of whether the prohibited act was done "directly or indirectly, overtly or covertly, or in cash or in kind" (Medicare–Medicaid Anti-Fraud and Abuse Amendments, 1977). The statute was revised again in 1980, because there was uneasiness regarding the application of the statute, to include what is known as a "scienter" requirement, which means that the person accused must have knowingly and willingly engaged in the prohibited conduct to be subject to criminal sanctions. This does not mean that the accused had to know that the conduct was illegal.

In 1987 Congress streamlined this statute into a single statutory scheme, 42 USC Section 1320a-7b(b). The current version of the statute provides in part:

> Whoever knowingly and willfully solicits or receives any remuneration (including any kickback, bribe, or rebate) directly or indirectly, overtly or covertly, in cash or in kind—
>> (A) in return for referring an individual to a person for the furnishing or arranging for the furnishing of any item or service for which payment may be made in whole or in part under a Federal health care program, or

(B) in return for purchasing, leasing, ordering or arranging for or recommending purchasing, leasing, or ordering any good, facility, service, or item for which payment may be made in whole or in part under a Federal health care program, shall be guilty of a felony and upon conviction thereof shall be fined not more than $25,000 or imprisoned for not more than five years, or both.

Providers can also be punished under state laws for accepting kickbacks.

Safe harbor regulations were issued by the DHHS in 1991 (42 CFR Section 1001.952 (a)-(m), 1992). DHHS explained that "[I]f a person participates in an arrangement that fully complies with a given [safe harbor] provision, he or she will be assured of not being prosecuted criminally or civilly for the arrangement that is the subject of that provision" (Background to Safe Harbor Provisions, 56 Fed. Register 35952, 35958, July 29, 1991). The safe harbor provision allowing for payments pursuant to personal services and management contracts provides as follows:

The following payment practices shall not be treated as a criminal offense under Section 1128B of the Act and shall not serve as the basis for an exclusion:

(d) Personal services and management contracts. As used in Section 1128B of the Act, "remuneration" does not include any payment made by a principal to an agent as compensation for the services of the agent, as long as all of the following six standards are met.

(1) The agency agreement is set out in writing and signed by the parties.

(2) The agency agreement specifies the services to be provided by the agent.

(3) If the agency agreement is intended to provide for the services of the agent on a periodic, sporadic, or part-time basis, rather than on a full-time basis for the term of the agreement, the agreement specifies exactly the schedule of such intervals, their precise length, and the exact charge for such intervals.

(4) The term of the agreement is for not less than one year.

(5) The aggregate compensation paid to the agent over the term of the agreement is set in advance, is consistent with fair market value in arms-length transactions and is not determined in a manner that takes into account the volume or value of any referrals or business otherwise generated between the parties for which payment may be made in whole or in part under Medicare or a State health care program.

(6) The services performed under the agreements do not involve the counseling or promotion of a business arrangement or other activity that violates any State or Federal law.

For purposes of paragraph (d) of this section, an agent of a principal is any person, other than a bonafide employee of the principal, who has an agreement to perform services for, or on behalf of, the principal.

[42 CFR Section 1001.952(d), 1992].

Kickbacks can be a major issue for nursing case managers because of the nature of their practice, which involves making referrals and procuring goods and services for clients. It is imperative to refuse to accept any type of gift or payment that depends on your making referrals of federally insured patients. If such gifts or payments are offered to you, your facility's risk manager or in-house attorney should be contacted at once.

References

Allen, S. (1994). Medicare case management. *Home Healthcare Nurse, 12*(3), 21-27.

Bower, K. (1995). Collaborative care: two effective strategies for positive outcomes. In K. Zander (Ed.), *Managing outcomes through collaborative care: The application of caremapping and case management* (pp. 1-38). Chicago: American Hospital Publishing.

Cantone, L. (1999). Corporate compliance: Critical to organizational success. *Nursing Economics, 17*(1), 15-19.

Department of Justice (Oct. 1997). Qui Tam cases filed and recoveries. Available at www.taf.org/taf/docs/pub.html.

Department of Justice (Apr. 18, 2003). Press release: Poudre Valley Health Care, Inc. pays $2.9 million to settle fraud suit.

Department of Justice (Jun. 26, 2003). Press release: Largest health care fraud case in U.S. history settled, HCA investigation nets record total of $1.7 billion.

Department of Justice (Mar. 6, 2003). Press release: San Diego hospital to pay U.S. $6.2 million to settle false claims allegations.

Elizondo, A. (Dec. 1994). Nursing case management in the neonatal intensive care unit, part 1: Pioneering new territory. *Neonatal Network, 13*(8), 9-12.

False Claims Act. 31 USC Section 3279.

Federal provisions regarding exclusion from Medicare and Medicaid. 42 USC Sections 1320 a-7.

Federal sentencing guidelines, 2002.

Gibbs-Brown, J. (1997). Results of operation restore trust audit of medicare home health services in California, Illinois, New York and Texas (A-04-96-02121) (pp. 4-22) (Report sent to HCFA from OIG). Washington, D.C.: U.S. Government Printing Office.

Harshad v. DeBuono (1997). 661 NYS 2d 66.

Health Care Financing Administration (1998). *Financial report for fiscal year 1997*. Washington, D.C.: US Department of Health and Human Services, The Administration.

Health Care Financing Administration (1989). *Health insurance manual-11 (HIM-11). Revision 222*. Washington, D.C.: The Administration.

Department of Health and Human Services and Department of Justice (Apr. 2002). *Health care fraud and abuse control program annual report for FY 2001*. Washington, D.C.: The Departments.

Kleiman, M. (Jun. 1999). The False Claims Act. *JONA's Healthcare Law, Ethics, and Regulation, 1*(2), 17-22.

Knollmeuller, R. (1993). The role of prevention in home health care nursing practice. *Home Healthcare Nurse, 11*, 21-23.

Kurlander, S. (1997). Liability under the false claims act for inadequate care of nursing facility residents. *Advances in Wound Care, 10*(5), 47-49.

McCallum, R.D. (2002). Remarks to the American Health Lawyers Association Meeting, September 30, 2002.

Medical Necessity of Medicare Services. 42 USC Section 1320.

Medicare Law. 42 USC Sections 1395 et. seq.

Medicaid Law. 42 USC Sections 1396 et. seq.

Medicare–Medicaid Anti-fraud and Abuse Amendments, Pub.L. No. 95-142, 91 Stat. 1179, 1181 (1977).

Medicare report. Washington, D.C.: The Bureau of National Affairs, Inc., 1998, 9:9:220.

Mitchell, E. (Spring 1997). Medicaid, Medicare, and managed care: Case management for dually eligible clients. *Journal of Case Management, 6*(1), 8-12.

National Association for Home Care (1992). *Home care management and evaluation: Understanding and documenting*. Washington, D.C.: The Association.

Office of the Inspector General (Dec. 11, 2002). Press release: OIG saves taxpayers record $21 billion.

Saucier, P. (1995). *Federal barriers to managed care for dually eligible persons*. Portland, Me.: National Academy for State Health Policy.

Schorr, B. (1998). OIG knocks DME claims for documentation & HHA claims for lack of necessity. *Home Health Line, 23*(18), 9.

Schwartz, R. (Feb. 1998). OIG targets nursing homes—again. *Nursing Homes*, pp. 10-11.

Social Security Amendments Act, Pub. L. No. 92-603, Sections 242 (b) and (c), 86 Stat. 1419, 1972.

Stahl, D. (1998). Consolidated Billing and Compliance Program Part 2. *Nursing Management, 29*(6), 12-15.

U.S. Department of Justice (1997). *1997 Annual report*, Washington, D.C.: U.S. Department of Justice, p. 27.

White, J. (Mar. 1998). How provider fraud flattens corporate profits. *Business & Health*, p. 28.

VIII

EVALUATION, OUTCOMES MEASUREMENT, AND RESEARCH

Important Components of Decision Making

One of the most commonly overlooked areas in the process of designing and implementing case management is the evaluation component. While often neglected, it is by far among the most critical elements. Today's organizations are data driven, and case management evaluation and research data are among the most robust data available in health care delivery settings. What makes these data unique and beneficial are their focus on the combination of clinical, financial, and quality issues. Unlike much of the data collected before case management, these data do not compartmentalize the information but place it in a context that makes it of use to practitioners, administrators, and regulatory bodies. Finally, outcomes data seek to answer many of the questions being raised in health care today in terms of efficacy and cost of care. Unit VIII provides a unique look into this complex and growing area of case management.

Key Functions and Direct Outcomes of Case Management

Sherry L. Aliotta

CHAPTER OVERVIEW

This chapter describes the four key functions of case management and how they can be used to identify and measure the direct outcomes of case management. The chapter presents the Spectrum of Accountability model developed by the Council for Case Management Accountability (CCMA) and how that model will be used to link case management outcomes to the end outcomes of the health care system. The implications of this model on the practice of case management are presented.

FOUR KEY FUNCTIONS OF CASE MANAGEMENT

The Standards of Practice for Case Managers list four key functions of a case manager: assessor, planner, facilitator, and advocate.

Assessor

Without a thorough assessment, the probability of accurately identifying issues that can benefit from case management intervention is drastically diminished. Assessment by a case manager forms the database of information for the patient. The case manager should complete a comprehensive review of the key aspects of the patient and the situation. The case manager must be skilled in interviewing and gathering data. The manager must also be able to identify sources of information to obtain a detailed picture of the problems, issues, and barriers that may be present. In addition, the case manager must identify the strengths and resources that the patient possesses. The actual gathering of the information is just the first step of the process. The case manager must synthesize the information obtained to anticipate the problems, issues, or barriers and how these will impact the patient's progress toward the achievement of their goals. The case manager must also recognize where the patient's strengths, talents, and abilities can be used and where support, education, or further intervention is required. This requires critical thinking and analytical skills on the part of the case manager. Many a case has stalled due to information not acquired during the assessment. For example, it was several weeks into unsuccessful rehabilitation that the case manager learned the young boy with the traumatic brain injury had been diagnosed with emotional and behavioral issues before the injury.

Planner

The information gained and the analysis performed during the assessment phase form the foundation for the planning phase. The case manager collaborates with the patient, the patient's family and significant others, and all treating professionals to develop a case management plan. The plan contains the long-term

415

and short-term goals, the problems to be addressed, the pieces of the plan that are already in place, and the interventions necessary to achieve the established goals. The interventions in the plan should address the problems, issues, and barriers identified as a part of the comprehensive assessment and those revealed through joint planning with the patient. The plan should reflect where the patient is in relationship to the desired goals and anticipate the pitfalls and milestones to evaluate the success of the plan. Timing is a important piece of the planning process and is critical to the outcomes measurement. Case managers are often hesitant to attach time frames to the care plans. Some worry that they will be judged harshly if they fail to accomplish the plan in the specified time. In reality, time can be an important clue to evaluate the effectiveness of the plan and the likelihood of achieving the outcomes. For example, if the case manager expects that the patient should have learned to give the insulin in 2 weeks, and 4 weeks has passed, the case manager has a very strong sign that the plan needs modification in some way.

Facilitator

The case manager implements or ensures implementation and coordination of the care plan. The case manager maintains communication with all the parties. She or he looks for opportunities to prevent duplication, delays, and miscommunications in the care of the patient and intervenes when possible. The case manager is the "trouble-shooter" to resolve conflicts and expedite care. Case managers often accomplish the extraordinary on a routine basis. Part of the facilitation role includes establishing the accountabilities among the other team members. Cases involving a case manager are typically too complex for one person to hold all the accountability. This involves team involvement in the planning phase above. People are more likely to support and follow through on a plan they helped create. It also requires clear communications of the goals. People must know how their actions will affect the outcome. Obviously, clear goals and expectations increase the ease of outcome measurement at plan completion.

Advocate

The case manager advises the patient of the available options and ensures that the patient's interests are identified and supported. Where possible, the case manager provides the patient with the information needed for the patient to be an effective advocate of his or her own requirements. The advocacy role of the case manager includes ensuring that the patient and significant others are the key architects of their own life and lifestyle choices. Often case managers decide what the patient's problems are, what the patient is going to do to solve them, and which problem the patient will tackle first. The fact that the patient later agrees to the case manager's plan does not mean the patient was a participant in the care planning. Such practices, although commonly used, do not fulfill the potential of the case manager as an advocate.

It is important that the case manager not confuse advocacy with fulfilling each request made by the patient. For example, a novice case manager was working aggressively to get a patient her 120 Vicodin tablets without considering that a true advocate may want to explore other issues. Such issues include whether the patient's pain had been properly evaluated, whether the current medication was the correct option, whether the patient had developed a substance abuse issue, and other unexplored topics that may better serve the patient's interest.

THE KEY FUNCTIONS OF CASE MANAGEMENT AND OUTCOME MEASUREMENT

Outcome measures for case management need to demonstrate two things:
1. Case managers are effective in performing the four key functions.
2. Effective performance of the four key functions has a positive impact on overall outcomes.

Much of the research published to date (Wagner et al., 1999) regarding the outcomes of case management have focused on indicators such as reduction in inpatient days, improved health status, and decreased in costs. These items and other related outcomes are more accurately described as "end outcomes." The challenge for case managers lies in quantifying exactly how its key functions affect the end outcomes.

END OUTCOMES OF THE HEALTH CARE SYSTEM

The major end outcomes reported by the health care system include the following:
- *High quality care*—This is often measured using proximate measures such as patient satisfaction, readmission rates, complications, morbidity and mortality, or adherence to recognized treatment standards. As with the key functions of case management, these proximate measures are based on assumptions. Sometimes the assumptions are supported by research evidence, and sometimes they are not. For example, in their landmark article on a nurse-led multidisciplinary intervention, Rich et al. (1995) used an instrument that was found to be responsive in measuring quality of life in patients with congestive heart failure. This measure is supported by research evidence.
- *Decreased or appropriate costs*—Measurements for costs include reductions in hospital admissions, emergency department visits, and overall "per-case" costs. For example, researchers in Australia used their hospital's inpatient and outpatient costing systems to compare the costs of the study interventions with the costs of usual care (Stewart et al, 1998). Some measurements are obtained using "pre-post" comparisons where costs are measured before the case management intervention and then after the case management intervention. The before and after measurements are compared and the cost reductions calculated. Using measurements of appropriate costs is more difficult. It is often difficult to state what the cost of care *should* be. When these types of measurements are done, they are usually based on comparison with recognized standards or actuarial data and are often correlated with quality or health status measures.
- *Improved health status*—This is often measured via use of questionnaires or surveys that examine the patient's perception of the impact their health has on their quality of life. Other indicators could include the absence of symptoms, resumption of employment, or other aspects of the patient's chosen lifestyle. As with quality of care, there are numerous proximate measures that are used as verification of improvement in health status.

If case management is to be able to conclusively establish a correlation between what the case manager does and the desired end outcomes of the health care experience, they must achieve clear definitions. Case management must define both the interventions and the impact of those interventions.

DIRECT IMPACT OF CASE MANAGEMENT

The first question that had to be answered was, "What are the direct outcomes of case management?" This question was proposed to case management leaders and to customers, recipients, purchasers, and colleagues of case management by the CCMA. The three leading answers were as follows:
- Improved adherence
- Improved coordination of care
- Enhancement of patient empowerment and involvement

The Spectrum of Accountability from the CCMA (Figure 37-1) describes and illustrates the relationship between the key functions of case management, the direct outcomes of case management, and the end outcomes of the health care system.

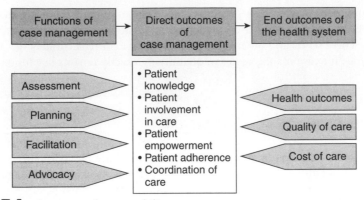

FIGURE **37-1**   Spectrum of accountability.
(Courtesy *Case Management Society of America Council for Case Management Accountability, Little Rock, Arkansas* © *1997. Used with permission.*)

The Spectrum of Accountability is the model that the CCMA developed to guide their approach to the development of outcome measures for case management. The model illustrates the functions of case management (assessment, planning, facilitation, and advocacy) resulting in the direct outcomes of patient knowledge, involvement and empowerment, increased adherence, and coordination of care. The final piece of the model depicts the direct outcomes of case management as contributing to the end outcomes of case management.

IMPROVED ADHERENCE

Improving adherence has long been a key focus for case management. In many case management models, nonadherence is a "trigger" to initiate an assessment by a case manager. All of the key functions of case management are applied to the problem of nonadherence. In the assessment the case manager specifically seeks information that will offer cues as to the cause of the nonadherence. As a planner, the case manager identifies the problem and collaborates with the patient to establish goals relating to better adherence and interventions to help the patient achieve the goal. In the role of facilitator the case manager helps to eliminate or minimize barriers to adherence. Finally, as an advocate the case manager offers solid, factual information on the impact of the nonadherence and supports the patient in the decision-making process. Which of these actions is most likely to enhance adherence? Which strategy is the one that all case managers should implement? Which of these examples is not as effective as the others? All of these questions remain unanswered without effective outcome measurements.

In adherence, as with the other "top three" case management outcomes, there is already a significant amount of information in the literature. Glenys A. Hamilton authored a paper for The Case Management Society of America and the CCMA entitled "Patient Adherence Outcome Indicators and Measurement in Case Management and Health Care." The paper details the results of Dr. Hamilton's comprehensive review of several hundred articles on adherence. The paper substantiates several concepts key to the development of case management outcomes. First, there are factors and interventions that enhance adherence. The presence of evidence in the literature documenting the ability to improve adherence is crucial for case management outcomes because it proves that adherence is a "modifiable" problem, issue, or barrier. If it was discovered that adherence could not be improved, then it would not be possible for case management to address nonadherence effectively. The second concept the Hamilton paper confirms is that there are barriers to adherence. This is important because it supports the idea that there are interventions that can minimize or eliminate the barriers to adherence. The final assumption validated in the Hamilton paper is that adherence can be measured. The impact of these three concepts—(1) adherence can be enhanced, (2) there are barriers to adherence, and (3) adherence can be measured—provides the evidentiary backing needed to establish the linkages between case management functions and the direct outcomes (impact) of case management. The final linkage to the end outcomes of cost savings, quality of care, and improved health status are also established.

IMPLICATIONS FOR PRACTICE

Using adherence as a model, case management can begin to develop the initial body of research that conclusively links case management actions with outcomes that affect the overall cost, quality, and health status of the individual. How might this work in clinical practice? First, valid and reliable measurements of adherence would be developed and tested. Once these measures are determined to be accurate, the case manager would include these measurements in the initial assessment of the patient. A specific set of interventions would be culled from the literature. The case manager would include these interventions in the care plan. As the plan was executed, the case manager would record the results of each intervention. At the conclusion of the case management episode, the case manager would administer the measures of adherence again. The improvement in the scores, or lack there of, would help to determine the effectiveness of the interventions and the case manager. Finally, overall end outcomes would be measured to demonstrate the impact of improved adherence on end outcomes. Once the link is firmly established, case managers could simply measure their own direct outcomes. Although the state of the science papers on empowerment and involvement and coordination of care have not been completed, similar findings are expected.

IMPLICATIONS FOR CASE MANAGEMENT

Case managers will need to develop a "measurement orientation." The days of "good faith" belief are rapidly coming to an end. A standard line in most any educational program for a health care professional is the phrase, "If it isn't documented, it wasn't done." The new mantra for case managers will be, "If we didn't measure it, it didn't make a difference." Of course, we all know things were done even if they were not written down, and we all know that we are having an impact even if we do not measure the impact. The key element in both of these expressions is the ability to prove the action was taken or the impact was observed. Case managers will need to incorporate measurement into all key aspects of their practice.

The second key implication for practice lies in the ability to link interventions and outcomes. Case managers frequently initiate various interventions to help resolve or improve an identified problem. Anecdotal reports indicate that in most circumstances the case manager can impact the problem positively. What is often missing is the knowledge of which intervention or combination of interventions resulted in the positive outcome. In the quest to measure and demonstrate outcomes, we cannot forget process. It is obligatory to clearly delineate the processes employed to reach the outcome. Recently, a friend was having a computer problem that would result in having to redo a large and complicated spreadsheet. We both tried everything we could think of to resolve the problem. After I made one desperate move, the problem went away. My friend exclaimed, "How did you do that?" I had no idea what I had done, or why it worked. The immediate problem was resolved, but I had no way of reproducing the result because I did not define my intervention. Furthermore, I had no understanding of why it worked. Case management has a history of being apparently successful without clearly understanding why. Our future depends on reversing that trend.

Once we can measure our results and describe our interventions and rationale, standardizing of practice can be accomplished. Case managers can begin to base practice on proven interventions. Imagine the power of being able to measure a patient's level of nonadherence and identify this patient's barriers to adherence. Now imagine implementing a series of interventions proved to be effective in improving adherence where these particular barriers exist. Think of the savings in time when trial and error methods are eliminated and envision obtaining authorization for needed services and equipment when the outcome achieved by using that service is well documented. These are just two examples of what could be accomplished with solid outcome measurements. An additional benefit of standardized practice is the ability to perform comparisons and benchmarking.

Another barrier to outcome measurement for case management has been the numerous variations of interventions, outcome measurement, evaluation methodologies, and terminology. This variation has prevented across-the-board comparisons. Without the ability to compare, it is difficult to identify best practices and innovation. When there is marked variation, differences in outcomes may result from the methodology used to calculate the outcomes, the intervention, or any number of other factors. This often drives people or organizations assigned to evaluate the value of programs to force comparisons. This can result in conclusions based on incomplete or inaccurate comparisons.

With all of this uncertainty, the industry is reluctant to endorse standards of care for case management problems. However, the ability to benchmark and compare data would allow for the identification of best practices and the establishment of standards of care. This process resembles what happened when the Standards of Practice for Case Managers began to forge the requirements for the practice of case management and for what constitutes case management. Standards of care may serve to quell the debate over who is a case manager. Once the controversies over who case managers are, what they do, and what their qualifications should be are resolved, the efforts of case management can focus on shaping and improving practice.

The CCMA was formed by the Case Management Society of America in 1995. The objectives are to establish a framework for accountability and define consistent mechanisms for reporting and comparing performance measurements industry-wide and to disperse those measurements to key stakeholders. They are seeking to identify existing measures and indicators that can be linked to those currently available and used and to identify where there are gaps and no measurements exist.

PATIENT INVOLVEMENT AND PARTICIPATION

Another key outcome attributed to case management is increasing a patient's involvement and participation in their care. In the second State of the Science Paper, Carrie Jo Braden, PhD, RN, FAAN, and editors Gerri Lamb, PhD, RN, FAAN, and Mary Koithan, PhD, RN, report on the role of case managers in involving patients and gaining their participation. They define two distinct concepts of patient engagement. Involvement represents inviting the patient to participate once the problem has been identified, and participation suggests engaging the patient in the identification of the problems and issues that are present.

In most of the literature, case managers write of their desire to have the patient participate, but most of the models describe involvement. In fact, most of the literature discusses interventions that seek to either increase involvement for patients who are perceived as not being sufficiently involved or decreasing involvement for patients designated as overly involved. The concept of patient empowerment is in the very early stages in case management literature. There is little discussion of specific empowerment interventions, and most of the articles achieved little more than simple definitions and references to practice applications.

The chapter indicates that case management is currently in an evolutionary period of shifting values regarding the roles of patients and professionals. Case management is at a crossroads where we will need to determine how to move from what we value (participation and empowerment) to what we implement in practice (involvement). As we shape practice and evaluate outcomes, we need to specifically examine actions case manager take to increase participation and how increased participation is of value to the patients and the health care system.

COORDINATION OF CARE

Coordination of care is a cornerstone of case management practice. The third CCMA State of the Science paper is currently in an unpublished draft form. It is being authored by Madeline H. Schmidt, PhD, RN, FAAN, and Nancee L. Bender, MSN, RN. In the early draft of the work, the authors describe the work of Hesook Kim, which they refer to as the most sophisticated and conceptually advanced definition of care coordination. Hesook uses the concept of the "three Cs." The three Cs are cumulation, complementarity, and contiguity.

- Cumulation is additive rather than repeated activities that build over time without much duplication or overlap.
- Complemetarity are almost transparent. They mutually supply each other's lack without canceling each other.
- Contiguous care is linking pieces in the optimal order that are moving forward in sequential order.

These rationale and systematic connections by different providers progress systematically instead of haphazardly. This definition helps us understand that coordination is a very complex concept. In fact, many times there is confusion. Sometimes people think that the concepts that are related to coordination of care as the definition. The authors compare cooperation, coordination, and collaboration. These concepts progress from cooperation, the most informal, to collaboration, the most complex concept.

The author cites various sources that assert that coordination and communication among those directly involved with the patient's care seem logically important in outcomes. They cite that collaboration and care coordination are among the many variables that are postulated to affect outcomes beyond disease-specific treatment.

Clearly, coordination is a very important variable. Ironically, while coordination of care is very important, it may be the most difficult to quantify directly. Coordination of care has powerful implications for case management practice and outcomes. The levels and complexities of coordination described here offer both opportunities and challenges for our future work in this area.

CONCLUSION

Outcome measurement is critical to the future of case management. In addition to proving the case for case management to the stakeholders, it is necessary for the growth and improvement of case management practice. This imperative for outcome measurement has sparked the industry and even the federal government to embark on a serious quest for reliable measurements of case management impact. The next 5 years will likely generate numerous credible methods to validate case management's role in cost-effective, quality health care.

References

Braden, C.J., Lamb, G., Koithan, M., Council for Case Management Accountability, Case Management Society of America (2002). *State of the Science Paper: Involvement/participation, empowerment and knowledge outcome indicators of case management.* Little Rock, Ark.: Case Management Society of America.

Council for Case Management Accountability, Case Management Society of America (1998). *Informational brochure.* Little Rock, Ark.: Case Management Society of America.

Council for Case Management Accountability, Case Management Society of America (1997). *A framework for case management accountability.* Little Rock, Ark.: Case Management Society of America.

Hamilton, G.A., Council for Case Management Accountability, Case Management Society of America (1999). *State of the Science Paper: Patient adherence outcome indicators and measurement in case management and health care.* Little Rock, Ark.: Case Management Society of America.

Rich, M.W., Beckman, V., et al. (Nov. 2, 1995). A multidisciplinary intervention to prevent the readmission of elderly patients with congestive heart failure. *The New England Journal of Medicine, 333*(18), 1190-1195.

Schmitt, M., Bender, N., Council for Case Management Accountability, Case Management Society of America (2002). *State of the Science Paper: Coordination of care.* Unpublished draft. Little Rock, Ark.: Case Management Society of America.

Case Management Society of America (1995). *Standards of practice for case managers.* Little Rock, Ark.: Case Management Society of America.

Stewart, S., Pearson, S., et al. (1998). Effects of home-based interventions on unplanned readmissions an out-of-hospital deaths. *Journal of the American Geriatric Society, 46,* 174-180.

Wagner, E.H., Davis, C., et al. (1999). A survey of leading chronic disease management programs: Are they consistent with the literature? *Managed Care Quarterly, 7*(3), 56-66.

Case Management

Life at the Intersection of Margin and Mission

Kathleen A. Bower

CHAPTER OVERVIEW

Clinical outcomes. Length of stay and cost per case management. Denial management. Observation status. Patient and family satisfaction. Physician interaction. Revenue cycle enhancement. These are just a few of the issues that case managers address on a daily basis, making it one of the most pivotal and crucial roles in today's complex healthcare environment. Effective financial management is inexorably linked with effective clinical management, and case managers have a role in both. Life in the intersection of margin and mission is frenetic, charged with tension, politically ensnaring . . . in short, hectic. This chapter will highlight some of the strategies that case managers and others use to optimize their organizations' financial outcomes while *simultaneously* maximizing clinical outcomes for their patients. It will emphasize the work of case managers in the financial arena of health care, including revenue cycle management, and outline key strategies for optimizing financial as well as clinical outcomes.

In its most basic form, case management is "a process that efficiently and effectively aligns patient needs/issues with resources to meet quality, clinical and cost outcomes." This definition reinforces the intimate link between the financial and clinical natures of the role. The intersection of margin and mission is a potential "combat zone," with each side vigorously pressing its agenda. Outstanding case managers have the skill and ability to weave between the agenda of all involved parties.

THE FINANCIAL ENVIRONMENT

The financial environment in which health care organizations operate is complex and becoming increasingly so. Pressures from commercial payers are mounting. Government-funded health programs at both the state and national levels are threatened with reductions or closure. Individuals with no insurance or insufficient insurance are presenting themselves to hospitals and other health care providers in staggering numbers. Operating margins have declined from 6.7% in 1996 to 4.6% in 2000, led by reductions in Medicare and Medicaid margins. For example, the average Medicare margin declined from just under 4% in 1997 to below 1% in 2000. In addition, uncompensated care rose from 18% in 1995 to almost 21% in 1999 (American Hospital Association, 2000).

At the operational level, all of this translates into pressures to manage revenue cycles more effectively, reduce length of stay and cost per case, prevent denials, and more. Case managers are in a position to "manage the bottom line . . . one patient at a time." By optimizing clinical efficiencies, they simultaneously enhance the financial viability of the organization and clinical effectiveness.

In addition, revenue cycle management is receiving increased attention by chief financial officers and other members of the executive team. It is a complex process involving all downstream activities that have a direct bearing on the collection of revenue. It means legitimately maximizing the revenue realized on *each* patient and minimizing the amount of time between care provided and revenue billed, and monies received. As a result, it is a process that influences and is influenced by almost all departments and services within a health care organization. Common revenue cycle issues include: Denials, high numbers of days in accounts receivable, and delays between service and billing.

Enhancing financial outcomes and optimizing revenue cycle management require attention to all processes along the patient experience beginning with registration and admitting procedures. For example, case managers have a significant role in timely and effective communication with payer representatives about ongoing need for care. Further downstream, achieving desired outcomes requires careful nurturing of referral sources to facilitate the safe and effective discharge of patients. The admitting and registration processes are additional examples of high-profile departments because the revenue cycle is enhanced when *all* patient information is accurate. This in turn has multiple effects, including (1) bills can be dropped more efficiently, reducing the length of time that bills are in accounts payable; and (2) case managers can more efficiently and effectively initiate discharge plans using the correct payer information to initiate referrals to network postacute providers.

WORK OF CASE MANAGEMENT

Case management is a relationship-based role, linked to almost every department in the organization. At the individual patient/family level, case managers use a clinical reasoning process (assessment, goal setting, planning, implementation, and evaluation) to carefully coordinate patient care and move patients through the care trajectory. The steps of the clinical reasoning process significantly influence both clinical care and financial outcomes. The steps are highlighted below:

1. *Assessment.* This is a comprehensive procedure in which the case manager examines a wide range of patient aspects such as resources (financial, insurance, and community), barriers, impact of the illness, advance directives, capacity to return to the patient's previous living situation, availability of caregivers, and severity of illness/intensity of services. A timely assessment early in the care trajectory alerts the case manager to potential discharge issues and to patient problems that require expedient referrals to other services, particularly social work.

2. *Goal setting* and the definition of desired clinical outcomes with the patient and caregiver(s). The case manager integrates the expected outcomes related to the patient's disease or procedure with the patient's personal goals. Goals become the foundation on which discharge rests and congruence among the goals of the patient/caregiver, the health care team and the case manager minimize struggles over the discharge date. Alignment of expectations regarding length of stay enables patients and their caregivers to anticipate discharge.

3. *Interventions* are planned and implemented; this includes a variety of interventions to facilitate the patient's clinical progression. Case managers are *active* members of the health care team and their

interventions include proactive planning for the next level of care, discharge plan A and plan B (and sometimes C), negotiations with payers, convening meetings with the health care team and/or the patient and family, facilitating patient/family education, engaging ethics consultation as needed, and communicating with and coordinating team activities.

4. *Evaluation.* In this phase, case managers assess the degree to which clinical outcomes are met, the status of financial outcomes (at both the organization and patient/family levels), and levels of satisfaction with the process from among the patient/family as well as involved physicians. The ongoing evaluation of whether outcomes are met positions the case manager to expedite movement of patients through the care trajectory. It also cues the case manager to situations that require the plan to be revised to better achieve desired outcomes.

The clinical reasoning process is an essential component in the case manager's skill set, supporting effective and efficient patient care management. There are additional strategies to optimize this process, and they will be addressed in the next section.

PRIORITY STRATEGIES FOR OPTIMIZING CLINICAL AND FINANCIAL OUTCOMES

There are a number of strategies that have demonstrated efficacy in enhancing the achievement of clinical and/or financial outcomes. Each also has a role to play, whether direct or indirect, on revenue cycle enhancement. Priority strategies are outlined in this section.

Work Toward 100% Accuracy in Registration

Case managers depend on this information to be timely and correct. It is also an important component in revenue cycle enhancement; 100% accuracy involves attention to both roles and procedures within the admitting and registration departments for both scheduled and emergency admissions. Individuals in registration roles must be exceptionally precise and detail oriented. They must also have the capability to obtain information from patients and/or their families in very difficult and sensitive situations. Procedural components include rigorously enforcing a review of each patient's insurance information at *every* admission, even if the patient was "just discharged a few days ago." Dramatic events in patients' lives occur in days, if not hours, that can change an individual's insurance coverage.

Inaccurate patient information can create significant delays and rework for case managers. Incorrect payer information leads to the development of postdischarge plans that are not consistent with the patient's payer network. In turn, often this leads to prolonged length of stay as the correct payer and corresponding network providers. If inaccurate registration information is a consistent issue, it should be quantified to provide a base for discussions between case management and the admitting/registration department focusing on resolving the issue. In many organizations this is a process that begins with the director of case management and the director of admitting/registration acknowledging, in a nonpunitive manner, that there is an issue and making a commitment to address it using an objective, problem-solving (versus blame-finding) approach. The mutual goal is 100% accuracy in patient information.

Use of Criteria

Established and validated criteria should be used on a regular basis to confirm that *all* patients are at the appropriate level of care; this includes Medicare patients as well as commercial payers. When patients do not meet criteria, the day(s) are at risk for being denied. Even if the days are not denied, capacity issues are aggravated. Although case managers must be intimately familiar with the use of criteria, it is also important for other key individuals, including physician advisors and nursing management staff, to have a working knowledge of the process. This makes them more sensitive to the urgency created when patients no longer meet an acute level of care. Effective case managers are skilled in using criteria-based patient review findings in negotiating with physicians and payers.

Pay Close Attention to Observation Status Patients

Observation status is a very complex issue throughout the nation and, as such, requires careful management. That management is best founded on a detailed and current operational observation status policy and procedure for Medicare patients as well as commercial patients. This serves as the foundation for consistently applying this outpatient designation.

How the management of observation status is included in the case managers' role is also a consideration within each organization. Some organizations establish one (or more, depending on the size of the facility) case manager to focus on all observation status patients; others incorporate the management of observation status into the caseload of all case managers. In either model, patients on observation status must be a high priority for daily case manager interactions.

In addition to establishing a policy and procedure, data regarding the application of observation status must be carefully trended, analyzed, and addressed. In particular, the following data points should be monitored: Volume of Medicare patients with a 1- or 2-day length of stay; number of observation status patients compared with the total number of admissions; and denials related to observation status. These data points will provide important cues regarding the appropriate use of observation status and where the procedure and its operationalization should be strengthened.

Anticipate Denials and Work Proactively to Prevent Them

The best way to manage denials is to prevent them. These is a simple statement but requires vigilant case manager efforts to accomplish. As noted earlier, when patients no longer meet acute care criteria, there is a risk for denials. From a quality point of view, prolonged hospitalization can also lead to increased risk of complications and/or deterioration in functional status, particularly in the elderly and disabled. Awareness of a potential denial is a cue for case managers to intensify their efforts toward discharge planning or transfer to postacute care.

This is another situation that mandates the development of an operational procedure. When a payer representative concurrently indicates that a denial will be issued, case managers are triggered to intervene. The first intervention is to thoroughly review the case, keeping the appropriate criteria in mind. When case managers disagree with the payer decisions, they request the payer case managers/representatives to clearly articulate, using criteria, the nature of the denial. A negotiation ensues and if the issue cannot be resolved, the hospital case manager should document the status of the patient per criteria on the worksheet and notify the attending physician of the pending denial. In some situations it is also advisable to notify the director of case management and the physician advisor about the pending denial.

Establish a Tight Appeal Management Process

Denials have a significant impact on the financial situation of an organization. The care has already been provided and so expenses have been incurred. Denials also negatively influence the revenue side. As a result, the appeal process must be carefully managed. This includes the following:

- Contractually clarifying with payers the circumstances under which denials may be issued. Case managers need that information as it is updated, keeping in mind that case managers manage payer contracts one patient at a time.
- Establishing a central point for denial notifications to be received in the organization.
- Logging in all denials as they are received and then dispersing them for review, action and a timely response.
- Creating a process by which denials are appealed within established timeframes.
- Involving physicians in the appeal process. In many situations, denials may be overturned through direct physician communication with the payer.
- Writing detailed, accurate, compelling letters of appeal.
- Trending the organization's denial experience by days and dollars at the following levels: case type, diagnosis-related group (or DRG), physician, payer, nursing unit, and case manager. As trends are identified, strategies can be developed to address issues and problems.
- Tracking the success rate in the denial appeal cycle. For example: How much money has been recovered through the appeal process; with which payers have appeals been most successful? This information is very useful in contract negotiations with third-party payers as well as revising internal procedures.
- Providing a careful orientation regarding denials and their appeal to case managers as well as others in the organization (including the nurse manager level).

Tighten the Discharge Planning Process

Keep in mind that discharge is not the outcome; it is the result of meeting clinical outcomes. Timely discharge planning is a critical strategy for effective patient care management and ultimately for achieving desired clinical and financial outcomes. This requires more than tokenism and must be founded on concrete structures and processes. Those structures and processes include the following:

- Identifying family and others who are willing, able, and *available* to provide needed postdischarge support to each patient by day 2.
- Establishing an anticipated discharge date for each patient by day 2.
- Collaborating with physicians to create realistic outcome criteria for high-volume case types and for individual patients. Those outcome criteria become the basis for negotiations with physicians, patients, and their families as well as payers.
- Expecting that case managers go see, smell, touch, and listen to each patient to minimize surprises. Functional status and mental status are frequently identified problem areas in moving patients toward discharge.
- Optimizing discharge planning rounds; discharge planning rounds should occur *daily* with the case manager, social worker, and a member of the unit's nursing staff. The goals of discharge planning rounds are to (1) identify actual or potential barriers to patient discharge; (2) identify who will be accountable for addressing those issues; and (3) establishing the next step(s) for moving the patient to discharge. To maximize the effectiveness of rounds, it is useful to establish a format for presenting patients and for proceeding through issue identification and resolution.

There are six questions to *routinely* ask in discharge planning rounds about each patient:

1. What is the anticipated discharge date?
2. Could care be provided in another level of care or setting?
3. What are the anticipated postdischarge needs?
4. What are the actual or potential barriers to discharge or transfer?

5. Who will be accountable for addressing identified barriers?
6. What are the next steps?

- Creating and documenting discharge *plan A* and *plan B* for each patient. This provides back up when the primary plan falls through, which usually happens on Friday afternoons. The ensuing chaos can be alleviated if there is a reasonable backup plan in the works.
- Treating Thursday as the most important day of the week for discharge planning. Friday is often too late to establish a firm discharge plan, particularly for more complex patient situations. Instead of focusing on Fridays as the discharge day, shift to Thursdays and use Fridays to confirm and/or finalize the plans.
- Working toward a goal of having 45% of all discharged patients referred to a postacute provider (home care, rehabilitation, SNF, TCU, etc.). This will also have the positive effect of reducing readmission rates.

Nurture the Organization's Post-Acute Referral Base

This has a profound effect on an organization's ability to smoothly and efficiently transfer patients to the next level of care. In particular, establish letters of agreement with providers about when patients can be admitted, including weekend admissions. Develop working relationships with members of high-volume referral organizations to facilitate "special occasion" transfers. Regular meetings with the organization's primary postacute providers can be a forum for identifying ongoing issues in transitioning patients from one location to another and establishing strategies to resolve them.

Establish Medicare and Medicaid as Equal Payers with All Other Payers

Because Medicare and Medicaid do not provide external reviews, it is up to the provider to be disciplined about managing this population. As a result, Medicare patients often slip to the bottom of the case managers' priority lists, allowing unnecessary days to slip in. Vigor in optimizing the management of Medicare patients translates into (among other activities) reviewing Medicare patients on a regular basis, managing the issuance of HINNs (hospital-issued notices of noncoverage), and managing observation status. The outcome is generally reduced length of stay, more appropriate administration of HINNs, and fewer denials related to inappropriate designation of observation status versus inpatient status.

Pay Attention to the Status of Clinical Outcomes and Critical Indicators

Clinical outcomes and critical indicators are anchors for case management practice. They represent important landmarks for planning discharge and for negotiating with patients, physicians, payers, nursing staff, and others.

Clinical outcomes describe the usual, desired condition of the patient at discharge or at the end of treatment; they reflect the patient's response to treatment. Case managers work within five categories of clinical outcomes: health status (the patient's physiological response to treatment), comfort (including pain, anxiety, inspiratory effort, etc.), patient/caregiver knowledge and skills regarding self-management of the disease process, functionality (including ambulation and activities of daily living), and management of actual or potential complications anticipated in the diagnosis. Agreement on clinical outcomes in an important step in effectively transitioning the patient to the next level of care.

Critical indicators are a subset of interventions and outcomes per case type, patient population, or sometimes individual patient that represent significant turning points in the care trajectory. They incorporate interventions and/or outcomes that, if not met within a specified timeframe, may lead to a longer length of stay, poorer outcomes, and/or increased resource use. There are a *limited* number of critical indicators in each case type or patient situation. Ideally critical indicators are evidence based or consensus driven. Critical indicators represent essential components of care for individual patients as well as patient populations. They are invaluable case management tools and serve as an effective foundation for process improvement initiatives.

Create a Paid Physician Advisor Position

This is an important resource to the case managers, particularly in interacting with physicians and payers around difficult patient situations. The physician advisor must be available to the case managers on a regular basis to review cases and situations, to identify consistent issues and problems that require physician input, and to develop realistic departmental goals. The physician advisor is an important participant in the long-stay review process, identifying issues where physician input is likely to eliminate or reduce barriers.

This position has a direct, positive effect on revenue cycle enhancement, length of stay, long-stay patients, and cost per case. This is particularly true if the individual in this position has a combination of political savvy, clinical knowledge, good communication and negotiation skills, and knowledge about payer requirements. Belief in the necessity for stewardship of medical resources is a strong foundation for incumbents as they interact with case managers, peer physicians, and payers. A list of useful activities for physician advisors is included in Box 38-1. When selecting a physician advisor, knowledge about payer requirements is a plus, but keep in mind that it is a topic about which the physician can be educated fairly quickly. It is important that the advisor interact with physicians in noncrisis situations rather than only dealing with urgent issues. In particular, the director of case management and the physician advisor need to develop a strong working relationship to facilitate problem solving and goal setting.

Pay Special and Consistent Attention to Long-Stay Patients

Long-stay patients are medical/surgical patients who have been hospitalized for 7 or more days in acute care. They usually represent intense and/or complex issues that require in-depth interventions by case managers and social workers. Because complex patients almost always present cues early in the hospital

---

BOX 38-1   TEN SIMPLE RULES FOR PHYSICIAN ADVISORS

1. Develop a working knowledge about utilization management processes, including review criteria, processes, principles, rationale, and application; observation status, and denials.
2. Develop a working knowledge about levels of care and community resources.
3. Identify length of stay and clinical resource issues for the organization's top diagnoses (by volume, cost, and/or loss), highlighting benchmarks and best practices.
4. Develop a first-line response to hearing "I've always done it this way" or "I tried it once before and got in trouble" from physician colleagues.
5. Get as much information as possible about problem patient situations from case managers, social workers, and/or nursing staff.
6. When addressing issues related to multiple physicians, become the platform from which physician interaction and communication occur as needed. Call a team meeting as needed; have the issues outlined, the desired goals articulated, and a time-limited agenda.
7. Interact with peer physicians about nonurgent issues as well as urgent ones.
8. Round with case managers and social workers on problem and/or high-risk patients.
9. Optimize the use of internal resources, including the ethics consultation service and social workers (especially for complex family situations).
10. Ask two questions on a routine basis: (1) What is keeping this patient in acute care? (2) What is needed to move the patient to the next level of care?

stay, case managers and social workers should pay particular attention to days 2 and 3. By this point, sufficient data have usually been amassed about the patient and the nature of the illness has begun to emerge. As patients are identified to be potential long-stay patients, the case manager–social worker team must establish a plan to closely monitor the patient's progress or lack thereof, intervening as needed. This is a patient who cannot fall off the team's radar screen.

In addition to increased attention by the case manager and social worker, a weekly, organization-wide long-stay review meeting should be established. This involves a weekly meeting that is attended by all case managers and social workers, the director of case management, and the physician advisor. Members of the executive team, particularly the vice president for finance, also find it helpful to attend on a regular basis to gain insight into internal and external barriers to patient care, to the movement of patients through the health care trajectory, and to the impact of physician practice patterns on length of stay.

Address End-of-Life Issues Early On

An unfortunate number of patients spend the last few days of their lives in intensive care and/or acute care. In some cases, this is in direct opposition to their expressed wishes. Case managers and social workers are often called on to reconcile the wishes of the patient, his or her family, the physician(s), and other members of the health care team. This creates a true impetus for case managers and social workers to carefully explore the advance directives of individual patients and to establish a working relationship with patients and their support system. While this is true for all patients, it is particularly important when dealing with the elderly and the chronically ill. Negotiating care within the individual's preferences necessitates a high level of skill for both case managers and social workers. It is a skill that requires ongoing development through case discussions and role play.

Organizational structures are critical, including a strong ethics consultation service that is available to all. Data monitors important in this situation include the number of "no code" patients who die in intensive care and the number of patients who are resuscitated yet have a "no code" advance directive. This information provides important cues to situations in which earlier case review and consultation may have been useful.

Work Toward Positive Relationships with Physicians

Successful management of clinical and financial outcomes is directly related, in part, to the relationship that evolves between case managers and physicians. Positive physician relationships are based on a number of factors, including the case manager's clinical knowledge, communication skills, and ability to create options for individual patients as well as patient populations. In conjunction with the Physician advisor, effective case management directors and case managers develop strategies to optimize relationships, including identifying core issues, concerns, and needs of the physicians with whom they work. In some organizations, aligning the case manager assignments to physicians (individual and/or groups) provides the foundation to create more effective relationships. Case manager participation in physician meetings (such as department/specialty) is another approach that has demonstrated efficacy in strengthening case manager–physician relationships.

Strengthen Relationships with Nursing Colleagues

Case managers share patients with the clinical nursing staff. It is critical for success that case managers be actively engaged with those nurses versus being seen as "paper pushers" or "data miners." Collaboration with clinical nursing staff will facilitate early referrals of high-risk patients to case managers. It will also facilitate communication of plans and issues from one shift to the next and from one day to the next.

Nursing managers and administrative staff are powerful allies as well. There are some key points of convergence that should be optimized:

1. Establishing mutual goals. It is essential that the nursing management staff and the case managers have mutual goals vis-à-vis patient management. The mutual goals may incorporate length of stay, denials, readmissions, and cost per case.
   a. This will require regular forums for discussing the existing goals and highlighting future goals.
   b. The discussions should lead to identifying data points that will be used to evaluate the extent to which the goals are met and discussed on a consistent basis.
2. Optimizing care management structures such as identifying high-risk patients, defining long-stay patients, intershift report, and discharge planning rounds.
   a. Collaboration between case managers and nursing management staff enhances the identification of high-risk patients and provides a consistent response to the question that is often posed, "Why is this patient still here?" The desired response is an immediate call to the case manager.
   b. Management staff can increase the likelihood that patient management information such as anticipated discharge dates, expected outcomes, and discharge plans are communicated in intershift report.

Carefully Monitor and Analyze Readmissions

For case managers, readmissions are an indication that something has not gone as planned. In this manner, they become a critical quality indicator for case management. The readmission may be a patient who is hospitalized for the same or related condition within 31 days of a previous hospitalization. However, it is equally important to identify and address the needs of patients who experience three or more inpatient admissions in a 12-month period. Readmissions have a potential financial effect. They also influence capacity, a common problem in today's health care environment.

Readmissions are related to a variety of issues, including system, clinician, and patient/family. An example of a system issue is the patient for whom home services are arranged but do not materialize in a timely way. Clinician issues include inadequate teaching of patients and their families about the essentials of caring for their condition or disease. Incomplete assessment of the patient's situation is also a clinician issue. For example, patients who cannot afford to purchase needed medications are often reluctant to express this problem; gaining this knowledge requires skillful interviewing and relationship building by the case manager and social worker.

When a patient is readmitted, a careful, comprehensive assessment is essential to unearth root causes of the admission. Noncompliance is often mentioned as a point of fact and cited as a cause of patient readmissions, most often referred to in diagnostic terms. However, success in reducing readmission rates in individual patients as well as patient populations (such as for congestive heart failure patients) means revising how noncompliance is viewed from a diagnosis to a symptom. Approaching noncompliance as a symptom leads to further investigation about the underlying cause; is the problem related to finances, cognition, social support, an exacerbation of comorbidities, conflict with cultural or religious beliefs, or a myriad of other potential causes? Each cause requires a distinct strategy.

Create an Emergency Department Case Manager Role

The emergency department is usually the entry portal for the majority of inpatient admissions. Its importance is magnified by the consideration that patients experiencing frequent visits to the emergency department also experience a high number of inpatient admissions. This is a difficult cycle to break and requires an individual who can focus on the needs and issues of these patients to reduce recidivism.

Emergency department staff primarily concentrate on stabilizing the patient for discharge to home or preparing them for an inpatient admission. This group of professionals usually do not have the knowledge or time to explore other options for patients, even though there may be legitimate alternatives such as home with services and/or a geriatric assessment unit.

Case managers in the emergency department can provide a vital direct service by creating options other than an inpatient admission. They also provide support and education about appropriate decisions regarding observation status, which are almost always made for these patients in the emergency department. Finally, emergency department case managers can be invaluable in establishing programs and plans of care for patient populations experiencing high readmission rates, such as pain management or sickle cell anemia.

SUMMARY

Case managers are pivotal in reaching effective clinical and financial outcomes. Their success depends on sound processes and procedures. It also depends on establishing a network of relationships with internal and external entities. Internal entities include physicians, nursing staff, social workers, admitting/registration staff, administrators, and other members of the health care team. External entities include payers and community based resources.

The case manager role requires simultaneous attention to the needs and progress of individual patients and families as well as populations. Knowledge of and integration of clinical outcomes and critical indicators anchor case management practice to reality and provide a safety net for patients and the organization. Case managers attend to the needs of multiple constituencies and must therefore possess a wide range of skills in addition to their knowledge about clinical processes. Those skills include negotiation, inclusion, time management, priority setting, interviewing skills, and team skills.

Because the health care environment is constantly evolving, effective case management departments review their processes, relationships, and strategies on a regular basis—at least annually. The 15 strategies outlined in this chapter may be pertinent for an organization this year but may need extensive revision next year. Creating alignment between the needs of individual patients and internal and external environments is a constant challenge. All of this creates a role that is often complex, conflictive, and political but certainly never dull.

Reference

American Hospital Association (2000). Hospital statistics. Chicago, Ill: American Hospital Association.

39

Maximizing Reimbursement Through Accurate Documentation and Coding

Toni G. Cesta

CHAPTER OVERVIEW

Each year hospitals lose millions of dollars in unreimbursed revenue because of their inability to code medical records into the most appropriate DRG that reflects the actual care rendered. This chapter reviews strategies for educating physicians in documentation and coding, and processes for monitoring documentation, coding, and reimbursement in any organization.

INTRODUCTION

In 1983 the U.S. Congress mandated a prospective payment system (PPS) for all Medicare inpatient stays based on the diagnosis-related group (DRG) system. This system applies to all inpatient acute care facilities except psychiatric facilities, children's hospitals, cancer care hospitals, and other specialty hospitals. The DRG system is a model developed to aggregate patients with similar pathology who use similar amounts of hospital resources and have similar length of stay patterns. It is used to determine appropriate utilization of services and to calculate financial reimbursement.

Each DRG is assigned a relative weight, which is used to calculate the prospective payment for an inpatient stay. The relative weight is based on the average resources used to treat Medicare patients in that DRG compared with the average resources used to treat Medicare patients in all DRGs. The relative weight is multiplied by the "hospital pay rate" for a specific hospital to calculate the hospital's reimbursement for a Medicare patient's hospital stay. The relative weights are calculated around an "average" weight of 1.0. Therefore weights noted to be greater than 1.0 are considered to reflect DRGs representing case types that have a higher resource utilization and average length of stay. Relative weights below 1.0 reflect case types that are less resource consuming and have a shorter length of stay in the aggregate.

Many states also use DRGs for their Medicaid programs. The relative weights under each state's prospective payment system may be different than the Medicare weights, as each state bases its weights on patterns it notes in its own patient population. In some cases the DRG is used for per diem rate setting. States with these rate-setting programs use the DRGs to adjust per diem rates. In addition, there are some DRG-exempt categories in some states.

The DRGs lump together "like" patients. Patients are considered alike if they demonstrate similar resource utilization and length of stay. Resource utilization is defined by the product or personnel resources used to care for that type of patient. *Product resources* refer to diagnostic and therapeutic interventions such as use of medications, laboratory tests, radiology, and so on. *Personnel costs* refer to the use of nursing hours per case or other personnel. Length of stay refers to the number of days that the patient remains in the hospital.

MAJOR DIAGNOSTIC CATEGORIES

The DRGs are categorized into major diagnostic categories (MDCs). The number of DRGs in each MDC varies from 1 to 20 or more. The MDCs are consistent with anatomical or pathophysiological groupings and/or the ways in which patients would be clinically managed. Examples include diseases of the central nervous system, diseases of bone and cartilage, and diseases and disorders of the kidney and urinary tract. The major diagnostic categories are broken down into either medical or surgical, meaning the presence or absence of a surgical procedure.

HOSPITAL PAYMENT

Hospital payment is calculated by multiplying the relative weight with the hospital's assigned base rate. Each hospital is assigned a base rate for reimbursement by the federal government, that is, the Centers for Medicare and Medicaid Services (CMS). The base rate is determined based on the specific hospital (teaching, academic, community), geographic location, population served, cost of living in that area, and types of services provided. CMI and base rates are reviewed periodically by the CMS and adjustments made as needed based on actuarial data (Cesta and Tahan, 2002). In addition, the DRG system is reviewed and updated on an annual basis. The results of this review are published in the federal register. Each year some DRGs are added, whereas others may be deleted.

THE CASE MIX INDEX

The CMI is the sum of all DRG-relative weights divided by the number of cases (patients) cared for over a period of time, usually 1 calendar year. The higher the CMI, the higher is the assumed case mix complexity of the hospital. Case mix is affected by the following:
- Severity of illness
- Prognosis
- Treatment difficulty
- Need for intervention
- Resource intensity
- Presence of complications and comorbidities

MEASURING THE ELEMENTS IN CASE MIX

Severity of illness and prognosis reflect the complexity of services or the types of services provided. Severity of illness is made up of objective, clinical indicators of the patient's illness that reflect the need for hospitalization. Prognosis indicates the patient's likelihood of recovering and to what extent. Treatment difficulty, need for intervention, and resource intensity comprise the intensity of service or the number of services per patient day or hospital stay. The case mix influences hospital costs. It is not the number of patients that affects the costs incurred by the hospital but rather the types of patients and their use of resources.

ASSIGNING THE DRG

Assignment of a DRG is made based on the documentation in the medical record. For the proper information to be obtained, the record must be comprehensive and complete. The documentation must be timely, legible, thorough, and proper.

Finally, documentation in the medical record, although always important, carries even greater weight under this system. Because reimbursement is contingent on the diagnoses and surgical procedures, charting must be complete and accurate. In some hospitals an individual monitors the medical record documentation to ensure that it is accurate, timely, and reflective of what is currently happening in the case. Hospitals with case management programs sometimes assign this function to the case manager.

DRG ASSIGNMENT

After discharge, the medical record coders review the patient's record. The DRG assignment requires a thorough accounting of the following:
- Principal diagnosis
- Secondary diagnosis
- Operating room procedures
- Complications
- Comorbidities
- Age
- Discharge status

The principal diagnosis (or primary diagnosis) is the condition determined to have been chiefly responsible for the admission to the hospital. The major diagnosis is that which consumed the most hospital resources. The principal diagnosis and the major diagnosis are not necessarily the same. The secondary diagnosis is prioritized next in terms of resource consumption. Principal procedures are those performed to treat the chief complaint or complication rather than those performed for diagnostic purposes. If more than one procedure is performed, then the one most closely related to the principal diagnosis will become the principal procedure. Any other surgical procedures are considered as secondary. Operating room procedures other than those performed for diagnostic purposes are also considered as principal procedures. Complications and comorbidities, as defined earlier, are also considered. Age is a determining factor for about one fifth of the DRGs. Age 65 is a demarcation line for some. For a small number of DRGs, the patient's discharge status is considered. Discharge status refers to the final patient destination after discharge, such as nursing home, home, or home with services.

MEDICAL RECORDS CODING

One DRG is assigned to each medical record for a particular hospital stay by the hospital coding staff, based on an abstraction of the information documented by physicians, nurses, and others in the patient's medical record. The coders are not allowed to interpret anything in the medical record that is not explicitly documented by a physician. This makes it vital that physician documentation is complete and accurate. During their chart reviews, the coders obtain information on the principal diagnosis, secondary diagnoses (up to eight) and procedures (up to six), which are used to assign the appropriate DRG. The DRG is also affected by the age and gender of the patient, discharge status, and the presence or absence of "complications or comorbidities."

A *complication* under the PPS system is defined as a condition that arises during the hospital stay that prolongs the length of stay by at least 1 day in approximately 75% of the cases (Lorenz and Jones, 2002).

A *comorbidity* is considered a preexisting condition, that, because of its presence with a specific diagnosis, causes an increase in length of stay at least one day in 75% of the cases (Lorenz and Jones, 2002).

Documentation of complications and comorbidities is critical to accurate and appropriate reimbursement. In many instances, the DRG relative weight is doubled with the addition of a complication/comorbidity (CC) designation. This means double the reimbursement to the hospital. The CC allows for additional reimbursement for cases that had a higher cost or length of stay, attempting to compensate the hospital for the additional cost these conditions may represent. Neither a complication nor a comorbidity can be coded unless there is clear documentation supporting that designation.

MEDICAL RECORD DOCUMENTATION

Documentation in the medical record serves multiple purposes. Documentation is a means of communication between the members of the interdisciplinary team; it is used as a mechanism for evaluating the appropriateness and adequacy of patient care; and it provides supportive data to ensure reimbursement, legal protection to patients and health care providers and organizations, and clinical data for education and research.

Multiple regulatory organizations provide standards regarding documentation in the medical record. Medicare's Conditions of Participation require that medical records be written accurately, be completed promptly, be properly filed and retained, and accessible. In addition, records must document as appropriate, complications, hospital-acquired infections and adverse drug reactions. The final diagnosis must be documented in the medical record within 30 days of the patient's discharge from the hospital.

The Joint Commission on Accreditation of Healthcare Organizations (JCAHO) (2000) states in its standards that the medical record must contain sufficient documentation to identify the patient, support the diagnosis, justify the treatment, document the course and results, and promote continuity among health care providers. All of these data and information are ultimately used by the coders as the basis for the selection of the *ICD-9* codes for reimbursement purposed under the DRG system. With accurate and complete documentation, the medical records coders are able to analyze, code, and report the required information. This ensures proper reimbursement to the hospital.

THE CODING PROCESS

The coders in the medical records department are trained professionals who have studied the *ICD-9* coding system and how to identify *ICD-9* codes in the patient's medical record. Within each DRG, there are large numbers of *ICD-9* codes, many of which represent a diversity of clinical conditions. The *ICD-9* codes designate diagnoses and procedures. The coders extrapolate all relevant *ICD-9* codes that are placed into a computer system. The system then follows an internal decision tree using the *ICD-9* codes to arrive at the DRG assignment.

THE RELATIONSHIP BETWEEN DOCUMENTATION AND CODING

Physician documentation is critical to accurate coding. It is expected that physicians and coding professionals work together to ensure that documentation is accurate and complete. This relationship is based on the collaboration of the physician, with his or her clinical knowledge, and the coding professional, with his or her expert knowledge of the coding classification system.

Coded data are used for more than just reimbursement purposes. It is used to:
- Improve the quality and effectiveness of patient care
- Expand the body of medical knowledge through education and research
- Assist in making decisions regarding health care policies, delivery systems, funding, and expansion of services
- Monitor resource utilization
- Improve clinical decision-making
- Facilitate the monitoring of fraud and abuse
- Provide comparative data to consumers regarding cost and outcomes of care

IMPROVING PHYSICIAN DOCUMENTATION

The coders cannot accurately code without complete and legible documentation. Many physicians are unaware of the impact that slight changes in the verbiage they document can make on the reimbursement to the hospital. Improving documentation and therefore coding is a process that can mean significant financial gains to a hospital that finds its case mix index below that of similar organizations with like types of patient groupings. Typically, the hospital can extrapolate pairs of similar DRGs that represent comparable types of patients but significantly different amounts of reimbursement. For example, urinary tract infection and septicemia may appear to be clinically similar, but in coding language they represent very different clinical types and different amounts of reimbursement (Box 39-1). Similarly, simple pneumonia and respiratory infection code differently and represent different levels of reimbursement (Box 39-2); another pair might be angina and coronary artery disease (Box 39-3).

To the practicing physician, a urinary tract infection, or urosepsis, may be considered one and the same, and therefore the physician may not differentiate this adequately in his or her documentation. *Urosepsis* is defined as bacteria in the blood, as confirmed by culture, which may be transient and denotes

---

BOX 39-1 ▶ URINARY TRACT INFECTIONS AND SEPTICEMIA

DRG 320 Kidney and urinary tract infections, age greater than 17, with complication/comorbidity
Medicare reimbursement = $5187*
DRG 416 Septicemia, age greater than 17
Medicare reimbursement = $14,706*

* Based on national average, actual reimbursement may vary.

BOX 39-2	SIMPLE PNEUMONIA VERSUS RESPIRATORY INFECTION

DRG 89 Simple pneumonia with complications or comorbidities
   Medicare reimbursement = $9586*
DRG 79 respiratory infection
   Medicare reimbursement = $14,898*

*Based on national average, actual reimbursement may vary.

BOX 39-3	ANGINA AND CORONARY ARTERY DISEASE

DRG 140 Angina without documented coronary artery disease
   Medicare reimbursement = $4951*
DRG 132 Angina with known coronary artery disease
   Medicare reimbursement = $6039*

*Based on national average, actual reimbursement may vary.

a laboratory finding. *Septicemia* denotes an acute illness. Urosepsis progresses to septicemia only when there is a more severe infectious process or an impaired immune system. Septicemia, or generalized sepsis, is caused by leakage of urine or toxic byproducts into the general vascular circulation.

If the physician, in his or her medical record documentation, differentiates the diagnosis as above, the coder can code as septicemia, which by DRG relative weight pays considerably more than bacteremia. Nothing has changed in the care of the patient or in the patient's actual clinical condition. The physician is simply providing the necessary language, which will allow the coder to apply the more highly weighted DRG and ensure the more enhanced and appropriate reimbursement to the hospital.

Simple pneumonia with either a complication or comorbidity would include any of the following:
- Pneumonia (not otherwise specified)
- Viral pneumonia
- Bronchopneumonia
- Pneumococcal pneumonia
- *Streptococcus*
- *Haemophilus influenzae* pneumonia
- *Mycoplasma* pneumonia

Respiratory infection with complications or comorbidities would include any of these diagnoses:
- *Klebsiella* pneumonia
- *Pseudomonas*
- *Haemophilus parainfluenzae*
- *Staphylcoccus aureus* pneumonia
- *Escherichia coli* pneumonia
- Aspiration pneumonia
- Probable gram-negative pneumonia

BOX 39-4 EXAMPLE OF A COMORBID CONDITION

Primary diagnosis: Chronic cholecystitis with cholelithiasis
Secondary diagnosis: Coronary artery disease
                    Stable angina
Procedure: Laparoscopy to open cholecystectomy
DRG 198 Open cholecystectomy without complications/comorbidities = $11,270*
DRG 197 Open cholecystectomy with complications/comorbidities = $22,868*

*Based on national average, actual reimbursement may vary.

Inclusion of these organisms in the medical record will provide the necessary documentation to allow the coder to apply the most appropriate DRG and ensure the appropriate level of reimbursement.

In the example of angina with and without coronary artery disease, the inclusion of the documentation indicating the finding of coronary artery disease will mean an increase in reimbursement of $1088 per admission.

Surgical diagnoses can also be monitored for adequate documentation. In many of these instances, adequate documentation of the patient's comorbidities (Box 39-4) can result in the assignment of a much higher weighted DRG.

The following broad categories can be used to assist physicians in ensuring that their documentation is accurate and complete.

1. Address the clinical significance of abnormal test results. Coders cannot draw conclusions or make assumptions based on laboratory or other findings in the medical record. The physician must discuss the findings in the record and their significance to the patient's clinical condition.
2. The documentation must support the level of services and the intensity of services being provided. This would include the evaluation and treatment being provided as well as describing the thought processes and complexities involved in the decision making process.
3. Include a discussion of all diagnostic and therapeutic procedures, treatments, and tests performed, with their results included and discussed.
4. Include any changes that have occurred in the patient's condition, such as psychosocial or physical symptoms.
5. Include any conditions that coexisted at the time of the patient's admission to the hospital, or that developed after admission, or that affect the treatment received or the length of stay. This would include all conditions that affect patient care in terms of requiring clinical evaluation, therapeutic treatment, diagnostic procedures, extended length of hospital stay, or increased nursing care or monitoring.
6. Update as necessary to reflect all diagnoses relevant to the care or services being provided.
7. Be consistent and discuss and reconcile any discrepancies.
8. The document must be legible, written in ink, or typewritten or electronically signed and printed.

Following these standards for documentation can better ensure that the physician's documentation can be optimally used by the coding professionals. At the same time, the coders have responsibilities that complement those just listed for the physician. Coding professionals are expected to support the accurate, complete, and consistent coding practices in the production of quality health care data. They follow a standard within the American Health Information Management Association (AHIMA) Code of Ethics (1996). The Code of Ethics stipulates that health information management professionals promote high standards for health information management practice, education, and research and that health information management professionals strive to provide accurate and timely information.

Coding professionals are required to maintain data accuracy and integrity. They are expected to use practices that produce complete, accurate, and timely information to meet the health and related needs of individuals. They must follow the guidelines set forth by the organization's compliance plan and HIPAA (Health Insurance Portability and Accountability Act) regarding the reporting of improper preparation, alteration, or suppression of data. Finally, they must not participate in any improper preparation, alteration, or suppression of health record information or any other organizational data.

Coding professionals can only assign and report codes that are clearly and consistently supported by physician documentation in the medical record. A checks and balance system must be in place to reassess physician documentation to ensure that it supports the diagnosis and procedural codes reported.

CODERS AND PHYSICIANS MUST WORK TOGETHER

Open communication and a mutual understanding are critical to the successful collaboration between coders and physicians. The coder's clinical knowledge and understanding are improved through these communications, and the physician's knowledge and understanding of coding principles are improved. Coding professionals are expected to consult with physicians when they require clarification and additional documentation before the code assignments are made. This is particularly critical when there are conflicting or ambiguous data in the medical record. Coding professionals can assist and educate physicians by advocating for proper documentation practices and greater specificity in the physician's documentation. The coders can also assist and educate physicians by instructing them in the resequencing, or inclusion of diagnoses or procedures when needed, which will more accurately reflect the acuity, severity, or occurrence of events.

It is improper for coders to misrepresent the patient's clinical picture through incorrect coding or by adding diagnoses or procedures unsupported by the documentation to maximize reimbursement or to meet insurance policy coverage requirements. They cannot inappropriately include or exclude diagnoses or procedures.

THE PHYSICIAN QUERY PROCESS

Each hospital should have a policy and procedure in place for physician querying. The process of physician querying can be a highly successful means to improving the quality of the documentation and the coding. Query processes can be designed in a number of different ways. These differences may be dependent on the organization's resources with which to carry each of them out as well as the specific needs of the organization in terms of its documentation deficits and requirements for improvement. Because physicians are not taught these essential elements of documentation and its relationship to coding in medical school, most organizations will find that there are opportunities for improvement that they can address and incrementally improve on.

A query process can be done through the use of query forms. These forms are used as tools for communication between a coder, a chart reviewer such as a case manager, and the physician. Such tools must be used before the completion of the coding process. The goals of query forms are to improve documentation and enhance coding as it relates to that documentation, not to inappropriately enhance reimbursement.

A policy and procedure must be developed to guide the coders and/or case managers in obtaining clarification from the physician on documentation that will affect the coding assignment. The AHIMA's

Standards of Ethical Coding should be used to guide this process. It is expected, as per the ethical standards, that the process be a patient-specific process, not a general process. It is not acceptable for the coder to ask generic-type questions; the coder must ask patient-specific level questions.

Physicians should not be asked to provide clarification of the specific medical record without the opportunity to review that medical record. The query process can take place either concurrently while the record is open, or retrospectively, after discharge. If the hospital has a concurrent coding process, then most likely the query process will be conducted by a coding professional. If they do not have a concurrent coding process, then a specific individual may be assigned to review open medical records for accurate and complete documentation. This may be a coding specialist, a registered nurse such as a case manager, or another appropriately educated and trained individual. Charts may also be reviewed retrospectively in medical records by a coding specialist, a physician, or a case manager. Either method is acceptable. It may be somewhat easier from a process perspective to correct documentation while the patient is in the hospital and the physician is available and accessible. Querying while the patient is still in the hospital can also assist in improving the quality of patient care.

In some cases, conflicts may arise between the physician and the coding professionals. In these instances, the hospital may want to designate a physician liaison who can resolve any conflicts between the coder and the physician. Appropriate use of the physician liaison should also be included in the policies and procedures for the query process.

There are specific formats to be used for the query process. Scrap paper or "sticky notes" are not acceptable formats. The query form should be developed by the hospital and be included in its policies and procedures. A proper query form should:
- Be clearly and concisely written
- Contain precise language
- Present the facts from the medical record and identify why clarification is needed
- Present the scenario and state a question that asks the physician to make a clinical interpretation of a given diagnosis or condition based on treatment, evaluation, monitoring, and/or services provided. Open-ended questions should be used that allow the physician to document the specific diagnosis. A query that appears to lead the physician to provide a particular response may give the appearance of improper coding practice.
- Be phrased so that the physician is allowed to specify the correct diagnosis. It should not indicate the financial impact associated with the query. The form should not be designed as a pre-printed documentation tool that the physician simply has to sign.

Box 39-5 provides appropriate elements for inclusion in a query form. Box 39-6 outlines the elements that should not be included in a query form.

BOX 39-5 ▶ ELEMENTS TO BE INCLUDED ON A QUERY FORM

- Patient name
- Admission date
- Medical record number
- Name and contact information of the coding specialist
- Specific question and rationale
- Place for physician to document his response

BOX 39-6 ▸ ELEMENTS NOT TO BE INCLUDED ON A QUERY FORM

- Phrases that lead the physician
- Phrases that sound presumptive, directing, prodding, probing, or as though the physician is being led to make an assumption
- Questions that can be responded to in a yes or no format
- Indication of the financial impact of the response to the query
- Be designed so that only a physician signature is required

BOX 39-7 ▸ DOCUMENTATION REQUIREMENTS FOR CARDIAC CHEST PAIN (ANGINA)

- Type of angina
- As completely as possible, the cause of the angina
- Comorbidities, especially those associated with cardiovascular disease. Examples include severe hypertension, arrhythmias
- History of coronary artery disease, myocardial infarction, coronary artery bypass graft, or other contributory diagnosis
- Arrhythmias, electrocardiographic findings
- Signs and symptoms of angina
- Failure of outpatient management
- Plan of care on a daily basis
- High-risk status
- Functional status

WHEN TO MAKE A QUERY

The physician should be queried whenever there is conflicting, ambiguous, or incomplete information in the medical record regarding any significant condition or procedure. Querying the physician only when reimbursement is affected can lead to the skewing of national data and might lead to allegations of upcoding.

FOCUS ON SPECIFIC DRG PAIRS

Each hospital may find that its performance is better with certain DRGs than with others.

Hospitals can identify many such pairs of similar DRGs that may represent significantly different amounts of reimbursement. By properly documenting in the medical record, the hospital increases its likelihood of being reimbursed for services and care that were legitimately rendered. In no way does this process suggest that the physician document beyond the actual care provided or clinical condition of the patient; he or she must simply document in a manner that will provide sufficient accurate information to the coders so that the most appropriate DRG assignment can be made. Many organizations are

| BOX 39-8 | PROPER DOCUMENTATION FOR NONCARDIAC CHEST PAIN |

- The suspected etiology of chest pain, within progress note
- Plan of care on a daily basis
- Signs and symptoms of chest pain, including
  - Type and duration
  - Frequency
  - When pain occurs (at rest, exertional, nocturnal)
  - Location
  - Radiation of pain
- History of chest pain, myocardial infarction, coronary artery bypass graft
- Comorbidities
- High-risk status
- Functional status
- Plan for follow-up testing
- Any refusal for inpatient work-up or management

providing physicians with documentation "prompts." Such prompts should serve only as a guide to the physician, to aid them in completing their medical record documentation. Prompts should never be used to dictate the physician's documentation.

For example, chest pain (a lower weighted DRG) versus cardiac-related angina (a higher weighted DRG) are two distinct diagnoses that, when not documented properly, can result in under-coding. As illustrated in Boxes 39-7 and 39-8, lack of proper documentation for angina will result in a coding to chest pain. This will result in an underreporting of the higher weighted DRG and a reduction in appropriate reimbursement.

By providing documentation prompts to physicians, hospitals can better ensure that their coding will reflect the appropriate DRG as well as more accurate reporting of the case mix of patients cared for in that organization.

References

AHIMA Coding Policy and Strategy Committee (1996). Practice brief: data quality. *Journal of AHIMA, 67*(2), 2.

Cesta, T.G., & Tahan, H.A. (2002). *The case manager's survival guide: Winning strategies for clinical practice*, 2nd ed. St. Louis: Mosby.

Joint Commission on Accreditation of Healthcare Organizations (2000). *Comprehensive accreditation manual for hospitals: The official handbook*. Oakbrook Terrace, IL: Joint Commission on Accreditation of Healthcare Organizations.

Lorenz, E.W., & Jones, M.K. (2002). *St. Anthony's DRG guidebook*. Reston, Va.: St. Anthony's Publishing.

The Data-Driven Health Care Environment

Methods of Gathering and Presenting Relevant Data About Health Care Systems

Amy J. Barton
Diane J. Skiba

CHAPTER OVERVIEW

Being information poor and data rich is a common phenomenon in health care. Health care professionals collect volumes of data but are unable to extract valuable information from these data. Clinical data represent an underutilized resource, yet they have the potential to make the greatest impact on the delivery of health care. According to Zielstorff, Hudgings, and Grobe (1993), the underutilization of data results from the current inability to manage large volumes of data and to determine patterns that will be useful in predictions. Rose (1999) uses the term *informaciation* to represent the phenomenon of having inadequate patient information and evidence to make patient decisions and guide choices for quality, cost-effective care. He believes that data toxicity, an overload of redundant, inaccurate, uninformative, or confusing facts, led to poor decision-making.

How do we interpret data, and how do we prepare data so we can transform them into meaningful information? These key questions need to be addressed by all case managers. Generally, data alone do not provide adequate information for decision-making. Data are facts that must be summarized and displayed in meaningful ways for interpretation.

This chapter provides a foundation for data-driven decision-making. In the world of best practices, evidence-based practice (EBP), and benchmarking, it is imperative that data-driven decision-making is part of the case manager's role. In this chapter we view data-driven decisions from three interrelated lenses. The first view of data is through a traditional statistical lens, the second view of data is through an informatics lens, and the final view is through a continuous quality improvement (CQI) lens. This chapter consists of three major sections. The first section defines data and highlights the issues related to data necessary for decision-making, the second section focuses on data collection methods, and the final section highlights techniques for analysis and presentation of data.

WHAT ARE DATA?

First, what are data? According to Bauer (1996), "Data are the recorded and reported measures of real-world phenomena—the values of variables, which are the possible numeric measures of an event or experiment" (p. 42). This definition represents a statistical or research frame of reference. Data by themselves are not considered useful and must be viewed within a quantification framework. There are several frameworks proposed to view the quantification process that leads to data-driven decisions. One such model (Cleveland, 1985) conceptualized quantification as a five-step interactive process:

Thought (initial stage characterized by conjecture, hypothesis, and curiosity)

Data (undigested observations or unvarnished facts)

Information (numbers put into useful form, organized data)

Knowledge (organized, internalized information)

Wisdom (integrated knowledge that can be used to make decisions) (pp. 22-23)

In this model, according to Bauer (1996), descriptive statistics are the tools used for organizing data and creating information. Accordingly, inferential statistics are necessary for translating information into useful knowledge. Bauer (1996) considers wisdom as the art of being a good decision maker. Statistics provide the knowledge, but it is the wise human who makes the decisions.

In the world of statistics, there are two types of data related to four levels of measurement (Table 40-1). Statisticians classify data as either parametric or nonparametric, and these distinctions are related to the levels of measurement. Parametric data are observations on variables that are consistent in their measure of distance between points on a scale. In other words, parametric data have consistent units of measure and have a uniform distribution of values. Interval and ratio levels of measurement are related to parametric data. On the other hand, nominal and ordinal data are related to nonparametric data. These data are not consistent, are arbitrarily measured, and are considered distribution free. Consequently, there is no uniform distance between units of measure, and the magnitude of the scale varies across and within groups. Definitions of the levels of measurement help to clarify the two types of data.

Each level of measurement corresponds to specific descriptive and inferential tools to translate data to information and information to knowledge.

Another model from the informatics field presents a comparable quantification continuum. Graves and Corcoran (1989) view data as the initial stage of the continuum that eventually leads to discoveries and decisions. They use Blum's (1986) definitions as a basis for their continuum:

Data are discrete entities that are described objectively without interpretation.

Information consists of data that are interpreted, organized, or structured.

Knowledge is information that is synthesized, so relationships are identified and formalized.

Accordingly, a *datum* is a fact about a variable that has the attributes of both value and type. *Value* is an attribute because datum represents a discrete entity in the real world. The attribute of *type* refers to this

TABLE 40-1	**LEVELS OF MEASUREMENT**		
Level of Measurement	**Definition**	**Data Type**	**Example**
Nominal	Numerical naming; numbers do not represent quantity or degree	Nonparametric	Gender (male/female)
Ordinal	Rank-ordered numbers	Nonparametric	Patient acuity rating
Interval	Equal differences between numbers represent equal differences in the variable	Parametric	Length of stay
Ratio	Numbers represent equal amounts to form an absolute zero	Parametric	Kelvin temperature scale

representation in terms of a restricted set of values and a restricted set of operations to manipulate or alter its values. Data types include *numbers* (integer or real), *character strings* (text), or *media* (sound, photo, etc.). Depending on the data type, certain mathematical operations are possible. For example, it is not possible to perform addition and subtraction on text, but you can do so on numeric data.

Data, information, and knowledge are considered three states of the phenomena generically termed information (Graves & Corcoran, 1989). To understand how data are viewed in the continuum, it is important to first define *nursing informatics:*

> "Nursing informatics is a specialty that integrates nursing science, computer science, and information science to manage and communicate data, information, and knowledge in nursing practice. Nursing informatics facilitates the integration of data, information and knowledge to support patients, nurses and other providers in their decision-making in all roles and settings. This support is accomplished through the use of information structures, information processes, and information technology" (ANA Scope and Standards of Nursing Informatics Practice, 2001, p. vii).

Given this definition, the management component is the ability to collect, aggregate, organize, move, and represent information, whereas the processing is viewed as the transformation of one state (data) to a more complex state (information). The progression of information to knowledge leads to the final transformation of knowledge into decisions or discoveries.

Let's take this view of data on the quantification continuum and apply it to health care. Stead (1991) defines five categories of health care data: historical data (about a particular patient or device), encounter patient data, subgroup data of a specified population or set of events, work-flow management data, and knowledge databases for use in decision-making. Three primary users (administrator, support personnel, and direct care providers) retrieve these five categories of health data. In nursing, patient care data are of central concern and thus become the basic information unit. Atomic-level data, as defined by Zielstorff et al. (1993), are the elemental, precise data captured at the source in the course of clinical practice. These discrete, uninterpreted data are then available for processing. The processing of this atomic-level data allows it to be analyzed, combined, aggregated, and summarized with the end result of being transformed into information and knowledge. Transforming data from one state to a more complex state adds meaning and value to the data. In Figure 40-1 (Zielstorff et al., 1993), one can see how atomic-level data can be abstracted, aggregated, and summarized for use by other health care professionals. For example, outcome measures at the patient level can be aggregated and summarized by diagnosis for presentation to quality managers.

From an informatics point of view, the goal of moving along the continuum from data to knowledge is considered the process of *informatting*. This term, coined by Zuboff (1991), describes a key consequence of information technologies on organizations. According to Zuboff (1991, p. 3), to *informate* means to "translate or make visible as explicit information." In health care, there has been limited success in making the data elements of nursing visible.

Data from a CQI lens build on the atomic level and move up the pyramid to present cross-sectional data over time and across populations. Quality managers incorporate not only patient-level data but also financial and population-based data to make decisions. When applied to case management, the case management plan serves as a foundation for data collection and analysis according to Cohen and Cesta (1997). They state the case management plan provides patient care data, length of stay (LOS) information, and resource utilization data.

Data Issues

The quality of the data is also an issue for decision makers. Without good data, it is hard to move along the continuum to decision-making. Two concepts are used as a measure of data quality: validity and reliability. *Validity* refers to the meaningfulness of the data. It is the extent to which the data represent the

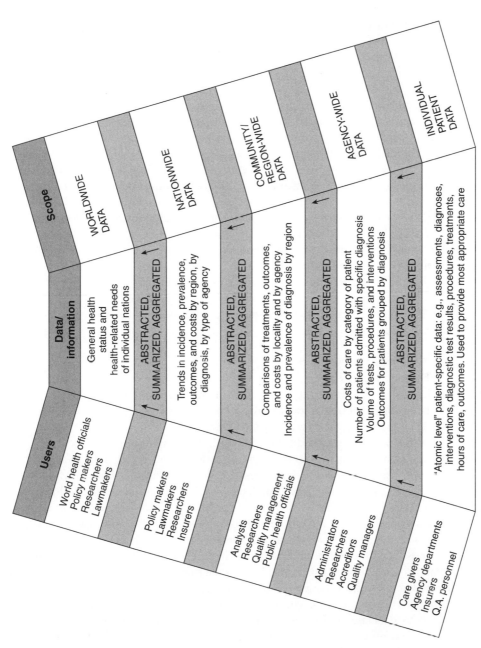

FIGURE **40-1**   Examples of uses of atomic-level patient data collected once and used many times. (Reprinted with permission from *Zielstoff, R.D., Hudgings, C.I., Grobe, S.J., & the National Council Implementation Project Task Force on Nursing Information © 1993 American Nursing Publishing. American Nurses Foundation/American Nurses Association, Washington, D.C.*)

phenomena. *Reliability* refers to accuracy of the data, that is, the repeated precision of the quantification process (Bauer, 1996). All three lenses use these concepts as indicators of quality data.

Health care is an information-intensive activity. One difficulty with health care data, in particular, nursing data, is its dependence on textual information. It has long been a tradition to record narrative notes. These textual notes are extremely rich in nature but difficult to transform across the quantification continuum. According to Ozbolt and Graves (1993), "Nurses have traditionally recorded narrative notes whose information content and form were as varied as the nurses authoring them" (p. 409). In many instances, the lack of consistent and atomic-level patient data has fostered the invisibility of nursing.

There have been many attempts to make visible the data elements related to nursing practice. Werley and Lang (1988) first addressed this issue in an invitational conference to identify approaches for delineating data elements essential for diagnosis, nursing intervention, and evaluation of care. The work eventually identified 16 data elements that would constitute the Nursing Minimum Data Set (NMDS). The NMDS identified patient demographic and other service data elements, but there was still work needed in the four nursing care elements: diagnosis, intervention, outcomes, and intensity of nursing care. To this end, several efforts were made to develop vocabularies and classification systems for these data elements. The 13 vocabularies and classification schemes recognized by the American Nurses Association are as follows:

- North American Nursing Diagnosis Association: http://www.nanda.org
- Home Health Care Classification: http://www.sabacare.com
- Omaha System: http://www.omahasystem.org
- Nursing Intervention Classification: http://www.nursing.niowa.edu/centers/cncce
- Nursing Outcomes Classification: http://www.nursing.niowa.edu/centers/cncce
- Patient Care Data Set (PCDS): http://www.nursingworld.org/nidsec/classlst.htm
- Nursing Management Minimum Data Set (NMMDS): http://www.nursingworld.org/nidsec/classlst.htm
- Perioperative Nursing Dataset: www.aorn.org/
- SNOMED RT: http://www.snomed.org
- Nursing Minimum Data Sets (NMDS): http://www.nursingworld.org/nidsec/classlst.htm
- International Classification for Nursing Practice (ICNP): http://www.icn.ch/icnp.htm
- Alternative Link (ABC Codes): http://www.alternativelink.com
- Logical Observation Identifiers Names and Codes (LOINC): http://www.loinc.org

Although these efforts are making major strides in providing meaning to nursing data, there is still no one existing vocabulary or classification system that represents all that nurses do (Henry & Mead, 1997). No single terminology has emerged as a de facto standard. However, there are several techniques we could use to resolve unnecessary differences between nursing terminologies while accepting motivated diversity. One of the major motivations behind current terminology work is to provide a basis or standard for the comparison and interchange of data recorded using diverse terminologies. A reference terminology is just one possibility for a standard. Hardiker, Hoy, and Casey (2000) discuss terminology standards in more detail and outline an approach used in Europe that is based on a terminology model or terminology schema. For more information about terminology standards, visit the International Standards Organization (ISO) (http://www.iso.ch/iso/en/ISOOnline.frontpage).

Another issue related to databases is the lack of information related to transactions that could describe the cost of nursing services as well as represent diagnoses, treatments, and outcomes from other disciplines. This is of particular importance for case managers who are using critical pathways designed to capture patient care using terminology across health care disciplines. Jones (1997) indicates that transaction databases used by health care purchasers, policymakers, and health care organization administrators exclude information about the quality, type, or cost of nursing services. The national health care transaction databases consist of the *International Classification of Diseases, Ninth Revision* (ICD-9-CM), *Current Procedural Terminology* (CPT), and the National Drug Code (NDC).

Data Management Issues

Data-based decision-making in case management requires collecting the right information at the outset to manage outcomes appropriately. Outcomes management is "the enhancement of patient outcomes through development and implementation of exemplary health practices and services, driven by outcome assessment" (Luquire & Houston, 1997, p. 5). Even though the process is driven by outcomes assessment, it is imperative to collect the input and process data to determine the factors associated with outcomes achievement.

Outcomes management is rooted in the quality framework introduced by Donabedien (1966) who used systems theory to evaluate care. In his model, structures or inputs give rise to processes that influence outcomes. Holzemer and Reilly (1995) expanded this framework to add the dimensions of client, provider, and setting. The resulting matrix (Table 40-2) broadly illustrates the types of data required to facilitate outcomes management. For example, to evaluate the process of clinical pathways as a model of care delivery, you may monitor patient (LOS), provider (cost of practitioner services), and/or institutional (patient satisfaction) outcomes.

One difficulty associated with outcomes assessment is that the data required are often dispersed throughout an organization, requiring "considerable time and energy to find, collect, and organize the data. Negotiation with the 'owners' of the databases is required" (Schriefer, Urden, & Rogers, 1997, p. 18). To deal with this obstacle, Meistrell and Schlehuber (1996) propose the concept of a corporate database. They further describe the corporate database as providing the following:

"1. Accessibility by a broad community of legitimate users, including clinicians, researchers, decision makers, and policy makers
2. Accountability for the accuracy of the data
3. Accessibility to definitions of the data elements, entities, and their relationships
4. Accessibility to definitions of the context in which the data are generated, including documentation of the operating assumptions of those responsible for data collection" (p. MS93).

A second difficulty associated with outcomes assessment concerns collecting data at multiple levels within an organization. "The current challenge among persons charged with outcomes projects in nursing appears to lie in a lack of awareness of the difficulties in mixing levels of data, planning studies in which the resulting data will meet the statistical assumptions, and using the available techniques" (Minnick, 2000). Collecting data at the individual patient level would allow for aggregating the data in such a way as to permit testing of statistical assumptions.

It is important to distinguish between two database types that are commonly referred to in the health care literature: data warehouse and clinical data repository (Waldo, 1998). A *data warehouse* contains clinical and financial data and is used by managers and analysts for population-based management. Data are comparative, trended, and aggregate. A clinical *data repository*, on the other hand, is designed to facilitate a clinician's decision-making concerning individual patients. The focus of the repository is on operational and clinical data that are available in real time.

"The goal of clinical decision support is to present the 'right information' to the 'right person' at the 'right time,' in the 'right format' " (Broverman et al., 1996). Key choices regarding design of an effective clinical support system include the following:

- Passive versus active systems
- Aggregate versus individual patient-based
- Concurrent versus retrospective

TABLE 40-2   THE OUTCOMES MODEL FOR HEALTH CARE RESEARCH

	Inputs	Processes	Outcomes
Client (individual, family, school, community)	Personal characteristics, cultural values and beliefs, social support networks, personal strengths, concerns and needs, well-being, functional status, quality of life, and sociodemographic factors (level of education, ethnicity, income per capita, disability rates, and unemployment rates)	Self-care activities	Mortality, complications, length of stay, readmission rates, physiological status, functional status, behavior, knowledge, symptom control, quality of life, home functioning, family strain, goal attainment, safety, and resolution of nursing diagnosis
Provider (physicians, nurses, social workers, nontraditional healers)	Technical competence, interpersonal skills, level of experience specialty certification, level of education, and personal characteristics	Critical paths, care maps, standardized care plans, clinical practice guidelines	Costs of health practitioner services, provider satisfaction, provider intent to stay or leave, and level of ongoing continuing education
Setting (formal and informal organizations of care delivery)	Values, attitudes, and beliefs of the organizations, as well as available resources, including financing, equipment, number and type of providers, size, ownership status, customers, average volume of service, facility type, and environmental and health conditions of communities Staff mix, staffing levels, professional practice models, and patient acuity Medical care resources, number of physicians per capita, percentage of physician specialists, number of beds per capita	Implementation of total quality improvement principles, strategic planning, implementation and evaluation of policies and procedures, governing activities, communication among providers and different departments, evaluation of operational systems, decision making, and organizational interventions	Patient satisfaction, provider turnover, morbidity, mortality, malpractice rates, costs of care, and readmission rates Appropriateness, availability, continuity, effectiveness, efficacy, efficiency, respect and caring, safety, and timeliness

Adapted from *Holzemer, W.L., & Reilly, C.A. (1995). Variables, variability, and variations research: Implications for medical informatics. Journal of the Medical Informatics Association, 2, 183-190.*

- Systems integrated with patient database versus stand-alone systems
- Proprietary versus standards-based encoding

Ideally, the decision support system should be active, patient-based, concurrent, integrated, and standards-based. The decision support system should be active in that it processes information prospectively as opposed to waiting for input from the user. The system should be designed to facilitate decision-making regarding specific individuals when they require care as opposed to decision-making about a group of patients based on retrospective information. "Clinical decision support is intended as a front-line process that actively defines critical data required for real-time analysis and reporting. Specifically, the information is relevant to the provider within the context of the patient visit" (Orlando, 1998).

It is also important that the information system be integrated across the care continuum. This means that the system should do the following:

- Facilitate data exchange among all system components
- Track patients from cradle to grave
- Provide real-time information to support clinical and administrative decision making
- Monitor quality of service, clinical outcomes, resource use, and financial performance measures (Kennedy, 1996)

Such a system must incorporate a data repository linked with a knowledge base and a user-friendly decision-support interface. The system must be enterprise-wide. Patient data must be linked from outpatient, acute, community-based, and home settings.

DATA ANALYSIS AND PRESENTATION

> Where is the knowledge that we have lost in the information?
> — *T.S. Eliot*

This section presents three different approaches to analysis and presentation techniques. The first approach is a traditional statistical approach. The second approach introduces data mining from an information-processing perspective. The final approach presents data analysis through a continuous quality performance lens.

Statistical Approach

The first traditional method uses statistical techniques to analyze nursing data and standard graphing techniques to present data. Statistical techniques are tied to the research or evaluation questions generated by the decision-makers. To ask appropriate questions, the decision maker must understand the data set and recognize the data sources required to answer the questions. If these conditions are met, the decision maker can use statistical techniques. These techniques can use either descriptive or inferential tools on either parametric or nonparametric data. Let's review the various tools available.

Descriptive statistical techniques are used when one wants to describe aggregated data. Depending on the level of data (nominal to ratio), different measures are used to describe these aggregates. Two specific measures, central tendency and variability, describe aggregated data. With interval-level data, the mean and the standard deviation are the specific measures. For nominal-level data, the mode and the range are considered the appropriate measures.

Let's take an example from case management: LOS as a standard outcome measure. In this case, LOS is considered an interval-level measure, so the mean and standard deviation can be used to describe aggregated LOS data. For example, the mean LOS was 2.34 days with a standard deviation of 1.37 days. To best view these data, one could plot the frequency distribution of the data and examine the distribution (Figure 40-2).

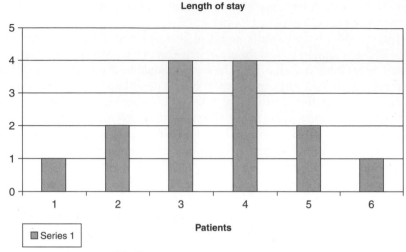

FIGURE **40-2**   Length of stay with normal distribution.

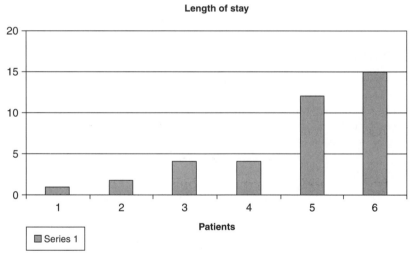

FIGURE **40-3**   Length of stay with skewed distribution.

In the second case, the distribution is skewed with one or two cases exceeding the average LOS and thus inflating the mean and positively skewing the distribution. The mean of this distribution is 6.34 with a standard deviation of 5.75 and a median of 4. In this case, the median is the appropriate measure of central tendency (Figure 40-3).

According to biostatistician Nina Kohn of North Shore University Hospital (Bean, 1995), the most effective method to display LOS is through the use of box plots. Kohn stated that most people report the average LOS when this does not give the most precise picture, because there is no zero point. Most LOS distributions are skewed, and it would be more appropriate to report the median value and the interquartile range as the measures of central tendency and variability. In a box plot, sometimes called a box and whisker plot, a box is drawn to represent the middle half of the scores, with the lower hinge

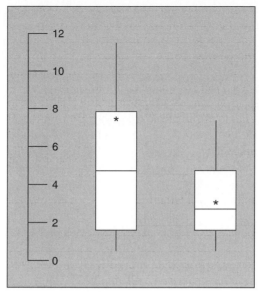

FIGURE **40-4**   Box and whiskers plot.

being the 25th percentile and the top hinge being the 75th percentile. The median is represented as a line across the box and the mean is the plus sign (+). The whiskers are drawn from the box to represent the lowest and highest values. In Figure 40-4, pre– and post–case management LOS is compared in two plots. Plot A represents the preimplementation data. Plot B represents postimplementation data of the care management intervention. Before implementation, the distribution was positively skewed with the LOS varying from 1 to 12 days with a mean of 7 and a median of 4. For the postimplementation phase, the LOS decreased and varied less (1 to 7 days) with a mean of 3 and a median of 2.8.

Another set of statistical tools is used for inferential statistics in which the decision makers ask questions about comparisons, relationships, or causality. Again, various statistical techniques are related to levels of measurement. For example, if a case manager wanted to compare the outcomes of two different critical pathways for a specific chronic condition, one could use analysis of variance or *t* test techniques to compare cost outcome data. If one wanted to compare the satisfaction of two different groups of clients using a nominal level satisfaction scale (1 = happy, 2 = not happy), one would use a chi-square analysis for the comparison. The results of these inferential statistics can be graphed to demonstrate comparison or relationships.

Presenting results of statistical analyses is a complex task requiring decision makers to use their knowledge of both statistics and the art of graphic design. There are several resources that are invaluable for any case manager who wants to present statistical results in the most meaningful and reader-friendly manner. The first are two books available from the American Psychological Association. Nicol and Pexman (1997) provides specific guidelines for the creation of statistical tables for a wide range of techniques. The second one by Nicol and Pexman (2003) extends beyond the statistical tables to a wide variety of presentations including figures for articles, posters, and presentations. Another resource is a book by Lang and Secic (1997) that focuses on reporting statistical results in medicine. An outstanding resource by King, Tomz, and Wittenberg (2000) provides exceptional guidelines to improving her interpretation and presentation of your statistical findings. In this article, their goal is as follows.

to show one how to convert raw data of any statistical procedure into expressions that: (1) convey numerically precise estimates of the quantities of greatest substantive interest, (2) include reasonable measures of uncertainty about those estimates and (3) require little specialized knowledge to understand (p. 347).

In addition to this article, the authors had a computer program that is designed to implement the methods described in the article. Their software, CLARIFY (Software for Interpreting and Presenting Statistical Results), can be viewed at website http://gking.harvard.edu/clarify/docs/clarify.html.

Another resource for the presentation of data is Tufte (1983), who believes that "graphics reveal data" (p. 13). Data graphics, according to Tufte, visually display measured quantities through the use of various objects like points, lines, numbers, symbols, and color. He believes that graphics are tools for quantitative reasoning. In his book on the visual display of quantitative data, Tufte outlines his principles of graphic excellence. His principles are as follows:

Graphic excellence:

- Is the well-designed presentation of interesting data—a matter of substance, of statistics, and of design.
- Consists of complex ideas communicated with clarity, precision, and efficiency.
- Gives the viewer the greatest number of ideas in the shortest time with the least ink in the smallest space.
- Is nearly always multivariate.
- Requires telling the truth about the data.

In a more recent text by Tufte (1997), he provided principles for the display of evidence for making decisions. He believes that both principles of scientific and design reasoning should guide visual representations. If making comparisons as evidence, Tufte (1997, p. 51) recommends the following:

- Document the sources and characteristics of the data.
- Insistently enforce appropriate comparisons.
- Demonstrate mechanisms of cause and effect.
- Express those mechanisms quantitatively.
- Recognize the inherently multivariate nature of analytic problems.
- Inspect and evaluate alternative explanations.

Information Processing Approach

In the previous approach, the decision maker's questions dictated the statistical analysis of the data to make decisions. The statistics served as a method to summarize data to make decisions. The decision maker as an analyst was able to query the data and summarize the results of the question. This approach rapidly breaks down as the quantity of data grows and the number of dimensions increases (Fayyad & Uthurusamy, 1996). As health care organizations collect voluminous data in large data warehouses, it is impossible for anyone to understand all the data sets and to make reasonable sense of the data. To this end, there are a growing number of researchers and computer scientists who are interested in the problem of automating data analysis and have labeled these attempts as data mining and knowledge discovery in databases (KDD). This growing field, whose core disciplines are from statistics and database management, is joining forces to extract useful knowledge from the volumes of data in warehouses. According to Fayyad, Piatetsky-Shapiro, & Smyth (1996), finding useful patterns in data is known by different names in different communities; terms such as *knowledge extraction, information discovery, information harvesting, data archeology,* and *data pattern processing* are but a few examples. To understand this concept, Fayyad, Piatetsky-Shapiro, & Smyth (1996) declare that KDD is the term used to describe the overall process of discovering useful knowledge from data. Here is a diagram of the KDD process:

DATA $\rightarrow$ Target DATA $\rightarrow$ Preprocess DATA $\rightarrow$ Transform DATA/Patterns $\rightarrow$ Knowledge

The KDD process is both interactive and iterative. In the first step, the decision maker learns about the data set and the goals. The creation of a targeted data set or subset on which the KDD is performed is the next step. Data cleaning and preprocessing, such as extraction of outliers, is the third step. Data reduction and other transformational methods are used in the next step to reduce the effective number of variables. Data mining, the application of specific algorithms for extracting patterns or models of the data, is the fifth step. In this step, one must choose the appropriate model to match the KDD process. Once the data are mined, the interpretation phase occurs in which patterns are examined for redundancy and irrelevance. The last phase is using the discovered knowledge and incorporating previous knowledge and proper interpretation. The one caution is data dredging, the blind application of data mining models to the data, which results in the discovery of meaningless patterns. To compare the statistical with the KDD approach, it is important to remember these following assumptions. The traditional statistical approach is predicated on hypothesis testing. In this approach, one is testing a conjecture against a body of data to confirm or reject that hypothesis. In many cases, the data drive the discovery. In KDD, particularly in data mining, the end-user draws conclusions from the data, allowing the data to suggest the conclusion. Many propose that KDD is a combination of hypothesis testing and data-driven discovery.

There are several excellent resources to help you understand data mining within a health care context. First, Cheung, Moody, and Cockram (2002) describe the use of data mining of electronic databases and the implications of this to shape nursing and health policy agendas. This article describes the data mining techniques, various existing databases, and advantages and limitations of these strategies. Second, SPSS and co-author Philip Baylis produced a white paper on better health care with data mining. This white paper introduced the Clementine Data Mining Systems and provided examples of how this system can be used to examine a variety of health care decision-making in hospitals, especially in United Kingdom. For more information about this system, go to the website www.fes.uwaterloo.ca/crs/gp555/dataminingspss.pdf.

A final resource is a booklet available on the Web from IBM: *Mining Your Own Business in Health Care: Using DB2 Intelligent Miner for Data.* This booklet describes the use of the DB2 miner and provided examples of its use in health care. To retrieve this booklet, you can go to the website http://publib-b. boulder.ibm.com/redbooks.nsf/redbookabstracts/sg246274.html.

Data visualization tools are used to facilitate KDD. *Data visualization* is the visual interpretation of complex relationships in multidimensional data using a host of graphic tools. These graphic tools include *map* (data displayed on a geographic map), *scatter* (data points shown in one to three dimensions), and *tree visualizers* (data are mapped to see hierarchical breakdowns). An example might be to use a map visualization to represent the incidence of particular patient characteristics in a community of interest; an example of this is shown as Figure 40-5. The use of a geographic information system permits analysis of community needs. In the illustration provided, the median household income for clients from an indigent care clinic clearly identifies a pocket of need within an otherwise affluent community. Data or information visualization (Walker, 1995) helps "to bridge the gap between the abstract, analytical world of the digital computer and the human world."

This relatively cursory view of KDD and data mining is merely an example of another approach to data-driven decisions. The intent was not to provide a detailed description of KDD and data mining but rather to raise awareness of other techniques that can be used to facilitate decision-making in organizations. Here are some exceptional examples using data mining techniques to examine several different topics in health care. In nursing, there has been extensive data mining conducted by Goodwin (Goodwin & Iannacchione, 2002) and her team (Prather, Lobach, Goodwin, Hales, Hage, &

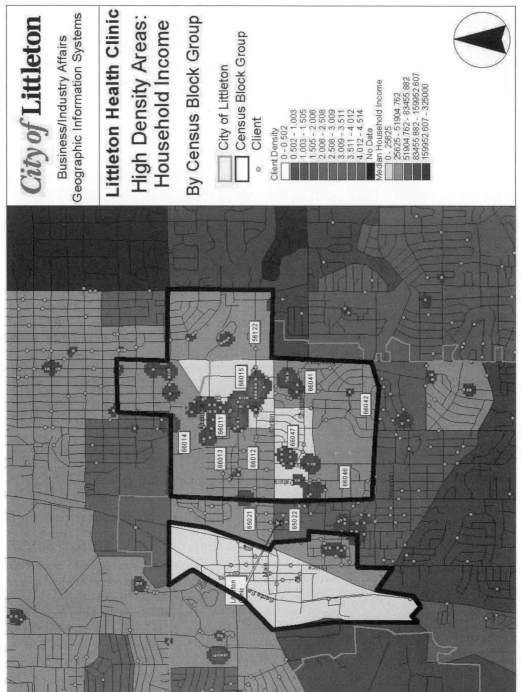

FIGURE **40-5**   Median household income within a community.

Hammond, 2000) at Duke University. Their focus is the examination of an extensive clinical database of obstetrical patients, and their goal is to improve birth outcomes by identifying predictors of full-term versus preterm deliveries. A nursing administration example of using data mining was described in several case studies of executive dashboards used by administrators at Hartford Hospital. Rosow, Adam, Coulombe, Race, and Anderson (2003) described how administrators can use "user-defined virtual instruments and dashboards that connect to hospital databases" (p. 58) to make important decisions. Another example used data mining techniques to identify medication errors in terms of near misses and adverse drug events (Rudman, Brown, Hewitt, Carpenter, & Campbell, 2002). In this study, the person administering the drug and proximal cause predicted near misses, whereas drug type, proximal cause, and place predicted adverse drug effects (Rudman et al., 2002).

Continuous Quality Improvement Approach

From a CQI perspective, data presentation techniques include those concerning idea generation (e.g., brainstorming, boarding, multivoting, decision matrices), portrayal of beliefs (flow diagrams, fishbone diagrams), display (check sheets, histograms, run charts), and analysis (Pareto charts, control charts, pie charts, scatter diagrams) (Wagner, 1995). For purposes of this chapter, display and analysis techniques are discussed.

Display techniques for data presentation include check sheets, histograms, and run charts (Wagner, 1995). Check sheets are used to facilitate recording the frequency of an activity or event (McLaughlin & Kaluzny, 1994). For example, in case management this may be used to track prolonged LOS reasons for a population of patients. A sample check sheet for total hip arthroplasty patients is presented in Table 40-3.

The histogram is simply a bar chart that graphically presents the data from a check sheet. The categories are placed on the x-axis at equal intervals. The length of the bar on the y-axis represents the number of observations within that interval (Figure 40-6).

A run chart (Figure 40-7) allows for visualization of observations over time (Gaucher & Coffey, 1993). Assessing performance over time allows one to "(1) see what the temporal behavior of the process is and (2) establish the time of process performance changes so that they can be linked to the time of other possibly related events" (Gaucher & Coffey, 1993).

Of the analysis techniques for data presentation, Pareto charts and control charts are discussed here. Pareto charts are named after a seventeenth-century Italian economist who noted that the greatest amount of wealth was distributed among a small group of people (McLaughlin & Kaluzny, 1994).

TABLE 40-3	CHECK SHEET ILLUSTRATING REASONS FOR EXTENDED LENGTH OF STAY (LOS)			
Reason for Increased LOS	**Week 1**	**Week 2**	**Week 3**	**Week 4**
Preexisting chronic condition	3	5	2	4
Surgical complication	1	3	2	1
Delay in ambulation	2	3	1	4
Lack of home support	1	2	2	1

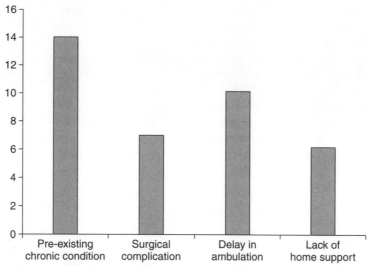

FIGURE **40-6**   Histogram representing causes of delay in discharge.

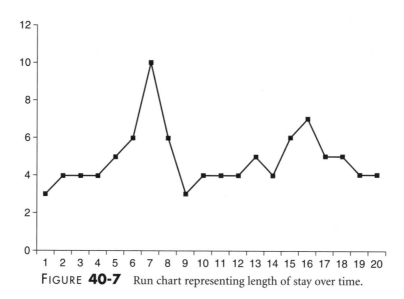

FIGURE **40-7**   Run chart representing length of stay over time.

"A Pareto chart (Figure 40-8) is used to display visually the significance of different factors, to separate the many from the vital few. This is similar to the '80-20 rule,' which ascribes 80 percent of the potential improvement to 20 percent of the issues" (Gaucher & Coffey, 1993).

A control chart is similar to a run chart, with the added feature of upper and lower control limits at three standard deviations above and below the mean. Control charts facilitate determining whether a variation is due to a special cause or a common cause (Gaucher & Coffey, 1993). For example, in the chart displayed (Figure 40-9), even though the average LOS is 4.7 days, only a value of 10 falls outside the upper control limit and requires further analysis to the cause of the variation.

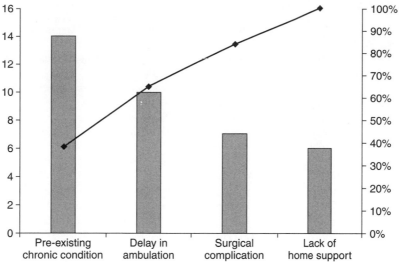

FIGURE **40-8**   Pareto chart representing the most frequently occurring reasons for discharge delay.

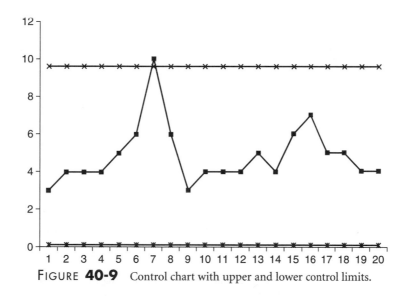

FIGURE **40-9**   Control chart with upper and lower control limits.

SUMMARY

We have provided three perspectives on which one may consider when building an infrastructure to support data-based decision-making. The first method is use of traditional statistical theory, the second is use of an informatics perspective, and the third is through a CQI perspective. Regardless of approach, it is essential to carefully define the data to be collected before beginning.

References

American Nurses Association (2001). *Scope and standards of nursing informatics practice.* Washington, D.C.: American Nurses Publishing.

Bauer, J. (1996). *Statistical analysis for decision makers in healthcare: Understanding and evaluating critical information in a competitive market.* Chicago: Irwin Professional Publishing.

Bean, B. (1995). *Issues in evaluating a clinical pathway program. Issues and outcomes: The newsletter for mapping and managing care* (pp. 9-11). South Natick, Mass.: Center for Case Management.

Blum, B.L. (Ed.) (1986). *Clinical information systems.* New York: Springer-Verlag.

Broverman, C.A., Clyman, J.I., Schlesinger, J.M., & Want, E. (1996). Clinical decision support for physician order-entry: Design challenges. *AMIA,* 572-576.

Cheung, RH., Moody, L.E., & Cockram, C. (2002). Data mining strategies for shaping nursing and health policy agendas. *Policy, Politics & Nursing Practice, 3*(3), 248-260.

Cleveland, H. (1985). *The knowledge executive: Leadership in an information society* (pp. 22-23). New York: Dutton.

Cohen, E.L., & Cesta, T.G. (1997). *Nursing case management: From concept to evaluation,* 2nd ed. St. Louis: Mosby.

Daly, J.M., Maas, M.L., & Johnson, M. (1997). Nursing outcomes classification: An essential element in data sets for nursing and health care effectiveness. *Computers in Nursing, 15*(suppl 2), S82-S86.

Donabedien, A. (1966). Evaluating the quality of medical care. *Milbank Quarterly, 44,* 166-206.

Fayyad, U., & Uthurusamy, R. (1996). Data mining and knowledge discovery in databases. *Communications of the ACM, 39*(11), 24-26.

Fayyad, U., Piatetsky-Shapiro, G., & Smyth, P. (1996). The KDD process for extracting useful knowledge from volumes of data. *Communications of the ACM, 39*(11), 27-34.

Fields, W., & Siroky, K. (1994). Converting data into information. *Journal of Nursing Care Quality, 8*(3), 1-11.

Gaucher, E.J., & Coffey, R.J. (1993). *Total quality in healthcare: From theory to practice.* San Francisco: Jossey-Bass.

Goodwin, L.K., and Iannacchione, M.A. (2002). Data mining methods for improving birth outcomes predictions. *Outcomes Management for Nursing Practice, 6*(2), 80-85.

Graves, J.R., & Corcoran, S. (1989). The study of nursing informatics. *IMAGE: Journal of Nursing Scholarship, 21,* 227-231.

Grier, M., & Foreman, M. (1989). In I. Abraham, D. Nadzan, & J. Fitzpatrick (Eds), *Statistics and quantitative methods in nursing: Issues and strategies for research and education.* Philadelphia: Saunders.

Hardiker, N., Hoy, D., & Casey, A. (2000). Standards for nursing terminology. *Journal of the American Medical Informatics Association, 7*(6), 523-528.

Henry, S.B., & Mead, C.N. (1997). Nursing classification systems: Necessary but not sufficient for representing "what nurses do" for inclusion in computer-based patient record systems. *Journal of the American Medical Informatics Association, 4,* 222-232.

Holzemer, W.L., & Reilly, C.A. (1995). Variables, variability, and variations research: Implications for medical informatics. *Journal of the Medical Informatics Association, 2,* 183-190.

Jones, L.D. (1997). Building the information infrastructure required for managed care. *IMAGE: Journal of Nursing Scholarship, 29,* 377-382.

Kennedy, M. (Mar. 1996). Building information systems to manage care and improve clinical quality, *The Quality Letter,* 2-11.

King, G., King, M., & Wittenberg, J. (2000). Making the most of statistical analyses: Improving interpretation and presentation. *American Journal of Political Sciences, 44*(2), 341-355.

Lang, T.A., & Secic, M. (1997). *How to report statistics in medicine: Annotated guidelines for authors, editors, and reviewers.* Philadelphia: American College of Physicians.

Luquire, R., & Houston, S. (1997). Outcomes management: Getting started. *Outcomes Management for Nursing Practice, 1*(1), 5-7.

McLaughlin, C.P., & Kaluzny, A.D. (1994). *Continuous quality improvement in health care: Theory, implementation, and applications.* Gaithersburg, Md.: Aspen Publications.

Meistrell, M., & Schlehuber, C. (1996). Adopting a corporate perspective on databases: Improving support for research and decision making. *Medical Care, 34*(3), MS91-MS102.

Minnick, A. (2000). Levels of data: The whys and hows of selection and analysis. *Outcomes Management for Nursing Practice, 4*(3), 106-109.

Nicol, A., & Pexman, P.M (2003). *Displaying your findings: A practical guide for creating figures, posters and presentations.* Washington, D.C.: American Psychological Association.

Nicol, A., & and Pexman, P.M. (1999) *Presenting your findings: A practical guide for creating tables.* Washington, D.C.: American Psychological Association.

Orlando, M.L. (1998). Outcomes: Essential information for clinical decision support: An interview with Ellen B. White. *Journal of Health Care Finance, 24*(3), 71-81.

Ozbolt, J. (1996). From minimum data to maximum impact: Using clinical data to strengthen patient care. *Advanced Practice Nursing Quarterly, 1*(4), 62-69.

Ozbolt, J., & Graves, J. (1993). Clinical nursing informatics: Developing tools for knowledge workers. *Advances in Clinical Nursing Research, 28*(2), 407-425.

Prather, J., Lobach, D., Goodwin, L.K., Hales, J.W., Hage, M.L., and Hammond, W.E. (1997). Medical data mining: Knowledge discovery in a clinical data warehouse. *Proceedings of the American Association of Medical Informatics Annual Symposium,* 101-105.

Rose, J.S. (1998). *Medicine and the information age* (p. 28). Tampa, Fla.: Hillsboro Printing.

Rosow, E., Adam, J., Coulombe, K., Race, K., & Anderson, R. (2003). Virtual instrumentation and real-time executive dashboards: Solutions for health care systems. *Nursing Administration Quarterly, 27*(1): 58-76.

Rudman, W.J., Brown, C.A., Hewitt, C.R., Carpenter, W.O., & Campbell, B. (2002). The use of data mining tools in identifying medication error near misses and adverse drug events. *Topics in Health Information Management, 23*(2), 94-103.

Schriefer, J., Urden, L.D., & Rogers, S. (1997). Report cards: Tools for managing pathways and outcomes. *Outcomes Management for Nursing Practice, 1*(1), 14-19.

Stead, W.W. (1991). Systems for the year 2000: The case for an integrated database. *MD Computing, 8*(2), 103-110.

Tufte, E. (1997). *Visual explanations: Images and quantities, evidence and narrative.* Cheshire, Conn.: Graphics Press.

Tufte, E. (1983). *The visual display of quantitative information.* Cheshire, Conn.: Graphics Press.

Wagner, P.S. (1995). Guide to identifying, collecting, and managing data. In J.A. Schmele (Ed.), *Quality management in nursing and health care* (pp. 408-458). Albany: Delmar.

Waldo, B. (1998). Decision support and data warehousing tools boost competitive advantage. *Nursing Economics, 16*(2), 91-93.

Walker, G. (1995). Challenges of information visualization. *British Telecommunications Engineering, 14,* 17-25.

Werley, H.H., & Lang, N.M. (Eds). (1988). *Identification of the nursing minimum data set.* New York: Springer.

Zielstorff, R.D., Hudgings, C.I., Grobe, S.J., & the National Commission on Nursing Implementation Project (NCNIP) Task Force on Nursing Information Systems. (1993). *Next-generation nursing information systems: Essential characteristics for professional practice.* Washington, D.C.: American Nurses Publishing.

Zuboff, S. (Summer 1991). Informate the enterprise: An agenda for the twenty-first century. *Phi Kappa Phi Journal,* 3-7.

The Importance of Research in the Evaluation Process

CHAPTER OVERVIEW

Implementation of a case management model should include establishment of a nursing research methodology. Nursing research data provide the framework for evaluating and justifying the efficacy of the overall model.

This chapter explores methods for designing the research and provides samples for data analysis, including patients, staff, and length of stay for selected diagnosis-related groups (DRGs). Each organization must determine its own research design based on its goals for the model, but some sort of research base is recommended to provide a framework for evaluation.

DATA TALKS

Someone once said, "In God we trust. When all else fails, use data." Creating change in any organization is never an easy task. Obtaining the support and cooperation of hospital administration is necessary for complete integration of a nursing case management model. With such support, the model can be viewed as both a nursing and a multidisciplinary model.

Perhaps the best way to obtain the support of the institution as a whole is through the use of data; this includes collecting, analyzing, and disseminating the results of a statistical data analysis as well as any anecdotal data collected. Some data will already exist and be available in the organization. Other data will need to be collected.

Obtaining the administration's support is only part of what is needed as the change to case management proceeds. A sound, valid evaluation process must be implemented to provide ongoing support as the model continues to develop and become part of the institution. It is imperative therefore that the elements to be monitored and evaluated be determined before any changes are implemented (Jennings & Rogers, 1986).

Case management provides an opportunity for nursing to conduct research, as well as to quantify the case management model. *Research*, broadly defined, is an attempt to find the solution to a problem so that it may be predicted or explained (Treece & Treece, 1973). *Research* has also been described as a formal method for carrying on the scientific method of analysis, which in turn involves the use of several problem-solving steps. These include problem identification, hypothesis formation, observation, analysis, and conclusion (Polit & Hungler, 1983).

These basic elements are no less important in the analysis of a case management model and all the changes that come about as a result of the integration of this system (Jennings & Rogers, 1986). Generally, research is divided into two categories. The first is basic research, the goal of which is to obtain knowledge for the sake of knowledge. The second category is applied research, which takes this process one step further as it seeks to apply the research to everyday situations (Nachmias & Nachmias, 1981). Case management research is applied research in its truest sense. Everyday questions concerning the efficacy of the model are asked, answered, and applied as the case management research data are collected and analyzed.

The methodology used for case management analysis can take several forms and can encompass several different elements. It need not be limited to one particular process but can include several steps and processes. Nursing research includes the clinical elements of the nursing profession, such as the steps of the nursing process: assessment, diagnosis, outcome identification, planning, implementation, and evaluation. Nursing research also involves the preparation and evaluation of practitioners and studies the systems in which nurses work and apply the steps of the nursing process (Corner, 1991).

EVALUATION VERSUS EXPERIMENTAL RESEARCH

Research involving case management can be approached as evaluation research. It can also be designed as an experiment or quasi-experiment. In evaluation research, data are collected and analyzed to evaluate or assess the effects of some project or change. This type of research helps to evaluate how well implementation of the program is going.

Experimental research tests the relationships between the variables being manipulated. A control group and an experimental group are used in classic experimental research. The control group symbolizes a normal representation of subjects, and the experimental group consists of those subjects for whom at least one variable has been altered.

In case management research it is difficult to devise a classic experimental design. If patients are compared, the researcher must be sure that the cases are similar enough to justify comparison. Some examples of factors to be controlled when choosing subjects are severity of illness, concurrent problems, gender, and age. In addition, random assignment to each group must be conducted. This process involves the admitting office, which ensures that certain previously evaluated patients are placed on particular units.

If nurses on nursing units are being studied for job satisfaction, for example, it would be impossible to separate those nurses who had been affected by the model from those who had not. Comparing nurses between nursing units can lead to some of the same methodology questions that arise when comparing some patients with others (Schaefer, 1989). The registered nurses could be matched only if differences were controlled in some way.

Even comparing one nursing unit with another is difficult. There are few institutions in which nursing-unit patient populations are so similar, and yet so randomized, that nurses' and patients' experiences could be said to be similar from one to the next. It is more likely that comparing one nursing unit with another is like comparing apples with oranges. Nursing units are often designated by specialty, and physicians will usually, whether formally or informally, prefer that patients be sent to a particular nursing unit because the physicians believe that unit is most suited to meeting their patient's nursing needs.

The Quasi-Experimental Approach

Because of the difficulties in matching subjects for control and experimental groups, it becomes practical to use each nursing unit as its own control. Once this takes place, the methodology becomes quasi-experimental. Unit data, including staff satisfaction, length of stay, and so on, are compared before and after implementation. Additional postimplementation data are collected and analyzed at predetermined intervals. A longitudinal approach of this kind cannot guarantee that the same staff members will be compared from one time frame to the next (Kenneth & Stiesmeyer, 1991). Whenever possible, the same nurses and staff members should be compared from one time period to the next. For those staff members who come and go during the study, global score comparisons can be made.

Certain intrinsic factors affecting internal validity are impossible to control (Lederman, 1991). One such intrinsic factor that always affects longitudinal studies is maturation. The nurses tested may have either an increase or a decrease in job satisfaction solely because of the passage of time. For some workers the passage of time provides a certain comfort that increases job satisfaction and sense of accomplishment. For others, longevity can lead to exhaustion, disillusionment, and decreased job satisfaction. In either case, these elements associated with maturation can probably not be controlled.

Another intrinsic factor is that of experimental mortality. One of the goals of case management is to decrease turnover rates among registered nurses, but there will always be a certain amount of turnover among any group of employees, no matter how happy they are with their work. Some may leave because they cannot deal with the changes accompanying the introduction of case management. In either case, it is clear that the researcher will not have the same sample at each stage of data collection. Dropouts from the study can prejudice the results. Unfortunately, this factor cannot be controlled.

One way to account for the issue of experimental mortality or dropouts is to statistically analyze the entire sample size as a global unit and then match subjects from a previous data collection period with those in the current period and study this group separately.

Subjects serve as their own controls in a pretest-posttest design (Nachmias & Nachmias, 1981). The advantage to this design is that the variable is measured both before and after the intervention. In other words, the variable is compared with itself.

As the first step in either process, preimplementation data and continuous data are obtained as the model goes forward. The provision of a solid nursing research base for evaluation lends credibility to the model for those evaluating it in 6 months, 1 year, 2 years, or longer (Rogers, 1992).

Typically when changes are made in nursing, very little data collection occurs during the implementation phase (Acton, Irvin, & Hopkins, 1991). This lack of data makes validation of results difficult, which in turn makes it difficult to maintain the momentum and support needed for change to progress.

To determine what to measure, the organization must first decide what it hopes to achieve by implementing the case management model. After identifying the goal of implementation, it will be easier to formulate the questions that should be asked. Based on these questions, the researcher can begin to form a hypothesis. The hypothesis indicates what the researcher believes to be the cause and effect of a given situation, and it states the relationship between the variables.

Basic research questions will not be affected by the type of methodology used, regardless of whether an evaluation or experimental methodology is chosen. These research questions are prospective and based on hoped-for outcomes. The outcomes will fall into several categories. Data collection will be longitudinal because it will probably be collected at predetermined intervals over a long period of time. The changes attempted in case management will take years to take hold, so choosing an evaluation time period that is too short may make it appear as if implementation has failed to achieve the desired outcomes. On the other hand, some measure of changing trends will need to be shown within the first year of implementation to prove that things are moving in the desired direction.

The areas affected by the implementation of a case management model are diverse and complicated. They range from patients to staff to finance. Many of the changes are obtuse, intangible, and anecdotal, but others can be validated through stringent data collection and statistical analysis. Those changes to be measured must be determined in advance so that baseline data can be collected. These data will provide the foundation for comparison.

If a case management model is being implemented, the focus of evaluation must be on patients, finance, length of stay, and quality of care. Therefore some outcomes may be measured against changes occurring within the care delivery systems and processes. Some may have to do with changes in care management clinical interventions. Some outcomes are actually measuring programmatic changes associated with the implementation of case management, while others are measuring the clinical effects on patients when protocols and/or resource utilization is altered.

Consider the following factors when identifying organizationally specific outcomes; outcomes should be
- Patient and family oriented
- Realistic and practical
- Clear and concise
- Measurable and observable
- Concrete and doable
- Time/interval specific

A non–unit-based case management model is broadly focused, and it may be difficult to prove a relationship between implementation of the model and level of staff satisfaction. Therefore this might not be a variable worth trying to measure.

In the unit-based case management model, certain changes affect particular nursing staff members in specific ways (Swanson et al., 1992). The response of these individuals can be measured and evaluated in terms of job satisfaction, turnover rates, absenteeism, and vacancy rates.

One of the most difficult but essential elements to measure in a case management model is quality of care. The basic tenet of case management is to move the patient through the hospital system as quickly and efficiently as possible. Because the hospital stay is being accelerated, some controls must be put in place to guarantee that quality care is not being compromised (Edelstein & Cesta, 1993; Mitchell, Ferketich, & Jennings, 1998).

Perhaps the most tangible measure, and possibly the most important in terms of hospital viability, is the length of stay. Decreases in length of stay have come to be associated directly with case management. It is difficult to address case management without also addressing the issues of hospital reimbursement and patient length of stay.

The prospective payment system provided the first and most potent incentive to hospitals to move toward reducing length of stay. Now with the rapid infiltration of managed care, other financial incentives are in the health care arena; these include capitation and negotiated per diem rates under managed care. These payment schemes provide for the same need to control cost and reduce length of stay as the prospective payment system did in the 1980s. These incentives are strictly financial. Shorter hospital stays mean increased profits. It is only a matter of time before every institution in the United States will be looking at measures for reducing length of stay as well as controlling other costs.

Caution should be taken when studying and reporting length of stay statistics. The prospective payment system and DRGs were designed to be used only as financial tools for determining reimbursement.

Because of a lack of other ways to tap into this information, the DRG has become the basis for studying length of stay and related clinical interventions. A serious analysis of many DRGs will reveal that the DRG is usually too broad and too heterogeneous to be used as a determinant of the effect of a particular clinical intervention.

To report this information with the utmost accuracy, it is more advantageous and appropriate to analyze the situation at a microlevel. For example, there is one DRG for chemotherapy, despite the fact that there are 1-day, 2-day, and 5-day chemotherapy protocols. The reimbursable length of stay is 2.6 days, no matter what the protocol. If a managed care plan is applied to a particular case for a specific chemotherapy protocol to determine the effectiveness of the plan, the researcher would have to identify more than just the DRG. If the plan is a 5-day plan, clearly the reimbursable rate is inadequate. But having this information would allow the investigator to determine, for example, whether the length of stay could have been shortened or whether quality care was provided.

Elements of Data Collection

One form of data collection is the questionnaire. Using questionnaires that have been previously determined to be valid and reliable can reduce or eliminate many of the problems associated with this technique. The content of the questions determines their ability to control bias, which could influence a respondent's answer in a particular way.

One way to test staff nurses is to compile packets of various questionnaires, including one on demographics, that the researcher can use to describe the sample itself. The questionnaires should take no longer than 15 to 20 minutes to complete (Kenneth & Stiesmeyer, 1991).

BOX 41-1 ▶ DATA COLLECTION MONITORS

1. Staff satisfaction outcome indicators
   a. Improved registered nurse job satisfaction
   b. Improved physician job satisfaction
   c. Improved nursing assistant job satisfaction
   d. Decreased registered nurse burnout scores
   e. Decreased absenteeism
   f. Decreased turnover rate
   g. Increased recruitment
2. Patient satisfaction outcome indicators
   a. Improved patient satisfaction
   b. Improved family satisfaction
   c. Reduction in patient/family complaints
3. Quality of care outcome measures
   a. Quality improvement data
   b. Improved patient satisfaction
   c. Reduction in readmission rate (24 hrs, 1 day, 1 week, 30 days)
   d. Uniform treatment of all cases
   e. Frequency and type of patient education
   f. Clinical outcome indicators
   g. Variance analysis data
4. Length of stay outcome measures
   a. Reduction in length of stay
   b. Reduction in pre-operative length of stay
5. Communication or collaboration among disciplines outcome measures
   a. Development of collaborative practice groups
   b. Opened lines of communication between all disciplines
   c. Development of case management plans
6. Financial outcome measures
   a. Reduced third party payer denials (initial and final)
   b. Improved resource use (both product and personnel)
   c. Reduced cost per day/case
   d. Decreased absenteeism, turnover, and vacancy rates
   e. Decreased delays in waiting for tests and procedures
   f. Uniform treatment within physician groups
   g. Alteration of registered nurse and ancillary staff mix

The consent form should clearly indicate that participation in the study will in no way affect the respondent's employment in the institution.

When questioning patients, nurses must ensure that patient care is not being disturbed. The researcher must also determine whether the patient is able to understand, read, and respond to the questionnaire appropriately. One way to do this is to provide questions on the demographic questionnaire that address the respondent's highest level of education, age, and ability to speak and understand English.

Box 41-1 presents some of the broad categories that an organization converting to a case management model might want to address when collecting data for determining success or failure of implementation. The list in the box is certainly not exhaustive. An organization on the brink of implementing case management may choose to study any or all of these questions. Questions may involve a multitude of benchmarks or only a few. There may be areas for study not listed in the box but still important to the organization in question. Each organization must decide for itself what is most important to measure and how it will be measured. The tools for measuring each of these expected outcomes are determined by the nurse researcher involved in the case management analysis. Valid and reliable tools exist to measure most variables, but others will have to be obtained from already-existing hospital information systems, DRG information, and managed care and hospital billing records. The areas from which to obtain the data vary from institution to institution. The finance department, the DRG office, and the managed care departments can be of great assistance to the nurse researcher evaluating a case management system. Each unit of analysis will require the use of the nurse researcher's expertise for selecting the most appropriate data with which to answer the research questions.

References

Acton, G.J., Irvin, B.L., & Hopkins, B.A. (1991). Theory-testing research: Building the science. *Advances in Nursing Science, 14*(1), 52-61.

Corner, J. (1991). In search of more complete answers to research questions. Quantitative versus qualitative research methods: Is there a way forward? *Journal of Advanced Nursing, 16*, 718-727.

Edelstein, E.L., & Cesta, T.G. (1993). Nursing case management: An innovative model of care for hospitalized patients with diabetes. *The Diabetes Educator, 19*(6), 517-521.

Jennings, B.M., & Rogers, S. (1986). Using research to change nursing practice. *Critical Care Nurse, 9*(5), 76-84.

Kenneth, H.K., & Stiesmeyer, J.K. (1991). Strategies for involving staff in nursing research. *Dimensions of Critical Care Nursing, 10*(2), 103-107.

Lederman, R.P. (1991). Quantitative and qualitative research methods: Advantages of complementary usage. *The American Journal of Maternal/Child Nursing, 16*, 43.

Mitchell, P.H., Ferketich, S., & Jennings, B.M. (1998). Quality health outcomes model. *Journal of Nursing Scholarship, 30*(1), 43-46.

Nachmias, D., & Nachmias, C. (1981). *Research methods in the social sciences.* New York: St. Martin's Press.

Polit, D., & Hungler, B. (1983). *Nursing research.* Philadelphia: J.B. Lippincott Company.

Rogers, B. (1992). Research utilization, *AAOHN, 40*(1), 41.

Schaefer, K.M. (1989). Clinical research: Gaining access to patients. *Dimensions of Critical Care Nursing, 8*(4), 236-242.

Swanson, J.M., Albright, J., Steirn, C., Schaffner, A., & Costa, L. (1992). Program efforts for creating a research environment in a clinical setting. *Western Journal of Nursing Research, 14*(2), 241-245.

Treece, E.W., & Treece, J.W. (1973). *Elements of research in nursing.* St. Louis: The C.V. Mosby Company.

Documentation of Quality Care

CHAPTER OVERVIEW

For health care organizations to improve delivery of services, they must first determine their definition of quality. Recently, quality issues have moved from an organizational perspective to a consumer-oriented one, in which the needs and concerns of the customer count.

Among the elements measured in defining quality is patient satisfaction. Patients can be questioned directly through focus groups or indirectly through written questionnaires.

Each organization must determine its measures in relation to the incorporated case management documentation system. Patient, health care provider, and operational variances can be used to continuously improve quality. The case manager serves an important role in this process.

WHAT IS QUALITY?

The meaning of quality takes on a new twist when introduced as a concept relevant to health care. Quality may be seen in terms of its effect on the health care delivery system or on specific dimensions of the system (Institute of Medicine [IOM], 1976). In 1997 the IOM defined *quality* as the degree to which health care services increase the likelihood that desired outcomes are consistent with professional knowledge available at the time care is provided to individuals and populations (Vladeck & Shalala, 1997).

On the larger scale of the entire health care system, quality may include the availability and accessibility of health care services, credentialing requirements and standards of the providers, comprehensive assessment and documentation, collaborative and informed relationships with the patient and family, minimal injuries or complications in hospitalized patients, evaluation of new technology and resources, and effective management of health care resources (McCarthy, 1987).

The advent of the prospective payment system forced health care institutions to focus on health care as a business. Leaving good-quality care to chance did not work and ultimately did not make good business sense. As organizations, regulatory agencies, and patient needs became more complicated, it became obvious that health care was no less a business than any other and that the product of the business was patient care. Increasingly, the value of that care depended on matching cost and quality. Before they could determine the value of the product, organizations had to know what the expected quality comprised.

Manufacturers, small-business owners, and large corporations have known for years that to provide quality, the organization or business must first determine its definition of quality (Davis, 1990). Discovering what attributes the organization wants to attain is one way to arrive at such a definition.

Health care organizations have already begun to realize that a change in the definition and measurement of quality is needed (Cesta & Tahan, 2002; Jones, 1991). The products of health care are often intangible items that are difficult to identify and measure. Quality assurance measures in the past have attempted to identify errors and then place blame on the individual who made the error (Joint Commission on Accreditation of Healthcare Organizations [JCAHO], 1994). However, one could argue that counting the number of bedsores or medication errors only partially helps to define quality health care. It also did not provide a mechanism for monitoring and then *improving* quality.

Consumer Focus

As in business, it became obvious that one useful technique for defining quality health care was to ask the recipients of that care how they defined quality. This technique of asking consumers what they want often highlights issues to which the health care practitioner is blind. In the past, our definition of *quality* was to count the number of patient falls. If the organization came in below the desired threshold, it was providing quality care. However, the patient's definition of *quality care* was care given by a competent, pleasant employee who was familiar with the patient and the patient's needs, providing a clean and quiet healing environment and good food!

Of course, the issue of falls is an important one in terms of ensuring quality, and patients will surely consider this equally important if they have ever fallen. The point is, once the customer's needs have been queried and identified, an entirely new area can be addressed. Invariably the necessary dimensions of quality that the consumer identifies focus on the business end of health care. This area has been ignored in the past. Organizations believed they knew what patients needed and supplied it to them within the constraints and needs of the organization. The patient had to conform to the organization. There are occasions when this approach is truly necessary. But remaining forever in this mindset eliminates the possibility of ever going beyond providing basic services, and it does not allow for an atmosphere of continual improvement. Case managers must work closely with the organization to assess, monitor, and analyze the delivery of care and the patient's response to the care to continuously improve the organization's quality performance (Flarey & Smith-Blanchett, 1996).

By determining what constitutes quality, it can be measured. Once measured, it can be managed. Managing care allows for a process of continual improvement toward excellence, and excellence is the definition of quality.

PATIENT SATISFACTION

With a renewed focus on patient needs, the issue of how to measure patient satisfaction has never been more important. Patient satisfaction is quickly becoming the benchmark for measuring quality health care (Cesta & Tahan, 2002; Roth & Schoolcraft, 1998). Customer needs not only are identified but also are the basis on which quality improvements are made. Within the mission statement of most health care organizations is a clause that cites patient satisfaction as a goal. Although the health care industry has always identified itself as a service industry, clearly this was a self-serving need. In most instances the attitude of health care providers was that the patient was lucky to be getting what he or she was getting.

How often have nurses used the following phrases in defense of a system that was obviously failing the patients and customers?

"You had to wait 5 days for a CAT scan? Well, Mrs. Jones had to wait 6 days. Aren't you lucky?"

"You haven't seen your surgeon since the operation? That is something you are going to have to accept if you want to have the best surgeon in this field."

The patients were certainly not lucky to be sick, to be in the hospital, or to be having surgery. When even minimal expectations are not being met, something is terribly wrong with the system.

Customer service will be what defines quality in the next decades. As patient consumers become more versed in the use of the Internet and access health care information, they will become greater advocates for themselves and their family members. Patient consumers will continue to access "report cards" on physicians and health care providers, which they will use to help them make informed decisions and choices regarding their health care services. Health care organizations that provide service to all customers, from physicians to patients to the community, will be the most successful. The focus must shift away from a purely organizational approach to one that blends consumer and organizational needs (Strasen, 1991).

Depending on the philosophy, resources, and goals of the organization, the approach for measuring patient satisfaction can be made in a number of ways. Generally a questionnaire is used to gauge the level of patient satisfaction. Such a survey can be administered while the patient is in the hospital or after discharge (Steiber & Krowinski, 1990). Generally an attempt is made to administer the questionnaire 24 to 48 hours before discharge. However, some patients may be intimidated by a questionnaire that is filled out while they are still in the hospital, fearing that if a bad report is given, one of the health care providers may retaliate with less-than-optimal care. On the other hand, patients' memories of their hospital stays will be most vivid if recorded while still in the hospital. Positive and negative impressions will be fresh in their minds, and these impressions can provide valuable information.

However, patients who are queried after discharge, in the safety and comfort of their homes, may be more likely to provide honest information because they have no fear of retribution. Unfortunately, positive and negative experiences can be quickly forgotten once the patient is home, which means valuable information can be lost if patients are questioned in this manner.

The pros and cons of each method must be evaluated by each organization. There is no perfect way, and it is possible that some form of patient satisfaction questioning is already in place. These data can be used both as preimplementation data and for ongoing studies.

If the questionnaires are administered to patients while they are in the hospital, someone who is not directly involved in the patient's care should administer the survey. This method will help to diminish any potential for bias.

Because people who are ill or who have been ill recently are being questioned, care should be taken to select a questionnaire that has short, understandable questions. The focus of each question should be clear to the patient. Patients who are questioned while still in the hospital are more likely to be experiencing increased anxiety or other physical conditions that may affect their ability to participate.

It is best to select instruments that have been identified previously as valid and reliable. Most instruments use closed-ended questions in which a series of possible choices are given. This format is easiest to score and analyze statistically. Open-ended questions provide the investigator with less control of response content and are more difficult to analyze. Even so, the open-ended format may provide the most meaningful information. It may be beneficial to design an instrument that combines both closed-ended and open-ended questions. This allows for some control over responses and the opportunity to elicit useful anecdotal information.

The focus of the survey also may depend on the philosophy and goals of implementing the case management system. Many patient satisfaction surveys focus on hygiene needs, such as food, room comfort, noise, and so on. Although these factors are important, they may not be capturing the elements that a case management system is attempting to change. Therefore it may be necessary to find a questionnaire that focuses more on the professional care provided. In some cases the institution may have to develop its own instrument that clearly questions the patients with regard to this unique switch to case management.

Developing an instrument can be difficult. The decision to develop a unique questionnaire should not be taken lightly. If the organization is looking for immediately valid and reliable results, the use of a pilot instrument is not the best route to take. The use of more than one instrument is one way to address this dual requirement so that the needs of both the organization and the researcher can be met. Previously established questionnaires allow for a rapid compilation of information with which to measure implementation. In the long run, however, a new questionnaire, aimed at determining specific effects of the case management system on the patient, will contribute a great deal to the validation of the model's efficacy. In addition, the questionnaire can be used by other organizations that implement case management systems.

Another technique is the qualitative method. Qualitative assessment is used to compile data that can be used later in a self-report or paper-and-pencil questionnaire. Patient-focused groups and interviews provide data for the development of written questions. Qualitative approaches allow the researcher to see the situation through the experience of the patient. The patient's perceptions are used to compile information that is later categorized. These categories are then transformed into specific questions.

The qualitative method is time consuming. Personal interviews or focus groups last from 1 to 2 hours, but the researcher must devote even more time to use this form of data collection. However, the information gained can be invaluable.

Determining which patients to question is really a matter of good research technique. The sample should be as heterogeneous as possible to allow for the greatest deal of generalizability. Random sampling will provide this.

Every health care organization compiles statistics that are fed back to regulatory agencies. This information is generally used to determine accreditation and licensing and to analyze mistakes, untoward effects, and outcomes. Information categorizing the number and type of falls, infections, and medication administration errors has been tracked for years. Analysis of these data helps identify patterns or frequent offenders. Such a system has been referred to as the "bad apple" approach. If a health care practitioner makes a mistake, that person is counseled. If the practitioner makes the same kind of mistake repeatedly, more serious intervention on the part of the employer might take place. This system does not take into account possible system issues that may contribute to the problem. Instead, one person is seen as the cause of the problem as well as the means for fixing it.

This approach not only looks for the bad apple but also lies in wait for the accident or error. The approach does not provide a mechanism for addressing the larger elements of the problem, and it does nothing to control the recurrence of this problem. Nevertheless, most institutions evaluating case management systems have turned to the bad-apple approach in an attempt to improve quality patient care. A reduction in patient falls or patient infections might be reported as a result of the introduction of a case management model. In reality, the factors leading to a fall or an infection go beyond a managed care plan or a case manager.

If the goal of data analysis is to improve the quality of care, a method other than the bad-apple approach must be selected. Patient care is simply too multidimensional to be analyzed effectively by this method. Identifying more appropriate data to measure will come as a direct result of establishing a definition of quality. Case management data are positive outcome data because they focus on the expected outcomes of the interventions in which we participate as health care providers. The case management plan provides all the expected outcomes of care during hospitalization, from patient teaching expectations to expected resource use to expected length of stay. It also provides for the expected clinical outcomes of care.

These expected outcomes provide the foundation for determining quality care. By delineating these outcomes, each discipline is identifying the quality issues around a particular diagnosis or procedure (Baker, Miller, Sitterding, & Hajewski, 1998).

Additional indexes of patients' perceptions of quality can be identified. These indicators should be incorporated into any measure of quality. Until the organization has converted to a case management system or until the new case management plans are in place, it may be necessary to continue to report the quality assurance data to obtain baseline indexes of quality. Ultimately this format can be abandoned or combined with other quality indicators.

Patient Safety

An example of the new consumerism in health care is demonstrated by the public outpouring following the reports from the IOM. In November 1999, the IOM reported on errors in health care. The initial report was followed up in 2000 with statistics indicating the extent of the medical errors, including 44,000 to 98,000 patient deaths reported annually associated with errors, representing the eighth leading cause of death in the United States, with an overall cost of about $38 billion each year. The IOM also reported that $17 billion of these costs are associated with preventable errors (IOM, 2000). The IOM report caught the attention of the news media, regulators, and the public at large.

The IOM's recommendation was that each health care organization establish a patient safety program with defined executive responsibilities that
- Are clearly focused on patient safety
- Implement nonpunitive systems for reporting and analyzing medical errors
- Incorporate well-understood safety principles
- Establish interdisciplinary team training for providers of patient care that incorporates proven methods of team training.

Other responses to the IOM report included President Clinton's response:
- Reduce errors by 50% over the next 5 years
- Quality Interagency Coordination Task Force
- Dissemination of evidence-based, best practices

The Centers for Medicare and Medicaid Services response:
- New condition of participation establishing requirements for patient safety programs in hospitals

The JCAHO (2000) implemented new patient safety standards:
- Six new standards
- Twenty-three revised standards
- "Speak Up" consumer campaign

As a case manager, you should familiarize yourself with the Speak-Up Campaign as it may play a part in your role as patient advocate.

THE JCAHO SPEAK-UP CAMPAIGN

The Speak-Up campaign is designed as a mechanism for the lay public to use in ensuring that they receive safe and appropriate health care. It encourages active participation in their care processes and an understanding of the services they are receiving or should be receiving. It includes the following principles to be followed by patients and family members:

Speak up if you have questions or concerns, and if you don't understand, ask again. It's your body and you have a right to know.

Pay attention to the care you are receiving. Make sure you're getting the right treatments and medications by the right health care professionals. Don't assume anything.

*E*ducate yourself about your diagnosis, the medical tests you are undergoing, and your treatment plan.

*A*sk a trusted family member or friend to be your advocate.

*K*now what medications you take and why you take them. Medication errors are the most common health care mistakes.

*U*se a hospital, clinic, surgery center, or other type of health care organization that has undergone a rigorous on-site evaluation against established, state-of-the-art quality and safety standards, such as that provided by JCAHO.

*P*articipate in all decisions about your treatment. You are the center of the health care team.

What Each Health Care Organization Should Do

Each health care organization should enact the following components in their patient safety plans:

- Develop a nonpunitive reporting culture.
- Ensure that appropriate mechanisms exist to report, intervene, and follow-up on events and near misses.
- Design a central, coordinating body that interfaces with all other related activities.
- Create a proactive risk reduction process to complement the reactive root cause analysis process for sentinel events and near misses.
- Establish a process for patient and family communication about occurrences.
- Outline a comprehensive education and communication plan to include board, leadership, physicians, and staff.
- Identify monitoring activities and outcomes and report to leadership at least quarterly.

CRITERIA FOR MEASURING OUTCOMES

Some of the outcomes identified on the case management plan can be tracked during hospitalization. These outcomes are the day-to-day clinical, psychosocial, and teaching interventions. The case manager addresses these on a daily basis and ensures that the patient is moving along the continuum of health care in a timely fashion. If any outcome is not achieved, the case manager is responsible for determining why and correcting the problem or changing the plan.

The unit of analysis within the case management plan will vary depending on the increments in which the hospital stay is measured. For example, while most case management plans are developed on the basis of the 24-hour day, others may have longer or shorter units of analysis. In the neonatal intensive care unit, where the expected length of stay can run from 1 to 3 months, daily measures are not appropriate. In this case the managed care plans are "time-lined" in 1-week intervals, during which the expected outcomes should be achieved.

In some cases, such as an emergency department setting, the time frames may be short. Then the case management plan time frames are set at 15-minute or 30-minute intervals. During these shorter time periods, specific outcomes are expected. Whatever the time frame, it should realistically correlate to the clinical situation being planned. Once a unit of analysis or time period is chosen, analysis can begin.

In case management, anything that does not happen when it is supposed to happen is called a *variance*. Variances alert practitioners to changes in the patient's condition, or they highlight problems in the health care delivery system itself. Any variances that occur are identified daily as well as retrospectively. Every expected outcome on the plan is a potential variance, and, unless the outcome is achieved within a predetermined time period, it falls into the variance category. There are four causes for variances: the patient, the health care provider, operations, or unmet clinical indicators.

There are two types of patient variances. The first is a patient variance, comorbidity, or a condition identified on admission. These conditions may or may not require an alteration in the usual plan for that diagnosis or procedure. For example, a patient allergy identified on admission might mean that a drug usually considered standard for that diagnosis or procedure cannot be administered. As a result, the plan of care must be discussed with the physician, who decides either to refrain from using the drug or to replace it with a suitable alternative.

In some cases the variance is noted, but no change is made to the plan at that time. An example of this is a patient who has diabetes. The person admitting this patient reviews the plan and notes that no changes are needed. The patient's condition still must be noted in the Patient Exception on Admission section of the case management plan. This section may also be labeled as preexisting conditions or comorbidities. This alerts all health care providers that the patient has diabetes. It also indicates that the plan was individualized at the time of admission.

The other type of patient variance is one that the patient causes. In other words, this type involves situations in which an expected outcome cannot be achieved because of the patient's condition or noncompliance.

For example, a tuberculosis case management plan might call for collection of sputum specimens on the first, second, and third days of hospitalization. If the patient cannot produce sputum on the second day, that outcome cannot be achieved within the anticipated time frame. In such a case, specimen collection is moved to the third and fourth days.

An example of a patient variance caused by noncompliance might occur on the second postoperative day, when the plan calls for the patient to dangle the legs over the edge of the bed. Because of pain, the patient refuses. Despite pain medication, the patient continues to refuse. This refusal results in an inability to achieve the desired outcome, and the patient's plan must be adjusted accordingly.

By reviewing the patient's progress throughout the day and anticipating the course of recovery for the entire hospital stay, the case manager can adjust the plan so that the variance does not change the length of stay. If the patient refuses to ambulate, the "dangling" and "out-of-bed-to-the-bathroom" goals can be combined into expected outcomes for the following day, when the patient is feeling better. Another possibility might be to try the dangling step again on the next shift, when the pain medication is more effective.

Regardless of the reason for the variance, the case manager and the staff nurse should be aware of the recovery protocol and should attempt to get the patient back on track as soon as possible. This method helps avoid unnecessary delays and makes the patient's progress and expected plan well known and easily tracked. This in turn means that potential problems will be less likely to continue for several days without being noticed.

A health care provider variance is caused by an omission or error made by a health care practitioner. Institutions have unique regulations regarding documentation, and employees must acquaint themselves with these policies. However, mistakes are bound to occur.

An example of a health care provider variance might involve a transcription error. If a physician order for a medication is not transcribed by the nurse but the error is detected on the next shift, the patient might have missed a dose of the medication. Other health care provider variances involve changes in practice patterns that alter the patient's predetermined case management plan.

Operational variances are probably the most common variances. Operational variances include those that happen within the confines of the hospital as well as some caused by a condition outside the hospital.

A large-system variance, one that occurs because of something outside the hospital, might involve discharge placement. These types of variance would fall within the operational category. Sometimes a patient is assessed as appropriate for nursing home placement, so all the paperwork is completed and the patient is clinically ready for discharge, but no nursing home beds are available. As a result, the patient remains in the hospital until a bed becomes available, and the extended stay is classified as a large-system variance.

The most typical large-system variances are postdischarge problems in which a proper discharge location is not available. This type of variance is difficult to control. The best prevention is for the case manager to attempt to identify those patients who will need placement as early in the hospital stay as possible and to begin to prepare the necessary paperwork so that delays can be avoided.

Other operational variances can occur because of the institution's infrastructure. Most health care institutions are large, complex places. Systems have developed over time, often without planning. Once these systems are in place, most workers are too busy to correct the operational problems. Instead, informal mechanisms are developed to work around the flaw in the system. Such operational problems can delay the patient's progress toward discharge. An inadequate patient-scheduling system may mean that the nursing unit is unaware of a scheduled procedure and the patient is not correctly prepped. Thus the procedure cannot be performed, which may increase the length of stay.

Other operational variances occur when equipment breaks. One such operational variance is an inability to complete a computed tomography (CT) scan because the machine is not functioning. Any equipment malfunction results in a delay, which in turn takes the patient off the case management schedule. Clinical quality indicators are those expected clinical indicators identified by the physician that may include intermediate and discharge outcomes. These indicators are used to assess clinical progress and quality of care. See Chapter 31 for more information on variances.

Any of these variances require the input of the case manager, whose responsibility it is to identify the variance and intervene to correct it. The goal is to minimize the effect the variance will have on the patient's length of stay.

The other responsibility of the case manager is to document the variance. Retrospective analysis of operational variances results in the identification of frequently occurring, but rectifiable, problems. It is important that variances also be documented for the purposes of utilization review and reimbursement.

OUTCOME DATA AND CONTINUOUS QUALITY IMPROVEMENT

Outcome measurement data, including variance data, is used as the foundation for continuous quality improvement (CQI) efforts. Data are used to identify performance improvement opportunities, to analyze the improvement areas associated with those opportunities, and to identify strategies to correct them. Case managers should participate as active members of CQI teams whenever possible.

The outcomes management process includes the following steps (Cesta & Tahan, 2002):
- Review strategic goals.
- Match goals to outcome indicators.
- Design clear, measurable, time-oriented outcome indicators.
- Select appropriate outcomes measurement tools.
- Collect data.
- Analyze data.
- Communicate findings.
- Identify, design, and implement improvements.
- Repeat the process.

The case manager plays an important part in all steps of this process. As part of their role of outcomes or quality manager, many case managers are responsible for collecting and documenting much of the data used in these processes. Their perspective is vital to both operational and clinical performance improvement projects and initiatives. A discussion of the CQI process continues in Chapter 43.

References

Baker, C.M., Miller, I., Sitterding, M., & Hajewski, C.J. (1998). Acute stroke patients: Comparing outcomes with and without case management. *Nursing Case Management, 3*(5), 196-203.

Cesta, T.G., & Tahan, H.A. (2002). *The case manager's survival guide: Winning strategies for clinical practice,* 2nd ed. St. Louis: Mosby.

Davis, W.W. (1990). Quality care and cost control? *The Case Manager, 1*(3), 24-29.

Flarey, D.L., & Smith-Blanchett, S. (1996). *Handbook of case management.* Gaithersburg, Md.: Aspen Publications.

Institute of Medicine (1976). Assessing quality in health care: An evaluation. DHEW Publication No. 282-75-0437 PM. Washington, D.C.: National Academy of Sciences.

Institute of Medicine (2000). *To err is human: Building a safer health system.* National Academy Press. Available at www.books.NAP.edu/books/039068371/html132.html.

Joint Commission on Accreditation of Healthcare Organizations (1994). *Lexicon dictionary of health care terms, organizations, and acronyms for the era of reform,* Chicago: Joint Commission on Accreditation of Healthcare Organizations.

Joint Commission on Accreditation of Healthcare Organizations (2000). *Hospital accreditation standards, 2000-2001.* Oakbrook Terrace, Ill.: Joint Commission on Accreditation of Healthcare Organizations.

Jones, K.R. (1991). Maintaining quality in a changing environment. *Nursing Economics, 9*(3), 159-164.

McCarthy, C. (Feb. 1987). Quarterly health care inches closer to precise definition. *Hospital Peer Review,* 19-20.

Roth, T.A., & Schoolcraft, M. (1998). Patient satisfaction: The survey says. *Nursing Case Management, 3*(5), 184-189.

Steiber, S.R., & Krowinski, W.J. (1990). *Measuring and managing patient satisfaction.* Chicago: American Hospital Publishing.

Strasen, L. (1991). Redesigning hospitals around patients and technology. *Nursing Economics, 9*(4), 233-238.

Vladeck, B., & Shalala, D. (1997). Medicare and Medicaid Programs: Use of the OASIS as part of the conditions of participation for home health agencies, 42 CFR, Part 484, *Federal Register 62,* 11035-11064.

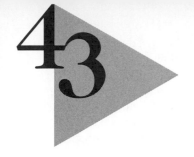

The Link Between Continuous Quality Improvement and Case Management

CHAPTER OVERVIEW

The continuous quality improvement (CQI) process has gradually been adapted to the health care setting to improve quality without increasing costs. In traditional quality assurance models, quality is measured by the number of accidents or errors occurring. No provision is made for improving the conditions under which the errors occurred.

However, CQI focuses on the processes used to achieve a goal. These processes may be clinical, financial, or operational issues. Each step in the process is analyzed; then a plan for improvement is tested and refined.

The three leaders in the CQI process are Deming, Juran, and Crosby. Each has made unique contributions toward improving the quality of work performed in the industrial setting. Now their concepts are being applied in the health care arena.

Case management and CQI are linked in philosophy and process. The steps of the CQI process can be applied to managed care plans from both clinical and financial perspectives.

INTRODUCTION TO CONTINUOUS QUALITY IMPROVEMENT

The CQI process was officially introduced in 1991 as a more effective approach to improving the quality of health care. In that year the Joint Commission on Accreditation of Healthcare Organization (JCAHO) announced that it would be introducing new standards requiring all chief executive officers of hospitals to be educated on CQI methods (*Hospitals*, 1991). This mandate went into effect for accreditation surveys as of January 1, 1992.

This seemingly abrupt switch from traditional quality assurance methods to an approach that had had tremendous success in the business arena was timely. Quality had become the promotional tool for many health care organizations as they adopted a more consumer-oriented approach (Naisbitt, 1982).

At the same time the prospective payment system had changed the speed and scope of health care delivery. Techniques that had been successful in the past were no longer financially feasible. Change, once considered something to be avoided, was hailed as the way to financial viability for the industry (Kanter, 1983). The changes included new and more effective management styles that could provide quality under a cost-containment umbrella.

Another force driving the need for change was an emerging consumerism (Naisbitt, 1982). The average person had become an educated health care consumer who expected quality care. Consumers wanted to be involved in their care, which included participation in decisions involving treatment, cost, and self-care (O'Connor, 1984).

477

CQI falls in the realm of total quality management, a concept originated by W. Edward Deming (*Hospital Peer Review*, 1988). Quality improvement involves an analysis, understanding, and improvement of the processes of care. In the case of the health care industry, these processes include the hospital system, the personnel, the clinical management, and the financial structure surrounding each patient case.

In this format, *quality* is defined as the meeting or exceeding of customer requirements (Marszalek-Gaucher & Coffey, 1990). In other words, the customer defines quality. Suppliers and customers are involved in each of the above-mentioned processes. The supplier is the one who passes on the patient, information, or equipment, and the customer is the one who receives the patient, information, or equipment.

One of the first steps in CQI is the identification and study of the individual steps that make up each of the processes of health care. This CQI extends beyond individual departments because the exchanges between departments are usually the areas that yield difficulties. Each process can be broken down into its working parts in various ways. One way involves use of a flow chart. The flow chart pictorially describes each step and helps identify where bottlenecks or overuse of resources is occurring. Figure 43-1 is a simplified example of how a computed tomography (CT) scan scheduling process is broken down into its major steps.

Root causes of problems are identified through the flow chart. Once the root causes have been determined, more data can be gathered and the team can begin selecting solutions. It is necessary to pick the root cause that may result in the greatest initial improvement of the process. Additional

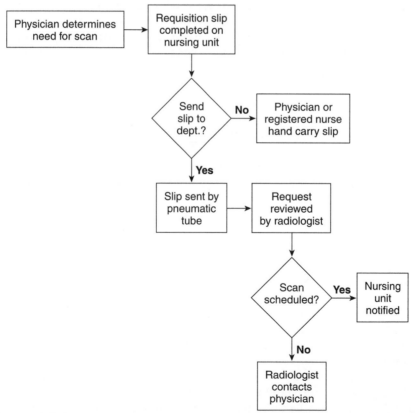

FIGURE **43-1**   Flow diagram of computed tomography (CT) scan scheduling process.

causes can then be addressed after one solution has been tried. At this point, more data should be collected to evaluate whether the solution was given enough time to take hold and whether it was effective.

TRADITIONAL QUALITY ASSURANCE

The health care industry has been crippled by waste and misuse of resources (Marszalek-Gaucher & Coffey, 1990). Within this wasteful environment, quality care has always been difficult to measure (Goldfield & Nash, 1989). Compounding this difficulty is the unabated growth of industry inspection, which has resulted in an adversarial relationship between health care organizations and inspection agencies. Sanctions mandating quality as defined by agencies, such as the Peer Review Organizations (PRO), the Joint Commission on the Accreditation of Healthcare Organizations (JCAHO), the state licensing agencies, and others, have resulted in measures designed to ensure minimum expectations rather than continuous improvement (Laffel & Blumenthal, 1989).

Relatively arbitrary thresholds have been established within organizations. These thresholds define minimum expectations and identify bad apples but do not provide any mechanism for finding causes or suggestions for improvements. These techniques for ensuring quality do not address health care's increasing need for improvement in all processes of the industry (Donabedian, 1980). It is clear that while quality must be maintained, systems have to be designed for improving business at all levels.

The traditional quality assurance process provides a system for identifying opportunities to improve care or solve problems. These opportunities are based on the collection of information regarding incidents or errors that have surpassed a predetermined threshold (Box 43-1). Factors affecting the occurrence of the incidents, the systems affecting the errors, or processes for improvement are not identified.

BOX 43-1 ▶ QUALITY ASSURANCE MONITORING AND EVALUATION

THE 10-STEP PROCESS
Assign responsibility for monitoring and evaluating activities.
Delineate the scope of care provided by the organization.
Identify the most important aspects of care provided by the organization.
Identify indicators (and appropriate clinical criteria) for monitoring the important aspects of care.
Establish thresholds (levels, patterns, trends) for the indicators that trigger evaluation of the care.
Monitor the important aspects of care by collecting and organizing the data for each indicator.
Evaluate care when thresholds are reached in order to identify either opportunities to improve care or problems.
Take actions to improve care or to correct identified problems.
Assess the effectiveness of the actions and document the improvement in care.
Communicate the results of the monitoring and evaluation process to relevant individuals, departments, or services and to the organization-wide quality assurance program.

In addition, errors or incidents are identified through individual finger-pointing based on the mistake of one person. Therefore each quality issue appears to be the fault of one particular person, acting independently. This focus removes all accountability from the organization or the systems within which the individual practitioner is working.

THE NEW HEALTH CARE AGENDA

Quality has become paramount on the health care agenda. Industrial models of quality improvement have been adopted and used successfully in the health care arena. Industry's goals, the reduction of costs and the improvement in the quality of the product, match those of health care. More than a decade ago, industrial leaders realized that to compete and survive in a world economy, quality improvement techniques were needed that would yield significant operational improvements (Drucker, 1991; Hickman & Silva, 1984; Naisbitt & Aburdene, 1985; Tichy & Devanna, 1986).

The three individuals most closely associated with these processes are Philip B. Crosby, W. Edwards Deming, and Joseph M. Juran. Crosby is probably the best known of the three quality experts. His approach is based on his *14 steps* for the quality improvement process (QIP) (Crosby, 1979):

1. Management commitment
2. Quality improvement team
3. Measurement
4. Cost of quality
5. Quality awareness
6. Corrective action
7. Zero defects planning
8. Employee education
9. Zero defects
10. Goal setting
11. Error cause removal
12. Recognition
13. Quality councils
14. Do it all over again

Crosby (1979) explains that his efforts differ from those of Juran or Deming in that these *14 steps* provide a complete process. This process, says Crosby, provides a methodology for improving quality, not just a series of quality improvement techniques.

W. Edward Deming is the leading figure in quality improvement. It was Deming who, working with Japanese manufacturers in the 1950s, was responsible for the tremendous improvements made in Japanese manufacturing. To make improvements, Deming relies on technical expertise as well as statistical analysis. His work helped place the Japanese in a completely different class of manufacturing.

Deming's (1986) approach places emphasis on 14 points, which have been used in the transformation of American industry:

1. Create constancy of purpose for improvement of product service.
2. Adopt a new philosophy.
3. Cease dependence on inspection to achieve quality.
4. End the practice of awarding business on the basis of price tag alone. Instead, minimize total cost by working with a single supplier.
5. Improve constantly every process for planning, production, and service.
6. Institute training on the job.

7. Adopt and institute leadership.
8. Drive out fear.
9. Break down barriers between staff areas.
10. Eliminate slogans, expectations, and targets for the work force.
11. Eliminate numerical quotas for the work force and numerical goals for management.
12. Remove barriers that rob people of pride of workmanship. Eliminate the annual rating or merit system.
13. Institute a vigorous program of education and self-improvement for everyone.
14. Put everybody in the company to work to accomplish the transformation.

Deming (1986) may be best known for his work in involving the employee in the quality improvement system. Concepts such as the "quality circle" or the "QC circle" grew out of the development of these processes, which involved groups of employees in problem identification and solving. Perhaps most relevant in adapting Deming's work to the health care industry is its focus on implementing intervention strategies to improve quality and reduce cost. Other aspects applicable to health care are the continuous improvement in quality and the use of employee teams trained in problem-solving techniques (Deming, 1986).

Juran was with Deming in the 1950s in Japan and had previously worked with Deming in the 1920s at the Hawthorne Western Electric Plant in Chicago. Juran, like Deming, is considered a pioneer and an expert in quality improvement technology. Best known for his *quality trilogy* (Juran, 1987, 1988), Juran broadened the quality approach to a wider operational or managerial perspective:

Quality planning: The process of developing the products and processes required to meet customer needs

Quality control: The regulating process through which actual performance is measured and compared to standards and the difference is acted on

Quality improvement: The organized creation of beneficial change

The structure, process, and outcome approaches of these quality issues can be operationalized and evaluated for continuous improvement. With the patient as the focus, quality is identified as those factors most important to patient and family. If asked, the patient might identify many of the factors outlined in Figure 43-2 as important to his or her care.

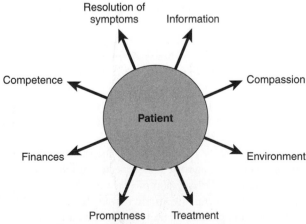

FIGURE **43-2** Patient care concerns.
(Courtesy *A. Ron & M. Holtz.*)

THE LINK TO CASE MANAGEMENT

Data for analysis in traditional quality assurance methods have focused on "unquality" or "disquality," such as infections, falls, medication errors, returns to the operating room, and deaths.

Some of these elements focus on the institution, such as global indicators of quality within the hospital. Examples of global indicators include morbidity and mortality and generic risk-management indicators. The focus of these elements has been on those identified as outliers.

Another traditional data base has been financial data and analysis, which tracks the cost of specific procedures or diagnosis-related groups (DRGs). The finance department uses this information to determine case mix index, which in turn helps determine the reimbursement rate.

Data related to individual practitioners have been more loosely followed. Utilization review evaluators and other quality management departments have focused on specific practice patterns.

Within case management, each of these elements can be followed more comprehensively. The data, once collected, are linked to CQI methods. The first step in a CQI process such as this is to identify problems that appear to be more than isolated events and to identify all of the issues that may be affecting the outcome. These issues might be linked to a DRG cost analysis as well as to individual practice patterns. In a case management framework, all practitioners are monitored for quality, use of resources, and length of stay. (Walrath, Owens, and Dziwulski, 1998.)

The case management plan is the foundation for this kind of data collection and analysis. The case management plan provides a guideline for administering care to a particular patient type. These plans take into consideration not only length of stay but also resource use. During the development of the case management plan the optimal treatment plan, one that streamlines care without compromising quality, is identified.

If planned correctly, these collaborative guidelines are agreed on by the group of practitioners for whom the guidelines are relevant. These plans, in essence, describe the one best treatment plan for a particular patient problem. By following these guidelines, quality issues are easily tracked. The case management plan provides the collection and evaluation of variances or complications or both. These data may or may not reveal the need to alter the plan to improve quality (Deming, 1986).

For example, a plan for the treatment of pneumonia may indicate that more than 50% of the patients managed by this plan develop some complication on the third or fourth day. This pattern is seen when retrospectively analyzing the variances documented on the case management plan. A review of this information may indicate the need for a change in the protocol. This may mean providing some element of the plan either earlier or later in the hospital stay.

The cost of the hospital stay can also be followed through the use of the case management plans. Performance within a particular DRG can be tracked financially or through a quality perspective. Comparing case-managed patients to similar patients who are not case managed is one way to do this tracking. Another method is to compare physicians' practice patterns and any deviations from the care plan. This information then can be evaluated for both quality and cost.

Monitoring length of stay or cost before and after implementation of the case management system allows particular nursing units to be their own controls.

If nursing documentation is a part of the managed care plan, the documentation is reviewed for completeness. The registered nurse documents against each expected outcome as it appears on the plan. Thus the documentation more accurately reflects the plan of care and the expected outcomes.

In any case, the processes surrounding the quality issue become the main focus when a CQI approach is taken. Theoretically this process makes continuous analysis and improvement possible because it pinpoints every imperfection in the process and opens the door for change (Berwick, 1989).

THE COST OF QUALITY

Poor quality is costly (Marszalek-Gaucher & Coffey, 1990) and can be assessed by the following:

Cost associated with giving wrong medications or treatments

Increased costs related to misuse of personnel or product resources

Cost of delays

Loss of sales because of dissatisfied patients or physicians

Crosby stresses a "cost of quality" determination as part of the quality improvement process (*Quest for quality*, 1989). His outline parallels actions used when developing a managed care plan. However, the development of the managed care plan takes Crosby's process one step further because it addresses issues and incorporates solutions into the plan of care:

Audit medical records to determine medically unnecessary tests, treatments, or procedures and other factors contributing to increased cost or length of stay.

Meet with a quality assurance or utilization review representative and review incident reports to determine opportunities for improvement.

Interview key members of the organization to identify barriers to the smooth operation and coordination of care.

Interview the medical staff to identify areas for improvement.

Review and analyze patient records to identify costs that can be eliminated.

Evaluate current reporting procedures, information related to operations, and data related to patient satisfaction.

The cost-of-quality analysis identifies a number of potential opportunities for quality improvement. From a case management perspective, the information may lay the foundation for managed care plans by taking into account the best, most cost-effective method available.

THE CONTINUOUS QUALITY IMPROVEMENT PROCESS

The CQI process consists of a number of specific steps. Although it is not necessary to follow the steps in a precise sequence, all steps should be evaluated and addressed (Marszalek-Gaucher, & Coffey, 1990). The achievement of quality care and cost savings is the foundation of both case management and CQI. The process is a cycle that continuously repeats itself.

As with the case management implementation process, the first major step in the CQI process is that of planning and preparing to improve; the second step is to implement; and the third step is to innovate.

Preparing to improve involves seven essential steps (Marszalek-Gaucher & Coffey, 1990). Once again, it is not necessary to follow them in precise order, but each should be addressed in some manner:

1. *Find a process.* The first step is to find a process that needs quality improvement, cost control, or both. These processes may be within a clinical, operations, or financial setting from admitting, to medication distribution, to billing.
2. *Assemble a team who knows the process.* It has been said that those who know the process best are those working the front line or those who work within the process on a day-to-day basis. Therefore a large percentage of the team should be those directly involved in health care delivery. Management should also be included because this division can remove obstacles and facilitate change and improvement. The members of the team should know the process they are evaluating.
3. *Identify the customers and the process outputs and measure the customer expectations of these outputs.* Quality has been defined as meeting or exceeding customer expectations (*Hospital Peer Review,*

1988). Because of the complexity of health care, each process may be made up of several smaller processes. The first thing the team should do is identify its customers, the outputs of each process, and the customer expectations regarding these outputs. In some cases, such as clinical settings, the expectations may not be those of individuals but of the profession as a whole. These expectations may be based on profession-wide standards for the practice of nursing and medicine.

4. *Document the process.* The process consists of a series of steps or inputs, each of which is working toward a particular output. Each step can usually be broken down into subsets, which are hierarchical. A fundamental knowledge of the process is necessary to identify each of the steps accurately, and this is why the input of the front-line worker is so important. A process cannot be managed or improved without this fundamental knowledge.

5. *Generate output and process specifications.* Specifications are measurable, explicit attributes expected of the process and the output. Output specifications may involve the expectations of the customers, which are considered expectations external to the process. However, process specifications are the key internal process factors. Each of the specifications must be measurable. When these specifications are achieved, quality is achieved. Quality is maintained by conforming to these specifications, which is precisely what the managed care plan facilitates. The expected outcomes, if met, ensure quality care has been delivered for that particular problem. As these processes and outputs are evaluated, the process is adjusted to continuously improve it.

6. *Eliminate inappropriate variation.* The sixth step involves implementation. Each specification denotes a measurement point, which is evaluated. One major goal is to prevent quality failures or variations. Two types of variations will occur. The first is random variation. These variations result from factors inherent in the process, and they occur each time the process is played out. The other form of variation is the specific variation, which is a variation that occurs because of one specific component within the process. Once the processes for improvement are implemented, specific variation frequency should be reduced. The goal of the CQI process is to eliminate as many specific variations as possible (Deming, 1986). This results in consistently high-quality output. Within case management, the managed care plans allow for the documentation of variations in clinical practice. By working as a team, the health care professionals can differentiate between random variation and specific variation. The elimination of inappropriate variations results in an approach to health care delivery in which only random variations occur. Random variations are inherent within every process because every patient is different, and every response to treatment is slightly different. These "noises" in the system occur for every process and affect every output.

7. *Document continuous improvement.* This is the final process and the one that makes continuous improvement possible. Once the opportunities for specific or nonrandom variations have been reduced or eliminated, improvements or innovations are introduced. Team members can make changes that result in improved quality or increased productivity. Because the opportunity for variation has been reduced, it is easier to evaluate the impact of the innovation. After such evaluation the change either becomes permanent, or the team discontinues its use.

Walter A. Shewhart described this method of using a stable process to test innovations as the *plan-do-check-act cycle* (PDCA) (Deming, 1986). First developed in the 1930s, this process has become known as the *Shewhart cycle* (Deming, 1986) (Figure 43-3).

JCAHO (1994) introduced the PDSA *(plan-do-study-act)* cycle into the accreditation process. A slight variation from the PDCA cycle, it is expected that organizations seeking accreditation use approaches that incorporate the elements of PDCA/PDSA process in their performance improvement activities.

The PDCA cycle is applied to the process used in case management for addressing and improving health care delivery for particular patient types. Planning involves the identification of specific clinical areas for improvement. As discussed earlier, these areas involve either patients in a specific DRG or nurses in a particular unit chosen to undertake the switch to case management.

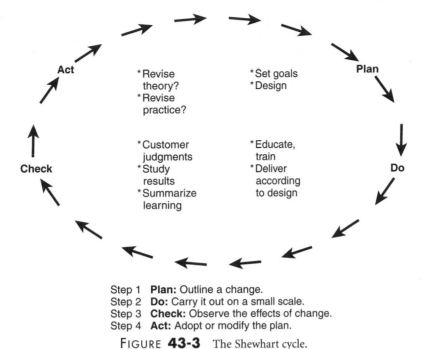

Step 1 **Plan:** Outline a change.
Step 2 **Do:** Carry it out on a small scale.
Step 3 **Check:** Observe the effects of change.
Step 4 **Act:** Adopt or modify the plan.

FIGURE **43-3**   The Shewhart cycle.

The *plan* step involves determining the best case management plan. The *do* step involves implementation of the case management approach. The third step, *check,* involves the analysis of variances that hinder efficient use of the plan. The effects of such variances can be observed by changes in length of stay, patient satisfaction, staff satisfaction, or costs. In some cases the plan might need further revisions until these tangible results are noted.

The *act* step is for modifications if needed. Minimal case management variances indicate that the plan is usable and can be adopted at that point as the standard. If the variances are not minimal, the process begins again with the plan changed, tested, checked, and finally adopted.

The aim of the team is to continuously improve the process. In health care, the process may never be brought to a conclusion because of the evolutionary nature of the treatment of disease. Changing technology, an aging patient population, and economic considerations all have a prolonged effect on the delivery of health care. Therefore the process probably will remain open ended and continuous.

In any case, each process should be seen as one that unremittingly moves forward because today's goals may be tomorrow's standard.

THE NURSE CASE MANAGER IN THE CONTINUOUS QUALITY IMPROVEMENT PROCESS

The case manager can play a vital role in the quality improvement efforts of any organization. CQI can occur through the use of formal teams or through case by case clinical process changes made at the patient level. The case manager plays a vital role in both.

Identification of CQI teams can be done through analysis of the variance data collected by the case manager and analyzed by the case management department. Generally the systems-related variances are most helpful in identifying opportunities for quality improvement efforts. By noting recurring, aggregated variances related to the system, the case manager identifies opportunities for process improvement teams or projects. On the other hand, patient- or family-related variances will generally not provide data for process improvement but may provide data needed for revisions of an existing guideline or pathway.

A case manager should always be part of any process improvement team, particularly those that originate from the variance collection process. The leader of the team should be an individual who has the greatest familiarity with the process being studied. This may be the director of a department or, in the case of clinical processes, a physician. The case manager will play an important role as either the facilitator of the team or a member. The facilitator is responsible for organizing the entire improvement process, including setting up meetings, taking minutes, and providing any data that the team may need during their assessment process. Team members should have a working knowledge of the process and be active participants on the team, bringing their clinical insights to the process.

An important mechanism for facilitating this process is through variance collection and analysis. The case manager identifies quality improvement opportunities through anecdotal discoveries as well as through aggregated data. The facilitation/coordination function of the case manager opens the door to the discovery of system patterns that may need analysis or improvement. In addition, the aggregate of these noted variances will support the discovery and provide the foundation for a quality improvement effort. CQI, therefore, has its basis in the variance collection and analysis process, a fundamental component of case management.

References

Berwick, D.M. (Jan. 5, 1989). Sounding board. *The New England Journal of Medicine, 53-56.*

Bryce, G.R. (Feb. 1991). Quality management theories and their application. *Quality*, 23-26.

Crosby, P.B. (1979). *Quality is free: The art of making quality certain.* New York: McGraw-Hill.

Deming, W.E. (1986). *Out of the crisis.* Cambridge, Mass.: Center for Advanced Engineering Study, Massachusetts Institute of Technology.

Deming's philosophy improves quality. (1988). *Hospital Peer Review, 13*(10), 12-24.

Donabedian, A. (1980). *Explorations in quality assessment and monitoring. Vol. 1: The definition of quality and approaches to its assessment.* Ann Arbor, Mich.: Health Administration Press.

Drucker, P. (Nov.-Dec. 1991). The new productivity challenge. *Harvard Business Review*, 67-79.

Goldfield, N., & Nash, D.B. (Eds.). (1989). *Providing quality care.* Philadelphia: American College of Physicians.

Hickman, C.R., & Silva, M.A. (1984). *Creating excellence: Managing corporate culture, strategy, and change.* Ontario, N.Y.: New American Library.

Joint Commission on Accreditation of Hospitals (1990). *Quality assessment and improvement proposed revised standards.* Chicago: Joint Commission on Accreditation of Hospitals.

Joint Commission on Accreditation of Healthcare Organizations (1994). *Framework for improving performance: From principles to practice.* Oakbrook Terrace, Ill.: Joint Commission Publications.

Juran, J.M. (1987). *Juran on quality leadership: How to go from here to there.* Wilson, Conn.: Juran Institute.

Juran, J.M. (1988). *Juran on planning for quality.* New York: Free Press.

Kanter, R.M. (1983). *The change masters: Innovations for productivity in the American corporation.* New York: Simon & Schuster.

Laffel, G., & Blumenthal, D. (1989). The case for using industrial quality management science in health care organizations. *Journal of the American Medical Association, 262*(20), 2869-2873.

Marszalek-Gaucher, E., & Coffey, R.J. (1990). *Transforming healthcare organizations.* San Francisco: Jossey-Bass.

Naisbitt, J. (1982). *Megatrends: Ten new directions transforming our lives.* New York: Warner Books.

Naisbitt, J., & Aburdene, P. (1985). *Reinventing the corporation.* New York: Warner Books.

New JCAHO standards emphasize continuous quality improvement. (Aug. 5, 1991). *Hospitals*, 41-44.

O'Connor, P. (1984). Healthcare financing policy: Impact on nursing. *Nursing Administration Quarterly, 8*(4), 10-20.

Quest for quality and productivity in health services. (Sept. 1989). Excerpts from the 1989 Conference Proceedings. Washington, D.C.

Tichy, N.M., & Devanna, M.A. (Jul. 1986). The transformational leader. *Training and Development Journal*, 27-32.

Walrath, J.M., Owen, S., & Dziwulski, E. (1998). Case management: A vital link to performance improvement. *Nursing Economics, 14*, 117-122.

44

Job Satisfaction

CHAPTER OVERVIEW

Many variables affect job satisfaction in the workplace. Among these variables, autonomy, professional status, and socialization are consistently and positively related to increases in job satisfaction for registered nurses. Job satisfaction has also been positively related to retention of nurses.

Case management models integrate many of the elements associated with greater job satisfaction, including autonomy, a feeling of connectedness on the job, and professional status.

Two case studies show the relationship between a case management model and job satisfaction. The Nursing Initiatives Program at Long Island Jewish Medical Center in New York demonstrated that the introduction of the case manager role on three pilot units increased job satisfaction and reduced vacancy rates for registered nurses. This study was replicated at Beth Israel Medical Center in New York City. Data on three pilot units were collected before start-up and after 9 months. Outcomes demonstrated improved job satisfaction for staff registered nurses and case managers and reductions in vacancy and turnover rates.

JOB SATISFACTION AS A VARIABLE

Among the variables affected by the implementation of a case management model is staff job satisfaction. The introduction of a case manager to a nursing unit can improve the work environment and thus the level of job satisfaction of nurses working there.

The case manager plans and organizes the care of patients who have the most complex cases, assists with patient teaching, and follows through with discharge planning. In an era when many nurses complain that they spend more time documenting patient care, meeting regulatory documentation requirements, filling out requisitions, or making telephone calls than they do with patients, this model allows nurses to remain at the bedside while ensuring that all peripheral patient needs are met. Because the case manager relieves staff nurses of some of the indirect nursing functions related to their patients' care, many staff nurses report that they are able to spend more time in direct contact with their patients.

Clearly the case management model builds in a support system to help busy practitioners meet complex patient needs. The model promotes independent practice in those nurses providing the direct patient care, but it does not expect these same nurses to function in a vacuum without the proper support systems to meet all their patients' needs in a rapid-paced, complicated health care environment.

Job satisfaction has been related to nurses' job turnover rates (Curry et al., 1985; Reich, 1984; Slavitt, Stamps, Piedmont, & Haase, 1978). Choi et al. (1989) demonstrated that nurses' overall dissatisfaction with their work was the strongest predictor of intent to leave the place of employment or current position. Job satisfaction has been directly related to nurse retention and turnover (Hinshaw & Atwood, 1982; Weisman, Alexander, & Chase, 1981). Therefore the importance of this variable should not be overlooked when a new nursing care delivery system is being designed or evaluated.

A case management model affects the staff nurses providing direct patient care as well as the case managers. The model takes a team approach to care. The team consists of the patient, the family, the physician, the case manager, the direct nursing care provider, the social worker, and others as needed. The model brings all members of the team together with a common focus. Whereas primary nursing led to feelings of isolation and separation for the direct care providers, the case management model does just the opposite. The model's structure works to bring everyone together. Each member supplies information relevant to the care of the patient, and value is placed on every member's input.

As a highly socialized model, case management allows for combined work units organized around a common goal: good patient care. Communication and conflict resolution become needed skills for each team member. If the members of the team cannot function as a group, the outcomes of care will not be achieved in a timely and efficient manner. Because these are among the primary goals of case management, group dynamics play a significant part in the success or failure of the model.

The case manager role, which fosters teamwork, also provides the nurse with an autonomous job that requires independent thought and action. The support provided by the case manager to the other nurse providers reinforces similar feelings of autonomy and independence in them (Alexander, Weisman, & Chase, 1982). It does this by positioning the direct-care provider in a strategic position. A team must rely on the information provided by each of its members, and it is the nurse responsible for direct patient care who provides the information that determines the clinical course of treatment, the teaching needs, and the discharge plan.

This enhanced role for nurses builds feelings of professionalism and self-esteem because nursing's input is valued and deemed important to the patient's progress. In the past, communication was of a hierarchical nature, with the physician dictating to the other members. In the case management model the nurse case manager serves as the thread that links all members of the team. Each member's input is needed so that appropriate and timely outcomes of care are achieved. In this system the staff nurse providing direct care at the bedside supplies the case manager and the rest of the team with valuable information.

A case manager position allows clinically expert, educated, experienced nurses to take on increased responsibility while remaining close to the patient. This position provides a new set of job responsibilities and new wage scale that takes into account all these factors.

The case management model incorporates those elements that have been correlated to increased job satisfaction and decreased turnover. These elements include autonomy, a feeling of connectedness on the job, and salary (Johnston, 1991; McCloskey, 1990; Pooyan, Eberhardt, & Szigeti, 1990).

Some institutions have attempted to measure the satisfaction of their nurses when implementing a case management tool. Although it may be said that other factors can affect the nurses' feelings of satisfaction or dissatisfaction with their work—such as the physical work environment, the presence of a computerized clinical information system, the hours of work, or the fringe benefits—some of these other variables can be controlled by testing the same nurses before and after implementation.

CASE STUDIES

In 1988 as part of the United Hospital Fund's Nursing Initiatives Program, five hospitals—The Brooklyn Hospital Center, Long Island Jewish Medical Center, The Neurological Institute of the Presbyterian Hospital, The New York Hospital, and New York University Medical Center—were selected to orchestrate innovative methods for addressing the nursing shortage. Four of the sites proposed and tested new methods of structuring nursing care providers' work, with the goals of increasing nursing productivity, satisfaction, and retention. The fifth site, New York University Medical Center, introduced a stress reduction program with similar goals (Gould & Mezey, 1991).

Long Island Jewish Medical Center, New York

At Long Island Jewish Medical Center a new nursing position was created as part of the United Hospital Fund's program. The new position was titled patient care manager and became part of a case management delivery model. The position was designed specifically to match the nurse's expertise with the patient's needs and the severity of the illness. One of the reasons for the new position was to keep nurses at the bedside. The position provided the patient care manager with a challenging and rewarding role (Gould & Mezey, 1991).

Three data collection points were used to gauge nurses' job satisfaction. The first point was before implementation, the second at 1 year, and the third about 18 months into the project. Job satisfaction was measured by the Nursing Job Satisfaction Scale (Atwood & Hinshaw, 1981, 1984). The instrument, which has been tested for validity and reliability, was given to all nurses on all shifts at each collection point (Ake et al, 1991).

The medical center's implementation strategies were as follows:

Selecting expert registered nurses as patient care managers

Assigning patient care managers to coordinate care

Decentralizing unit decision-making to registered nurses and physicians

Upgrading nursing attendant tasks

Establishing walking rounds

Registered nurse vacancy rates and registered nurse hours per patient were evaluated in addition to tracking nurse job satisfaction.

Nurses were chosen as patient care managers based on their clinical expertise and willingness to participate in what was, at that time, an experimental role.

The three units participating in the project were a 39-bed medical unit, a 32-bed surgical unit, and a 40-bed neonatal intensive care unit (NICU). At the end of the first 18 months of implementation, 20% of the registered nurses on each unit involved were patient care managers. They managed the care provided for one to three patients in addition to their regular direct care functions.

After about 1 year, the patient care managers on the medical unit reported that this dual role was too difficult and stressful. At that time, one patient care manager was recruited to take on the role full-time and was removed from direct nursing role functions. This individual functioned in a truly autonomous and independent case management role.

Average nursing hours per patient remained relatively consistent throughout the project. However, the number of registered nurse hours per patient and the number of registered nurses on the unit decreased from 119.8 full-time equivalents (FTEs) at the start to 113.7 FTEs at 18 months, indicating an increase in productivity.

The registered nurse vacancy rate also improved during the 18-month period. On the medical unit, the rate decreased from 8% to 0%; on the surgical unit the vacancy rate decreased from 23% to 0%; and in the NICU it remained constant at 0%.

Among the most dramatic findings was the improvement in nursing job satisfaction, particularly comparing start-up scores with those at 18 months for nurses functioning as patient care managers and those working as staff nurses on the units (Table 44-1).

TABLE 44-1	REGISTERED NURSE SATISFACTION BY SERVICE AND BY TITLE ON CASE-MANAGED PILOT UNITS AT LONG ISLAND JEWISH MEDICAL CENTER 1988-1990					
	At Start-Up (1988)		At 12 Months (1989)		At 18 Months (1990)	
	N	Average Score	N	Average Score	N	Average Score
UNIT						
Medicine	20	87	26	90	19	94
Surgery	13	92	16	98	15	97
Neonatal intensive care unit	79	103	69	105	59	105
Total	112		111		93	
TITLE						
Staff PCMs	26	99	17	104	15	110*
Other registered nurses	86	99	94	100	78	100
Total	112		111		93	

*Patient care managers (PCMs) include all full-time and part-time PCMs.

Note: $p = .008$; lowest possible score: 23; highest possible score: 115.

From Gould & Mezey, 1991.

Beth Israel Medical Center, New York, New York

The findings of the Nursing Initiatives Program at Long Island Jewish Medical Center pointed to a relationship between nurse roles and responsibilities and job satisfaction. The study was replicated at Beth Israel Medical Center in New York City to determine if the case manager role did indeed play an important part in the job satisfaction of registered nurses.

At the time of implementation of the three pilot units at the Beth Israel Medical Center in January 1991, all patient care managers were employed on a full-time basis, carrying a case load of 15 to 20 patients. Three pilot units were chosen for the study; these units included a 38-bed neurosurgical unit, a 12-bed acquired immunodeficiency syndrome (AIDS) unit, and a 45-bed medical/surgical unit for the chemically dependent. One case manager was employed on each unit on a full-time basis, meaning that all three were removed from direct care responsibilities.

Indirect care responsibilities included coordination and facilitation of services to the patient, multidisciplinary care planning, patient and family teaching, and discharge planning.

It was anticipated that the introduction of a case management model would increase employee job satisfaction. The case managers, working as staff nurses, remained close to the bedside. Relieved of any administrative responsibilities or direct nursing functions, the case managers were better able to provide not only indirect care to the patients but also assistance to other staff nurses.

The case manager was the only staff nurse working a 5-day-a-week schedule. The case manager was able to fill the information gaps caused by flextime schedules, which were fragmenting care. This built-in continuity factor allowed the staff nurse to spend more time in direct patient contact rather than in reviewing reports or trying to catch up on what happened to the patient in the nurse's absence.

It was also hypothesized that a case management documentation system would enhance registered nurse job satisfaction. With the new system, involving the use of multidisciplinary action plans (MAPs), the nurse could anticipate care needs on a daily basis. In addition, nursing documentation was collapsed onto the form itself, eliminating the need for long, narrative notes. Instead of paragraph notation, the nurse responded to a series of implementation strategies designed to achieve the goals outlined on the plan. Each 24-hour period was attended to separately, and sufficient room was provided so that all nurses caring for the patient within that period could document patient progress and outcomes.

The management of patient care provides a structure that addresses length of stay as well as quality of care. Because the case manager is not geographically bound within the nursing unit, this person is the primary caretaker for the patient and family from admission to discharge from the unit. The case manager's lack of geographic constraints and the 5-day-a-week schedule provide for continuity of care for the patient and family.

The case management system, which improves communication between staff members, leads to a greater feeling of teamwork and collegiality. In addition, the enhanced information base from which nurses function provides a greater level of autonomy in their practices.

All registered nurses working on the pilot units were tested for job satisfaction via the Nursing Job Satisfaction Scale (Atwood & Hinshaw, 1981, 1984). Testing took place before implementation and about 9 months after implementation of the case management model. Thirty registered nurses, or 70% of all nurses filling out questionnaires, completed the questionnaire at both data collection points. Of those 30, 3 were case managers and 27 were staff nurses. All three shifts were represented in the sample.

Job satisfaction scores before start-up and after 9 months indicate that there was a statistically significant increase in satisfaction for those nurses working on case-managed care units who were there for both data collection periods (Table 44-2). Comparisons of case managers to other staff nurses at both collection points indicated an increase for both groups (Table 44-2).

For all three units, both registered nurse vacancy rates and turnover rates decreased over the period of the pilot project (Table 44-3).

On neurosurgery the vacancy rate decreased from 17.33% at start-up to 6% at the end of 9 months. The turnover rate decreased from 21% to 12.5%. On the AIDS unit the vacancy rate went from 11% at start-up to 7% at the end of 9 months, and the turnover rate went from 9% to 7%. The medical/surgical unit for chemically dependent patients achieved a reduction in the vacancy rate from 9% to 0% and a drop in turnover from 17% to 12% at the end of 9 months.

While largely anecdotal, there have been some recent studies measuring the work satisfaction of case managers in various settings. Lancero and Gerber (1995) studied the job satisfaction of nurse case managers as related to their control over nursing practice and their perceived job stress. These comparisons were made on two separate groups of nurse case manager, those working in a "within-the-walls" model, and those working in a "beyond-the-walls" model of case management. The within-the-walls model studied was the acute care delivery (ACD) model practiced at Tucson Medical Center at Tucson, Arizona. The Carondelet community-based (CCB) model was used to measure satisfaction within a beyond-the-walls model.

The ACD model, designed as a typical hospital-based model, had as its major goal to standardize the appropriate use of resources using standardized care planning methods. Case managers, with extensive clinical experience functioned either as unit-based case managers or across multiple in-patient units. The CCB model, a community-based model, links case managers to high-risk patients with the goal of assisting them in achieving and maintaining their maximum level of wellness.

Both groups, the ACD and CCB, were tested on the 21-item Control Over Nursing Practice Scale (CONPS), the NCM Job Stress Index (NCMJSI), and the 29-item Work Satisfaction Index (WSI/NCM). Both groups were correlated positively with work satisfaction and negatively with job stress. A high

| TABLE 44-2 | REGISTERED NURSE SATISFACTION BY UNIT AND BY TITLE ON CASE-MANAGED PILOT UNITS AT BETH ISRAEL MEDICAL CENTER, NEW YORK, NEW YORK |

	At Start-Up (12/90)		At 9 Months (9/91)	
	N	Average Score	N	Average Score
UNIT				
Neurosurgery	11	82	11	82
AIDS	9	88	9	91
Medical-surgical for chemical dependency	10	84	10	90
Total	30		30	
TITLE*				
Patient care managers	3	78	3	86
Other registered nurses	27	84	27	89
Total	30		30	

Note: $T = 2.57$, $df = 29$, $p = 0.0157$. Not significant at the .05 level. Lowest possible score: 23; highest possible score: 115.
*Data at both points.

| TABLE 44-3 | REGISTERED NURSE VACANCY AND TURNOVER RATES AT BETH ISRAEL MEDICAL CENTER BEFORE AND AFTER CASE MANAGEMENT INTRODUCED |

Unit	Time	Vacancy Rate	Turnover Rate
Neurosurgery	Start-up	17.33%	21%
	9 Months	6%	12.5%
AIDS	Start-up	11%	9%
	9 Months	7%	7%
Medical/surgical for chemical dependency	Start-up	9%	17.6%
	9 Months	0	12%

degree of control over practice was highly correlated with positive work satisfaction. Both groups perceived the same amount of control over practice, whether they were working within the hospital or beyond the walls. One conclusion drawn by the investigators was that the role itself contributed to the sense of satisfaction rather than the setting in which the case manager was working. Interactions with physicians also contributed to higher job stress. The major conclusion of the study was that the high degree of autonomy in the role of case manager does contribute to less stress and greater job satisfaction.

Tonges (1998) studied the hypothesized differences between the characteristics of nurse case manager and staff nurse jobs, including intended positive effects and unintended negative effects. Nurse case managers reported significantly higher levels of autonomy, job identity, and collaboration with physicians. Conversely, they reported significantly more required interactions, which resulted in higher job stress, greater amounts of role conflict, ambiguity, and overload.

Goode's (1995) research demonstrated greater job satisfaction for staff engaged in multidisciplinary care map process and who provided care under a case management practice model. The effects indicated greater collaboration, autonomy, and satisfaction with quality of care. In addition, patients surveyed communicated increased satisfaction with their care and greater participation in decision-making.

References

Ake, J.M., Bowar-Ferris, S., Cesta, T., Gould, D., Greenfield, J., Hayes, P., Maislin, G., & Mezey M. (1991). The nursing initiatives program: Practice based models for care in hospitals. In *Differentiating nursing practice: Into the twenty-first century.* Kansas City, Mo.: American Academy of Nursing.

Alexander, C.S., Weisman, C.S., & Chase, G.A. (1982). Determinants of staff nurses' perceptions of autonomy within different clinical contexts. *Nursing Research, 31*(1), 48-52.

Atwood, J., & Hinshaw, A. (1981). Job stress: Instrument development program results. *Western Journal of Nursing Research, 3*(3), 48.

Atwood, J., & Hinshaw, A. (1984). Nursing job satisfaction: A program of development and testing. *Research in Nursing and Health.*

Choi, T., Jameson, H., Brekke, M.L., Anderson, J.G., & Podratz, R.O. (1989). Schedule-related effects on nurse retention. *Western Journal of Nursing Research, 11*(1), 92-107.

Curry, J., Wakefield, D., Price, J., Mueller, C., & McCloskey, J. (1985). Determinants of turnover among nursing department employees. *Research in Nursing and Health, 8,* 397-411.

Goode, C. (Nov./Dec., 1995). Impact of a CareMap and case management on patient satisfaction and staff satisfaction, collaboration, and autonomy. *Nursing Economics, 13*(6), 337-348.

Gould, D.A., & Mezey, M.D. (1991). *At the bedside: Innovations in hospital nursing.* New York: The United Hospital Fund of New York.

Hinshaw, A.S., & Atwood, J.R. (1982). Anticipated turnover: A preventive approach. *Western Journal of Nursing Research, 4,* 54-55.

Johnston, C.L. (1991). Sources of work satisfaction/dissatisfaction for hospital registered nurses. *Western Journal of Nursing Research, 13*(4), 503-513.

Lancero, A.W., & Gerber, R.M. (1995). Comparing work satisfaction in two case management models. *Nursing Management, 26*(11), 45-48.

McCloskey, J.C. (1990). Two requirements for job contentment: Autonomy and social integration. *Image, 22*(3), 140-143.

Pooyan, A., Eberhardt, B., & Szigeti, E. (1990). Work-related variables and turnover intention among registered nurses. *Nursing and Health Care, 11*(5), 255-258.

Reich, P.A. (1984). *The relationship between Jungian personality type and choice of functional specialty in nursing.* Unpublished master's thesis. Adelphi University, Garden City, N.Y.

Slavitt, D.B., Stamps, P.L., Piedmont, E.B., & Haase, A.M. (1978). Nurses satisfaction with their work situation. *Nursing Research, 27,* 114-120.

Tonges, M.C. (1998). Job design for nurse case managers. *Nursing Case Management, 3*(1), 11-23.

Weisman, C.S., Alexander, C.S., & Chase, G.A. (1981). Determinants of hospital staff nurse turnover. *Medical Care, 19,* 431-443.

Nurse Case Manager Job Characteristics and Effects on Well-Being*

Mary Crabtree Tonges

CHAPTER OVERVIEW

As managed care expands, nursing case management is becoming increasingly widespread. Yet little is known about the characteristics of the case manager (CM) job and its effects on the workplace well-being of nurses. This study investigated hypothesized differences between the characteristics of the nurse case manager (NCM) and staff nurse (SN) jobs, including both intended positive and unintended negative effects associated with changes incorporated in the NCM job. NCMs reported significantly higher levels of autonomy, job identity, feedback from agents, and collaboration with physicians than SNs; however, they also reported higher levels of required interaction, role conflict, overload, and ambiguity. These findings have important implications for NCMs and the organizations that employ them, in relation to job design, career/candidate selection, and orientation and ongoing development.

Introduced in the mid-1980s (Ethridge, 1987; Zander, Ethridge, & Bower, 1987), hospital-based nursing case management is a relatively new innovation that has been widely implemented during the past decade (Sherer, 1993; Wake, 1990). Most hospitals currently have or are in the process of implementing some form of case management. With continued growth in managed care, particularly capitated contracts, this trend can be expected to continue.

Despite the growing popularity of nursing case management, however, little is known about the characteristics of this job and its effects on the workplace well-being of nurses. Most of the studies that have been conducted focus on patient and organizational outcomes rather than on the effects on nurses (Lamb, 1992). Although patient and organizational outcomes are clearly important, it is also recommended that hospital managers monitor and evaluate the effects of changes in organizational design and nursing jobs on nursing personnel themselves (Institute of Medicine, 1996).

This chapter presents summary findings from a study of the motivational characteristics of nursing jobs that examined links between these characteristics and nurses' job satisfaction, stress, and burnout.

Note: This research was partially funded by the American Organization of Nurse Executives Nursing Administration Research Award.
*Adapted with permission from Tonges, M.C. (1998). Job design for nurse case managers: Intended and unintended effects on satisfaction and well-being. *Nursing Case Management, 3*(1), 11-23.

Building on these results, the study evaluated differences in the perceived characteristics of the NCM and SN jobs, which is the primary focus of this discussion.

SIGNIFICANCE AND NEED FOR STUDY

As our nation's largest group of health professionals, nurses play an important role in the quality and cost of health care. Moreover, nurses can be part of the solution to key problems within the existing system by, for example, managing patients' care to achieve clinical outcomes more quickly and cost-effectively. Thus nurses' workplace well-being is a significant issue.

Job design theory directs "the design of the work itself—that is, changing the actual structure of the jobs that people perform" (Hackman & Oldham, 1980, p. 44). These changes are intended to increase the quality of employees' work experience as well as their performance. Many adults spend most of their waking hours at work, and workplace well-being has important personal consequences (Locke, 1983; Maslach, 1982; Motowidlo, Packard, & Manning, 1986).

From an organizational perspective, negative workplace well-being outcomes, including burnout (Maslach, 1982) and stress (Motowidlo, Packard, & Manning, 1986), are related to poor performance. Dissatisfaction (Price & Mueller, 1981, 1986) and burnout are also linked to turnover. In nursing specifically, job satisfaction is related to patient satisfaction, which is in turn associated with patients' compliance with care regimens (Weisman & Nathanson, 1985).

The Job Characteristics Model (JCM) developed by Hackman and his colleagues (Hackman & Lawler, 1971, Hackman & Oldham, 1976, 1980) is the most influential paradigm in contemporary job design theory and research. The JCM has provided the theoretical framework for hundreds of studies, and reviews of this evidence suggest that specified motivational characteristics of jobs are reliably related to personal and work outcomes (Berlinger, Glick, & Rodgers, 1988; Fried & Ferris, 1987). Yet it is important to note that the JCM grew out of research with industrial workers, which means that our current understanding of job design is rooted primarily in the study of manufacturing jobs. Given the transformation to a service economy, our knowledge of job design may no longer provide an adequate explanation of relationships between job characteristics and workers' responses.

In addition to the shift from manufacturing to service employment, other important changes are occurring in the world of work, including the redesign of existing jobs (Hammer & Champy, 1993). Based on a growing recognition of the need to focus on business processes rather than on functional activities, many firms are reorganizing to enable one individual to ensure continuity in the performance of a series of tasks (e.g., fulfillment of a customer's order from beginning to end) (Davenport & Nohria, 1994; Hammer & Champy, 1993). This new approach, known as *case management*, redesigns business processes at the customer interface (Tonges, 1989) and is characterized by the creation of a quintessential service role, in which CMs buffer clients from the difficulties of dealing with complex organizational structures and processes (Hammer & Champy, 1993).

Davenport and Nohria (1994) pointed out that the CM job includes a number of elements, such as autonomy, that work motivation theorists identify as desirable. Yet they cautioned that the potential for satisfaction in these jobs may be paradoxically low. Potential sources of dissatisfaction include conflict with functional departments and existing procedures and a loss of face-to-face interactions in jobs mediated through a telephone or computer workstation. What these authors described is a common, yet underresearched, phenomenon. Although real-life job design changes are often complex and may not create simple effects, our knowledge of how job dimensions combine to influence perceptions and reactions to work is limited.

Case management structures have been observed in various different industries, including banking (customer relationship management), insurance (underwriting and issuing new policies), and health care (patient care management) (Davenport & Nohria, 1994). Hospitals have been on the forefront of this trend. The change to prospective payment, coupled with nursing leaders' desire to enrich the SN job, led to the creation of the NCM job (Tonges, 1989; Zander, 1988). Given its growing popularity and intended function as an enriched job, there is a pressing need to examine NCM job characteristics and links to nurses' well-being.

PURPOSE OF STUDY

This study was designed to achieve the following: (1) test an extended model of job characteristics for human service professions and (2) investigate the characteristics of case management as a new job design expected to have mixed motivational consequences. Development and testing of the extended model have been reported in detail elsewhere (Tonges, 1997). This chapter focuses on the second component of the study—CM job characteristics—and provides an overview of the model testing component to create a context for presenting the CM findings.

Literature Review

As illustrated in Figure 45-1, the JCM identifies five core job dimensions (skill variety, task identity, task significance, autonomy, and feedback) that evoke three critical psychological states (CPSs) (experienced meaningfulness of the work, experienced responsibility for outcomes of the work, and knowledge of the

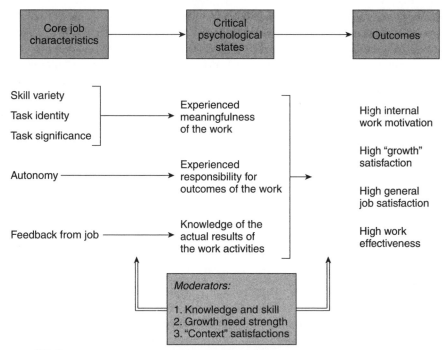

FIGURE **45-1**   The complete job characteristics model.
(From *Hackman, J.R., & Oldham, G.R. [1980]. Work redesign. Pearson Education Inc., Upper Saddle River, N.J. Reprinted with permission.*)

actual results of work activities). The CPSs, in turn, lead to four desirable personal and work outcomes (high levels of internal work motivation, general job satisfaction, growth satisfaction, and work effectiveness) (Hackman & Oldham, 1976, 1980).

EXTENSION OF THE JOB CHARACTERISTICS MODEL

The JCM is generally a well-supported theory (Berlinger, Glick, & Rodgers, 1988; Fried & Ferris, 1987; Loher, Noe, Moeller, & Fitzgerald, 1985; Taber & Taylor, 1990); however, theory development is an evolutionary process, and a number of authors have recommended that job characteristics theory be modified or extended. Beginning with the characteristics and moving across the model, key recommendations concerning each set of constructs and responses to these potential limitations are summarized here.

Task Characteristics

Many researchers have suggested and/or found evidence that the five core dimensions of the JCM may not represent an exhaustive list of possible attributes (Sims, Szilagyi, & Keller, 1976; Stone & Gueutal, 1985; Taber & Taylor, 1990). Examples of additional job content characteristics that appear to have consequences for motivation and redesign efforts include speed, time, and physical danger (Jermier, Gaines, & McIntosh, 1989), as well as a service versus production orientation (Stone & Gueutal, 1985).

Other authors have called for an integration of job characteristics theory with role theory (Abdel-Halim, 1981; Loher, Noe, Moeller, & Fitzgerald, 1985; Tumulty, 1992). Such an integration would combine the narrower considerations of task design with more global aspects of role design, to gain a better understanding of individuals' reactions to their work, particularly in the service sector.

In addition to the five characteristics of the work itself specified by the JCM, this research evaluated the effects of an expanded set of interpersonal relationship and work role characteristics, thought to be especially relevant in service jobs (Mills, Hall, Leidecker, & Marguiles, 1983). These characteristics are defined as follows:

1. *Required interaction*—The degree to which the job requires an individual to work closely with other people (coworkers and/or clients) in carrying out the work activities (Hackman & Oldham, 1975)
2. *Collaboration with physicians*—The degree to which the interactions of nurses and physicians enable synergistic influence of patient care (Weiss & Davis, 1982)
3. *Influence with other disciplines*—The extent to which other professionals (e.g., social workers, discharge planners, and dietitians) consider the nurse's ideas in making decisions about patient care
4. *Social integration*—The degree to which an individual has close friends among organizational members within the immediate work unit (Price & Mueller, 1986)
5. *Feedback from agents*—The degree to which the individual receives clear information about her or his performance from supervisors or coworkers (Hackman & Oldham, 1975)
6. *Role conflict*—The extent to which different members of a role set communicate disparate expectations that arouse motivational forces within the individual toward different behaviors (Kahn, Wolfe, Quinn, & Snoek, 1981)
7. *Role overload*—A specific type of role conflict in which members of a role set hold legitimate expectations that are compatible in the abstract but impossible for the individual to completely fulfill because of time constraints (Kahn, Wolfe, Quinn, & Snoek, 1981)
8. *Role ambiguity*—The extent to which an individual lacks information required to perform the job (Kahn, Wolfe, Quinn, & Snoek, 1981)

Critical Psychological States

Investigators have also proposed and/or found evidence that other psychological states, not specified by the JCM, may mediate relationships between characteristics and outcomes (Fried & Ferris, 1987; Renn & Vandenberg, 1995). A new psychological state, *experienced attachment to coworkers*, has been incorporated in the model to link the effects of close, supportive relationships with coworkers to outcomes (Baumeister & Leary, 1995; Korman, 1992).

Outcomes

Researchers have found links between job characteristics and/or psychological states and outcomes that are not included in the JCM. Riordan and Griffeth (1995), for example, found that friendship opportunities at work were strongly related to job involvement. Mental health has also been evaluated as a dependent variable and was meaningfully related to the three CPSs, especially experienced meaningfulness ($r = 0.39$) (Wall, Clegg, & Jackson, 1978).

In addition to general job and growth satisfaction from the JCM, this study included burnout and perceived job stress as dependent variables. *Burnout* refers to a "syndrome of emotional exhaustion and cynicism that occurs frequently among individual who do 'people-work' of some kind" (Maslach & Jackson, 1981, p. 99). *Psychological stress* occurs when a person has made an evaluation that external or internal demands tax or exceed her resources (Lazarus, 1991). These two workplace well-being constructs are particularly salient to the study of human service professionals (Maslach, 1982; Motowidlo, Packard, & Manning, 1986) and enhance our understanding of this type of job.

These characteristics, psychological state, and outcome constructs and their proposed interrelationships are depicted in Figure 45-2.

JOB CHARACTERISTICS RESEARCH WITH STAFF NURSES

Nursing has been the subject of a number of JCM studies (Holaday & Bullard, 1991; Joiner, Johnson, Chapman, & Corkrean, 1982; Roedel & Nystrom, 1988). A consistent pattern of findings has emerged (Joiner et al., 1982; Roedel & Nystrom, 1988) that shows that SNs perceive higher levels of significance and variety, about the same levels of autonomy and feedback from work, and lower task identity than those in other professional/technical jobs (Hackman & Oldham, 1980).

In their sample of 135 nurses, Roedel and Nystrom found statistically significant correlations between all five of the core dimensions and general satisfaction, ranging from a high of $r = 0.30$ ($p < .01$) with feedback from work to a low of $r = 0.12$ ($p < .10$) with significance (Roedel & Nystrom, 1988).

NURSING CASE MANAGEMENT JOB DESIGN RESEARCH

Review of the nursing case management literature suggests two general conclusions, which are supported by the findings of other reviewers: (1) this literature is largely anecdotal (Marschke & Nolan, 1993) and, as previously noted, (2) the research that does exist focuses primarily on patient and institutional, rather than nurses' outcomes (Erkel, 1993). A small body of relevant research was located, however, and descriptions and key findings from these studies are summarized in Table 45-1.

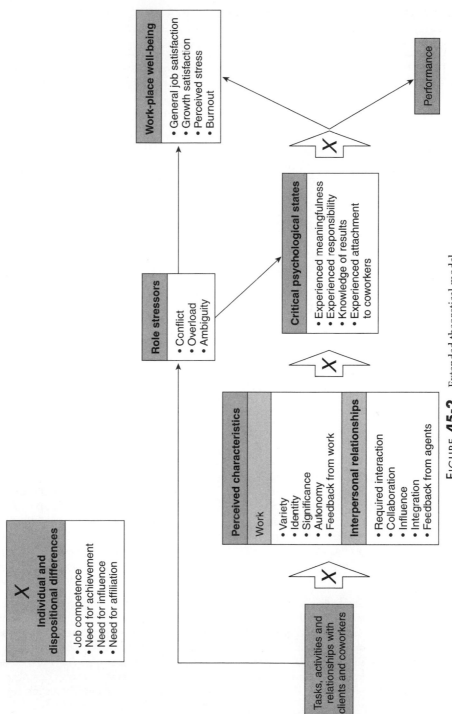

FIGURE **45-2** Extended theoretical model.

TABLE 45-1	NURSING CASE MANAGEMENT STUDIES AND KEY FINDINGS	
Author and Date	**Description**	**Key Findings**
Ethridge, 1987	Quantitative evaluation of Carondelet model	Nurse case managers (NCMs) (n = 7) reported significantly higher levels of autonomy, enjoyment of work, and professional status than staff nurses (n = 72).
Newman, Lamb, and Michaels, 1991	Qualitative study of nursing case management practice at Carondelet	Nurses experience something different when practicing as NCMs. Specifically, NCMs (1) are not bound by time and space and establish ongoing partnerships with clients and (2) are not organizationally empowered to carry out professional service. Relationships with hospital SNS were "sensitive" initially, but improved with time.
Van Dongen and Jambunathan, 1992	Qualitative pilot study examining role of psychiatric NCM in outpatient clinic	Both psychiatrists (n = 2) and NCMs (n = 5) described the NCM role as autonomous, yet collaborative with the psychiatrist.
Goode, 1993	Quantitative evaluation of hospital-based managed care (HBMC) intervention combining CareMaps and case management	Nurses who applied and were selected for NCM positions had higher levels of collaboration than other nurses, reported higher levels of job satisfaction with quality of care, and their autonomy increased with time in the NCM job.
		Multidisciplinary team members had higher levels of collaboration than other multidisciplinary staff on the experimental unit.
Lancero, 1994	Quantitative examination of perceived control over nursing practice, job stress, and work satisfaction among 30 NCMs in two different models	Satisfaction was positively correlated with control ($r = 0.65$, $p = 0.01$) and negatively correlated with stress ($r = 0.43$, $p = 0.01$). Stress scale items NCMs reported as most unique to NCM practice included "focusing on continuum rather than episode," "having independence and autonomy," and "long-term relationships with clients and families."
McGill, 1994	Qualitative evaluation of the impact of the NCM role on leadership development within a hospital setting, based on data from two focus groups of NCMs (n = 16)	NCMs' relationships changed with physicians and other disciplines positively, but relationships with staff nurses changed negatively. Specifically, NCMs reported more collaboration and communication with physicians and other disciplines; however, they also described a sense of being in an ambiguous job separated from other nurses.

TABLE 45-1	NURSING CASE MANAGEMENT STUDIES AND KEY FINDINGS—CONT'D	
Author and Date	**Description**	**Key Findings**
Rheaume et al., 1994	Qualitative study of the effects of case management on nursing practice, based on literature review and interviews with community-based NCMs (n = 17) in Canada	Case management has the potential to fundamentally alter usual lines of authority between nurses and MDs. Difficulties are encountered in relationships between NCMs and discharge planners and other nurses and health care workers, especially if the NCM role is not clearly understood. Despite the potential difficulties, however, case management appears to improve quality of working relationships in that it makes collaborative relationships feasible.

Motivational Characteristics of the Nurse Case Manager Job

The NCM job was developed in response to changes in hospital financing that presented an opportunity to enrich staff nursing and create a new job. Work redesign strategies focus on expanding the responsibilities of a job both horizontally, to increase characteristics such as variety and identity, and vertically, to increase autonomy.

These changes are intended to produce desired improvements in affective and behavioral outcomes, which have been reported in numerous studies (Fried & Ferris, 1987; Hackman & Oldham, 1980; Herzberg, 1966). Yet it has also been noted that the effects of work redesign initiatives are not always as intended (Joiner & van Servellen, 1984). I believe that the design of the NCM role has successfully introduced a number of theoretically important changes that should make it a more satisfying and motivating job. However, the design of this job is also expected to produce several unintended effects.

Unintended Effects from Job Redesign

Although not nearly as prevalent as reports of improved satisfaction and performance, there are occasional examples of unintended effects from job redesign scattered through the literature. Kopelman (1985) noted that job enrichment sometimes leads to decreased satisfaction with pay and supervision: employees may expect increased compensation for expanded responsibilities, and supervisors may interfere with the autonomy employees expect to receive. Moreover, because of the stimulating nature of highly motivating jobs, some employees may experience stress and mental overload.

Two studies identify the potential for unintended effects from job enrichment in nursing, specifically the transition to nurse managed care (Shigemitsu & Tsushima, 1990; Wolf, 1993). Wolf's (1993) dissertation research described a number of negative outcomes associated with the shift to a professional nursing practice model in which nurses assumed responsibility for managing the care of a caseload of patients, such as increased intensity of work and decreased work group cohesion.

As part of an evaluation of nurse managed patient care, Shigemitsu and Tsushima (1990) measured nurses' stress before and after implementation of a model that encouraged nurse–physician collaboration in managing patient care in accordance with predetermined protocols. Results suggested that a significant increase in nurse job stress occurred after the implementation of the care management program.

In summary, although these models appear to be extensions of primary nursing more than the type of formal nursing case management system in this research, it appears that there is a need for balanced consideration of potential unanticipated consequences, as well as intended effects, in assessing the motivational characteristics of the NCM job.

THE NURSE CASE MANAGER JOB

From the job characteristics and role theory perspectives, what is the NCM job? Its design appears to create changes in the SN job that affect characteristics of the work itself, relationships with colleagues, and the work role.

CHARACTERISTICS OF THE WORK. Staff nurse jobs are known to be high in significance and skill variety (Joiner et al., 1982; Roedel & Nystrom, 1988). The NCM job is likely to be similar in these characteristics; however, it is expected that NCMs experience more job identity, autonomy, and feedback in their work than SNs.

Compared with the traditional SN job, the NCM has an expanded scope in terms of both a broader perspective on patient care and a view across a longer continuum. NCMs see the system of patient care more broadly in that they manage the entire hospitalization, as opposed to just the nursing care component on one unit. They also follow the same patients longitudinally across unit and institutional boundaries.

McGill's (1994) and Lancero's (1994) studies with NCMs provide support for increased task identity in this job. CMs in McGill's study described a change in their focus to the total picture of patient care, and Lancero's findings suggested that one of the most unique aspects of NCM practice is focusing on a continuum of care.

Previous research also suggests that NCMs experience greater autonomy in their jobs. CMs in Lancero's study identified independence and autonomy as additional unique characteristics of their jobs. Ethridge (1987) explicitly demonstrated that NCMs report higher levels of autonomy than SNs, and Goode (1993) found that nurse autonomy increased over time in the NCM job. The jobs of NCMs are less structured by schedules and routines than the jobs of SNs, which allows NCMs greater latitude in organizing and managing their work. Because NCMs usually work with the most complex cases, they may also experience more independence in decision-making, as they are grappling with unique problems for which fewer standardized answers are available.

NCMs may also receive more feedback from their work, particularly if they are working with a clinical path/CareMap* system. These systems include concurrent and retrospective analysis of variances from the plan of care (Bower, 1993), which NCMs can use to assess effectiveness in facilitating a patient's progress through the hospitalization.

Bueno and Hwang (1993) described a sophisticated system developed at Robert Wood Johnson University Hospital that integrates variance analysis with the performance appraisal system for NCMs. Variance analysis data are entered into a database, and summary reports are prepared for each NCM that list the frequency for each case type and compare the average expected length of stay with the average actual length of stay. SNs generally do not receive this type of regular, quantitative performance feedback.

CHARACTERISTICS OF COWORKER RELATIONSHIPS. NCMs would be expected to have more influence with physicians and members of other disciplines because of their authority and responsibility for patients' movement through the hospital system. NCMs are in a better position to collaborate with physicians than are SNs because they can affect events that are important to physicians (e.g., arranging

---

*CareMap is a licensed trademark of The Center for Case Management, South Natick, Mass.

services that patients need) and have access to comparative information about physicians' practice patterns and outcomes. Thus although NCMs may not interact with physicians on a "level playing field," their relationships are more equitable. Descriptions of NCMs' interactions with physicians from McGill's (1994) research suggest a more balanced relationship in which nurses exert more control in relation to decisions about patient care (e.g., questioning a physician's assertion that a patient does not need a particular intervention).

McGill's findings also indicate that NCMs have influence with other disciplines in the management of patient care. For example, in relation to a question about relationships with members of other professions, the focus group facilitator commented, "I see you all nodding your heads, so would you pretty well agree that, as you become the recognized experts, other departments also approach you, not just your own area?" (McGill, 1994, p. 40). This was confirmed by the participants. Similarly, Goode (1993) found that members of multidisciplinary care management teams, including physicians, NCMs, a dietitian, and a pharmacist, reported higher levels of collaboration than other multidisciplinary staff on the unit.

NCMs perform an integrator/expeditor function within hospitals (Zander, 1994) and occupy what can be described as an intraorganizational boundary-spanning position (Adams, 1983). Because of their structural relationship to other roles, boundary positions have a number of unique properties. Boundary role individuals are more distant from other organizational members, may be viewed with suspicion, and must negotiate with multiple groups (Adams, 1983). Because NCMs move throughout the organization in the course of their work, they may have fewer opportunities to develop close relationships with coworkers in one geographic work area. In addition, the structure of their responsibilities may increase the potential for interpersonal conflict with other nurses and other professionals, such as social workers or discharge planners (McGill, 1994; Morse, 1991; Newman, Lamb, & Michaels, 1991; Rheaume, Frisch, Smith, & Kennedy, 1994).

In summary, nurses' jobs involve a great deal of interaction with others, and it is expected that both SN and NCM jobs are characterized by required interaction and feedback from agents; however, because of the design of their jobs, NCMs are expected to experience more collaboration and influence with other disciplines and less social integration than SNs.

WORK ROLE CHARACTERISTICS. The boundary spanning nature of NCMs' roles may also contribute to role conflict. NCMs link patients, physicians, and other disciplines to each other and to the organization. Dealing with these multiple constituencies places the NCM at high risk for intersender role conflict. The shift from a clinical to a more administrative role noted by Rheaume and colleagues (1994) may also create a form of intrapersonal role conflict in which the NCM feels torn because values as a clinician may suggest everything possible should be done for a patient regardless of cost, whereas role expectations require administrative attention to resource management. Thus it is predicted that NCMs will experience greater role conflict than their SN counterparts.

Work overload is an important factor in SNs' job dissatisfaction (Irvine & Evans, 1992). Similar to their colleagues in staff positions, NCMs report that they have difficulty completing their work within the time available (Lancero, 1994; McGill, 1994). It appears that role overload may characterize both jobs.

NCMs work in positions that are new and frequently incompletely defined. As previously noted, NCMs' jobs are also less structured by routines (e.g., medication administration schedules). In addition, NCMs are frequently at risk for role blurring and diffusion between their new roles and SN responsibilities (Tonges, 1993). McGill's subjects explicitly described the experience of repeatedly explaining their jobs to others (McGill, 1994). Thus it is expected that NCMs experience more role ambiguity than SNs.

Hypothesized differences between the characteristics of SN and NCM jobs that were evaluated in this research are summarized in Table 45-2.

TABLE 45-2	HYPOTHESIZED DIFFERENCES IN CHARACTERISTICS OF NURSE CASE MANAGER AND STAFF NURSE JOBS	
Job Characteristic	**Nurse Case Manager**	**Staff Nurse**
Autonomy	Higher	Lower
Job identity	Higher	Lower
Job feedback	Higher	Lower
Collaboration	Higher	Lower
Influence	Higher	Lower
Social integration	Lower	Higher
Role conflict	Higher	Lower
Role ambiguity	Higher	Lower

Method

A cross-sectional correlation design was used to collect data concerning relationships among perceived job characteristics and workplace well-being outcomes. More detailed descriptions of methodology are reported elsewhere (Tonges, 1997, 1998).

SUBJECTS, SAMPLE, AND SETTING
The sample comprised RNs employed as NCMs, unit-based care coordinators (CCs), and SNs; however, this report focuses on a comparison of NCMs and SNs. Nurses included in the sample (1) were female; (2) worked in acute care hospitals on inpatient units; (3) worked at least half-time; and (4) had a minimum of 2 years of registered nurse experience. NCM subjects also had to be employed in that position for at least 1 year.

Data were collected from eligible NCMs and a random sample of SNs from eight not-for-profit, acute care hospitals ranging in size from 238 to 1000 beds. A total of 413 subjects provided usable responses, which represented a 29% response rate.

The mean age of respondents was 40 years (SD = 9.2). Thirteen percent had a diploma in nursing; 30%, an associate's degree; 43%, a baccalaureate; and 13%, a master's degree or higher. Their mean years of experience was 14 (SD = 8.3). Distribution across clinical practice areas was as follows: 33% medical/surgical, 23% intensive care, 9% pediatrics, 6% obstetrics/nursery, and 28% other (does not total to 100% because of rounding and missing data).

INSTRUMENTS
Items from 11 instruments and a demographic data form were used to measure the variables in this study. Descriptions of their psychometric properties in previous research and this study are reported elsewhere (Tonges, 1997).

PROCEDURES
After receiving permission to access hospital staff, a list of eligible SNs and NCMs was obtained, and SN names were randomized. Surveys were coded and placed in envelopes labeled with subjects' names for internal distribution. Packets containing a cover letter, informed consent, demographic data form,

| TABLE 45-3 | DEMOGRAPHIC PROFILE OF RESPONDENTS FROM EACH JOB CATEGORY | | | | | | | | | | | | |

	Age		Education*				Years of Registered Nurse Experience		Clinical Area				
Job Title	M	SD	DIP	ADN	BSN	MSN or Higher	M	SD	M/S	CC	PEDS	OB	Other†
Staff nurse	40	9.8	17%	35%	46%	2%	14	8.4	29%	28%	10%	8%	25%
Case Manager	40	9.2	—	7%	37%	56%	17	6.2	47%	10%	14%	4%	25%

*Does not add to 100% due to rounding/missing data.
†"Other" includes inpatient specialties such as telemetry, oncology, and psychology.

questionnaire, and prepaid return envelope were mailed to an on-site coordinator to be delivered to subjects.

Results

Hierarchical regression analysis was used to evaluate hypotheses concerning relationships predicted in an extended model. Findings suggest that characteristics of interpersonal relationships and work roles explain significant increases in variance, beyond that explained by the core dimensions of the JCM, in general and growth satisfaction, burnout, and job stress. Again, a detailed description of these findings is reported elsewhere (Tonges, 1997).

INTENDED AND UNINTENDED EFFECTS OF NURSE CASE MANAGER JOB DESIGN

The demographic profile of the NCM and SN respondents who met criteria for inclusion in these comparisons is displayed in Table 45-3. One-way analyses of variance that compare the NCM and SN groups for age, education, and years of experience by job category indicated no significant difference in age at the 0.05 level. There were significant differences among the groups in education, with NCMs having more education than SNs. NCMs ($x = 16$) also had significantly more years of experience than SNs ($x = 14$). Effects of the demographic variables were controlled by entering the set of demographic covariates as step 1 in the regressions, and significant findings are reported here. The effect of site was evaluated in step 3 and reported elsewhere (Tonges, 1997).

Means and standard deviations for the job characteristic variables for NCMs and SNs are reported in Table 45-4. The number of subjects per category was further reduced because of missing data. A multivariate analysis of variance in job characteristics between job categories was significant at the $p < 0.01$ level. Based on this finding, analysis progressed to testing hypotheses concerning perceived differences in specific job characteristics between NCM and SN jobs.

TABLE 45-4	MEANS AND STANDARD DEVIATIONS FOR JOB CHARACTERISTICS BY JOB CATEGORY				

Variable	SN (n = 254)		CM (n = 53)	
	Mean	SD	Mean	SD
Autonomy	5.1	0.93	6.2	0.59
Job identity	4.2	1.10	4.8	1.10
Feedback from work	5.0	0.98	5.0	1.20
Collaboration	3.7	1.10	4.4	0.74
Influence	6.9	1.90	7.4	1.50
Social integration	3.7	0.69	3.7	0.79
Role conflict	3.4	0.99	3.7	0.92
Role ambiguity	3.4	0.77	3.9	0.94
Skill variety	5.7	0.90	6.0	0.75
Task significance	6.2	0.74	6.1	0.79
Feedback from agents	3.9	1.40	4.4	1.40
Required interaction	6.4	0.72	6.8	0.44
Role overload	3.7	1.60	4.6	1.30

Intended Positive Effects of Nurse Case Manager Job Design

Hypothesis 1 states that there is a significant relationship between working in the NCM job and perceived autonomy. For the sample of SNs and NCMs meeting the criteria for inclusion, the increment in R^2 for the variable representing the contrast coded vector for SN and NCM jobs was 0.144 ($p < 0.01$). This means that working as an NCM, rather than an SN, uniquely explains 14% of the variance in autonomy beyond that explained by demographic differences. Hypothesis 1 is therefore supported.

Hypothesis 2 states that there is a significant relationship between working in the NCM job and perceived job identity. The increment in R^2 for the contrast between SN and NCM jobs was 0.05 ($p < 0.01$), and hypothesis 2 is supported.

Hypothesis 3 states that there is a significant relationship between working in the NCM job and perceived job feedback. The increment in R^2 was 0.00001 ($p = 0.98$). This means that working as an NCM, rather than an SN, does not uniquely explain meaningful variance in feedback from work, and hypothesis 3 is not supported.

Hypothesis 4 states that there is a significant relationship between working in the NCM job and perceived collaboration with physicians. The R^2 for the set of covariates was 0.11 ($p < 0.01$). This means that demographic differences accounted for 11% of the variance in collaboration. Examining the β values for individual variables within the set revealed that the two strongest, significant explanatory variables were education (β = 4.1, $p < 0.01$) and working in intensive care (β = 3.36, $p < 0.01$).

The increment in R^2 for the contrast between SN and NCM jobs was 0.04 ($p < 0.01$). This means that working as an NCM, rather than an SN, uniquely explains 4% of the variance in collaboration, and hypothesis 4 is supported.

Hypothesis 5 states that there is a significant relationship between working in the NCM job and perceived influence with other disciplines. The increment in R^2 for the contrast was 0.002 ($p = 0.45$), and hypothesis 5 is not supported.

Unintended Negative Effects of Nurse Case Manager Job Design

Hypothesis 6 states that there is a significant relationship between working in the NCM job and perceived social integration. The increment in R^2 for the contrast between SN and NCM jobs was 0.002 ($p = 0.54$), and hypothesis 6 is not supported.

Hypothesis 7 states that there is a significant relationship between working in the NCM job and perceived role conflict. The increment in R^2 for the contrast was 0.03 ($p < 0.01$), and hypothesis 7 is supported. This means that working in the NCM, rather than the SN job, uniquely accounts for 3% of the variance in role conflict, beyond that explained by demographics.

Hypothesis 8 states that there is a significant relationship between working in the NCM job and perceived role ambiguity. The increment in R^2 for the contrast was 0.04 ($p < 0.01$), and hypothesis 8 is supported.

Although no differences were hypothesized between the NCM and SN jobs for the remaining five characteristics, contrasts were run to provide a comprehensive analysis. Findings from these regressions were as follows:

Variable	ΔR^2 for Covariates	ΔR^2 for Job
Skill variety	0.03 ($p = 0.23$)	0.01 ($p = 0.07$)
Significance	0.03 ($p = 0.25$)	0.003 ($p = 0.29$)
Required interaction	0.02 ($p = 0.49$)	0.035 ($p < 0.001$)
Feedback from agents	0.01 ($p = 0.83$)	0.016 ($p = 0.02$)
Role overload	0.07 ($p = 0.002$)	0.027 ($p = 0.002$)

These findings mean that for respondents in this study, working in the NCM job, as opposed to the SN job, uniquely explains significant increases in variance in required interaction, feedback from agents, and role overload, beyond that explained by differences in age, education, clinical area, and years of experience.

Regarding the other significant effects, all clinical areas except medical/surgical were significantly negatively related to role overload. This indicates that nurses working in the medical/surgical area reported significantly higher levels of role overload than nurses working in intensive care, pediatrics, obstetrics/nursery, and other inpatient areas.

DISCUSSION, CONCLUSIONS, AND FURTHER RESEARCH

Compared with staff nursing, the NCM job appears to combine higher levels of both positive and negative characteristics. Specifically, NCMs report significantly higher levels of autonomy, job identity, collaboration with physicians, and feedback from agents; however, they also report considerably more required interaction, which was significantly related to job stress, as well as higher levels of role conflict, ambiguity, and overload. Because these characteristics have opposite effects on outcomes and are significantly negatively related to each other, increasing them simultaneously would be expected to have mixed effects.

Work redesign changes the structure of people's jobs in an attempt to increase their perception of positive job characteristics. Although the identification of links between specific tasks and perceived characteristics has not been a major research focus, some evidence suggests that activities can be related to more than one characteristic (Tonges, Rothstein, & Kikiras, 1998). Thus changes designed to increase a particular positive characteristic may also increase a negative one.

As an example, consider the possibility that cross-training an employee to perform additional functions may increase perceptions of skill variety, but may also increase feelings of role overload. In this case, each characteristic would be expected to exert opposite effects on job satisfaction and burnout (i.e., variety is related positively to satisfaction and negatively to burnout, and overload has the opposite pattern of relationships). Ultimately, effects associated with increases in the positive may be offset by increases in the negative characteristic.

Three of the hypothesized differences between characteristics of NCM and SN jobs were not supported: higher levels of job feedback, higher levels of influence with other disciplines, and lower social integration. A possible explanation for NCMs reporting higher levels than SNs of feedback from agents, but not feedback from work, is that information about issues such as length of stay and cost management may be received in reports from supervisors. Thus although this information is about the results of the work of NCM, it comes through agents, rather than directly from the work itself.

Regarding the findings for influence, the wording of this scale asks about the frequency with which other disciplines ask and act on "nurses" opinions. Feedback was received from NCMs who completed the survey questioning which nurses' opinions to which the items referred—those of SNs or NCMs. It is possible that the general nature of this wording contributed to a lack of differentiation between jobs. Revising the items to refer to "my opinion" should clarify this issue.

Three of the significant differences between NCM and SN job characteristics were not predicted: higher levels of required interaction, feedback from agents, and role overload. There was limited prior research to guide these hypotheses, and the findings of this study should prove helpful to other researchers in this regard.

In summary, results of this study suggest that the NCM job is associated with differences in a number of motivational characteristics found to have positive and negative consequences for workplace well-being. Further study of nursing and other types of CM jobs is needed to continue to evaluate the characteristics and consequences associated with this job design.

IMPLICATIONS OF THIS RESEARCH

Given the growing popularity of the case management approach, results from this study have useful implications for individuals and organizations.

Implications for Individuals

Workplace well-being has important personal consequences. Work-related stress has been linked to depression (Motowidlo, Packard, & Manning, 1986), and burnout is characterized by a combination of negative feelings, including emotional exhaustion and low personal accomplishment (Maslach & Jackson, 1981). Clearly, it is in our best interests to know more about job characteristics and design and to use this knowledge to enhance workplace well-being.

The conclusions concerning negative and positive characteristics in the same job and mixed consequences of work redesign imply that individuals must think about the possible cons, as well as the pros, associated with job changes. The implication for individuals is to learn as much as possible about a job in its entirety when contemplating a change or, more specifically, to evaluate all the ways the new job differs from one's current position, not just how it is different in some particular positive way. Nurses specifically must be aware of the potential for problems with role overload, conflict, and ambiguity in the NCM job.

Implications for Organization

The implication for practice of the conclusions concerning negative and positive characteristics and mixed consequences of work redesign is that we need to learn more about the combined effects of job design changes. This knowledge could help us to enrich a job without introducing unintended negative characteristics at the same time.

In view of the turmoil within health care (Lumsdon, 1995), this is especially valuable and timely information for nursing and other health care professions. Conclusions about NCM job characteristics imply a specific need for attention to role stressors in this job. To address these concerns, however, it is necessary to have more information about the specific aspects of the job that give rise to perceptions of role overload, conflict, and ambiguity.

Rizzo, House, and Lirtzman (1970) suggested that role stressors are intervening variables that mediate the effects of various organizational practices. Specifically, *role conflict* is associated with violations of the principles of unity of command and single accountability, and *role ambiguity* is related to conditions such as lack of a clear idea of job scope and responsibility, vague task definition, inconsistent direction from a supervisor, and lack of clarification regarding the function of each member in a group.

Findings from an organizational stress study with a sample of 158 registered nurses, licensed practical nurses, and aides suggest that administrative efforts to establish goals, to plan and coordinate, and to resolve interdepartmental conflict are linked to lower levels of role conflict among staff (Gray-Toft & Anderson, 1985). The same study found that representation, consultation, and involving staff in decision-making (communication) directly and indirectly led to a significant reduction in role ambiguity among nursing staff.

Without more research concerning specific links between job activities and perceived characteristics, definitive recommendations for interventions to reduce perceived role stressors in the NCM job cannot be made. However, several suggestions are offered for evaluation.

There is a growing trend in hospitals to create NCM jobs by integrating utilization review/management, discharge planning, and, sometimes, quality improvement and social service functions into one position. Given the financial pressures hospitals are experiencing and the overlap among these jobs and case management, this approach is understandable; however, it appears to contribute to higher levels of role stressors.

For example, an NCM who is expected to inform patients that they need to go home because their insurance company is denying payment for further hospitalization (utilization review), while also trying to function as a patient advocate (clinical case management) may well experience feelings of role conflict. Similarly, adding the responsibility for responding to numerous calls from insurance companies for information (utilization review) to a day of seeing patients and families and working with other disciplines to expedite care (clinical case management) is likely to lead to feelings of role overload. The point is not that some additional functions cannot be integrated but rather that tasks must be consistent with the purpose of the job and the resulting workload must be realistic.

Although there may always be some ambiguity associated with a relatively new job, some possible interventions to clarify the NCM role include the following: (1) the development and distribution of a specific job description, (2) a thorough orientation, and (3) multiple opportunities for communication, including regular meetings with the manager and peer group.

The job description should include precise statements outlining the NCM's major responsibilities in the areas of clinical management, financial management, leadership, and self-development. Other essential functions may include performance improvement and consultation/education. This description should be augmented by a list of measurable cost/quality performance goals that are revised annually (e.g., "decrease length of stay for traditional DRG Medicare patients by 0.5 day" or "reduce readmission rates for COPD patients by 10%").

Orientation should focus on the desired behavioral outcomes of the job and include a combination of clinical, financial, and managerial content. If possible, introduction to the role should culminate in a precepted experience with a seasoned CM mentor.

Communication opportunities should be provided through a combination of regular one-on-one and group meetings with the case management supervisor. Group meetings should include case presentations and peer consultation. Again, however, specific sources of role ambiguity and the effectiveness of such interventions must be evaluated.

The findings of this study also have implications for selection of candidates for NCM jobs. In addition to knowledge and skills in the clinical and financial arenas, results suggest that serious consideration should be given to applicants' tolerance for ambiguity, time management abilities, and interpersonal skills.

In conclusion, a revolution is occurring in the world of work, and a combination of factors—including the shift to service employment and the emergence of case management job design—have created the need for an expanded job characteristics model and a better understanding of the characteristics of CM jobs. As work and assignments continue to evolve, the more we know about job characteristics and their links to workplace well-being, the better prepared we will be to design jobs that enhance personal and work outcomes. It is hoped that the results of this study will contribute to this goal.

References

Abdel-Halim, A.A. (1981). Effects of role stress–job design interaction on employee work satisfaction. *Academy of Management Journal, 24*, 269-273.

Adams, J.S. (1983). The structure and dynamics of behavior in organizational boundary roles. In M. Dunnette (Ed.), *Handbook of industrial and organizational psychology* (2nd ed.) (pp. 1175-1200). New York: Wiley.

Baumeister, R.F., & Leary, M.R. (1995). The need to belong: Desire for interpersonal attachments as a fundamental human motivation. *Psychological Bulletin, 117*, 497-529.

Berlinger, L., Glick, W., & Rodgers, R. (1988). Job enrichment and performance improvement. In J. Campbell & R. Campbell, and associates (Eds), *Productivity in organizations* (pp. 219-254). San Francisco: Jossey-Bass.

Bower, K.A. (1993). Case management: Work redesign with patient outcomes in mind. In K.J. McDonagh (Ed.), *Patient-centered hospital care: Reform from within.* Ann Arbor, Mich.: Health Administration Press.

Bueno, M.M., & Hwang, R. (1993). Understanding variances in hospital stay. *Nursing Management, 24*(11), 51-57.

Davenport, T.H., & Nohria, N. (1994, Winter). Case management and the integration of labor. *Sloan Management Review*, 11-23.

Erkel, E.A. (1993). The impact of case management in preventive services. *Journal of Nursing Administration, 23*(1), 27-32.

Ethridge, P. (1987). Nurse accountability program improves satisfaction, turnover. *Health Progress, 5*, 44-49.

Fried, Y., & Ferris, G.R. (1987). The validity of the job characteristics model: A review and meta-analysis. *Personnel Psychology, 40*, 287-322.

Goode, C.J. (1993). *Evaluation of patient and staff outcomes with hospital-based managed care.* Unpublished doctoral dissertation, University of Iowa, Iowa City, Ia.

Gray-Toft, P.A., & Anderson, J.G. (1985). Organizational stress in the hospital: Development of a model for diagnosis and prediction, Part I. *Health Services Research, 19*, 753-774.

Hackman, J.R., & Lawler, E.E. (1971). Employee reactions to job characteristics. *Journal of Applied Psychology, 55*, 259-286.

Hackman, J.R., & Oldham, G.R. (1980). *Work redesign.* Menlo Park, Calif.: Addison-Wesley.

Hackman, J.R., & Oldham, G.R. (1976). Motivation through the design of work: Test of a theory. *Organizational Behavior and Human Performance, 16*, 250-279.

Hackman, J.R., & Oldham, G.R. (1975). Development of the Job Diagnostic Survey. *Journal of Applied Psychology, 60*, 159-170.

Hammer, M., & Champy, J. (1993). *Reengineering the corporation: A manifesto for business revolution.* New York: HarperCollins.

Herzberg, F. (1966). *Work and the nature of man.* Cleveland: World Publishing.

Holaday, B., & Bullard, I.D. (1991). Pediatric staff nurses' reactions to job characteristics. *Journal of Pediatric Nursing, 6*, 407-416.

Institute of Medicine. (1996). *Nursing staff in hospitals and nursing homes: Is it adequate?* In G.S. Wunderlich, F.S. Sloan, & C.K. Davis (Eds), Washington, DC: National Academy Press.

Irvine, D., & Evans, M. (1992). Job satisfaction and turnover among nurses: A review and meta-analysis. *Quality of Nursing Worklife Research Monograph Series*, Toronto, Canada.

Jermier, J.M., Gaines, J., & McIntosh, N.J. (1989). Reactions to physically dangerous work: A conceptual and empirical analysis. *Journal of Organizational Behavior, 10*, 15-33.

Joiner, C., Johnson, V., Chapman, J.B., & Corkrean, M. (1982). The motivating potential in nursing specialties. *Journal of Nursing Administration, 12*(2), 26-30.

Joiner, C., & van Servellen, G.W. (1984). *Job enrichment in nursing.* Rockville, Md.: Aspen Publications.

Kahn, R.L., Wolfe, D.M., Quinn, R.P., & Snoek, J.D. (1981). *Organizational stress: Studies in role conflict and ambiguity* (Reprint ed.). Malabar, Fla.: Krieger.

Kopelman, R.E. (1985). Job redesign and productivity: A review of the evidence. *National Productivity Review, 4*, 237-255.

Korman, A.K. (1992). Seminar in organizational behavior: Work-place well-being. Baruch College of the City University of New York.

Lamb, G.S. (1992). Conceptual and methodological issues in nurse case management research. *Advances in Nursing Science, 15*(2), 16-24.

Lancero, A.W. (1994). *Work satisfaction among nurse case managers: A comparison of two practice models.* Unpublished master's thesis, University of Arizona, Tucson, Ariz.

Lazarus, R.S. (1991). Psychological stress in the workplace. *Journal of Social Behavior and Personality, 6*(7), 1-13.

Locke, E.A. (1983). The nature and causes of job satisfaction. In M. Dunnette (Ed.), *Handbook of industrial and organizational psychology* (2nd ed.) (pp. 1297-1350). New York: Wiley.

Loher, B.T., Noe, R.A., Moeller, N.L., & Fitzgerald, M.P. (1985). A meta-analysis of the relation of job characteristics to job satisfaction. *Journal of Applied Psychology, 70*, 280-289.

Lumsdon, K. (1995). Faded glory: Will nursing ever be the same? *Hospital and Health Networks, 69*(23), 30-35.

Marschke, P., & Nolan, M.T. (1993). Research related to case management. *Nursing Administration Quarterly, 17*(3):16-21.

Maslach, C. (1982). *Burnout: The cost of caring.* Englewood Cliffs, NJ: Prentice-Hall.

Maslach, C., & Jackson, S. (1981). The measurement of experienced burnout. *Journal of Organizational Behavior, 2*(2), 99-113.

McGill, R.L. (1994). *Nursing case management: Developing clinical leaders.* Unpublished master's thesis, College of St. Catherine, St. Paul, Minn.

Mills, P.K., Hall, J.L., Leidecker, J.K., & Marguiles, N. (1983). Flexiform: A model for professional service organizations. *Academy of Management Review, 8*, 118-131.

Morse, J.M. (1991). Negotiating commitment and involvement in the nurse-patient relationship. *Journal of Advanced Nursing, 16*, 455-468.

Motowidlo, S.J., Packard, J.S., & Manning, M.R. (1986). Occupational stress: Its causes and consequences for job performance. *Journal of Applied Psychology, 71*, 618-629.

Newman, M., Lamb, G.S., & Michaels, C. (1991). Nurse case management: The coming together of theory and practice. *Nursing & Health Care, 12*(8), 404-408.

Price, J.L., & Mueller, C.W. (1986). *Absenteeism and turnover of hospital employees.* Greenwich, Conn.: JAI Press.

Price, J.L., & Mueller, C.W. (1981). *Professional turnover: The case of nurses.* New York: SP Medical and Scientific Books.

Renn, R.W., & Vandenberg, R.J. (1995). The critical psychological states: An underrepresented component in Job Characteristics Model research. *Journal of Management, 21*, 279-303.

Rheaume, A., Frisch, S., Smith, A., & Kennedy, C. (1994). Case management and nursing practice. *Journal of Nursing Administration, 24*(3), 31-36.

Riordan, C.M., & Griffeth, R.W. (1995). The opportunity for friendship in the workplace: An underexplored construct. *Journal of Business and Psychology, 10*(2), 141-154.

Rizzo, J., House, R., & Lirtzman, S. (1970). Role conflict and ambiguity in complex organizations. *Administrative Science Quarterly, 13*, 150-163.

Roedel, R.R., & Nystrom, P.C. (1988). Nursing jobs and satisfaction. *Nursing Management, 19*(2), 34-38.

Sherer, J.L. (1993). Health care reform: Nursing's vision of change. *Hospitals, 67*(8), 20-26.

Shigemitsu, K., & Tsushima, G. (1990). Collaborative practice: Nurse managed care. *Straub Foundation Proceedings, 55*(3), 37-42.

Sims, H.P., Szilagyi, A.D., & Keller, R.T. (1976). The measurement of job characteristics. *Academy of Management Journal, 19*, 195-212.

Stone, E., & Gueutal, H.G. (1985). An empirical derivation of the dimensions along which characteristics of jobs are perceived. *Academy of Management Journal, 28*, 376-396.

Taber, T., & Taylor, E. (1990). A review and evaluation of the psychometric properties of the Job Diagnostic Survey. *Personnel Psychology, 43*, 467-500.

Tonges, M.C. (1998). Job design for nurse case managers: Intended and unintended effects on satisfaction and well-being. *Nursing Case Management, 3*(1), 11-23.

Tonges, M.C. (1997). *An extension of the job characteristics model for a service economy.* Unpublished doctoral dissertation. Baruch College of the City University of New York.

Tonges, M.C. (1993). Work designs: Sociotechnical systems for patient care delivery. *Nursing Management, 23*(1), 27-32.

Tonges, M.C. (1989). Redesigning hospital nursing practice: The Professionally Advanced Care Team (ProACT®) Model, Part 1. *Journal of Nursing Administration, 19*(7), 31-38.

Tonges, M.C., Rothstein, H.R., & Kikiras, H.C. (1998). Sources of satisfaction in hospital nursing practice: A guide to effective job design. *Journal of Nursing Administration, 28*(5), 47-61.

Tumulty, G. (1992). A model for nursing role redesign. In B. Henry (Ed.), *Practice and inquiry for nursing administration* (pp. 67-71). Washington, D.C.: American Academy of Nursing.

Tumulty, G. (1990). *The relationship of head nurse role characteristics, job satisfaction, and unit outcomes.* Unpublished doctoral dissertation, University of Texas at Austin.

Van Dongen, C.J. & Jambunathan, J. (1992). Pilot study results: The psychiatric RN case manager. *Journal of Psychosocial Nursing, 30*(11), 11-14.

Wake, M.M. (1990). Nursing care delivery systems: Status and vision. *Journal of Nursing Administration, 20*(5), 47-51.

Wall, T.D., Clegg, C.W., & Jackson, P.R. (1978). An evaluation of the Job Characteristics Model. *Journal of Occupational Psychology, 51*, 183-196.

Weisman, C.S., & Nathanson, C. (1985). Professional satisfaction and client outcomes: A comparative analysis. *Medical Care, 23*, 1179-1192.

Weiss, S.J., & Davis, H.P. (1982). Validity and reliability of the Collaborative Practice Scales. *Nursing Research, 34*, 299-305.

Wolf, K.A. (1993). *Professionalization at work: The case of nursing at Mill City Medical Center.* Unpublished doctoral dissertation, Brandeis University.

Zander, K. (1994). Case management series, Part I: Rationale for care-provider organizations. *The New Definition, 9*(3), 1-2.

Zander, K. (1988). Nursing case management: Strategic management of cost and quality outcomes. *Journal of Nursing Administration, 18*(5), 23-30.

Zander, K., Etheredge, M.L., & Bower, K.A. (1987). *Nursing case management: Blueprints for transformation.* Boston: New England Medical Center.

Measuring Cost-Effectiveness

CHAPTER OVERVIEW

Measuring cost-effectiveness is one of the most important tasks in the evaluation of nursing case management models. This chapter reviews various strategies for measuring cost savings in a case management system and provides examples of case studies using these approaches. In addition, suggestions for using these methods in further research are reviewed.

EFFECT OF CASE MANAGEMENT ON VARIANCES OF LENGTH OF STAY AND RESOURCE UTILIZATION

In a study done by the American Hospital Association titled *1990 Report of the Hospital Nursing Personnel Survey* (AHA, 1990), the case management model represented the largest increase of nursing care delivery systems most frequently used in the acute care setting. In light of this study and others, it is important to present some of the methods of evaluating the cost-effectiveness of nursing case management. The studies presented in this chapter represent some of the groundbreaking work done in measuring the cost-effectiveness of nursing case management and health care delivery approaches. In general, case management has been associated with reduced total costs per patient case, decreased patient length of hospital stay, increased patient turnover, and potential increase in hospital-generated revenues.

In a program instituted at Long Regional Hospital in Utah, cost savings were achieved through the use of a bedside-centered case management model (Bair, Griswold, & Head, 1989). With this approach the registered nurse controls the use of patient care resources, guides the outcomes of this care within acute care and community-based settings, and, as a member of a multidisciplinary care coordination team, monitors and evaluates the costs and quality components of hospitalization for patients within defined diagnosis-related group (DRG) categories.

The registered nurse was given the responsibility and accountability for assessing the inpatient and discharge care requirements and for developing and implementing the plan of care related to the prescribed length of stay and amount of patient care resources used. To determine actual costs, focus was placed on the clinical management of defined groups of patients within 10 DRGs or service lines. Each of these groups was analyzed with special emphasis placed on patient care services, length of hospitalization, treatment and educational outcomes, discharge and post-discharge care planning, and outpatient and community-based services. Some of the DRGs that were investigated included major joint procedures, angina, heart failure, chest pain, circulatory disorders, acute myocardial infarction, and pneumonia.

A cost-containment study that focused on reducing the average loss per DRG case type was implemented. A comparison was made of the actual cost per case and the average reimbursement for 10 DRGs. It was demonstrated that bedside case management resulted in cost savings associated with a decrease in length of stay of 0.4 day, an average hospital savings of $284 per case and overall cost savings of $94,572.

Additional savings were realized through strategic planning and better use of patient care resources as evidenced by a reduction in admissions to the intensive care unit by 0.7 day and through the accurate assessment and classification of Medicare reimbursement criteria related to inpatient and outpatient group status.

An investigation done by McKenzie, Torkelson, and Holt (1989) showed that interventions associated with nursing case management had a significant effect on patient resource consumption and expenditures.

Case management plans and critical paths were developed for specific high-volume DRGs associated with diseases and disorders of the circulatory system, coronary artery bypass, and catheterization. This study demonstrated an average cost saving per case that was equivalent to $350 for laboratory charges, $180 for radiology charges, and $766 for pharmaceutical charges for nursing case-managed patients. The average length of stay was also reduced by 1.1 days. Within a 1-year period, close to $1 million was saved by using the case management system of care.

Stillwaggon (1989) demonstrated the effect of a nurse model on the cost of nursing care and staff satisfaction. This study was conducted at Saint Francis Hospital and Medical Center in Hartford, Connecticut. An approach to the delivery of patient care called *managed nursing care* was developed and implemented. This model promoted collaborative practice arrangements, encouraged care based on individualized patient assessment and need, eliminated routine and non-nursing tasks, and established nursing practice guided by professional standards of care. In addition, the professional nurse was able to contract for services and care needed by the patient. This contracting eliminated the need for the traditional work schedule.

The study sample consisted of 100 cases of normal, spontaneous delivery without complication or comorbidity. Comparisons were made between the traditional nursing care delivery system and the new approach to patient care under the nurse managed care model. An assessment was made of the nursing care hours actually delivered and the staff's satisfaction with the nurse managed care model.

Results showed a reduction of 5 hours spent delivering nursing services and a $61.71 decrease in cost of care per case. Additional findings indicated a high level of nursing staff and patient satisfaction with the nurse managed care delivery system.

In another study, Cohen (1991) incorporated a cost-accounting methodology with a combined team nursing–case management model to investigate personnel factors and variable cost components such as pharmaceuticals and supplies under the nursing case management model. The purpose of this study was to substantiate the financial benefit of using the nursing case management model within the acute care setting.

It was predicted that cesarean section patients who received care under the nursing case management model would have a shorter length of stay than patients who received care under the existing practices. It was also predicted that the nursing case management system of care would result in an overall decrease in hospital costs and expenditures associated with the cesarean section patient (Cohen, 1991).

The study used a quasi-experimental design on the experimental and control units. The cesarean section case types, DRGs 370 and 371, were selected for study because of the high volume and long length of stay associated with these DRGs. The study sample consisted of 128 cesarean section patients who made up 768 total patient days in 1988. A nonrandom selection was used.

Because randomization was not used, homogeneity controlled for individual extraneous variables that may have affected patient length of stay. Restricting the patient sample to cesarean section helped to control for patient gender, type of diagnosis, and surgical operation.

The data needed for the study required the development and implementation of the nursing case management delivery system. Use of the case management model required thorough orientation for the nursing staff. This orientation period introduced nurses in the experimental group to care under a case management model and helped the case managers assume their roles. Those who were in the experimental group included registered nurses, licensed practical nurses, and nursing assistants. Critical paths and nursing case management care plans were also used.

Demographic data, length of stay, and comorbidity information were received and compiled from the patient subject group. An evaluation was made of professional staff mix as well as the amount of time spent by nurses in delivering patient care (Cohen, 1990, 1991).

Nursing staff members were expected to cooperate with the investigator of this hospital-based administrative research project. The implementation of the nursing case management model included the following guidelines:

1. The case manager (registered nurse) became responsible for the patient when she was admitted to the unit.
2. Case associates (co-case managers or primary registered nurses) and case assistants (licensed practical nurses and nursing assistants) were given responsibility for ensuring continuity of care and accountability throughout the patient's length of stay. Each of the co-case managers was assigned different schedules to avoid overlapping days on the unit. Each patient was designated one case manager whose caseload was covered by the co-case manager on the case manager's days off.
3. Each case manager was to collaborate with the attending physician in assessing and evaluating the outcomes of patient care and individualizing the case management plan and critical path.
4. Each case manager was trained to use the case management care plan and critical path to facilitate patient care.
5. The critical path was used for the change-of-shift report.
6. Variance from the case management care plan or the critical path required discussion with the attending physician and a nursing case management consultant.
7. The nursing case manager and physician were to communicate at least twice during the patient's length of stay.
8. The nurse case manager and the patient care coordinator (head nurse) were to collaborate daily to negotiate assignment planning that would optimize the use of nursing resources.
9. Daily documentation was to reflect the monitoring of patient progress and evaluation of outcomes specified in the case management care plan or variances on the critical path, or both (Cohen, 1990).

COST ACCOUNTING METHOD

One of the primary objectives of the nursing case management system is to develop a cost management information system that validates the patient's use of clinical resources and services and confirms the financial benefits of case management to the institution. In this investigative project a nursing case management concept was established with the cesarean section case type that incorporated the following fiscal priorities:

To maximize control over patient hospital stay by implementing definable and attainable patient goals within a short period of time.

To decrease service-related costs and enhance DRG reimbursement by reducing patient length of stay through anticipatory planning, early intervention, and the coordination and arrangement of services.

The cost accounting process used in this study involved the following four procedural steps.

Step I: Establishment of a Resource Use Profile on the Typical Cesarean Section Patient

A historical patient profile reflecting conventional practice patterns was developed from the hospital's management information system. This procedure involved a review of detailed charges based on the hospital's charge description and general ledger code reports. These charges were summarized and then compressed from 272 service codes into 14 major clinical use and expense categories. Those categories were then separated by sample group. The categories included routine care, delivery room, operating room, anesthesia, recovery room, laboratory or blood, radiology, respiratory physiology, general pharmacy, antibiotics, intravenous (IV) therapy, other pharmacy, routine treatment, and other.

A 2-month sample from 1988 medical records and bills was accessed so that clinical information, financial data, volume of tests and services, posted charge rates for room and board, and ancillary services could be analyzed. An average of the accumulated costs was obtained to arrive at the cost of a unit of service (i.e., patient day, tests, procedures, pharmaceuticals) for all clinically related resources used.

Step II: Establishment of a Resource Use Profile for the Cesarean Section Patient Based on the Nursing Case Management Concept

The historical data obtained from the patient profiles were used to develop a patient profile adjusted for nursing case management outcome standards. The major nursing, medical, and ancillary outcome indicators of care were derived from the cesarean section patients' critical paths and were used to assess the nursing case management model's efficacy and productivity. Cost standards were set by reducing patient length of stay by 2 days (from 6 to 4 days), streamlining tests and procedures, and initiating patient teaching early in the hospital stay.

Step III: Comparison of the Charge and Resource Use Associated with Comparable Cesarean Section Cases

A charge and clinical resource use comparison was made between the experimental (case management) and control (conventional practice) groups. The comparison involved correlating the average unit of service for both the experimental and control groups to establish the average clinical resource use for the cesarean section patient. For example, the following was identified: average number of tests incurred, average number of supplies used, average number of pharmaceuticals given, average number of nursing care hours provided, and average length of stay. This comparison established a mechanism for monitoring the change in resource use after switching from conventional practices to case management. Such monitoring helped ensure that efficient use of services was maintained. The results of this comparison substantiated the efficacy of the case management model.

Step IV: Determination of the Total Average Cost for the Nursing Case Management Model

The above analysis provided the total room and board charges. However, to more effectively determine the average cost of the nursing case management model as well as the required nursing care resources, the following methodology was used: (1) The total direct nursing care costs were computed for both sample groups; (2) nursing care was segregated from total room and board costs; and (3) the ratio of cost to charge (RCC) factor was applied. The comparisons in step III were then categorized by skill mix to determine the number of direct nursing care hours required under each system for the care of the cesarean section patient.

To determine the total direct nursing care costs associated with both the experimental and control groups, the following computation was completed:

$$\frac{\text{Average base salary per skill mix by sample group}}{1950 \text{ hours (the number of hours worked in a year by an employee)}} = \text{Average hourly wage rate}$$

$$\begin{array}{c} \text{Average hourly wage rate} \times \text{Sum total of direct nursing care} \\ \text{hours provided by skill mix (from the Nursing Case} \\ \text{Management Activity form)} \times 1.25 \text{ (average fringe benefits)} \end{array} = \begin{array}{l} \text{Total average costs of direct nursing} \\ \text{care for the cesarean section patient} \end{array}$$

The direct nursing care costs were then segregated from the total expenditures to arrive at the remaining room and board costs.

The method used for determining costs was the departmental RCC, which is the cost-accounting methodology most widely used by health care institutions. The RCC is delineated from the Institutional Cost Report, which is a cost statement used by the Medicare program for various reimbursement processes. This report contains revenue, cost, and clinical service use information by department.

The method involved taking the RCC for each major clinical use and expense category and applying it against the total charges to arrive at an approximate determination of the total cost per case. This provided the final pieces of data needed to establish the total average costs for the nursing case management model (Cohen, 1990, 1991).

Findings indicated that a significant reduction in patient length of stay was achieved. Length of stay declined by 1.16 days, or 19%, between the experimental and control groups ($p \leq 0.0001$). Expenditure and cost analysis showed an increase in direct patient-centered nursing care hours and intensification in use of inpatient services and treatments. This intensification of nursing time and resource use led to the reduction in patient length of stay and a decrease in total overall costs.

The analysis further demonstrated a savings of $930.40 per patient case and a general decrease in hospital costs and expenditures associated with the cesarean section patient. This profit was made possible because of the increase in patient turnover and the availability of additional patient beds. Potential savings and revenues of more than $1 million were identified for the hospital (Cohen, 1991; Health Care Advisory Board, 1990).

Although an analysis of the demographic data showed comparability between the experimental and control groups, the rigor of this investigation can be strengthened by using matched sampling to decrease the likelihood of extraneous variance and by using randomized assignment of the sample groups.

At Beth Israel Medical Center in New York City the case management model is used as a vehicle for reducing patient length of stay. Coupled with other initiatives such as CQI, reductions in the length of stay for selected diagnoses were realized in the first year of implementing the case management model (Table 46-1).

Nursing, medicine, social work, administration, patient representatives, operations, and finance were among the departments that participated in the change to a case management delivery system. In some cases, specific medical or surgical departments or specialties were targeted for the development of multidisciplinary action plans (MAPs). These plans incorporated all professional disciplines in management of the patient's care and ensured outcome-related quality services. In other cases, specific diagnoses or DRGs were targeted for significant reductions in length of stay (Table 46-1).

The Pareto chart, a statistical tool to determine which diagnoses or procedures to target, was used for the development of managed care plans and financial analysis (Figure 46-1). If an annual review is being conducted, the number of cases for the top volume DRGs can be tallied. These are then placed on the

| TABLE 46-1 | BETH ISRAEL MEDICAL CENTER CASE MANAGED INCREMENTAL REVENUE FOR SELECTED DIAGNOSES | | | | | |

Diagnosis	DRGs	ALOs 1990*	No. of Cases 1990	ALOs 1991*	No. of Cases 1991	Incremental Revenue†
Laminectomy	4/755/756/ 577/758/ 214/215	10.0	260	9.08	213	$238,000
Endocarditis	126	14.4	94	8.7	58	$900,000
Soft tissue infection	278	9.1	189	8.7	156	$28,000
Pneumonia	89	11.06 1/91-6/91	298 1/91-6/91	10.05 7/91-2/92	257 7/91-2/92	$196,000
Orthopedics	209/211/ 233/234/ 218/219/ 220/221/ 223/224	9.0	143	7/08	226	$489,000
11/11/91–1/31/92						
Diabetes team						
Principal diagnosis	294/295/ 296/297/ 566	9.9	300	3.45	37	
11/11/91–1/31/92						
Secondary diagnosis	—	11.8	—	10.5	29	
High-risk obstetrics	383	—	—	8.25	12	$438,000
					TOTAL	**$2,289,000**

*Average length of stay data compiled from an MIS download from the Charms systems.
†Incremental revenue calculated by Don Modzewleski, Assistant Vice President, Finance.

chart in the form of a bar graph in descending order. On the right side of the chart the percentage of the total cases that each number of cases represents is placed on a cumulative line graph. For example, DRG 707 represented 63 cases, or 31% of the total number of cases. The next highest volume, DRG 277, represented a total of 50 cases, or 24% of the total number of cases. These two percentages are represented cumulatively as 55% of all cases. This means that these two DRGs represented 55% of all cases admitted to the unit. In most instances, one would study the top 80%, in this case DRGs 707, 277, 708, and 89, which represent approximately 80% of all cases. In this way it is clear that a fair representation of all cases has been included.

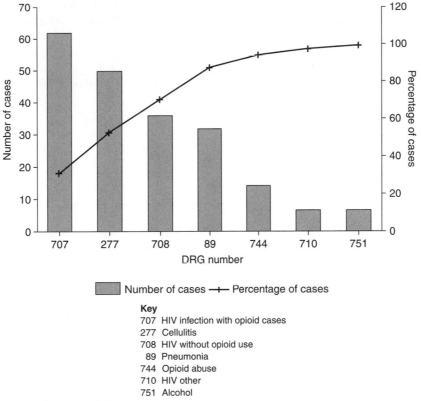

Key
707 HIV infection with opioid cases
277 Cellulitis
708 HIV without opioid use
 89 Pneumonia
744 Opioid abuse
710 HIV other
751 Alcohol

FIGURE **46-1**   DRG Pareto chart showing patient cases for 1991.

Non–unit-based case management teams are committed to following all patients of a specific case type who are admitted to the medical center. They are also responsible for monitoring length of stay, resource use, and quality. The teams also provide in-service training sessions to house staff and nursing personnel to maintain appropriate treatment of these patients.

Two teams, one for diabetes and one for asthma, consisted of several physicians, a nurse case manager, a nurse clinician, and other clinically relevant disciplines. In the case of the diabetes team a nutritionist was included and functioned as a full-time member who saw all patients assigned to the team.

The managed care plan is used to guide care and to provide a framework for keeping the length of stay in check. The length of stay on the plan is determined by studying the region, state, and federal lengths of stay for those DRGs relevant to the diagnosis or procedure. The physician practice patterns are then reviewed, and length of stay for the institution is established for that diagnosis.

Two groups for case management, unit-based case managers and non-unit-based case managers, were developed. The unit-based case managers assumed the same role as the non–unit-based case manager. However, the unit-based manager's primary responsibility was on an individual unit level and involved more than one diagnosis and many different physicians. The unit-based case manager can be equally effective because that person sees the patient several times during the day, intervening whenever necessary. The non–unit-based case managers, on the other hand, may spend a portion of the day traveling from one unit to another. Therefore their time with each patient is more limited.

Both groups, the non-unit-based case managers and the unit-based case managers, were able to demonstrate significant cost reductions within the first few weeks and months of implementation. Once the targeted diagnoses had been identified, the institution's prior length of stay history was obtained. These data allowed the team to determine what the expected length of stay would have been if the conventional model of patient care had been used.

After implementation of case management the length of stay was tracked on a monthly basis for those patients followed by the case management approach. Patients with certain diagnoses or surgical procedures were targeted and followed by the case manager.

Stringent data collection was necessary for accurate cost accounting. Preimplementation length-of-stay data provided the framework for determining whether the length-of-stay goals were achieved.

RELATIVE WEIGHTS AND FINANCIAL ANALYSIS

Some diagnoses fall within a single DRG. For example, pneumonia will almost always be coded within DRG 89. Conversely, many surgical procedures can be classified within a number of DRG categories. For example, laminectomy can be coded within as many as seven DRGs. Each of these DRGs may have a different financial weight.

The weights applied to each DRG are called *relative weights*. The relative weight is a value applied to the DRG based on the average complexity and resource consumption for patients within that DRG. The relative weight for carpal tunnel release will be much lower than the relative weight for major chest procedures, which is one of the most highly weighted DRGs. The relative weight will apply differently for Medicare versus other third party payers.

Institutions performing a larger number of procedures with higher relative weight values will see a higher overall reimbursement, reflected in the case mix index (CMI) for each department and ultimately the institution. The CMI provides an indication of the relative cost of providing care and is determined by taking an average of all the service intensity weights over all discharges for the institution. The service intensity weights are the average of all the weights of all DRGs seen on a particular service.

For example, transplants carry an extremely high relative weight. Therefore a large number of transplants will inflate the overall CMI, resulting in a better financial appearance. Complexity and intensity form the basis of the CMI system. Although there is no clear definition of complexity, it generally refers to the types of services rendered, while intensity refers to the number of services per patient day or hospital stay (Luke, 1979).

There is some incentive in this system for health care organizations to bring in larger numbers of patients whose DRG will be of a higher relative weight. Often hospitals emphasize these types of services to the detriment of lower paying groups.

Beth Israel Medical Center used the relative weight values as a basis for determining the financial gain or loss of each of the diagnoses or procedures tracked under the case management system. If the diagnosis being evaluated falls within one DRG, the process is much easier. In the case of endocarditis the length of stay for case managed patients decreased from 14.4 days in 1990 to 8.7 days in 1991. This length-of-stay reduction was analyzed against the number of cases at the shorter length of stay and the relative weight for the DRG.

A relative cost weight is obtained by dividing the adjusted national cost per DRG by the adjusted national cost per case for all DRGs. The larger the relative cost weight, the greater the relative costliness of a DRG (Grimaldi & Micheletti, 1983).

An assumption was made that for each day's reduction in length of stay, the bed was "back-filled" with a patient falling into a DRG with the same or greater relative weight. In this way, although the length of stay was decreased, available beds were used.

In other cases the surgical procedure being analyzed fell under more than one DRG, as in the case of laminectomies. In this circumstance the relative weight for all possible DRGs must be averaged.

With case management teams that potentially could be managing several DRGs, the same process would be followed. The average relative weight would be averaged for all possible DRGs, again assuming the beds would be back-filled with similar patients.

Although this type of cost-accounting system is not precise, it does give a good indication of the approximate incremental revenue savings for the diagnosis or surgical procedure under analysis.

More recent studies have shown similar results of decreased length of stay and costs (Blegen, Reiter, Goode, & Murphy, 1995).

IMPLICATIONS FOR FURTHER RESEARCH

All the studies reviewed share common implications for clinical and professional practice. One implication is in the area of assessing the quality of the critical path analysis and MAPs. Both the critical path and MAP were used to set clinical resource and cost standards and were responsible for most of the planning, coordination, and integration activities of the nursing case management model. Future research would be helpful for evaluating the critical path's and MAP's reliability and validity. Additional research should also focus on the treatment and practice protocols developed by the critical path and MAP analysis as they relate to patient care and clinical practice outcomes.

One other major implication is in objectively measuring the contributions of the nursing case management model to the quality of patient care, in particular, its effects on patient care resources, and in assessing patient and provider satisfaction. Additional research is needed to look at the effects of nursing case management on professional autonomy and decision-making opportunities for nurses, collaborative practice arrangements between nurses and physicians, nursing case management staffing and assignment allocations, payment and reimbursement mechanisms for nursing case management services, and the types of nursing case management interventions used and the effects of these interventions on patient outcomes. Other general implications for nursing follow:

- The changes in practice patterns associated with nursing case management can help to reduce overall expenditures related to hospitalization.
- Nursing case management can provide substantial improvements in the cost-effectiveness of patient care.
- Nursing case management focuses on collaborative practice arrangements between nurses and physicians to help shorten length of hospital stay and maintain effective use of money and materials, thereby having a significant effect on the hospital's fiscal bottom line and viability.
- Nursing case management has the potential to equate the effects of clinical nursing services and outcomes with resource allocation, costs, and reimbursement systems.
- Nursing case management has the potential to positively affect the present nursing care shortage by reorganizing delivery systems to maximize professional decision-making opportunities for nurses and allowing for continuity of patient care.
- Nursing case management can relate the cost savings of nursing interventions to specific patient populations in the acute care setting.
- Nursing case management can enhance the management of nursing services and substantiate the economic accountability and contribution of nurses to consumers of health care services.

Nursing case management provides the baseline for further research and evaluation of the functional competencies and uses of different skill levels in delivering nursing care services to patients and their families. This approach allows for more efficient integration of various levels of support staff by defining role expectations. Cohen's (1990) study successfully used the registered nurse as the case manager and case associate with the nursing assistants as support staff. The nurse case manager coordinated, assessed, evaluated, and participated with the case associates in the delivery of patient care. The nursing assistants carried out tasks associated with the patients' activities of daily living as delegated by the nurse case manager.

References

American Hospital Association. (1990). *1990 report of the hospital nursing personnel survey.* Chicago: American Hospital Association.

Bair, N., Griswold, J., & Head, J. (1989). Clinical RN involvement in bedside-centered case management. *Nursing Economics, 7*(3), 150-154.

Blegen, M.A., Reiter, R., Goode, C.J., & Murphy, R. (1995). Hospital based managed care: Cost and quality. *Obstetrics & Gynecology, 86*(5), 809-814.

Cohen, E. (1990). *The effects of a nursing case management model on patient length of stay and variables related to cost of care delivery within an acute care setting.* Dissertation Abstracts International, 51-07B, 3325 (University Microfilm No. 90-33878), Ann Arbor, Mich.: University Micro Films International.

Cohen, E. (1991). Nursing case management: Does it pay? *Journal of Nursing Administration, 21*(4), 20-25.

Grimaldi, P.L., & Micheletti, J.A. (1983). *Diagnosis related groups.* Chicago: Pluribus Press.

Health Care Advisory Board. (1990). Tactic #1 potential savings of more than $1 million from change in delivery system, use of critical paths for two DRGs. Superlative clinical quality: Special review of pathbreaking ideas, clinical quality (1) (pp. 23). Washington, D.C.: Advisory Board Co.

Luke, R.D. (1979, Spring). Dimensions in hospital case mix measurement. *Inquiry, 16,* 38-49.

McKenzie, C., Torkelson, N., & Holt, M. (1989). Care and cost: Nursing case management improves both. *Nursing Management, 20*(10), 30-34.

Stillwaggon, C. (1989). The impact of nurse managed care on the cost of nurse practice and nurse satisfaction. *Journal of Nursing Administration, 19*(11), 21-27.

Case Management Evaluation

The Use of the Cost-Effectiveness Analysis Method

Hussein A. Tahan

CHAPTER OVERVIEW

The widespread restructuring of health care has created an urgent need for strategies that optimize the health condition of the people, their access to a wide variety of care services, and the quality and cost-effectiveness of these services. One strategy that has gained considerable attention and recognition is case management. There is growing consensus that case management enhances the value of health services (i.e., cost and quality), accessibility to care services, and client (patient, family, and significant other/care giver) and professional (health care providers and staff) satisfaction. Yet the research data to support this conclusion are still limited. Increasingly, administrators of case management programs of care delivery are called on to provide evidence that their decisions are, in fact, contributing to strategic quality and cost goals. This chapter explores how case management evaluation studies should be conducted so that better decisions regarding effective patient care delivery systems, health services, and health policy can be made and the utility of the case management systems can be widely supported. A review of select case management research studies (Appendix 47-1) is also presented to support the discussion and recommendations made.

Case management is defined according to the American Nurses Association as follows:

> Dynamic and systematic collaborative approach to providing and coordinating health care services to a defined population. It is a participative process to identify and facilitate options and services for meeting individuals' health needs, while decreasing fragmentation and duplication of care and enhancing quality, cost-effective clinical outcomes. The framework for nursing case management includes five components: assessment, planning, implementation, evaluation, and interaction (1999, p. 3).

However, because the practice of case management is not limited to nursing, it is essential to include the definition of case management advocated for by the Case Management Society of America, an international, multidisciplinary, not-for-profit organization with members from various disciplines, including nursing, medicine, managed care organizations, workers compensation, social work, physical therapy, and durable medical equipment company representatives. The Case Management Society of America defines case management as a collaborative process which assesses, plans, implements, coordinates, monitors, and evaluates options and services to meet an individual's health needs through communication and available resources to promote cost-effective outcomes (1995, p. 8).

In examining these definitions, one may note that they are very similar and basically contain the same elements of the case management process, specifically, assessment, planning, implementation, facilitation, coordination and collaboration, monitoring, and evaluation. These elements are important when considering a research process for evaluating the effectiveness of case management programs. The variables studied should reflect these essential elements.

The case management research literature reviewed and critiqued in Appendix 47-1 shows that case management programs are rarely appropriately evaluated and, in some instances, variables are loosely defined or used. The research design methods, data collection, and sampling methodologies seem to be an "afterthought." These research studies are for the most part retrospective attempts at validating the value of case management programs and neglect the use of cost-effectiveness analysis methods despite the fact that they claim to evaluate cost. None of these studies discuss any confounding variables that may have influenced the results obtained. Therefore these studies are of minimal significance for health policy and health services decision-making practices. In addition, they are weak studies and can be deemed minimally effective if used by health care administrators to promote the practice of case management as a patient care delivery model. Issues of cost, quality, access to care, and scope of services should be examined when evaluating case management delivery systems so that their implications for health policy decisions can be heightened. Very rarely, more than one of these variables are examined in the studies shared herein. The following section discusses the extent to which different variables are examined in the reviewed studies.

THE PROCESS, STRUCTURE, AND OUTCOME VARIABLES

One of the most complex tasks is to design a study that evaluates the interconnectedness and relationships of the process, structure, and outcome variables of any care delivery system, not just case management. However, researchers should attempt to maximize the significance of their studies by including a mix of variables that address important process, structure, and outcomes variables of their care delivery systems. The reviewed case management studies were found to be lacking in this area. A select list of the most commonly examined variables in the case management studies reviewed and summarized in Appendix 47-1 is presented in Box 47-1. Most of the case management process variables were addressed in a descriptive and conceptual way (Edelstein & Cesta, 1993; Erkel et al., 1993; Ethridge & Lamb, 1989; Goode, 1995; Polinsky, Fred, & Ganz, 1991; Rubin, 1992; Trella, 1993), and the information shared was not based on research outcomes but rather on the case management model design at the specific institution where the study was conducted. Descriptive statistics (mean, median, standard deviation, frequency, and percentage) were primarily used in the analyses of these studies; regression analysis or other inferential techniques were seldom applied.

A few qualitative studies described the nurse case manager's activities and attempted to identify the case management process(es) of care delivery (Goodwin, 1994; Newcomer, Arnsberger, & Zhang, 1997; Sohl-Kreiger, Lagaard, & Schorrer, 1996; Van Dongen & Jambunathan, 1992; Williams et al., 1993). Researchers should rely on the results of these studies when they design quantitative studies for the evaluation of case management programs. A few other studies examined the structure of case management by evaluating the uncertainty and ambiguity of the work environment, extent of staff autonomy, collaboration with other providers, and role conflict and overload (Allred et al., 1995; Arford & Allred, 1995; Tonges, 1998).

As to the outcomes of case management services, many studies identified the effect of case management on patient satisfaction, staff satisfaction, length of stay, number of clinic visits, cost of care, complications, readmissions, and other variables (refer to Appendix 47-1 and Box 47-1). Some studies evaluated the relationships between two types of variables: either process or structure with outcome variables.

| BOX 47-1 | VARIABLES EXAMINED IN THE CASE MANAGEMENT STUDIES REVIEWED |

STRUCTURE
Case management team
Nurse case manager qualities
Collaboration
Autonomy
Need for transportation
Available housing
Availability of providers/service
Participation in decision making
Work environment (uncertainty, ambiguity, predictability)
Telephone-based case management
Hospital-based care
Clinic-based care
Community-based care
Client outreach programs
Use of advanced practice nurses/clinical nurse specialists
Role conflict, identity
Role overload
Interactions with other providers

PROCESS
Case management activities/process (assessment, planning, interventions, evaluation, monitoring, etc.)
Transfer to skilled nursing facility
Access to case managers/health care provider
Access to prenatal care
Access to immunization services
Discharge process
Telephone-based case management
Patient/family teaching
Client outreach process
Care coordination process
Referral process
Client advocacy
Information sharing

OUTCOMES
Length of stay
Blood glucose control
Patient satisfaction
Staff satisfaction
Social stability
Number of clinic visits
Length of time spent with the patient
Physical and functional abilities
Level of dependence/independence

Continued

BOX 47-1	VARIABLES EXAMINED IN THE CASE MANAGEMENT STUDIES REVIEWED—CONT'D

Emotional status
Physiological outcomes (blood pressure, respiration rate, ejection fraction, oxygen saturation, etc.)
Direct cost
Indirect cost
Cost per case
Cost per patient day
Hospital charges per case
Average daily charges
Discharge destination
Nosocomial infections
Adverse events (urinary tract infection, pressure ulcer, bacteremia)
Patient/family health knowledge
Number of telephone calls
Emergency department visits
Readmissions
Infant mortality and morbidity
Resource utilization
Estimated reimbursement
Nurse case management hours per patient day
Cost of nurse case management hours per patient day
Medications
Nutritional status
Weight loss
Pain

THE SCOPE, ACCESS, COST, AND QUALITY VARIABLES

Regardless of the setting where case management is practiced (e.g., ambulatory, acute, community, long-term), the type of health care professional (discipline or specialty) responsible for the case manager's role or the type of health care organization (e.g., private, academic, research, non-for-profit, etc.) and geographical location, the goals of case management remain the same. Case management care delivery models are basically implemented to the following:

1. Expand the scope of services provided to the population
2. Increase access to health care services
3. Reduce cost of health care services
4. Improve outcomes of the care delivered
5. Improve quality of care

The scope of services is considered a structure variable, whereas cost and quality are outcome variables. Access to health care services, on the other hand, may be a process or a structure variable. As a process, it entails the way a person accesses health care services, for example, via telephone or home care visit. As a structure, it is concerned with availability of services that enhance patient accessibility to care. None of the case management studies reviewed examined the relationships of these four types of variables at the same time. The combination of variables most commonly used was scope, cost and quality, or access, cost, and quality. This may have resulted from the difficulty of conducting a study that combines the four variables. Such studies are known to be complex, costly, and time consuming and require the coordination of a professional with a specialized knowledge base.

In the studies reviewed in Appendix 47-1, cost and quality are the most commonly examined outcome variables in case management. However, this does not mean that the quality outcomes of case management delivery systems are well supported by research and well documented in the literature. The most frequently examined variables are cost per case, length of stay, readmission rate, and complication rate. These variables are defined by some researchers as quality of care indicators and by some others as cost indicators. The confusion as to whether these indicators are quality or cost variables may have contributed to the present lack in the use of cost-effectiveness analysis (CEA) method in case management evaluation studies.

Studies that incorporate the CEA method in their evaluation enhance better decision making regarding health policy and health services practices. Thus conducting such research is a priority if case management is to be endorsed as a desired care delivery system. Health policy makers cannot and will not support such endorsement unless the cost-effectiveness of these systems is validated using health services research designs, that is, examining the relationship between cost and quality of case management delivery systems and demonstrating that these systems are more cost-effective than the standard/traditional care delivery approaches. Cost and quality variables are integral to CEA research. Eliminating the confusion surrounding which variables constitute quality and which ones constitute cost is important before conducting case management evaluation studies that have implications for health policy and health services research.

COST-EFFECTIVENESS ANALYSIS IN NURSING CASE MANAGEMENT

Late, interest in applying economic methods to the evaluation of health care interventions, options, and delivery systems has increased. CEA is one economic method commonly used to evaluate outcomes and costs of interventions and treatments or delivery systems designed to improve the person's state of health (Allred et al., 1998).

CEA is defined as a method for evaluating the health outcomes and resource costs of patient care treatments and interventions (Russell et al., 1996; Stone, 1998). Its central function is to show the relative value of alternative interventions implemented for improving the health condition of an individual patient or the health status of a population. Such analysis leads to information that can assist the decision maker weigh the alternatives and select the best one(s). Cost of the alternative interventions is measured in monetary values. However, outcomes effectiveness is measured using nonmonetary terms (e.g., health-related quality of life, life years gained) (Chan & Henry, 1999). Arford and Allred (1995) developed a quality index measure and used it to evaluate the effectiveness of nursing outcomes. It is feasible to use this quality index measure when applying the CEA method for the evaluation of case management systems.

Although the influence of CEA in the development of health care policy is not well documented (Allred et al., 1998; Chan & Henry, 1999), this method allows the making of more influential health policy decisions. The CEA framework is also an effective mechanism for making decisions regarding health care resource allocation, scope of services, accessibility of the public to health care, and especially those decisions that involve the delivery of nursing care and improvement of clinical care quality outcomes. Thus CEA as a case management evaluation method is perfectly appropriate because it facilitates and promotes a better decision-making process regarding the essential strategies that improve the scope of and access to health care services while maintaining or enhancing quality outcomes and reducing cost.

The CEA method is a preferred approach to evaluating the effectiveness of case management systems of patient care delivery because it does not necessitate the conversion of outcomes/benefits into dollar values, unlike the cost-benefit analysis method, which cannot be applied unless benefits are quantified using dollar amounts (Chan & Henry, 1999; Udvarhelyi et al., 1992). Outcomes of case management systems are not limited to cost. Quantifying some of the outcomes such as patient and family satisfaction, continuity of care, and quality of life in dollar amounts is a challenge.

The CEA method has been advocated widely since the early 1990s by federal agencies, including the Agency of Health Care Policy and Research (known today as the Agency for Healthcare Research & Quality [AHRQ]), the National Institutes of Health, the Health Care Financing Administration, and the Centers for Disease Control and Prevention (Chan & Henry, 1999). The use of this method in evaluating nursing case management has been lacking. Although the financial and quality-related variables and outcomes of nursing case management systems for patient care delivery have been widely studied, this method has been applied in few cases only (Allred et al., 1995; Arford & Allred, 1995; Erkel et al., 1993). In a review of medical, nursing, and health services literature for the years 1990 through 1996, Chan and Henry (1999) identified 88 articles that applied cost analysis methods, of which four were attributed to nursing. Of these articles, 36 used the CEA method, including only two studies conducted by nurses. The lack of CEA studies in the field of nursing may be attributed to the lack of knowledge and training in financial-cost analyses in nursing, and the difficulty and complexity of such evaluations. It was not until 1997 that cost analysis research was recommended as an area of study in nursing administration education (American Association of Colleges of Nursing, 1997).

In the evaluation studies reviewed in this chapter, the CEA method was applied on three occasions only, but it could have been appropriately used in 16 studies. To bring case management systems to the forefront of health care delivery and public/health policy decisions, health services research applying the CEA method is highly needed.

Often the goal of CEA is to compare the cost-effectiveness of a new alternate intervention (Allred et al., 1995; Russell et al., 1996; Stone, 1998) or care delivery system (in this case the use of case management care delivery system) to current/traditional standards. Cost-effectiveness studies of case management are influential in health policy making, because the goals of case management are similar to those of health policy, which are to increase accessibility to care services, improve quality of care, and reduce the incurred cost. Other goals that are integral to case management are services coordination, integration, and brokerage, as well as the use of preventive services such as wellness and health promotion programs. Studies addressing these goals are of interest to the payers, providers, and consumers of health care alike but especially to health policy makers, lobbyists, and public advocates.

OVERVIEW OF THE COST-EFFECTIVENESS ANALYSIS METHOD

Conducting case management evaluation studies using the CEA method must comply with the six principles of cost analysis identified and defined by Udvarhelyi et al. (1992) and Stone (1998), and applied by Chan and Henry (1999) in their review of the literature on cost analyses in the disciplines of nursing, medicine, and health services. These principles define the minimum acceptable standard (minimum requirement) for conducting and reporting a CEA study. Udvarhelyi and his colleagues (1992) designed these principles based on a review of the theoretical literature regarding the methods of cost analysis and the economic evaluation of health care practices. The six principles recommended are the ones found to be most commonly advocated for in the literature reviewed (Udvarhelyi et al., 1992). These principles help clarify any misunderstandings of the methodology applied, prevent faulty techniques, and avoid inconclusive or incorrect procedures. These principles are summarized here.

Principle 1

Explicit statement of the analytic perspective, which usually addresses who pays specific costs (e.g., payers such as managed care organizations and the federal government) and who benefits from an intervention (e.g., patients and society).

Principle 2

A description of the anticipated benefits, of the intervention (in this case the case management care delivery system). If the benefits are unproved, one can make explicit the assumed benefits. Examples of the anticipated benefits of case management systems may include reduced readmission/rehospitalization rates, patient and family satisfaction with care, and increased patient and family knowledge of illness, health condition, and health needs.

Principle 3

A specification of the types of costs used or considered that are carefully derived from the statement of the analytical perspective. Examples of costs as they relate to the practice of case management are cost of case managers (i.e., salaries), costs of services such as utilization reviews/managed care reviews, including the cost of the method used for communication, and costs of equipment (e.g., computers, fax machines) and supplies (e.g., paperwork). Cost can also be defined as the cost per case, that is, the cost incurred while caring for a particular patient.

Principle 4

Adjusting for differential timing, which is called *discounting*. This process is important when the costs and benefits studied accrue during significantly different time periods, usually greater than 1 year. Frequently the timing of costs and the noted benefits are different. It is essential to account for this difference in the analysis, so future costs and benefits are adjusted back to their present values. As for case management, discounting is necessary if the CEA evaluation is performed in a time period greater than 1 year.

Principle 5

Conducting a sensitivity analysis to test the robustness of conclusions to variations in the underlying assumptions and estimates. The sensitivity analysis usually explores whether alternative assumptions explain the costs and benefits noted. It reinforces the validity of the conclusions made.

Principle 6

Including a summary measurement of efficiency such as a cost-effectiveness (C/E) ratio. The use of a C/E ratio is essential to facilitate the comparison of the alternative interventions. The ratio is usually expressed using incremental cost-effectiveness terms to compare and prioritize one intervention with the next least expensive or the next least effective/beneficial. In case management, for example, the interventions compared can be the use of disease-based case managers versus patient care unit-based case managers (i.e., general case managers) or a fragmented case management role versus an integrated role (i.e., combined clinical management, utilization management, and transitional planning).

   The question that CEA is designed to address must be clearly stated. Often the goal is to compare the cost-effectiveness of one intervention or model with either the current standard or with one or more other variations on the model. The question asked delineates what outcomes should be included and evaluated in the analysis; therefore the question must be stated explicitly. In case management the practice of case management may be compared with the traditional way of delivering patient care or different variations of the case management system can be compared with each other. Either way, the purpose of the CEA evaluation and the question should be clearly asked before the data are collected and the analysis is performed. Different questions demand different types of cost and benefit data collection and analyses.

The benefits evaluated in case management CEA are the outcomes of the case management system as defined by the individual institution implementing this system of patient care delivery. The appropriate outcomes depend on the purpose of the analysis. Since outcomes of case management systems may not be considered society-based, quality-adjusted life years as an outcome is considered inappropriate. Developing a specific case management quality index (CMQI) measure based on the quality index developed by Arford and Allred (1995) can result in a better determined outcome measure for case management systems. The outcomes considered in the development of the Arford and Allred's quality index are occurrence of urinary tract infection, occurrence of bacteremia, skin breakdown, patient satisfaction, and length of stay. Two of these outcomes are appropriate for case management, specifically, patient and family satisfaction and length of stay. Other case management–based outcomes can be determined by the individual institution in relation to the specific goals of the case management system. Among these outcomes are staff satisfaction, readmission/rehospitalization rates, emergency department visits, unplanned primary care provider's visits, rate of reimbursement denials, rate of denied appeals, patient/family knowledge of illness and treatment regimen, carve-out days (these are hospitalization days the payer denies payment for), patient/family perception of health and quality of life, continuity of care, and others as desired.

To estimate the cost of resources incurred by the case management system, different types of costs must be considered. Traditionally, costs have been classified as "direct" or "variable" and "indirect" or "fixed." Direct/variable costs are those incurred in providing direct care for patients. Indirect/fixed costs, however, are those of overhead (e.g., salaries, utilities, etc.). Health care organizations determine these costs differently depending on specific factors such as payer mix, patient mix, staffing patterns, or the cost accounting system they use. In acute care case management, for example, determining the cost per patient is important when performing a CEA.

Arford and Allred (1995) identified a method for CEA incorporating a quality index. The quality index is multidimensional, hence, it captures the multidimensionality of the outcomes of case management systems. The steps involved in this method are outlined here.

STEP 1
Identifying the outcomes/benefits or indicators used to measure the effectiveness of case management systems.

Examples of these outcomes are presented in Table 47-1. It is important to determine the threshold of the indicators (desired level/criterion) that cannot be reported in a percentage figure. For example, patient and family satisfaction is reported as an average score based on a rating scale of 1 to 5, with 1 being poor and 5 being outstanding. A threshold for such indicator could be patient and family satisfaction with care ratings of 4 and above. Similar indicators can then be incorporated in the CMQI score as the percentage of patients meeting or exceeding the predetermined threshold; for example, percentage of patients reporting their rating of satisfaction with care as 4 or above. Other similar indicators that require building a threshold for are staff satisfaction, patient and family knowledge of illness and treatment regimen, and patient's perception of health and quality of life.

STEP 2
Weighing the outcomes in terms of importance to quality care and to measuring the effectiveness of case management systems.

TABLE 47-1	OUTCOME INDICATORS/ATTRIBUTES FOR THE CASE MANAGEMENT QUALITY INDEX		
Indicators/Attributes		**Average Assigned Weight**	**Standardized Weight**
a. Length of stay reduction (%)		8.6	0.0956
b. Patient and family satisfaction (% meeting the threshold)		9.3	0.1033
c. Staff satisfaction (% meeting the threshold)		8.5	0.0944
d. Rate of readmissions/rehospitalizations (%)		9.4	0.1044
e. Rate of reimbursement denials (%)		9.6	0.1067
f. Rate of emergency department visits (%)		8.9	0.0989
g. Rate of unplanned primary care provider visits (%)		8.6	0.0956
h. Patient and family knowledge of illness and treatment regimen (% meeting the threshold)		9.0	0.1000
i. Patient's perception of health and quality of life (% meeting the threshold)		9.1	0.1011
j. Carve-out days (%)		9.0	0.1000
Total		90.0	1.0

NOTE: The weights shared are hypothetical and presented for clarification purposes only.

Weights can be established using an expert panel of case management providers applying appropriate research methods. The expert panel can use a 10-point rating scale to rate their perception of the importance of each indicator in the benefits/outcomes of case management systems. The weights assigned to each of the outcome indicators correspond to the indicator's mean importance rating. The mean weights are then standardized by dividing each weight by the total value of all the assigned weights. For example, based on the hypothetical examples presented in Table 47-1, the mean rating (i.e., assigned weight) for length of stay is 8.6 and the total weight is 90.0, so the standardized weight for length of stay becomes 0.0956. The standardized weight is important for calculating the quality index.

STEP 3

Measuring the outcomes using appropriate methodologies as indicated by the type of outcome indicator.

For example, questionnaires are used to measure patient and family satisfaction, and length of stay can be determined based on data extracted from the Admit-Discharge-Transfer (ADT) automated system. It is important to be clear upfront regarding the best method(s) to be followed in outcomes data collection.

STEP 4

Calculating the CMQI score.

The quality index is calculated based on the unit of analysis identified in the purpose and question of the CEA study. In CEA the unit of analysis is related to the alternative ways of accomplishing the outcome indicators. The CMQI score (Box 47-2), for example, may include the environment of delivering patient care (i.e., case management versus no case management). The formula shared here is derived based on the formula developed by Arford and Allred (1995). The outcomes incorporated in the current formula compared with the ones found in the original formula are considered more reflective of the practice of case management.

BOX 47-2

FORMULA FOR CALCULATING THE CASE MANAGEMENT QUALITY INDEX (CMQI) SCORE

$$CMQI = \frac{\sum_{i=1}^{10} W_i \cdot n_{ti}/N_t}{\sum_{i=1}^{10} W_i \cdot n_{oi}/N_o}$$

Where:
$CMQI$ = the case management quality index for each of the practice environments (case management versus no case management)

n_{ti}/N_t = the proportion of patients, in the case management practice environment, who demonstrated the accomplishment of the quality attribute/indicator

n_{oi}/N_o = the proportion of the total patients in both practice environments that demonstrated the accomplishment of the quality attributes/indicators

W_i = the standardized weight for each of the quality attributes/indicators

Σ = summation across all 10 quality attributes/indicators (the number of attributes/indicators is adjusted based on the actual number of indicators measured)

NOTE: Modified from Arford, P., & Allred, C. (1995). Value = quality + cost. *Journal of Nursing Administration, 25*(9), 64-69.

The CMQI score is calculated as described in Box 47-2. As illustrated, the numerator is derived by determining the proportion of patients in the case management practice environment that demonstrated each of the 10 quality indicator/attributes and then multiplying the proportion of accomplishing each indicator by its associated standardized weight, shown in Table 47-1, and finally totaling the 10 products (i.e., resulting values). The denominator is calculated in the same way, however, the proportion of the total patients accomplishing the quality indicator/attribute is calculated based on both practice environments (i.e., case management and no case management). Table 47-2 presents a practical example on the application of the quality index. Data presented in this example are hypothetical and shared for clarification purposes only.

STEP 5

Calculating patient care costs (direct and indirect). Patient care costs are calculated differently in different health care organizations. The more sophisticated an organization is in its cost accounting system, the more accurate the resulting cost estimate is. However, because the environment of health care reimbursement is no longer based on fee for service, the calculated cost reflects a relative estimate rather than 100% accurate dollar amounts. In any case, it is important to determine the average cost per patient for both the case management and no case management practice environments. The average cost per patient is determined by dividing the total costs per environment accrued in a specific time period (usually the time period of the CEA study) by the total number of patients cared for in that environment during the same time period. These figures are needed for calculating the associated C/E ratios.

STEP 6

Calculating the cost-effectiveness ratio. The C/E ratio (Box 47-3) is a measure of value of case management. It is constructed with the cost as the numerator and the net benefits as the denominator (Arford & Allred, 1995; Stone, 1998). Therefore the average cost per patient forms the numerator and the CMQI forms the denominator. A lower C/E ratio is desired because such a ratio indicates better outcomes and lesser costs. The greater the C/E ratio, the lower is its associated value. The higher the CMQI, the lower becomes the C/E

TABLE 47-2	EXAMPLE OF CALCULATING THE CASE MANAGEMENT QUALITY INDEX (CMQI) SCORE

Sample A consists of 100 patients who received case management services, and sample B consists of 100 patients who did not receive case management services. All patients were cared for in an acute care setting. Assuming that the patients in both samples have similar case mix index and the following data on the 10 quality indicators prospectively determined as the attributes/benefits of case management services, calculate the CMQI. Note that the average length of stay before case management was 7.0 days.

Indicator	Sample A	Sample B	All
a. Length of stay reduction	2.8 (40%)	1.4 (20%)	2.1 (30%)
b. Patient and family satisfaction	89%	78%	83.5%
c. Staff satisfaction	95%	89%	92%
d. Rate of readmissions/rehospitalizations	3%	7%	5%
e. Rate of reimbursement denials	2%	5%	3.5%
f. Rate of emergency department visits	2%	3.5%	2.75%
g. Rate of unplanned primary care provider visits	4%	6%	5%
h. Patient and family knowledge of illness and treatment regimen	88%	79%	83.5%
i. Patient's perception of health and quality of life	85%	78%	81.5%
j. Carve-out days	1%	2.5%	1.75%

Quality Index for the Case-Managed Population (Sample A) =

$$QI = \frac{(0.0956)(0.4) + (0.1033)(0.89) + (0.0944)(0.95) + (0.1044)(0.03) + (0.1067)(0.02) + (0.0989)(0.02) + (0.0956)(0.04) + (0.1)(0.88) + (0.1011)(0.85) + (0.1)(0.01)}{(0.0956)(0.3) + (0.1033)(0.835) + (0.0944)(0.92) + (0.1044)(0.05) + (0.1067)(0.035) + (0.0989)(0.0275) + (0.0956)(0.05) + (0.1)(0.835) + (0.1011)(0.815) + (0.1)(0.075)}$$

QI = 1.0363

Quality Index for the Non–Case-Managed Population (Sample B) =

$$QI = \frac{(0.0956)(0.2) + (0.1033)(0.78) + (0.0944)(0.89) + (0.1044)(0.07) + (0.1067)(0.05) + (0.0989)(0.035) + (0.0956)(0.06) + (0.1)(0.79) + (0.1011)(0.78) + (0.1)(0.025)}{(0.0956)(0.3) + (0.1033)(0.835) + (0.0944)(0.92) + (0.1044)(0.05) + (0.1067)(0.035) + (0.0989)(0.0275) + (0.0956)(0.05) + (0.1)(0.835) + (0.1011)(0.815) + (0.1)(0.075)}$$

QI = 0.9676

ratio. The C/E ratio aids in determining which practice environment is relatively better: the case management or no case management environment. Box 47-3 presents an example of how to calculate a C/E ratio.

The CMQI and the C/E ratio can be used to evaluate the outcomes of case management systems over time. The application of these methods is not limited to comparing case management and no case management environments of care. Health care organizations that have implemented case management systems several years ago as their patient care delivery models can still apply these methods. However, a different type of comparison is used. The objective of using the CMQI and the C/E ratio in such organizations is shifted to studying the environment of care in terms of comparing the financial and quality

BOX 47-3 ▶	CALCULATING THE COST-EFFECTIVENESS (C/E) RATIO

Assume that in the same example presented in Table 47-2, the average cost per patient is $15,000.00 in sample A and $18,600.00 in sample B. Calculate the C/E ratios.

C/E ratio = Average cost per patient/Quality index

C/E ratio for the case-managed population (sample A) = $15,000/1.0363 = $14,474.57

C/E ratio for the non–case-managed population (sample B) = $18,600/0.9676 = $19,222.82

outcomes of the different services (e.g., cardiac, geriatric, obstetrics, oncology, pediatrics, pulmonary, etc.) or different case managers (e.g., cardiac case manager, geriatric case manager, obstetric case manager, oncology case manager, pediatric case manager, pulmonary case manager, etc.). In this case the C/E ratio is used to evaluate whether cost and quality outcomes are maintained or improved over time and how these ratios are compared across services and/or case managers. The same methods and formulas discussed in Table 47-2 and Box 47-3 are applied. However, the population of patients used to compute the values of the numerators and denominators of these formulas are defined differently and based on the patient populations of the particular services or who are cared for by the individual case managers.

If the cost-effectiveness comparative analysis is completed in relation to the different services, the numerator is computed for each of the services separately (i.e., cardiac), and the denominator is then computed, considering all the services combined, including cardiac. However, if the comparison is made in terms of the different case managers, then the numerator is computed for each of the case managers (i.e., cardiac patient population served by the cardiac case manager), and the denominator is computed for all the populations cared for by the case managers combined, including cardiac. After these values are computed, the results of the CMQI are used to compute the C/E ratios. The C/E ratios are compared and the service or the case manager who is most cost-effective is determined.

To use this comparison over time, it is important to determine the frequency of completing such CEA and the time period for which data are collected. Because the method is time consuming, a time interval of 4 to 6 months is recommended (i.e., two or three times per year). A threshold for the C/E ratio should also be predetermined. The value of the threshold communicates the minimum acceptable cost-effectiveness standard. This value is not arbitrary; it is determined based on the baseline data and the expectations of the health care organization. Usually it is desirable to have an observed C/E ratio that is lower than the threshold. This means that the performance of the case management system or case managers are more cost-effective. It is also desired to have a downward trend in the C/E ratios observed over time. Such a trend indicates improvement in cost-effectiveness.

Cost-effectiveness analysis allows health care organizations, decision makers, and health policy advocates to convey the value of case management services delivered based on cost information for an anticipated level of quality outcomes and health care benefits. CEA, especially, the use of the C/E ratio, facilitates a process of decision-making regarding what services to advocate for based on the relationship between their attached cost and quantifiable outcomes. Standardizing the CEA procedures can improve the quality and facilitate comparability of studies (Stone, 1998). The method described herein allows for such standardization and enhances a better way of analyzing the effectiveness of case management systems; thus providing a state of better health policy decisions considering the cost and value of case management services are better understood and measured.

Change today is very different. It is continuous and happening faster than ever before; it is more complex; its implications are more serious; and it is taking place on all levels: personal, professional, organizational, and societal. Applying the CEA method in case management evaluation practices presents a great challenge for all involved. It is an example of professional and organizational change that requires patience and perseverance. The results of such change affect the health of the society/population in that the outcomes of the CEA studies assist in making more appropriate decisions regarding access, scope, cost, and quality of health care services. The discussion and argument presented in this chapter make it clear that a revolutionary change in the way case management evaluations are done is necessary. It also provides a process for applying such analyses that can be used for expanding one's knowledge, alleviating fears and uncertainties, and reinforcing a positive attitude toward the necessity of such leap in nursing practice. The use of the CEA method in evaluating case management programs is essential for moving the practice of case management into a higher level of sophistication. The practical examples shared in this chapter can be used by health care administrators, executives, educators, and researchers as a step-by-step guide for applying the CEA method in case management program evaluations.

References

Allred, C., Arford, P., Mauldin, P., & Goodwin, L. (1998). Cost-effectiveness analysis in the nursing literature, 1992-1996. *IMAGE: Journal of Nursing Scholarship, 30*(3), 235-242.

Allred, C., Arford, P., Michel, Y., Dring, R., Carter, V., & Veitch, J. (1995). A cost-effectiveness analysis of acute care case management outcomes. *Nursing Economics, 13*(3), 129-136.

American Association of Colleges of Nursing. (1997). *Joint position statement on education for nurses in administrative roles.* Washington, D.C.: ANA.

American Nurses Association. (1999). *Modular certification examination catalog.* Washington, D.C.: American Nurses Credentialing Center.

Arford, P., & Allred, C. (1995). Value = quality + cost. *Journal of Nursing Administration, 25*(9), 64-69.

Baker, C., Miller, I., Sitterding, M., & Hajewski, C. (1998). Acute stroke patients: Comparing outcomes with and without case management. *Nursing Case Management, 3*(5), 196-203.

Case Management Society of America. (1995). *Standards of practice for case management.* Little Rock, Ark.: CMSA.

Chan, W., & Henry, B. (1999). Methodologic principles of cost analyses in the nursing, medical, and health services literature, 1990-1996. *Nursing Research, 48*(2), 94-104.

Cohen, E. (1991). Nursing case management: Does it pay? *Journal of Nursing Administration, 21*(4), 20-25.

Crawley, W., & Till, A. (1995). Case management: More population-based data. *Clinical Nurse Specialist, 9*(2), 116-120.

Edelstein, E., & Cesta, T. (1993). Nursing case management: An innovative model of care for hospitalized patients with diabetes. *Nursing Care Management, 19*(6), 517-521.

Eggert, G., Zimmer, W., Hall, J., & Friedman, B. (1991). Case management: A randomized controlled study comparing a neighborhood team and a centralized individual model, *Health Services Research, 26*(4), 471-507.

Erkel, E., Morgan, E., Staples, M., Assey, V., & Michel, Y. (1993). Case management and preventive services among infants from low-income families. *Public Health Nursing, 11*(5), 352-360.

Ethridge, P., & Lamb, G. (1989). Professional nursing case management improves quality, access and costs. *Nursing Management, 20*(3), 30-35.

Fitzgerald, J., Smith, D., Martin, D., Freedman, J., & Katz, B. (1994). A case management intervention to reduce admissions. *Archives of Internal Medicine, 154,* 1721-1729.

Fleishman, J., Mor, V., & Piette, J. (1991). AIDS case management: The client's perspective. *Health Services Research, 26*(4), 448-470.

Goode, C. (1995). Impact of a CareMap and case management on patient satisfaction and staff satisfaction, collaboration, and autonomy. *Nursing Economics, 13*(6), 337-348.

Goodwin, D. (1994). Nursing case management activities: How they differ between employment settings. *Journal of Nursing Administration, 24*(2), 29-34.

Helvie, C., & Alexy, B. (1992). Using after-shelter case management to improve outcomes for families with children. *Public Health Reports, 107*(5), 585-588.

Johnson, K., & Proffitt, N. (1995). A decentralized model for case management. *Nursing Economics, 13*(3), 142-165.

Lamb, G., & Stemple, J. (1994). Nurse case management from the client's view: Growing as insider expert. *Nursing Outlook, 42*(1), 7-13.

Lynn, M., & Kelly, B. (1997). Effects of case management on the nursing context: Perceived quality of care, work satisfaction, and control over practice. *IMAGE: Journal of Nursing Scholarship, 29*(3), 237-241.

Mahn, V. (1993). Clinical case management: A service line approach. *Nursing Management, 24*(11), 48-50.

Mawn, B., & Bradley, J. (1993). Standards of care for high-risk prenatal clients: The community nurse case management approach. *Public Health Nursing, 10*(2), 78-88.

McKenzie, C., Trokelson, N., & Holt, M. (1989). Care and cost: Nursing case management improves both. *Nursing Management, 20*(10), 30-34.

Micheels, T., Wheeler, L., & Hays, B. (1995). Linking quality and cost effectiveness: Case management by an advanced practice nurse. *Clinical Nurse Specialist, 9*(2), 107-111.

Morrison, R., & Beckworth, V. (1998). Outcomes for patients with congestive heart failure in a nursing case management model. *Nursing Case Management, 3*(3), 108-114.

Newcomer, R., Arnsberger, P., & Zhang, X. (1997). Case management, client risk factors, and service use. *Health Care Financing Review, 19*(1), 105-120.

Polinsky, M., Fred, C., & Ganz, P. (1991). Quantitative and qualitative assessment of a case management program for cancer patients. *National Association of Social Work, 16*(3), 176-183.

Rogers, M., Riordan, J., & Swindle, D. (1990). Community-based nursing case management pays off. *Nursing Management, 22*(3), 30-34.

Rubin, A. (1992). Is case management effective for people with serious mental illness? A research review. *National Association of Social Workers, 17*(2), 138-150.

Russell, L., Gold, M., Siegel, J., Daniels, N., & Weinstein, M. (1996). The role of cost-effectiveness analysis in health and medicine. *Journal of the American Medical Association, 276*(14), 1172-1177.

Sands, R., & Canaan, R. (1994). Two methods of case management: Assessing their impact. *Community Mental Health Journal, 30*(5), 441-456.

Sizemore, M., Bennett, B., & Anderson, R. (1989). Public hospital-based geriatric case management. *Journal of Gerontological Social Work, 13*(3), 167-179.

Sohl-Kreiger, R., Lagaard, M., & Schorrer, J. (1996). Nursing case management: Relationships as a strategy to improve care. *Clinical Nurse Specialist, 10*(2), 107-113.

Stone, P. (1998). Methods for conducting and reporting cost-effectiveness analysis in nursing. *IMAGE: Journal of Nursing Scholarship, 30*(3), 229-234.

Thompson, M., Curry, M., & Burton, D. (1998). The effects of nursing case management on the utilization of prenatal care by Mexican-Americans in rural Oregon. *Public Health Nursing, 15*(2), 82-90.

Tonges, M. (1998). Job design for nurse case managers: Intended and unintended effects on satisfaction and well-being. *Nursing Case Management, 3*(1), 11-23.

Topp, R., Tucker, D., & Weber, C. (1998). Effect of a clinical case manager/clinical nurse specialist on patients hospitalized with congestive heart failure. *Nursing Case Management, 3*(4), 140-145.

Trella, R. (1993). A multidisciplinary approach to case management of frail hospitalized older adults. *Journal of Nursing Administration, 23*(2), 20-26.

Twyman, D., & Libbus, K. (1994). Case management of AIDS clients as a predictor of total inpatient hospital days. *Public Health Nursing, 11*(6), 406-411.

Udvarhelyi, S., Colditz, G., Rai, A., & Epstein, A. (1992). Cost-effectiveness and cost-benefit analysis in the medical literature. *American College of Physicians, 116*(3), 238-244.

Van Dongen, C., & Jambunathan, J. (1992). The psychiatric RN case manager: Pilot study results. *Journal of Psychosocial Nursing, 30*(11), 11-14.

Williams, F., Warrick, L., Christianson, J., & Netting, F. (1993). Critical factors for successful hospital-based case management. *Health Care Management Review, 18*(1), 63-70.

APPENDIX 47-1

Summary of Selected Case Management Evaluation Studies

Author, Year	Aim(s)	Indicators			Services				Design	CEA	Findings	Limitations/Comments
		P	St	O	Sc	A	C	Q				
Ehridge & Lamb, 1989	Evaluate the impact of continuum-based nursing case management model			✔	✔	✔	✔		Retrospective review Varied patient population	N	Reduced cost and length of stay	Nonspecific procedure for data collection and instruments
McKenzie, Trokelson, & Holt, 1989	Evaluate the effectiveness of case management and its impact on cost and patient and staff satisfaction		✔	✔			✔	✔	Unclear design Retrospective MR review Comparative analysis of intervention and noninterventicn groups	N	Reduced cost and length of stay Improved satisfaction	Actual satisfaction data are not shared
Sizemore, Bennett, & Anderson, 1989	Examine the evidence of success of a geriatric case management program implemented in a large public teaching hospital	✔	✔	✔	✔	✔			Retrospective descriptive program evaluation	N/A	Elderly patients had serious multiple health and social problems Successful program implementation	Good program model Results are tentative No report of readmission or the need for institutionalization after hospital discharge Convenient sample

P, Process; St, structure; O, outcome; Sc, scope; A, access; C, cost; Q, quality; ✔, yes/related-indicators applied in the study; CEA, cost-effectiveness analysis.

Continued

Author, Year	Aim(s)	Indicators			Services				Design	CEA	Findings	Limitations/ Comments
		P	St	O	Sc	A	C	Q				
Rogers, Riordan, & Swindle, 1990	Examine the effectiveness of a community-based case management model	✓		✓			✓		Pre-/post-comparison	N	Reduced length of stay, admission rate, and cost of services	Only one process discussed: patient referral to community services Unclear data collection and sampling methods
Cohen, 1991	Study the effects of a nursing case management model on the care of patients hospitalized for cesarean section delivery		✓	✓			✓	✓	Quasi-experimental	N	Significant reduction in length of stay and cost Increased direct care hours in the experimental group	Nonexplicit content of case management intervention Nonrandom sample Excellent cost accounting method described
Eggert, Zimmer, Hall, & Friedman, 1991	Compare two types of community-based case management models: individual vs team approach	✓	✓	✓	✓		✓	✓	Randomized controlled trial	N	Team approach less costly, higher hospital admission rate, much lower length of stay	No report of reliability and validity of instruments Excellent study design

Study								Purpose	Study type		Findings	Comments
Fleishman, Mor, & Piette, 1991	✓	✓	✓	✓	✓	✓		Compare a community-based and clinic-based case management model for AIDS patients	Qualitative comparative	N/A	Clinic-based patients are more likely to be disadvantaged, some patients had no contact with case managers at all	Weak design Data reported quantitatively, although authors claim to use a qualitative approach
Polinsky, Fred, & Ganz, 1991	✓		✓		✓		✓	Evaluate a social work, telephone case management model	Unclear/unidentified Qualitative	N/A	Identified the needs, problems, and concerns of newly diagnosed cancer patients	Results reported in a quantitative format even though interviews were conducted for data collection
Helvie & Alexy, 1992	✓		✓		✓		✓	Examine the benefits of offering families after-shelter case management services	Descriptive	N/A	Case management services reduce length of stay in a shelter, increase housing stability after discharge	Unclear what made the difference; no description of the intervention Unspecified sampling method

P, Process; *St,* structure; *O,* outcome; *Sc,* scope; *A,* access; *C,* cost; *Q,* quality; ✓, yes/related-indicators applied in the study; *CEA,* cost-effectiveness analysis.

Continued

Author, Year	Aim(s)	Indicators			Services				Design	CEA	Findings	Limitations/ Comments
		P	St	O	Sc	A	C	Q				
Rubin, 1992	Review of eight studies conducted between 1987 and 1991 on case management to identify common, significant case management elements	✓		✓	✓			✓	Descriptive	N/A	Controversial and conflicting outcomes from the studies regarding quality of life, functional abilities, and social functioning	Research literature review found no common elements in case management models
Van Dongen & Jambu-nathan, 1992	Examine client satisfaction with RN case management		✓		✓				Pilot study Exploratory	N/A	Description of the qualities of nurse case managers and their most frequent interventions and services	Convenient sample No report of validity or reliability of instruments No quantitative data are reported
Edelstein & Cesta, 1993	Evaluate the effect of an acute care case management model on the outcomes of care for patients with diabetes	✓	✓	✓		✓		✓	Pre- and post-comparison Retrospective chart review	N/A	Team case management approach was found to have better outcomes: length of stay, readmission rate, and blood glucose control on discharge	Convenient samples No discussion of the comparability of the samples

Study	Purpose	P	St	O	Sc	A	C	Q	Design	CEA	Findings	Comments
Erkel, Morgan, Staples, Assey, & Michel, 1993	Determine the impact of case management services on use of child health clinic and immunizations in low-income families	✓	✓	✓	✓	✓	✓	✓	Quasi-experimental Retrospective record review	Y	Continuous case management was found to be better than fragmented approach and with better cost-effectiveness ratio	Nonrandom convenient sample Excellent application of the cost-effectiveness analysis method
Mahn, 1993	Examine the effectiveness of an acute care case management model for patients with coronary artery bypass surgery	✓		✓			✓		Comparative Intervention and nonintervention groups	N	Case management approach revealed better outcomes; length of stay, cost, readmission rate, and adverse events	Nonrandom convenient samples Patients matched based on preoperative risk using risk stratification guidelines
Mawn & Bradley, 1993	Describe the process of developing a risk stratification tool for use in case management programs				✓	✓		✓	Unclear	N/A	Work in progress Tool not shared	Excellent review of the literature No validity or reliability reporting

P, Process; St, structure; O, outcome; Sc, scope; A, access; C, cost; Q, quality; ✓, yes/related-indicators applied in the study; CEA, cost-effectiveness analysis.

Continued

Author, Year	Aim(s)	Indicators			Services				Design	CEA	Findings	Limitations/ Comments
		P	St	O	Sc	A	C	Q				
Trella, 1993	Evaluate the cost and quality outcomes of a geriatric acute care case management model	✓	✓	✓			✓	✓	Unclear, intervention and nonintervention and pre- and post-groups comparison	N	Case management group had better length of stay, cost per patient day, reimbursement index, and patient and staff satisfaction	No procedure for data collection shared No discussion whether the groups are comparable
Williams, Warrick, Christianson, & Netting, 1993	Identify the basic elements of case management models	✓	✓	✓	✓	✓	✓	✓	Unidentified phenomenology	N/A	Successful and unsuccessful characteristics of case management models are identified	Provide insights for successful program development Convenient sample Unclear the cost implications of each program
Goodwin, 1994	Examine the activities of case managers functioning in home health settings compared to other case management groups: insurance, independent, and HMOs	✓	✓		✓				Descriptive exploratory	N/A	The use of case management activities was identified by case manager type and setting	Nonrandom convenient sample, small size Unclear whether same patients were followed by more than one case manager (duplication)

Study	Purpose	P	St	O	Sc	A	C	Q	Design/method	N	Findings	Quality comments
Fitzgerald, Smith, Martin, Freedman, & Katz, 1994	Examine the effects of telephone case management program for patient after acute hospitalization	✔	✔	✔	✔	✔			Randomized controlled trial		Frequent contacts by case managers for patient/family education and care accessibility were not effective in reducing non-elective readmissions	Good study design Examining cost-effectiveness of the program could have been beneficial
Lamb & Stemple, 1994	Obtain patients' perspective and data regarding working with nurse case managers	✔	✔	✔					Grounded theory	N/A	Understanding the impact of case management on patient care Design of a model of how patients perceive case management	Solid design and data analysis method Results provide a perfect structure for future research in case management effectiveness
Sands & Canaan, 1994	Compare case management community treatment teams and intensive case management teams	✔	✔	✔					Comparative groups retrospective review	N/A	Similar outcomes in the two groups except for length of hospitalization, which was longer for community team	Random selection of subjects

P, Process; St, structure; O, outcome; Sc, scope; A, access; C, cost; Q, quality; ✔, yes/related-indicators applied in the study; CEA, cost-effectiveness analysis.

Continued

Author, Year	Aim(s)	Indicators			Services				Design	CEA	Findings	Limitations/ Comments
		P	St	O	Sc	A	C	Q				
Twyman & Libbus, 1994	Examine whether deceased AIDS patients who received case management services had shorter hospitalizations						✓	✓	Retrospective chart review Intervention and non-intervention Comparative groups	N	No significant differences were noted Only length of stay was examined	Random selection of the case management group only Convenient control group Quality and cost were not evaluated
Allred et al., 1995	Cost-effectiveness analysis of acute case nursing care management system	✓	✓	✓			✓	✓	Descriptive Exploratory	Y	Moderate environmental uncertainty is best factor for cost-effectiveness	Stratified random sampling technique Excellent application of the CEA method
Arford & Allred, 1995	Development of the quality index measure	✓	✓	✓			✓	✓	Descriptive Exploratory	Y	Case management is most cost-effective in an environment of moderate uncertainty	Random sampling Combines nurses and case managers in same group
Crawley & Till, 1995	Evaluate the cost and quality outcomes of case management	✓	✓	✓			✓	✓	Unidentified	N	Case management approach improved outcomes of care	Unclear sampling methodology No cost-effectiveness analysis

Author, year	Objective						Design/Methodology	N/A	Results	Comments
Goode, 1995	Examine the impact of a CareMap and case management systems on patient and staff satisfaction, collaboration, and autonomy	✓	✓	✓		✓	Patients: cohort pre- and post-intervention Staff: pre- and post-test		Results supportive of case management services in both groups; patients and staff—no difference in collaboration scores	No discussion of patient care outcomes (clinical) Confusing sampling methodology
Johnson & Proffitt, 1995	Examine the impact of an acute care case management model on cost and satisfaction (patient and staff)	✓	✓	✓	✓		Unidentified (?) Comparative	N	Reduction in length of stay and cost after case management No data on satisfaction	Unclear sampling method
Michaels, Wheeler, & Hays, 1995	Examine the relationships between advanced practice nurse case management, patient acuity, and length of stay	✓	✓	✓			Retrospective chart review Comparative groups	N	No significant differences between the two groups Those case managed by advanced practice nurse were of higher acuity and shorter length of stay	Small size, convenient samples

P, Process; *St,* structure; *O,* outcome; *Sc,* scope; *A,* access; *C,* cost; *Q,* quality; ✓, yes/related-indicators applied in the study; *CEA,* cost-effectiveness analysis.

Continued

Author, Year	Aim(s)	Indicators			Services				Design	CEA	Findings	Limitations/ Comments
		P	St	O	Sc	A	C	Q				
Sohl-Kreiger, Lagaard, & Schorrer, 1996	Examine the case management activities of clinical nurse specialists functioning as case managers	✓	✓						Unidentified	N/A	Description of the process of case management and its related activities	Unclear method and sample size. Cost data provided, but unclear implications. Very weak study
Newcomer, Arnsberger, & Zhang, 1997	To develop a typology of nurse case manager activities	✓	✓						Retrospective/ qualitative chart review	N/A	Typology of six major case management activity categories was developed	Probability sampling technique, large size. Excellent study design
Baker, Miller, Sitterding, & Hajewski, 1998	Examine the effectiveness of unit-based nursing case management model vs. standard nursing case	✓	✓	✓				✓	Retrospective chart review. Intervention and nonintervention comparison groups	N/A	Case-managed patient groups showed significantly better care outcomes and quality	Random sampling. Small groups. Pilot study. Unclear whether groups are comparable
Morrison & Beckworth, 1998	Describe the outcomes of care of patients with heart failure in a hospital-based nursing case management model	✓	✓				✓	✓	Descriptive Retrospective chart review	N	Descriptive results of several cost and quality variables are reported	Weak design. No report of nursing-sensitive outcomes, although one of the study goals was to do so

	Purpose	P	St	O	Sc	A	C	Q	Methodology	CEA	Findings	Limitations
Thompson, Curry, & Burton, 1998	Evaluate the effectiveness of prenatal nursing case management services for rural, low-income, Mexican-American families	✔	✔	✔	✔			✔	Quasi-experimental Retrospective chart review	N/A	Intervention group had more prenatal visits No statistical differences in initiation and number of visits	Secondary data analysis-type study Small sample size
Tonges, 1998	Test an extended model of nurse case manager's job characteristics Compare nurse case managers, care coordinators, and staff nurses	✔						✔	Cross-sectional correlation	N/A	Nurse case manager's job appeared to combine higher levels of positive (autonomy, identity, collaboration) and negative (role conflict, ambiguity, overload) characteristics	Random sample from eight large national hospitals
Topp, Tucker, & Weber, 1998	Evaluate the effect of case management on hospital length of stay and cost for patients with heart failure	✔	✔	✔	✔				Retrospective chart review Comparison groups	N	Case-managed patients had lower length of stay and lower hospital charges	Convenient sample No discussion of groups comparability

P, Process; *St*, structure; *O*, outcome; *Sc*, scope; *A*, access; *C*, cost; *Q*, quality; ✔, yes/related-indicators applied in the study; *CEA*, cost-effectiveness analysis.

Linking the Restructuring of Nursing Care With Outcomes

Conceptualizing the Effects of Nursing Case Management Using Measurement and Logic Models

Arthur E. Blank

CHAPTER OVERVIEW

Government, employers, and insurers are trying to restructure the delivery of health care. This restructuring of care has created opportunities for innovation as well as questions about the consequences of altering the delivery of health care. Nursing case management is one such innovation and as such needs to be studied. The Medical Outcomes Study (MOS) approach offers one conceptual framework for assessing the impact of nursing case management, but the MOS may not be specific enough to document adequately the consequences of nursing case management. To make the MOS approach more germane, nursing case managers need to accomplish three tasks: (1) identify how case managers change the structure and process of care, (2) identify what clinical, administrative, physiological, and patient outcomes are influenced by these changes, and (3) develop reliable and valid measures. Logic models are introduced as a mechanism for addressing these tasks and for helping to articulate the links between structure, process and outcomes. The development of these models should enable hospitals, nurses, and policy makers to assess whether nursing case management has "worked."

The delivery of health care remains in flux. National, state, and local governments continue to redefine the financing and delivery of health services. Employers continue to restructure employee benefits and premiums. And under pressure from patients and clinicians, employers, insurance companies, and government, health care providers are working to become more cost-effective without sacrificing quality.

Efforts to redefine how health care is provided and paid for have also engendered counter pressures. Employers, government, health care providers, and patients or consumers have started to question whether health care choices are being arbitrarily restricted, whether the quality of care is being sacrificed, and, in everyone's worst nightmare, whether lives are being unnecessarily jeopardized. These apprehensions remind us that change is taking place within another, more abstract context, one of uncertainty.

We are not trading one well-defined system of care for another; we are trading for a system of care whose basic parameters remain undefined and will, in all likelihood, remain fragmented.

As providers or consumers of care, we are in the midst of a societal, institutional, and personal struggle to balance opportunity and fear, or, more modestly, concern: opportunity, because the structural pressures to reconfigure the delivery of care supports leaders who are willing to innovate; concern, because the consequences of these changes, whether they be at a societal, institutional, or personal level, will not be known for some time.

How can we as health care professionals, as researchers, as policy makers, and as citizens assess the consequences, or outcomes, of these various and varied attempts to reconfigure the delivery of health care? One way is to undertake outcome studies. These studies describe how the structure and process of medical care have been refashioned and identify a set of measures—outcomes—that can be used to determine the consequences of those changes. When done well, these studies tell us how well opportunity and concern have been balanced, and the results become part of a broader social metric. But these studies can be part of the metric only if we identify and measure how components of the structure and process of care are conceptually linked with outcomes of care—health as well as financial—and at a societal as well as an institutional or personal level.

What has all of this to do with nursing case management? It suggests that the Medical Outcomes Study (MOS) approach be used as a *conceptual framework* for studying the consequences of nursing case management. After all, nursing case management is fundamentally an alteration in the structure and process of care.* As such it is an intervention, an opportunity to reshape the delivery of patient care—whether that care be in hospitals or primary care settings (Cohen & Cesta, 2001).† But more fundamentally, nursing case management is also an intervention whose benefits and harms are unknown (Lamb, 1995). The task then is not only to define and identify the organizational changes in the structure and process of care that nursing case management has brought about but also to articulate how structural and process changes are linked to what is of utmost concern—the effect of this restructuring of care with its consequences, with its outcomes (Aliotta, 2001).

Traditionally, clarifying the conceptual relationships between shifts in the organization of care and the outcome(s) of care is a critical step in designing a research study. However, there is a complementary step not often well attended to in health care: ensuring that our design appropriately measures the relationships and constructs we are interested in. At a technical level the challenge is about the *validity* of our measures: are they conceptually nuanced and robust enough to reflect the relevant dimensions of change introduced by nursing case management?‡ Unfortunately, designing valid measures is no less daunting a task than is designing a rigorous study (e.g., Issel, 1997; Mateo, 1998, 2001).

This chapter has five objectives: (1) to briefly review how valid measures are constructed, (2) to review how the MOS both conceptualized the structure, process, and outcomes of care and developed valid health status measures, (3) to raise questions about whether the definitions and measures used in the MOS research can be directly applied to the study of nursing case management, (4) to offer a mechanism, logic models, to help formally articulate the link among structure, process, and outcomes, and (5) to suggest some directions and issues for nursing case management research.

---

*Because *nursing case management* is not a term that means the same thing in every institution where it is practiced, these local variations are important to identify and document if we are to understand how the structure, process, and outcomes of care are linked.

†This chapter presumes nursing case management is being used in a hospital setting.

‡The concern in this chapter is with developing measures for, not the design of, outcome studies. Clearly both the study design and the measures will determine the scientific credibility of the results.

A PARTIAL* MEASUREMENT REFRESHER: DEVELOPING VALID MEASURES

For many years, the consequences of health care were assessed by measures of morbidity and mortality. Identifying the time of death, diagnosing whether the individual has an infection, or interpreting a particular laboratory result, for example, was—and is—relatively straightforward. When our measures were this concrete, little attention needed to be devoted to thinking about whether we were capturing what we intended to measure. But as health professionals' interest in the consequences of care became nuanced and abstract, such as quality-of-life and patient satisfaction, more attention had to be devoted to guaranteeing that we were successfully measuring the constructs we wanted to measure (Stewart, Hays, & Ware, 1992; Streiner & Norman, 1989), ensuring that we knew how to interpret the results (Kane, 1992; Messick, 1995; Streiner & Norman, 1989), and, more recently, knowing that the measures we use are sensitive enough to capture change (e.g., Patrick & Chiang, 2000). For example, measuring blood pressure is straightforward, as for the most part is the interpretation of the result. When we measure depression or patient or job satisfaction, we may be both less certain that we have accurately assessed the construct, less certain about how to interpret the resulting score, and unsure as to whether the measure is sensitive enough to capture change over time. Determining the nature of the construct is not easy, and experts may disagree. For example, some measures of inpatient satisfaction focus on hotel services such as the food, cleanliness of the room, and efficiency of the admitting or discharge process. Yet other measures focus on the nurses' responsiveness to pain, the clarity of information provided by physicians or nurses, and the compassion of the staff. Is one measure a more valid measure of satisfaction than the other? How do we measure and feel intellectually confident that we are correctly measuring and interpreting these more abstract consequences of health interventions?

As we approach our consideration of validity, it is essential to remember that there is a critical, inter-related step: to define, or more pointedly limit, what we are referring to when we talk about "outcomes." The concept of outcomes is broad and nonspecific and takes on a precise meaning only in the context of a particular intervention. In that context, outcomes must be defined in a way that is responsive to the intervention. This simple setting of boundaries, these definitional decisions, must not be made lightly. In the psychometric or scale development literature, defining the boundaries of the concept is usually treated as the purview of the expert. The expert's knowledge is based on his or her experience in the field as well as on knowledge of the literature. This expertise will help determine which conceptual domains should be included or excluded. For example, are measures of pain, patient satisfaction, functional status, well-being, cost of care, hospital readmission, and length of stay conceptually relevant when we want to document the effects of nursing case management?

If a peer-reviewed literature exists, experts are clearly beneficial. But they may be less helpful if the topic is new or if the literature is out of date. In this context, convening a panel of experts and "users" to discuss the concept's boundaries may help. This need to harness the experience of a diverse group of individuals can be important even in well-established areas of study. For example, the outcome measures discussed in the MOS have been criticized by some as capturing outcomes more sensitive to the work of physicians than of nurses (Kelly et al., 1994), which raises a caution and a simple reminder: definitions set limits. They decide what to include and exclude. These decisions should be explicit and public, not tacit and hidden.

Once we know the domains we want to assess, the issue of whether our scales and surveys measure what we intend them to measure falls under the rubric of validity (Crocker & Algina, 1986; Nunnally,

---

*This discussion is partial because it deals only with validity. There is no discussion of reliability, about how to write scale items, or about how to statistically assess the information collected.

1978; Portney & Watkins, 1993; Streiner & Norman, 1989; Thorndike, 1982). For abstract constructs, developing valid instruments is time consuming and difficult. In the field of psychometrics validity is usually discussed in terms of four different types: (1) face, (2) criterion, (3) content, and (4) construct validity.*

In developing measures of constructs, face validity is perhaps the easiest to use and develop. Face validity, however, is a weak form of validity. With face validity, items on a survey or questionnaire *appear* to address the question we are interested in. There is, however, no empirical test of this assumption. Content validity tries to ensure that the various *items* that comprise the measure, or which tap the conceptual domain, adequately *sample* the content of the concept or domain being measured. Some of the questions raised earlier about patient satisfaction surface here.

Should patient satisfaction include hotel services as well as the thoroughness and clarity of the information provided? Similar questions can be raised, and are, about quality of life measures and, more narrowly, health-related quality of life (HRQOL) measures—recognizing that HRQOL measures are multidimensional, what dimensions should be included, what items are considered as part of the construct, and how responsive are the measures to capturing change (e.g., Guyatt, 2000, and Testa, 2000). Part of the answer would be to review existing instruments, but it would also be useful to convene a panel of experts[†] to ensure that important items or concerns are not excluded inadvertently. But however the items are put together, content validity, like face validity, is still primarily subjective. The advantages of content validity are that it ensures that the item pool has been thoroughly documented and that the items reflect the concept being assessed *before* the measure is administered.

More rigorous—that is, more empirically based—tests of validity are possible with both criterion and construct validity. Criterion-related validity indicates that the test developed can be used in place of an already established test—a "gold standard." We may be interested, for example, in constructing a shorter version of a longer, more time-consuming scale. To determine whether the shorter test is valid, the long and the short tests are administered to the same set of subjects. If the two sets of scores are highly correlated, the shorter test is valid. Although this is an objective way to proceed, for many abstract constructs such as satisfaction or HRQOL a gold standard is not available. In these cases another approach, construct validation, is called for. Part of construct validity relies on content validity: that is, we have to have an item pool that adequately assesses the complexity of the concept. But the thrust of construct validity is to confirm that the measure accurately captures the construct by empirically ascertaining whether the new measure correlates with hypothetically related constructs.

Construct validity can be approached from a number of directions, but one common approach is that of convergent and discriminant validity (Cronbach & Meehl, 1955). Simply put, like measures should correlate highly with other measures of the same or similar theoretical constructs—convergent validity—but should not correlate, or show low correlations, with measures of dissimilar constructs— discriminant validity. If researchers are constructing a new measure to assess the impact of an illness on a person's life, the new measure should correlate highly with comparable illness burden measures but only minimally with measures of quite different constructs. The pattern of correlations documents whether the new measure is succeeding. In the absence of a gold standard, however, it is hard to

---

*Health care researchers have turned to the social sciences and in particular to psychometricians to help develop indices and measures of abstract constructs. A number of critiques of the psychometric approach exist, but are beyond the purview of this chapter. For the interested reader, one challenge to psychometrics has been raised by Feinstein's (1987) idea of clinimetrics, and another by Berwick (2000).

†Experts need to be thought of broadly. For example, the Picker Commonwealth Survey of Patient Satisfaction used patient focus groups to identify the dimensions of care that were important to them (Gerteis, Edgman-Levitan, Daley, & Delbanco, 1993).

absolutely know how well we have done. Consequently, for some researchers construct validity is an ongoing process, needing always to refine and test the measures (Messick, 1995; Stewart et al., 1992; Streiner & Norman, 1989). Within this framework, construct validity cannot be decided with the results of a single study.

THE MOS APPROACH: AN EXAMPLE OF LINKING THE STRUCTURE, PROCESS, AND OUTCOMES OF CARE

If we are to use the MOS approach as a guide for conceptualizing how to gauge the consequences of nursing case management, it is beneficial to review that study with two aims in mind: (1) to see how the components of structure, process, and outcomes were defined and (2) to see how a new generic measure of a patient's health status was validated.

The MOS was a "2 year observational study designed to help understand how specific components of the health care system affect the outcomes of care" (Tarlov et al., 1989). The study was conducted at multiple sites across the United States and sampled 502 physicians in group and solo practice, in health maintenance organizations (HMO), and in fee-for-service (FFS) systems of care. Information was collected from physicians using self-administered forms and telephone interviews. Patient data were collected using surveys, clinical examinations, and telephone interviews.

The MOS study was unique, in part, because of its explicit emphasis on developing measures that could capture the consequences of medical care from the patients' perspective (Stewart & Ware, 1992; Tarlov et al., 1989). In arguing for the need to supplement traditional clinical outcomes such as mortality, laboratory values, and symptoms and signs, the MOS study faced issues comparable to those case management research now faces: MOS researchers had to define outcomes, in this case from the patients' perspective, which should be conceptually responsive to changes in the structure and process of care. Of course, MOS researchers also had to clarify how the components of structure and process would be measured.

For the concept *structure of care*, three broad domains were identified: (1) system characteristics, (2) provider characteristics, and (3) patient characteristics (Tarlov et al., 1989). System characteristics identified five components, including financial incentives, access or convenience, and specialty mix. Provider characteristics included seven components: age, gender, specialty training, economic incentives, job satisfaction, preferences, and beliefs and attitudes; and the eight patient characteristics included age, gender, diagnosis, severity, comorbidity, health habits, beliefs and attitudes, and preferences. The *process of care* had two broad categories: technical and interpersonal style. Technical style included among its eight items medications, referrals, test ordering, expenditures, continuity, and coordination of care; and interpersonal style's four items were communication level, counseling, patient participation, and interpersonal manner. The *outcomes of care* had four components: clinical end points, functional status, general well-being, and satisfaction with care. As with the structure and process of care, each of these components was specified in more detail. For example, a patient's functional status was described by measuring a patient's physical, mental, social, and role functioning.

To develop and test the generic patient-centered health outcome measures being sought by the MOS, researchers built on scales that had been developed as part of RAND's Health Insurance Experiment (HIE) or by other researchers (Stewart & Ware, 1992). Over time the MOS staff examined the existing literature on measures of physical functioning, psychological distress or well-being, health perceptions, social and role functioning, pain, and physical and psychophysiological symptoms (Stewart & Ware, 1992). By incorporating new items and including a multitude of already developed measures into their study design, MOS researchers could test the validity of their measures.* Face validity was not discussed, and content validity was checked by assessing the literature to determine whether the relevant concepts were captured in the set of measures being used. Criterion validity was used, when available, to see how new measures compared to established old measures. For example, would a new shorter measure of depression correlate with a gold standard measure of depression (e.g., the Diagnostic Interview Schedule in the third edition of the *Diagnostic and Statistical Manual of Mental Disorders* [DSM-III] published by the American Psychiatric Association) or would a shorter measure of physical functioning correlate highly with a longer measure of physical functioning (Hays & Stewart, 1992; Stewart et al., 1992)?

Both convergent and discriminant validity were used to examine the construct validity of the measure. In principle, if we are developing new measures of well-being or pain, these measures should correlate highly with scales that measure similar constructs. But we would not expect these measures to correlate with those unrelated to either well-being or pain. More specifically, as the MOS authors indicate, "measures of physical functioning, mobility, and satisfaction with physical abilities were expected to correlate at least moderately with one another because they all assess physical functioning [and] physical functioning would not be expected to be highly related to a measure of depression or of loneliness" (Stewart et al., 1992, p. 315).

Under construct validity, Stewart et al. (1992) also discuss known-groups validity. Identified by Kerlinger (1973), known-groups validity involves comparing groups of individuals who should differ on the concept being measured. So, for example, on a measure of pain, mean scores should be higher for those patients known to be in pain than for those who are not.

This approach to developing an outcomes scale resulted in the MOS Short Form (SF-36). The MOS SF-36 is a generic 36-item measure of the patients' perception of their health status. This measure can be used across populations and across illness to measure the consequences of changes in the structure and process of care. The scale, demonstrated to be reliable and valid, captures eight health care concepts: (1) limitations in physical activities because of health problems, (2) limitations in social activities because of physical or emotional problems, (3) limitations in usual role activities because of physical health problems, (4) bodily pain, (5) general mental health (psychological distress and well-being), (6) limitations in usual role activities because of emotional problems, (7) vitality (energy and fatigue), and (8) general health problems (McHorney, Ware, & Raczek, 1993; McHorney, Ware, Rachael Lu, & Sherbourne, 1994; Ware & Sherbourne, 1992).

NURSING-BASED CHALLENGES TO THE MOS

Borrowing from Donobedian, the MOS's tripartite *conceptualization* of the delivery of health care has become an important framework for assessing the restructuring of health care. But while the framework is a useful guide to thinking about outcomes, we should not uncritically accept the specific details of the MOS approach without reassuring ourselves that the definitions of the structure, process, and outcomes of care are germane to studying the effects of nursing case management. Does the MOS approach define and capture what is unique to nursing case management?

Nursing-Based Criticisms of the MOS Outcomes

With the successful development and validation of the SF-36, changes in the structure and process of care can now, in principle, be captured from the patients' perspective. For those interested in the patients'

---

*The MOS covers more than the four types of validity identified in this chapter. Furthermore, it breaks down content, criterion, and construct validity in more detail than is offered here (Stewart & Ware, 1992). Even though there are important refinements that can be made, the general points and theme do not change.

perspective, the SF-36 is a valuable addition to a researcher's measurement tools. The question remains, however, as to whether the SF-36 is sufficiently sensitive to reflect the *specific* structural and process changes introduced by nursing case management. If we assume that nursing case management has some similarities to nursing care in general, the articles by Brooten and Naylor (1995), by Kelly et al. (1994), and by Naylor, Munro, and Brooten (1991) suggest the answer is no.

Two different concerns are raised in these articles: First, the SF-36 is dominated by outcome measures sensitive to physician practices. Consequently, there is a need to construct measures that can capture "nurse sensitive patient outcomes" (Brooten & Naylor, 1995). And second, because the research was begun before all the current changes in the health care environment took place, the MOS—as an approach to effectiveness research—neglects a number of important domains, especially the effects of provider mix, that is, that many different professionals care for the patient (Kelly et al., 1994). This latter point is critical. For we not only must identify what these nurse-sensitive measures are but also must assure ourselves that these measures reflect only what nurses offer and not what other providers of care offer. This chore becomes harder to accomplish, and perhaps is not even achievable, as patient care becomes more interdisciplinary.

Some Suggested Nursing Case Management–Sensitive Outcomes

In their discussion of how to measure the consequences of nursing care, Brooten and Naylor (1995) identify a number of potential indexes: functional and mental status (these two domains are captured on the SF-36), stress level, satisfaction with care, caregiver burden, and the cost of care. Brooten and Naylor expand their suggested list of nurse-sensitive outcomes by incorporating a number of outcome categories identified in Lang and Marek's review of outcomes: physiologic status, psychological status, behavior, knowledge, symptom control, quality of life, home functions, family strain, goal attainment, utilization of service, safety, resolution of nursing problems, patient satisfaction, and caring (cited in Brooten & Naylor, 1995). Tahan's (2001) review of case management studies suggests other possible consequences of nursing case management including, physical and functional abilities, emotional status, adverse events such as urinary tract infections, pressure ulcers, and bacteremia, as well as direct and indirect costs.

These suggested outcome measures continue in the tradition of developing clinical and patient-focused outcomes, but there are other outcomes introduced by nurses or nursing case management that also must be documented. Perhaps most basically, reconfigurations in health care have meant a redefinition of nursing responsibilities. What does this imply for nurses? Will they spend more or less time with patients? Will they be more or less integrated in the delivery of care? Will they feel less autonomous or more autonomous in their roles, more or less fragmented with their varied responsibilities? Will nurses leave their jobs more often? Will sick leave increase or decrease? These too are outcomes of changes in nursing case management and should not be slighted when we identify the range of outcomes to be studied.*

Of course, comparable questions could be asked of physicians, especially as their relationships with nurses change. It must be stressed that identifying outcome categories does not end the process; it starts it. The task is to move from the outcome categories to valid outcome measures.

Nursing Case Management and the Structure and Process of Care

Clearly, outcomes studies are critical, as they correct many past oversights. But particular outcomes should not be identified, or agreed to, without first specifying how they are conceptually linked to the structure and process of care. Functional status, mental status, and relief from pain are important

---

*The MOS approach characterizes provider satisfaction as a structural component, but in a dynamic environment it could also be considered as an outcome.

outcome measures because we expect them, under certain conditions, to be responsive to medical treatment, to the process of medical care. Similar efforts are needed for nursing case management: We must construct outcomes that are responsive to the specific changes introduced by nursing case management. So just as the MOS description of outcomes may not be fully germane for studying the effects of nursing case management, its description of the structure and process of care may also be deficient for studying case management. But Lamb (1995) has reminded us that there is a good deal of ambiguity regarding what nursing case managers do. Without knowing the specifics of what case managers do, it is unclear whether the nursing-sensitive outcomes listed above are sensitive to alterations in the structure and process of care introduced by nursing case management. And it is unclear whether these outcomes are, in the words of Brooten and Naylor (1995), "sensitive to nursing alone." How does nursing case management change the structure and process of care?

We can, in a sense, work backward to answer this question. The outcomes suggested by Brooten and Naylor, and Tahan, and others imply certain changes, or perhaps clarification, in some MOS definitions of the structure and process of care. For example, consider the process of care. If an outcome of case management is enhanced patient knowledge regarding his or her illness, we have presumed that nurses are educating their patients. Is this different from what is specified in the MOS component of interpersonal style, which "includes many aspects of the way clinicians relate to patients[?]. It encompasses friendliness, courtesy, respect, and sensitivity; the extent to which patients participate in making decisions and share responsibility for their treatment; whether the clinicians counsel patients about their health habits, the need to comply with treatment recommendations, and personal and emotional problems, and the overall level of communication" (Tarlov et al., 1989). Is nursing education distinctive enough to be considered a unique component of the process of care? Do nurses engage in this process differently from other clinicians? Furthermore, do nursing case management programs change how the process of care is organized, a topic that would fall under the MOS idea of technical style? Related questions could be asked about relief from stress, reductions in caregiver burden, or the cost of care? What is it about the process of care that would reduce a patient's stress level, alter a caregiver's burden, or reduce the costs of care?

These questions can also be used to inquire about needed modifications in how the MOS study defined the structure of care. The MOS study, under system characteristics, talks about specialty mix. But Brooten and Naylor's (1995) argument that nurses are working in environments where the skill mix of nursing staff has changed suggests that the idea of specialty mix must be expanded. In addition, the interdisciplinary nature of case management suggests that how care is organized may need to be amplified. Questions about team structure and about how well teams function may need to be incorporated into the MOS's definition of the structure and outcomes of case management.

LINKING PROCESSES OF CARE WITH THE OUTCOMES OF CARE: LOGIC MODELS

Working backwards, and trying to infer possible measures of structure, process, and outcomes from work written for other purposes is not, however, the best way to proceed. Measurement should be planned in advance, and the rationale for the measures chosen articulated. The rationale for the measure used should not only be that it is a reliable and valid outcome measure. We must also have a rationale that articulates why that particular outcome measure should be responsive to alterations made in the processes of care. One tool for helping to articulate these linkages comes from evaluation research, and has been termed logic or program models (Chen, 1990, Weiss 1997, Rogers, Hacsi, Petrosino, & Huebner, 2000).

Logic models serve many functions, but in the context of this paper it is intended to help a clinical team, with input from others, articulate the link between the structure, process, and outcomes of care.

The process of constructing the logic model can in itself be clarifying for the team-making tacit presumptions explicit for example- and serve as a template for use in other process changes. Developing a logic model is an iterative process, depends on team input and review, and requires open and honest discussion among team members. The process then involves a planning stage, an implementation stage, and a measurement and analysis phase.

The logic model is developed during the planning stage. As part of this process, the team, led by a facilitator, identifies its vision or ultimate goal. This is a general and abstract aim. After this lofty goal is articulated, you can identify those patients who will be the focus of the pending process change. (The target of the intervention can be broader than patients, but to keep the example simple, only patients are being considered.) Patients can be considered broadly or narrowly. For example, we can target elderly patients, or we can target elderly patients with congestive heart failure and cognitive impairment. Once the target group is identified, think about the vision you identified—e.g., improve the quality of patient care, and start to formulate what you think are the critical outcomes of these process changes. This list of outcomes usually, but not always, has a temporal or sequential dimension-some outcomes may occur soon after the process change whereas others may take time to develop. Consequently, outcomes can, and should, be separated into short-, intermediate-, and long-term categories. Clarifying the vision, outcomes, and target population can help the team realize that some of its desired outcomes cannot be realized in the time frame, or time constraints, they are working with.

Once the vision, outcomes, and the target of the intervention are identified the next step begins—and it can be a time consuming one: to reach consensus regarding the process changes and the activities that have to be engaged in and to articulate the reasons these changes can be expected to lead to the desired outcomes. To make the point again, and more directly, the list of changes and activities, must then be linked twice: first they have to be directly relevant to the identified patient group, and second they have to be conceptually linked to the outcomes identified by the team. The question that should always be asked is: Why are the planned changes expected to lead to the stated outcomes? Just as the prior steps may help clarify the goals, this step can help the clinical team clarify exactly what the team is doing, and why it expects these activities, and not others, to lead to the desired outcomes. This process may also result in recognizing that the activities and outcomes are not aligned, or that the planned activities do not address the desired outcomes. Should that occur the team has additional decisions to make—to redefine their proposed changes, to redefine their outcomes, or to decide that some desired outcomes will not be achieved through the proposed program changes. Logic models are sometimes presented in tabular form or as visual models.

Figure 48-1 presents a generic picture of an outline for a logic model. The Web page of the Centers for Disease Control and Prevention (www.cdc.gov) has examples of logic models should the reader want to see some concrete examples.

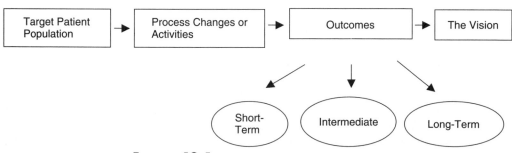

FIGURE **48-1**   Outline of a generic logic model.

Once the logic model is articulated, the measurement model can be put in place. While most of this chapter has discussed outcome measurement, the logic model makes it clear that having process measures is also important. If your intervention, for example, is dependent on a retraining of staff, you would want to know how many staff have been trained and whether there has been staff turnover. This will both help document that the processes you planned on were implemented and allow you to more directly show the link between the processes and outcomes of care. It can also be used to understand why you did not see anticipated outcomes; for example, all of the staff you trained resigned. Logic models can then also identify critical processes to measures—as well as identifying process or outcomes for which there are no measures. Logic models can also be used, as part of a QI effort, to monitor the implementation of the process changes. The logic model presented in Figure 48-1 is a simple, linear model—step A leads to step B. This is only a constraint of the example. Logic models can be nonlinear, and more complex-feedback loops can be considered and multiple target audiences identified, such as families, clinicians, insurers, policy makers.

PUTTING IT ALL TOGETHER: SOME FUNDAMENTAL QUESTIONS

Brooten and Naylor's (1995), Kelly et al.'s (1994), and Naylor et al.'s (1991) critiques are forceful, not because they question the conceptual framework of the MOS approach or the validity of the SF-36 but because they pose fundamental questions about definitional and conceptual boundaries regarding the structure, process, and outcomes of care as it relates to, in our case, nursing case management. These critiques suggest the need not only to augment the MOS categories but also to construct measures that capture the unique aspects of nursing case management, the unique role of nurses, and the unique nurse-sensitive outcomes that are conceptually distinct from those identified in the MOS approach.

In essence, just as the generic SF-36 should be used in conjunction with specific illness measures so that researchers can capture nuances not measured by the SF-36, the MOS conceptualization of structure, process, and outcomes must be modified according to the specific intervention being studied. To use the MOS approach to its full advantage, we need to formally conceptualize the linkages among the structure, process, and outcomes of care that are specific to nursing case management.

The need to articulate how nursing case management reshapes the delivery of patient care and the need to document the impact of those changes is underscored in Lamb's (1995) recent review of the case management literature, and by Aliotta's assertion that "The challenge for case managers lies in quantifying exactly how its key functions impact the end outcomes." As suggested here, via the use of logic models, quantifying these functions requires making the linkages among the structure, process, and outcomes of care explicit. Not articulating these linkages will leave us unclear as to the conditions that lead to successful, or unsuccessful, case management outcomes.

Lamb (1995) raised a series of questions for the research community about nursing case management:

> The task of researchers is complicated by the popularity and visibility of case management. As the number of professions and individuals with a stake in the future of case management expands, it is increasingly difficult to cut through the debate and rhetoric to get to some basic questions, such as: What is case management? Who needs it? Who provides it? For how long? What are its outcomes? What are its costs? Does it save money by keeping people from higher levels of care?

These questions bring us full circle: if we are to study the consequences of nursing case management, we must know what nurse case managers do. It is in the context of these questions that the discussion of measurement and logic models was raised. When the arguments raised in this chapter are put together to and used to specify the linkages among the structure, process, and outcomes of care, perhaps we will have moved forward in meeting Lamb's and Aliotta's challenge.

References

Aliotta, S.L. (2001). Key functions and direct outcomes of nursing case management. In Cohen, E.L., & Cesta, T.G. (Eds.), *Nursing case management* (pp. 417-422). St. Louis: Mosby, Inc.

Brooten, D., & Naylor, M.D. (1995). Nurses' effect on changing patient outcomes. *IMAGE: Journal of Nursing Scholarship, 27*(2), 95-99.

Chen, H.-T. (1990). *Theory-driven evaluation: A comprehensive perspective.* Newbury Park, Calif.: Sage Publications.

Cohen, E.L., & Cesta, T.G., Eds. (2001). *Nursing case management* (pp. 417-422). St. Louis: Mosby, Inc.

Crocker, L., & Algina, J. (1986). *Introduction to classical and modern test theory.* New York: Harcourt, Brace, Jovanovich.

Cronbach, L.J., & Meehl, P.E. (1955). Construct validity in psychological tests. *Psychological Bulletin, 52,* 281-302.

Feinstein, A.R. (1987). *Clinimetrics.* New Haven, Conn.: Yale University Press.

Gerteis, M., Edgman-Levitan, S., Daley, J., & Delbanco, T.L. (1993). *Through the patient's eyes.* San Francisco: Jossey-Bass.

Guyatt, G.H. (2000). Making sense of quality-of-life data, *Medical Care, 38*(9) Supplement II, II-175-II-179.

Hays, R.D., & Stewart, A.L. (1992). Construct validity of MOS health measures. In A.L. Stewart & J.E. Ware (Eds.), *Measuring functioning and well-being: The Medical Outcomes Study approach* (pp. 325-342). Durham, N.C.: Duke University Press.

Issel, L.M. (1997). Measuring comprehensive case management interventions: Development of a tool. *Nursing Case Management, 2*(4), 132-138.

Kane, M.T. (1992). An argument-based approach to validity. *Psychological Bulletin, 112*(3), 527-535.

Kelly, K.C., Huber, D.G., Johnson, M., McCloskey, J.C., & Maas, M. (1994). The Medical Outcomes Study: A nursing perspective. *Journal of Professional Nursing, 10*(4), 209-216.

Kerlinger, F.N. (1973). *Foundations of behavioral research* (2nd ed.). New York: Holt, Rinehart & Winston.

Lamb, G.S. (1995). Case management. In J.J. Fitzpatrick & J.S. Stevenson (Eds.), *Annual Review of Nursing Research, 13,* 117-136.

Mateo, M.A., Matzke, K., & Newton, C. (1998). Designing measurements to assess case management outcomes, *Nursing Case Management, 3*(1), 2-6.

Mateo, M.A., Matzke, K., & Newton, C. (2002). Designing measurements to assess case management outcomes, *Lippincott's Case Management, 3*(1), 261-266.

McHorney, C.A., Ware, J.E., Lu, J.F., & Sherbourne, C.D. (1994). The MOS 36-Item Short-Form Health Survey (SF-36): III. Tests of data quality, scaling assumptions, and reliability across diverse patient groups. *Medical Care, 32*(1), 40-66.

McHorney, C.A., Ware, J.E., & Raczek, A.E. (1993). The MOS 36-Item Short-Form Health Survey (SF-36): II. Psychometric and clinical tests of validity in measuring physical and mental health constructs. *Medical Care, 31*(3), 247-263.

Messick, S. (1995). Validity of psychological assessment. *American Psychologist, 50*(9), 741-749.

Naylor, M.D., Munro, B.H., & Brooten, D.A. (1991). Measuring the effectiveness of nursing practice. *Clinical Nurse Specialist, 5*(4), 210-214.

Nunnally, J. (1978). *Psychometric theory.* New York: McGraw-Hill.

Patrick, D.L., & Chiang, Y.P. (2000). Measurement of health outcomes in treatment effectiveness evaluations, *Medical Care,* 38(9) Supplment II, II-14-II-25.

Portney, L.G., & Watkins, M.P. (1993). *Foundations of clinical research: Applications to practice.* Norwalk, Conn.: Appleton & Lange.

Rogers, P.J., Hacsi, T.A., Petosino, A., & Huebner, T.A. (2000). Program theory in evaluation: Challenges and opportunities; New Directions for Evaluation, 87. San Francisco: Jossey-Bass.

Stewart, A.L., Hays, R.D., & Ware, J.E. (1992). Methods of validating MOS health measures. In A.L. Stewart & J.E. Ware (Eds.), *Measuring functioning and well-being: The Medical Outcomes Study approach* (pp. 309-324). Durham, N.C.: Duke University Press.

Stewart, A.L., & Ware, J.E. (1992). *Measuring functioning and well-being: The Medical Outcomes Study approach.* Durham, N.C.: Duke University Press.

Streiner, D.L., & Norman, G.R. (1989). *Health measurement scales: A practical guide to their development and use.* New York: Oxford University Press.

Tahan, H.A. (1989). The use of the cost-effectiveness analysis method. In Cohen, E.L., & Cesta, T.G. (Eds.). *Nursing case management* (pp. 503-524). St. Louis: Mosby, Inc.

Tarlov, A., Ware, J.E., Greenfield, S., Nelson, E.C., Perrin, E., & Zubkoff, M. (1989). The Medical Outcomes Study: An application of methods for monitoring the results of medical care. *Journal of the American Medical Association, 263*(7), 925-930.

Testa, M.A. (2000). Interpretation of quality-of-life outcomes, *Medical Care* 3(9) Supplement II: II-168-II-174.

Thorndike, R.L. (1982). *Applied psychometrics.* Boston: Houghton Mifflin.

Ware, J.E., & Sherbourne, C.D. (1992). The MOS 36-Item Short-Form Health Survey (SF-36): I. Conceptual framework and item selection. *Medical Care, 30*(6), 473-483.

Weiss, C.H. (1997). Theory-based evaluation: Past, present, and future. In Rog, D.J. & Fournier, D. (Eds.). *Progress and future directions in evaluation: Perspectives on theory, practice, and methods,* New directions in evaluation, San Francisco: Jossey-Bass.

An Overview of Assessing Health Through Quality of Life Indicators

Kathryn Nold

CHAPTER OVERVIEW

Various outcome indicators have been established as measurements of successful case management programs. Some of these indicators are resource utilization outcomes, institutions' economic outcomes, patient-centered outcomes, and process outcomes. As an additional outcome measure, quality of life indicators, or health status surveys, should be considered as essential tools for a case management program.

A population's health status, as defined by quality of life results, can be used externally by customers to purchase services or internally to improve outcomes. Customers, in this context, are payers, patients, and other health care providers and institutions. This Chapter describes the basics of quality of life measurements, outlines the selection of an instrument, and concludes with a case study using liver transplantation recipients.

WHY MEASURE QUALITY OF LIFE?

Quality of life (QOL) is an outcome measure that can document the effectiveness of medical interventions such as treatment of a disease, surgery, or use of drug therapy. It assesses patients' perceptions of their health, satisfaction with life, and/or general sense of personal well-being that can provide insights about the strengths and weaknesses of diagnostic and treatment therapies (Spilker, 1996). QOL can also be defined as "the gap between the patient's expectations and achievements" (Calman, 1984). The greater the gap, the lower is the quality of life. If the goal setting by the patient and the provider is realistic, the expectations of the patient may more closely align with the achievements.

One of the basic questions asked at institutions is, "Why measure quality of life (health status)"? Some health care providers have viewed QOL analysis as subjective psychosocial assessments that lack scientific methods (Spilker, 1996). Confusion comes in the assumption that something subjective cannot be as valid as physical measures. This narrow view of health does not account for today's complex environments. Both subjective and objective findings can be measured and meet reliability and validity standards. Some of the nonbiomedical model components that can be assessed in QOL data are values, beliefs,

Acknowledgments: Members of the Liver Transplant Program at the University of Colorado Health Sciences Center and Hospital who contributed to the case study are Tracy Steinberg, RN, MS (Transplant Coordinator and Case Manager), Michael Talamantes, LCSW (Transplant Team Social Worker), Igal Kam, MD (Professor/Chief of Transplant Surgery), Gregory Everson, MD (Professor/Director Hepatology), and Steve Hartwell, BS, MSEM (Database Administrator).

coping abilities, spiritual status, social networks, vocational status, cultural and religious opportunities, government and insurance policies, transportation and communication systems, and available medical facilities and services. Some researchers say that there are no perfect QOL instruments or surveys to measure the benefits of medical care, so it may not be possible to completely formulate definitive conclusions. Even with some controversy, the use of QOL measures is spreading and receiving increasing acceptance as an indicator for measuring effectiveness and efficacy and, therefore, accountability.

CATEGORIES OF QUALITY OF LIFE

The following categories are important to include in a QOL survey:
- Physical functioning (limitations attributed to physical problems)
- Social functioning (limitations attributed to social interactions/participation)
- Psychological functioning (limitations attributed to emotional problems)
- General well-being (general health perceptions)
- Economic resources (costs and access to care)

Various studies have been published using only one or two of these categories, sometimes referred to as domains (Granger et al., 1990; Lloyd et al., 1992). Without knowledge of the instrument's validation process, the novice should be cautioned about making an assessment of QOL by aggregating results across all domains. One single overall score for QOL may not reflect the differences in the domains. The physical functioning category may reflect improved outcomes, whereas the psychological category exhibits decreased outcomes. It is essential to understand the properties and limitations of the measurement tool being used.

SPECIFIC INSTRUMENTS

A broad range of health status data are being collected and reported in clinical trials. Clinicians and researchers use disease-specific, general non–disease-specific, population-specific (age), function-specific, problem-specific, or psychologically specific tools. Generic instruments address various domains and can identify aspects that are affected by the disease or therapy. Generic measures, however, may fail to examine detailed aspects such as symptoms or functions. Disease-specific instruments have the advantage of addressing areas that are unique to a population. The disadvantages of disease-specific surveys are not providing a comparison of QOL between populations with or without other diseases and the potential for eliminating a domain. For example, if physical functioning is decreasing, what effect does this have on emotional functioning? Or did the decreasing emotional functioning lead to the decreasing physical functioning?

Examples of QOL instruments are as follows:
1. Non–disease-specific (generic): Short Form-36-Health Survey (Ware, 1996)
2. Disease-specific: Arthritis Impact Measurement Scales (Mccnan, 1996)
3. Population-specific: The OARS Multidimensional Functional Assessment Questionnaire (OARS Duke University, 1996)
4. Function-specific: The Rapid Disability Scale (Linn, 1996)
5. Problem-specific: The McGill Pain Questionnaire (Melzack, 1996)
6. Psychologically specific: The Psychological General Well-being Scale (Dupuy, 1996), Rand Mental Health Inventory (Ware, 1996)
7. Psychosocially specific: Sickness Impact Profile (Bergner, 1996)

There are varying opinions as to the use of disease-specific surveys versus general surveys. Some clinical studies have used general and disease-specific scales for comparison. Choosing the instrument(s) where the expected differences are greatest in the domains measured by that instrument may lead to biases or overestimate the benefits of a therapy.

SELECTING AN INSTRUMENT

The number of surveys available is vast, and they differ in acceptability by experts in this field. The choice of a measure must be determined by the purpose and needs of the population and provider. Variables to consider are as follows:

What population(s) are you surveying? What are their characteristics?

How many subjects will participate in the assessment? Does this represent an adequate number for the outcome question you are asking?

How are you going to access this population?

Will your population(s) have special needs in completing a survey? (task perseverance, comprehension)

What outcomes are you measuring?

What is your purpose? (describe, predict, evaluate)

How many domains will you measure?

What "unit" are you interested in profiling? Patient? Family? Community?

What is in the current literature? (surveys and results for comparison data)

Will you use normative QOL measures where floor/ceiling effects could be encountered?

Will you use one or more surveys?

How are data reliability and validity tested? Has the survey been shown to be valid for your application? (measuring mortality, measuring functional ability)

What time treatment phases are you interested in surveying? (pre- and post-treatment, intervals of months or years)

How will the data be collected? (technical issues of collection)

Who will be the data collectors?

How are you going to handle missing data?

Is a scoring method defined? How will you analyze and report the data?

What are the costs?

How will feedback be given to the patients and providers?

McDowell and Newell (1996) have published a guide that can assist in selecting a credible instrument. These authors offer a review of over 80 surveys or instruments and address the measurement purpose and the reliability and validity results of each instrument. *Reliability* or *consistency* measures the reproducibility in obtaining the same results when the test is repeated, and *validity* measures the accuracy in measuring what it is supposed to measure. When available, an example of the instrument and the scoring method is included to aid clinicians in selecting the appropriate survey for their population. McDowell and Newell (1996) suggest that validated and reliable surveys should be used in clinical studies and that the creation of a new survey may not be necessary when an existing instrument is obtainable.

CASE STUDY: QUALITY OF LIFE AFTER LIVER TRANSPLANTATION

In measuring the success of surgical treatment, it is important to judge the results both in the traditional terms of operative mortality and operative morbidity, and in terms of the side effects that may impair function and health. Clinical decisions are often based on the patient's subjective feelings or physical abilities. This descriptive study summarizes the investigation of the biopsychosocial status of patients who have undergone orthotopic hepatic transplantation at a single institution. The results have not been published, so the findings reported are limited to preliminary observations. The purpose of this QOL review is to compare and describe, not to predict or evaluate.

The population reviewed is patients admitted for liver transplantation at the University of Colorado-University Hospital. Numerous factors contribute to their experiences and can impact results, including life-threatening illness, major surgery, financial issues, medications, and hepatic encephalopathy. These areas are additional opportunities for future research.

The National Institute of Diabetes and Digestive and Kidney Diseases (NIDDK) Liver Transplant Database (LTD) QOL questionnaire published by a multicenter study was selected as the instrument for measurement at the University of Colorado. Its selection was based on the published study and potential comparability to this population (Belle et al., 1997). A few demographic questions were added for this institution's analyses. The following domains were represented in the questionnaire: measures of disease, psychological status, personal function, social and role function, and general health perception.

The initial observations evaluated the outcome of 43 patients who completed a pretransplant baseline questionnaire and a 1-year posttransplant questionnaire. Data were obtained at the time of transplantation listing and 6 and 12 months after liver transplantation. An additional follow-up survey is planned after 2 years. The greatest improvements were shown in the posttransplant 1-year scales measuring physical symptoms (measures of disease) and psychological complaints. The University of Colorado results were equivalent to those of the multicenter study (Belle et al., 1997), which had over 300 patients enrolled. The changes in number and severity of physical symptoms (Tables 49-1 and 49-2) and psychological complaints (Tables 49-3 and 49-4) were statistically significant. Moreover, a generalized improvement in all

TABLE 49-1	MEASURES OF DISEASE: AVERAGE PRESENCE OR ABSENCE OF 21 PHYSICAL SYMPTOMS*		
		Pretransplantation	Posttransplantation
University of Colorado		14 symptoms	9.51 symptoms
Multicenter study		13.8 symptoms	10 symptoms

Multicenter study reported by Belle et al., 1997.
*Results were significant at <.001.

TABLE 49-2	MEASURES OF DISEASE: AVERAGE SEVERITY OF PHYSICAL SYMPTOMS*†		
		Pretransplantation	Posttransplantation
University of Colorado		29.62 severity	15.66 severity
Multicenter study		32.1 severity	17.8 severity

Multicenter study reported by Belle et al., 1997.
*Results were significant at <.001.
†Scale: 0, Not at all, sequentially to 4, extreme; maximum score of 84.

TABLE 49-3 PSYCHOLOGICAL STATUS: AVERAGE PRESENCE OR ABSENCE OF FIVE PSYCHOLOGICAL SYMPTOMS*		
	Pretransplantation	**Posttransplantation**
University of Colorado	3.87 symptoms	2.38 symptoms
Multicenter study	3.7 symptoms	3 symptoms

Multicenter study reported by Belle et al., 1997.
*Results were significant at <.001.

TABLE 49-4 PSYCHOLOGICAL STATUS: AVERAGE SEVERITY OF PHYSICAL SYMPTOMS*†		
	Pretransplantation	**Posttransplantation**
University of Colorado	7.91 severity	3.53 severity
Multicenter study	8.1 severity	5 severity

Multicenter study reported by Belle et al., 1997.
*Results were significant at <.001.
†Scale: 0, Not at all, sequentially to 4, extreme; maximum score of 84.

domains was found when compared with the same individual's pretransplant status, a finding to be viewed as preliminary. Overall, most liver transplant recipients were satisfied with their QOL even with considerable economic strains and occasional personal distress.

FUTURE DIRECTIONS

Marketing Quality of Life

The University of Colorado Hospital has been asked to quantify and qualify our services for prospective buyers. As our clinical databases grow, we believe we will be able to include QOL data in contract negotiations. Because we believe QOL is an important evaluative element and effective categorizing element, combining these outcomes with severity of illness adjustments might result in a marketing advantage. A template should be established for pricing based on the predicted value to patients (efficacy) or on cost-effectiveness. This value is the increase in or maintenance of the patients' QOL. The payer may ask at what cost is this increased QOL? A standard that assists in weighing the economic advantages and disadvantages of treatment is the quality-adjusted life-years (QALY) (Glasziou et al., 1998). This standard can be calculated by using symptom reports or QOL surveys to show correlations of cost, effectiveness, and QOL gains. An example is the Veterans Administration Cooperative Study (Takaro et al., 1976), which estimated that net cost per QALY gained from coronary artery bypass graft surgery (CABG) ranged from $3,500 in left main artery disease to $30,000 in one-vessel disease. Subsequent studies have revealed that the medical management costs and medication usage of not having CABG can result in higher costs than those associated with surgery (Rogers, 1985).

Case Management

If your case management program has not assisted in the development, measurement, and assessment of QOL at your institution, you may be forgetting a valuable professional resource. It is important to reiterate that QOL can be defined as "the gap between the patient's expectations and achievements" (Calman, 1984). The case manager is in an ideal position to assist in narrowing that gap through realistic goal setting. QOL results can be used by case managers to predict outcomes for patients, identify patient needs and services and meet those needs, and advise providers of systems improvements. For example, if joint replacement patients' psychosocial domains (ability to adequately perform social, occupational, and domestic roles) are lower immediately postoperatively than preoperatively, the case manager can provide patients with information and/or services to improve this outcome and advocate for systems development.

References

Belle, S.H., Porayko, M.K., Hoofnagle, J.H., Lake, J.R., & Zetterman, R.K. (1997). Changes in quality of life after liver transplantation among adults. *Liver Transplantation and Surgery, 3*(2), 93-104.

Bergner, M. (1996). Sickness impact profile. In I. MacDowell & C. Newell (Eds.). *Measuring health: A guide to rating scales and questionnaires* (pp. 431-437). New York: Oxford University Press.

Calman, K.C. (1984). Quality of life in cancer patients: An hypothesis, *Journal of Medical Ethics, 10,* 124-127.

Dupuy, J. (1996). The psychological general well-being schedule. In I. MacDowell & C. Newell (Eds.). *Measuring health: A guide to rating scales and questionnaires* (pp. 206-213). New York: Oxford University Press.

Glasziou, P.P., Cole, B.F., Gelber, R.D., Hilden, J., & Simes, R.J. (1998). Quality adjusted survival analysis with repeated quality of life measures. *Statistics in Medicine, 17,* 1215-1229.

Granger, C.V., Cotter, A.C., Hamilton, B.B., et al. (1990). Functional assessment scales: A study of persons with multiple sclerosis. *Archives in Physical Medicine and Rehabilitation, 71,* 870-875.

Linn, M.W. (1996). The Rapid Disability Rating Scale. In I. MacDowell & C. Newell (Eds), *Measuring health: A guide to rating scales and questionnaires* (pp. 82-88). New York: Oxford University Press.

Lloyd, C.E., Matthews, K.A., Wing, R.R., & Orchard, T.J. (1992). Psychosocial factors and complications of IDDM. The Pittsburgh Epidemiology of Diabetes Complications Study, VIII. *Diabetes Care, 15,* 166 172.

McDowell, I., & Newell, C. (Eds.). (1996). *Measuring health: A guide to rating scales and questionnaires.* New York: Oxford University Press.

Meenan, R.F. (1996). The Arthritis Impact Measurement Scales. In I. MacDowell & C. Newell (Eds.). *Measuring health: A guide to rating scales and questionnaires* (pp. 383-391). New York: Oxford University Press.

Melzack, R. (1996). McGill Pain Questionnaire. In I. MacDowell & C. Newell (Eds.). *Measuring health: A guide to rating scales and questionnaires* (pp. 346-351). New York: Oxford University Press.

OARS Duke University. (1996). The OARS Multidimensional Functional Assessment Questionnaire. In I. MacDowell & C. Newell (Eds.). *Measuring health: A guide to rating scales and questionnaires* (pp. 464-472). New York: Oxford University Press.

Rogers, W.J. (1985). Medical vs. surgical management of ischemic heart disease: Implications of the coronary artery surgery study. *Alabama Journal of Medical Science, 22,* 416-422.

Spilker, B. (Ed.). (1996). *Quality of life and pharmacoeconomics in clinical trials,* Philadelphia & New York: Lippincott-Raven.

Stewart, A., & Ware, J. (1992). *Measuring functioning and well-being, The medical outcomes study approach.* Durham & London: Duke University Press.

Takaro, R., Hultgren, H.N., Lipton, M.J., et al. (1976). The VA Cooperative Randomized Study of Surgery for Coronary Occlusive Disease. II. Subgroup with significant left main lesions. *Circulation, 54*(Suppl. III), 107-117.

Ware, J.E. (1996). Short Form 36 Health Status. In I. MacDowell & C. Newell (Eds), *Measuring health, a guide to rating scales and questionnaires* (pp. 446-456). New York: Oxford University Press.

Ware, J.E. (1996). The Rand Mental Health Inventory. In I. MacDowell & C. Newell (Eds), *Measuring health, a guide to rating scales and questionnaires* (pp. 213-219). New York: Oxford University Press.

Ware, J.E., Kosinski, M., & Keller, S.D. (1994). *SF-36 Physical and Mental Health Summary Scales: A user's manual.* Boston: The Health Institute.

50

Effective Management Tools for Case Management Leaders

*Strategy Maps and Balanced Scorecards, A Case Study**

Elizabeth Falter

Health care service providers face extraordinary business challenges in addressing the needs of the markets they serve. Their revenues often derive from cumbersome reimbursement mechanisms, which generally lag behind market conditions. Key elements of their cost structure, over which they have little or no control, have been increasing at rates substantially above inflation for the past several years. Finally, the very nature of the services they provide, health care to individuals, requires that their internal operations meet the highest standards of quality. *Strategy maps* and supporting *balanced scorecards*, components of the Balanced Scorecard concept developed by Robert S. Kaplan and David P. Norton (1996, 2001) can be powerful tools for unraveling complex relationships and issues to achieve and implement new strategies that will successfully address these and other issues.

- *Balanced Scorecard:* Translates an organization's mission and strategy into a comprehensive set of performance measures that provides the framework for a strategic measurement and management system.
- *Vision and Strategy:* Vision is a compelling statement of what the organization seeks to accomplish, readily understandable by every employee in the organization. Strategy provides the overall blueprint in the form of specific goals and objectives designed to achieve the organizational vision.
- *Strategy Map:* A graphic representation of key objectives and goals (for organization, unit, or individual) arranged in a series of hypothetical cause and effect relationships that outlines steps required to achieve an overall strategy.
- *Financial Perspective:* Focus on contribution of strategy, implementation, and execution to bottom-line improvement.
- *Customer Perspective:* Focuses on the customer and the market segments in which the organization will compete and the measures of performance in these targeted segments.
- *Internal Processes Perspective:* Focuses on the internal processes in an organization that will have the greatest impact on customer satisfaction and achieve an organization's financial objectives.
- *Learning and Growth Perspective:* Focuses the infrastructure (people, systems, and organizational procedures) that the organization must build to create long-term growth and improvement.

This case study is about a large physician practice whose participating physicians were given the opportunity to buy back their practice. At the time, MedPartners, Inc. owned the practice. To accomplish

---

*Copyright owned by Elizabeth Falter, © 2003.

the repurchase, the practice required outside financing, which in turn was contingent on their getting their financial house in order. This case study is about the need for a successful group of physicians, well regarded by patients and providers alike, to reorganize their own practice to manage high overhead costs. Changes associated with this shift were felt throughout the organization, some painful.

CASE STUDY

At first glance, it appeared to be a case of revenue versus overhead, the simple answer being to cut overhead to reduce costs. If this strategy were to be adopted, it would mean experienced, highly competent, cardiology nurses who were critical to the success of the practice would have to go. In a *capitated system* (defined as a set amount or a flat rate to cover a person's medical care for a specified period), these nurses were a gold mine. In the current reimbursement system, they were overhead. The board of directors, practice administration, and the cardiologists were all committed to quality patient care. To eliminate these nurses without careful thought would risk that commitment.

A thorough analysis of the existing internal processes of the practice revealed a very intricate, well-executed telephonic case management system for managing patients on complex cardiology drugs. In collaboration with the physician, nurses would manage patient inquiries, most of which dealt with medications, over the phone. Often, these conversations saved the patients a trip to the office and, sometimes, even to the hospital. The patients loved the nurses, and the cardiologists were able to devote a larger share of their time to other patients. Had they been under capitation, this process would have had a positive impact on practice profitability. Under current reimbursement processes telephone contacts required written records evidencing calls totaling at least 30 minutes in duration and did not allow for the inclusion the multiple telephone calls usually involved, nor the time spent tracking down all of the participants.

The task was to come up with a new strategy, which would transform a cost center into a revenue generator and then manage its implementation while maintaining quality patient care. Effective performance management requires two elements: communication and measurement. Strategy maps and balanced scorecards provided both. This case study demonstrates the merging of the strategy map for the larger physician practice with that of the smaller cardiology group. It also compares measurements identified by the physicians and nurses to measure success. While I worked with five teams to redesign multiple internal systems, including pacemaker clinic and lipid management, for purposes of this case study, we will focus on one of the solutions: a nurse-run, physician-managed Coumadin clinic.

As most health care providers know, Coumadin is the DuPont Pharmaceutical brand of warfarin sodium used as an anticoagulant that helps reduce clots forming in the blood. Two major complications exist around management of patients on this therapy. First, for many of the patients, the dosage is not the same every day. Second, patients need to have their blood drawn to make sure their blood is not being anticoagulated too little or too much. Furthermore, any time a patient has any kind of surgical or dental procedure, they must temporarily suspend their use of the drug. The mission of the Coumadin clinic is to effectively manage this patient population and to ensure high-quality care and in-depth patient education. The clinic resides in the physicians' office and is not for the treatment of routine or urgent problems. Patients of the clinic are seen by registered nurses and sent to the cardiologist when necessary.

I was not called in specifically to implement the balanced scorecard or even develop nurse-run clinics. Strategy maps and the balanced scorecard helped me to articulate what the practice needed to do and then integrate the new goals and measures of the full practice with the smaller practice. The complexities and contradictions of the situation required strong management tools. The idea for the clinics came from the cardiologists who were remarkably proactive during the entire process. The practice's board of directors, the practice administrator, and the individual cardiologists were all committed to maintaining quality patient care even in the face of lowering costs. The maps and scorecards helped me look at multiple issues, measure what was important to all the stakeholders and most importantly make the connections among all the objectives.

Continued

CASE STUDY—CONT'D

My first task, after analyzing the problem, was to draw a strategy map for the larger physician practice. I knew whatever solution was identified, it had to be in concert with the larger strategy of the entire physician practice group, which included a number of other medical specialties. Equally important, a significant part of the challenge here was ensuring that the larger group fully understood the workings of the cardiac practice. The strategy map was extremely useful in improving this level of communication (Figure 50-1).

As the first map shows, the strategy of the full practice group is focused on buying back their practice. To accomplish this, they needed to increase revenue and decrease overhead. At the same time, and equally important in this strategy map, they would have to meet and/or exceed the high standards of quality they set for themselves. Without succeeding along the customer dimension, the financial objectives could not be attained. Implementing this strategy required that they improve internal processes relating to internal referrals and patient management, as well as implement an internal quality improvement effort. Those objectives were all supported by learning and innovation to engage physicians in new ownership responsibilities and educate the staff to their new identity. I worked closely with the quality improvement director to link my approach to the work she was doing elsewhere.

To better understand these maps, let's focus on my second task, which was to create a separate strategy map for the cardiology group's innovative ideas. The map in Figure 50-2 includes the main goals within each key area. Discussion around each of these areas will be general, as specifics are proprietary to the practice.

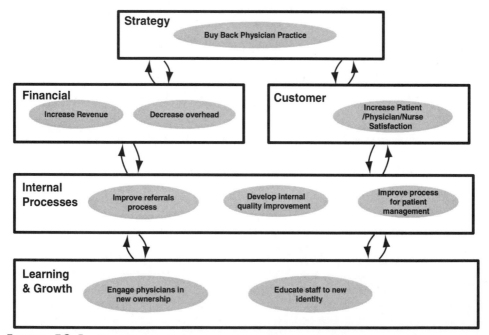

FIGURE **50-1**   Physician practice group strategy map.
(Adapted from *Kaplan, R., & Norton, D. (1996). The balanced scorecard. Boston: Harvard Business School Press and Kaplan, R., & Norton, D. (2001). The strategy focused organization. Boston: Harvard Business School Press.*)

CASE STUDY—CONT'D

Their strategy was two-fold: to cover the costs of these excellent nurses while meeting and/or exceeding physician, nurse, and patient satisfaction. They were so committed to this that nearly every staff member served on a team and I served as facilitator. Our *financial perspective* had two major goals. We needed to tie nurse work to reimbursement and increase physician revenue. The nurses on this team actually did the financial analysis. To this end they looked at the number of patients in the cardiology practice currently on Coumadin, which was around 550. Not every patient would move to this new approach to care, but could approximate how many might come each day. They also looked at the costs of running the clinic to include nurse time and test costs. (Vendors supplied computers and software.) Because most of the patients in the practice were on Medicare, visits would qualify for level I reimbursement. The finance department provided us with cost and reimbursement specifics. Each patient visit required one nurse for a 15-minute face-to-face. A physician was on site while the clinic was in operation. The physician or the nurse practitioner saw patients with more complicated issues, at the higher-level visit.

As in the larger map, the *customer perspective* looked at patient, physician and nurse satisfaction. Patient surveys already indicated high satisfaction. Physicians and nurses working together demonstrated the loyalty they had for each other. Communication was quite open so all verbalized their opinions though this was not measured formally.

Continued

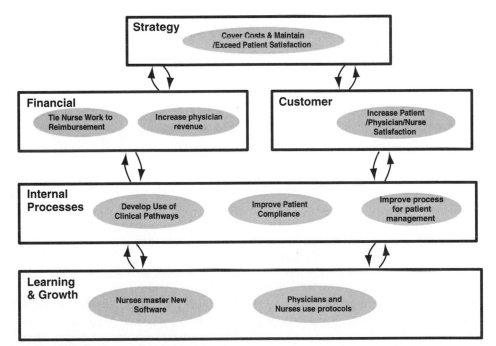

FIGURE **50-2**   Coumadin clinic strategy map.
(Adapted from *Kaplan, R., & Norton, D. (1996). The balanced scorecard. Boston: Harvard Business School Press* and *Kaplan, R., & Norton, D. (2001). The strategy focused organization. Boston: Harvard Business School Press.*)

CASE STUDY—CONT'D

Financial and customer goals are not met unless underlying process are efficient and support quality outcomes. Therefore our *internal process perspective* focused on designing three key internal processes: develop clinical pathways for management of patients on Coumadin; improve patient compliance in taking their medication through improving how the patient managed themselves at home; and improve the process for managing these patients in the clinic. The clinical pathways were the most difficult process to design since the practice had not yet developed guidelines and were use to daily conferences on these patients. Without the guidelines, the visits would become more complicated, involving more people. In terms of patient self-management, the software provided a printout that was easy to read and follow. Also, the face-to-face encouraged the patients to come to clinic , thus meeting their responsibilities. The nurses continued to set up the clinic so that it was efficient but personal and private as well. They were given an office to set up equipment, counters, computers, and so on, that met both their needs and that of the patients. This also included opening the clinic at 7 AM for patient convenience.

Neither financial, customer, nor processes are successful without an underlying foundation of *learning and growth* within the practice. Fortunately, this foundation was already present in the practice. For the Coumadin clinic, there were two major areas of learning that were required. Nurses and physicians needed to use the clinical pathways and, more important, act independently of each other. Conferences were needed only when a patient was outside of the protocols. Nurses also needed to learn to operate the automated laboratory equipment and controls in addition to the computer software. Sufficient time was allocated for training.

To summarize, the map serves as a guide for necessary steps to succeed at a strategy. When developing a map, four questions should be asked. What do I need to do to meet financial goals? To do that, I need customers. I must ask myself what I must do to make them happy. To make customers happy and meet financial goals, which processes must I design and continuously improve? To have good processes, what learning and innovation must happen within my business unit or organization? One component builds on the other. Without all four, your strategy most likely will not succeed.

It is important to note here that the physicians and nurses developed an extensive list of outcome measures for the clinic not seen in the map. They included the following:

- Improve patient outcomes, defined as fewer hemorrhagic and thromboembolic episodes
- Increase patient care compliance
- Increase efficiency of use of physician and registered nurse time
- Increase the percentage of instances that patients blood measures were within therapeutic range
- Minimize "no shows" (patients not showing up for laboratory tests)
- Increase patient knowledge of potential drug interactions and side effects
- More efficiently manage the large number of patients on Coumadin
- Screen for problems to avoid hospitalization

The balanced scorecard in Figure 50-3 is just a simple way of comparing measures associated with the four components of the strategy maps. It is not meant to include all measures.

The scorecard has more specific measurements than the strategy map, but is directly related to the four areas. For example, under learning and growth, the goal was to have physicians use clinical guidelines. This would be measured by how many of the cardiologists and nurses were using the guidelines. Measurement is a major communication tool. It is meant to guide, not punish. More importantly, the team or business unit using them must also develop measurements. The ones presented here are examples only and may or may not be helpful to another group developing a clinic.

Financial	Internal Processes
• Clinic revenue versus Plan • # Patient visits vs. Plan • % Patient visits achieving reimbursement target	• Avg time to complete process • # No shows for blood work appointments decreased • % Patients achieving target compliance
Customer	Learning & Growth

• % Increase in satisfaction
   • Patients
   • Cardiologists
   • RNs
   • Referring physicians
	• % Target MDs/RNs using protocols
	• % Target nursing staff using software
	• # New protocols

FIGURE **50-3**   Scorecard measures.
(Adapted from *Kaplan, R., & Norton, D. (1996). The balanced scorecard. Boston: Harvard Business School Press and Kaplan, R., & Norton, D. (2001). The strategy focused organization. Boston: Harvard Business School Press.*)

There are currently 800 patients coming to the clinic per month. The clinic is going so well, that internists are sending their patients to be managed by the nurses. Patient, nurse, and physician satisfaction is higher because of the new processes that make their work easier. For example, in the old process, patients would go to the laboratory and have their blood drawn. The laboratory would call the nurses who would find the doctors, evaluate therapy levels, call the patients, and so on. This cumbersome process resulted in a lot of telephone time and a lot of frustrated people. The new process involves one trip for the patient and one 15-minute visit. In that time, they receive one finger prick for blood. A computer reads the blood and prints out results along with recommended dosages.

Education is enhanced with an in-person visit. The nurses have the clinical guidelines to manage the patients. They no longer have to interrupt the busy physicians except for patients who need a higher-level visit because of other complications. A nurse practitioner is also on site to handle more complicated cases. Process improvement continues as the team continuously redesigns the clinic to make the patient and nurse more comfortable. Satisfaction has been extremely high. The clinic also has been recognized as a regional leader for Coumadin care, receiving the Roche Diagnostic's "DREAM" award.

Both nurses and physicians are now comfortable with the clinical guidelines and have expanded them to include guidelines for patients going to surgery. Together they attend an annual conference on managing patients on anticoagulants.

To summarize, a 2- to 3-day process has been reduced to a mere 15 minutes, with better outcomes for patients and revenue to support registered nurses. Although it is a privilege to tell the story of these good doctors and nurses, the case study is also about using management tools such as strategy maps and balanced scorecards to improve quality in a very difficult reimbursement health care environment.

References

Kaplan, R., & Norton, D. (1996). *The balanced scorecard.* Boston: Harvard Business School Press.

Kaplan, R., & Norton, D. (2001). *The strategy focused organization.* Boston: Harvard Business School Press.

Outcomes Effectiveness and Evidence-Based Practice

Colleen J. Goode

CHAPTER OVERVIEW

Evidence-based practice is conceptually defined as the use of current best evidence when making patient care decisions. When patient care interventions are based on the best evidence available, optimal outcomes are more likely to occur. Effectiveness is the degree to which the desired outcomes are achieved. Heater, Becker, and Olson's (1988) meta-analysis demonstrated that evidence-based practice produced more effective outcomes. The purpose of this Chapter is to help case managers understand evidence-based practice, its influence on outcomes, their role in practicing from an evidence-based practice framework, and how they can be leaders, by example, in evidence-based practice.

EVIDENCE-BASED DECISION-MAKING

Gray (1997) believes decisions about groups of patients or patient populations are made by combining evidence, values, and resources. These three factors also influence individual patient care decisions made by case managers. Evidence related to a specific intervention's effectiveness or management of a disease should drive the clinician's decision-making process, but sometimes the values of either the health care provider or the patient drive it, sometimes the availability of resources (i.e., money, staff, and equipment) is the motivating factor, and often a combination of all three factors influences decision-making. Berwick (2003) reminds us that even though health care is rich in evidence-based innovations, successful implementation in one organization does not guarantee dissemination to others. Case managers should be early adopters of evidence based interventions and help to accelerate the diffusion of interventions.

Case managers provide evidence-based care because quality is enhanced and outcomes are improved. Payers and policy makers have become interested in evidence-based clinical practice because of a desire to identify health care costs that do not result in benefit to the patient, thereby freeing resources for other uses. Case managers provide care from a quality perspective, linking practice to outcome. Evidence-based practice reduces variation in practice patterns. Tanner (1998) defines the aim of evidence-based practice as reducing wide variations in individual clinician practices, eliminating worst practices, and enhancing best practices, thereby improving quality and reducing costs. Case managers, payers, and policymakers must ensure that the best value is obtained from the resources available. A number of surveys have demonstrated that clinical decisions are often not based on the best evidence (Brett, 1987; Coyle & Sokop, 1990; Gibbs, Mead, Hager, & Sweet, 1994;

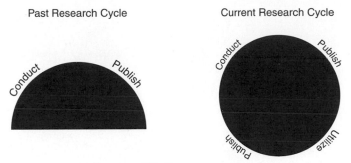

FIGURE **51-1**   Research cycle.

Institute of Medicine, 1992). The current health care climate emphasizes cost reduction but also demands positive patient outcomes. Evidence-based practice is an important vehicle for achieving these goals.

THE RESEARCH CYCLE

The evolution to a scientific basis for nursing practice has been slow. Figure 51-1 demonstrates the research cycle that was part of this evolution. In the early years the focus was on conducting and publishing research. Most of the research was done by those in academia, and it was often focused on studies related to nursing students, administration, or education, with few clinically focused studies. Today nursing research is very clinically focused and the cycle has expanded to include utilization of findings and publishing of outcomes when findings are used in practice.

The body of knowledge needed to conduct research differs from that needed for utilization of research. For example, utilization of a new research-based intervention on a busy medical surgical unit requires knowledge related to how to educate the providers about the change and convince them that there is value in changing their practice. Gathering support for the practice change, sustaining the change, and evaluating the effect of the change on patient outcomes are also parts of the utilization process. Changing behavior is complex, involves many systems, and usually cannot be achieved solely by education (Thomson, 1998). This process requires skills and knowledge that are not traditionally included in research courses that focus on conducting research.

EVIDENCE-BASED PRACTICE MODEL

Health care providers have evolved beyond research utilization to include other forms of evidence as a basis for practice. Figure 51-2 depicts a multidisciplinary evidence-based practice model. The first step in using the model is to obtain evidence from the synthesis of knowledge obtained from research. When there is no research available to guide decision-making, the clinician uses the other sources of evidence depicted in the model; retrospective or concurrent chart review; quality improvement and risk data; international, national, and local standards; infection control data; pathophysiology; cost-effectiveness analysis; benchmarking data; patient preferences; and clinical expertise. Even when there is research available, the additional sources of evidence can supplement the research evidence. The process of

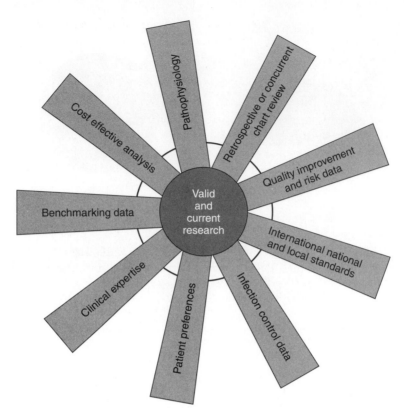

FIGURE **51-2**   Evidence-based multidisciplinary practice mode. (Courtesy *University of Colorado Hospital, Denver, Colorado.*)

evidence-based practice involves critically analyzing the evidence, selecting appropriate evidence-based interventions, implementing them, and evaluating outcomes.

Exploration of the evidence begins in the center or core of the model. Case managers should use current and valid research as the basis for clinical decision-making whenever there is an adequate research base available to guide practice. Evaluating clinical studies to determine if they are valid involves critically appraising both the merits and the limitations of the studies. All types of research should be evaluated for their contributions to the evidence. Results from experimental, nonexperimental, and qualitative studies may be synthesized to form the research base. No one would want to begin a drug regimen that had not been determined to be safe and effective in a randomized controlled trial. However, if we only use randomized controlled trials as the basis for our practice, we are missing important evidence. For example, descriptive research that focuses on the stresses and problems of caregivers of patients with Alzheimer's disease provides evidence that can be used to improve care to this vulnerable patient population. In addition, analysis of the cost-effectiveness of care models designed to meet the needs of the Alzheimer's patient and their family can guide public policy related to this problem.

Research skills and knowledge of statistics are required to evaluate and interpret a study. The clinician must look for the most current research so the latest evidence is included in the review. Haller, Reynolds, and Horsley's (1979) criteria for selecting studies to be used in the research base include using studies that are scientifically sound, replicated, and cause no harm to patients. Changes in practice should not be based solely on one study with one small sample.

THE NINE EVIDENCE SOURCES

The nine sources of evidence attached to the research core can supplement evidence obtained from research. When research is not available, these provide the best available evidence.

Pathophysiology is a frequent source of evidence used by the case manager. The science of the function of cells, tissues, and organs and how these functions are altered by disease is evidence that helps the case manager plan for the appropriate level of care for the patient. For example, understanding the type of stroke the patient has had and what portion of the brain is affected will help the case manager understand the type of services and level of care the patient will need to aid in recovery.

Cost-effectiveness analysis aids the case manager in determining whether the benefit is sufficient relative to the risks and costs. Effectiveness alone does not imply that an intervention should be adopted. The neonatal case manager may decide it is more cost effective to send a newborn home on an apnea monitor and have the hospital absorb the cost of the monitor rental than it is to keep the baby in the hospital for an extended length of stay. The case manager must clearly assess the skills and abilities of the parents and the risk to the infant in making this decision. Having the baby in the home environment rather than the sterile environment of the hospital might enhance bonding and improve outcomes.

Benchmarking data provide evidence related to best practices. Some institutions have better quality and cost outcomes than others for certain patient populations. For example, hospitals that belong to the University Health System Consortium, an organization comprised of academic health centers, share clinical data and costs. The case manager learns that hospital X's pulmonary unit has a shorter length of stay, lower costs, and fewer complications for patients with chronic obstructive pulmonary disease (COPD) than similar facilities caring for patients with the same diagnosis. These data are adjusted for severity and regional variation in costs. By studying the evidence from the "best practice" hospital, the case manager can determine what must be changed to improve outcomes in his or her practice setting.

Clinical expertise involves clinical judgment based on reflection and knowledge of the patient and is an important source of evidence. Whether an intervention can be applied to a specific patient cannot always be deduced from the evidence. There may be biological, social, or other differences that influence the effect of an intervention. Clinicians move from a status of novice to expert as they acquire proficiency and judgment through clinical experience. Clinical expertise must be integrated with other sources of evidence. For example, the oncology case managers should use their clinical expertise when selecting nondrug interventions to prevent nausea and vomiting. The expert knowledge may be based on the patient's past history or based on what has systematically worked with other patients with a similar diagnosis and treatment.

Infection control data provide evidence related to the incidence of infections, the organisms involved, and methods to prevent transmission. As case managers work with patients in their homes, they need this evidence to prevent spread of the infection to other family members. Case managers who work with patients who are positive for human immunodeficiency virus (HIV) infection rely heavily on evidence provided by infection control to plan appropriate care and provide needed education to prevent transmission.

International, national, and local standards of care often provide evidence that guides practice. The oncology case manager will draw on the standards from the Oncology Nursing Society when working with a patient who is receiving chemotherapy. Another example is using the Centers for Disease Control and Prevention (CDC) standards when planning for intravenous (IV) therapy in the home. Standards from the American Association of Critical Care Nurses will provide evidence related to appropriate care of arterial lines. The trauma case manager is guided by local community standards that determine where trauma patients will be cared for and the level of care those patients can expect to receive.

Quality improvement and risk data provide evidence to the case manager that can be used to support implementation of protocols to address problems. For example, if risk data indicate an increase in fall injuries in the neurosurgery population, the case manager can act on this evidence by providing instruction to caregivers and family members related to interventions to prevent falls. If quality data show an increased incidence of skin breakdown in the intensive care unit (ICU), the ICU case manager can use this evidence to support implementation of a new evidence based protocol to reduce skin breakdown.

Retrospective or concurrent chart review provides a wealth of evidence such as patient allergies or changes in vital signs. The record provides the case manager with a rich history telling how the patient responded to a specific medication, procedure, or treatment in the past. Evidence related to response to current interventions and diagnostic testing influences decision-making. The patient record also provides the payer source, and this information can drive decision-making. In today's market, it is essential that the case manager seek this piece of evidence when doing discharge planning. Often the patient's health plan will dictate where the patient may receive skilled care, the home care agency that may provide care, and the approved pharmacy where the patient must obtain prescriptions. If the patient is sent to an agency not covered in the health plan, he or she may pay large out-of-pocket expenses.

Patient preferences, such as religious or cultural preferences or treatment preferences, and other patient information such as living wills and advance directives are an essential source of evidence. Case managers must respect the preferences of the patient and family and provide ample opportunity for the patient to have input into the decision making process. The patient is no longer a passive participant allowing the clinical provider to make all of the decisions. In contrast, many patients are quite vocal about their desire to participate in decisions affecting their health. This is a positive change, but one that some providers may have trouble accepting. Patient preferences contribute significantly to evidence-based practice.

These are just some examples of how the nine sources of evidence can contribute to decision making. Finding the best evidence, critically appraising it, integrating it with the case manager's clinical expertise and the patient's unique preferences, and applying the results to practice is what evidence-based case management is all about.

PROVIDING EVIDENCE FOR PATIENTS AND FAMILIES

Nurse case managers must communicate evidence-based information to patients and their families so they can make informed decisions about their plan of care. Whenever there is a research base for an intervention, it is helpful to share that information with the patient and family. For example, the case manager who works with patients with acquired immune deficiency syndrome (AIDS) must share research evidence related to the effectiveness of combined medications in the treatment of HIV infection. The neonatal case manager should encourage parents of a low birth weight infant to participate in kangaroo care and should share with the parents the research related to this intervention. Obviously, clinicians must present information in a form that can be understood by the patient. Recipients of care are becoming very informed about health and illness and are asking thoughtful questions. It is possible that those who use the Internet to seek health information may be well informed about the current best evidence.

Case managers should provide information to support patients' participation in choosing treatments and strategies to manage their health. The information must be in concert with available evidence and be presented in a form that is understandable and useful if patients are to be active participants in decisions about their care. Educational pamphlets should be used to supplement and reinforce information provided by the case manager, but the information must conform to the highest standards of scientific accuracy. In most handouts, benefits of interventions are emphasized and risks and side effects often glossed over. The growth and wider availability of the Internet will greatly increase access to health information. It is quite possible that the patient will bring to the attention of the case manager the most current evidence related to a health problem. Accurate evidence-based information has the potential to enhance the quality and appropriateness of health care.

EVIDENCE-BASED CLINICAL PRACTICE GUIDELINES

Case managers have a significant role to play in the development and use of evidence based clinical practice guidelines. They should participate in multidisciplinary teams that develop, implement, and evaluate guidelines. Practice guidelines that are evidence based are highly valued because their efficacy is greater. Cardiovascular case managers should be extremely concerned that only 70% of ideal candidates for thrombolytic therapy after acute myocardial infarction receive it (Cronenwett, 2002). They should be champions for seeing that the evidence based clinical practice guideline for thrombolytic therapy is implemented in the patients they case manage. Case managers working with elders need to realize that only 52% of elders receive annual influenza vaccines and only 28% receive pneumococcal vaccines, even though the need for these vaccines is well documented in evidence-based clinical practice guidelines. Case managers must take accountability for implementing these guidelines in the elderly.

EVIDENCE RELATED TO ORGANIZATIONAL FEATURES

Organizational contextual variables (nonclinical variables) interact with specific treatments to influence patient care outcomes. We know more about the effectiveness of specific treatments than we do about the effectiveness of the health care system. Aiken, Sochalski, and Lake (1997) have demonstrated that nurse autonomy, nurse accountability, and registered nurse–physician relations affect patient care outcomes. Blegen, Goode, and Reed (1998) demonstrated that registered nurse skill mix affects outcomes related to adverse occurrences. Attention must be paid to the context in which patients receive their care because this knowledge will help to improve quality and patient outcomes (Aiken et al., 1997). Drawing on this research, it would seem that better outcomes might be achieved by case managers who work collaboratively with physicians, who are autonomous, and who are accountable for their actions.

When case managers work in an organization where evidence-based practice is valued, they are more likely to base their practice on the current best evidence. The literature indicates that organizational factors explain 80% to 90% of the variance in research utilization, environmental factors account for 5% to 10% of the variance, and individual characteristics contribute only 1% to 3% (Thomson, 1998). It appears that unless nurses work where evidence-based practice is an expectation, the likelihood of nurses using research is minimal. The organizational characteristics associated with evidence-based practice include administrative support; education related to evidence-based practice, including expectations for evidence-based practice in job descriptions and performance evaluations; rewarding and recognizing staff who use research in their practice; linking these activities to quality improvement; and providing time and resources for staff to participate in evidence-based projects. Case managers, when functioning at an advanced practice level, must be leaders in the evidence-based practice movement (Stetler et al., 1998).

MEASURING OUTCOMES FROM EVIDENCE-BASED PRACTICE

The outcomes from evidence-based practice are determined by the strength of the evidence and by the management and delivery of the interventions. If the interventions are not carried out as intended, the expected outcomes may not occur. The research and other supporting evidence may indicate the intervention is extremely effective, but if the intervention is not carried out appropriately, the positive outcomes may not occur. We see this sometimes in interventions related to pain management. An evidence-based pain management protocol may not be effective because providers are not assessing pain appropriately and intervening in a timely manner, or there may be resistance from providers or system issues that make it difficult to implement the evidence-based pain management intervention.

Gray (1997) indicates that an intervention designed to prevent mortality was initially expressed only in terms of the number of extra years of life. Evidence later indicated that quality of life was also important, which lead to a formula for "quality-adjusted life-years." Case managers should support the collection of patient satisfaction data, quality of life data, and specific clinical outcome data for the patients they manage. Case managers can evaluate outcomes related to the appropriateness of moving the patient to the next level of care by measuring the rate of returns to a higher level of care. A tracking system should be in place to record the case manager interventions implemented to allow a patient to return home in a timely manner.

When an evidence-based practice change is made, it is essential that a plan is in place to evaluate the expected outcomes (Goode, 1995). It is important to gather baseline data related to current practice. Sometimes these data come from quality improvement monitoring. The outcome variables to be measured are determined from the original research base. Horsley and Crane (1983) recommend that at least two dependent variables from the original research base be included as a measure of effectiveness. For example, when implementing an evidence-based guideline for the treatment of asthma, it would be important to gather data about current practice such as what drugs and treatments are currently being ordered. After the guideline is implemented, it would be important to measure whether the new guideline was used by the providers and whether it was effective in treating the asthma.

SUMMARY

Case managers must learn about evidence-based practice, embrace it, and help to create a culture where there is an expectation that care will be based on the best available evidence. Patient care should be based on evidence and not on tradition, opinion, or custom. Evidence-based care encourages a questioning and reflective approach to clinical practice and emphasizes the importance of life-long learning. Incorporating the current best evidence into the case manager's decision making will increase the proportion of patients to whom current best care is offered.

References

Aiken, L.H., Sochalski, J., & Lake, T.L. (1997). Studying outcomes of organizational change in health services, *Medical Care, 35*(suppl. 11), NS6-NS18.

Berwick, D.M. (2003). Disseminating innovations in healthcare. *JAMA*, 289 (15), 1969-1975.

Blegen, M.A., Goode, C.J., & Reed, L. (1998). Nurse staffing and patient outcomes, *Nursing Research, 47*(1), 43-50.

Brett, J.L. (1987). Use of nursing practice research findings. *Nursing Research, 36*(6), 344-349.

Coyle, L.A., & Sokop, A.G. (1990). Innovation adoption behavior among nurses. *Nursing Research, 39*(3), 176-180.

Cronenwett, L.R. (2002). Research, practice and policy: Issues in evidence based care. *Online Journal of Issues in Nursing.* Available http://www.nursingworld.org/ojin/keynotes/speech_2.htm

Gibbs, R.S., Mead, P.B., Hager, W.D., & Sweet, R.L. (1994). A survey of practices in infectious diseases by obstetrician-gynecologists. *Obstetrics & Gynecology, 83*(4), 631-636.

Goode, C.J. (1995). Evaluation of research-based nursing practice. In M.G. Titler & C.J. Goode (Eds.). *Nursing clinics of North America.* Philadelphia: W.B. Saunders.

Goode, C.J., & Blegen, M.A. (1993). Developing a CareMap for patients with a cesarean birth: A multidisciplinary process. *The Journal of Perinatal Neonatal Nursing, 7*(2), 40-49.

Gray, J.A.M. (1997). *Evidence-based healthcare.* New York: Churchill Livingstone.

Haller, K.B., Reynolds, M.A., & Horsley, J.A. (1979). Developing research based innovation protocols: Process, criteria and issues. *Research in Nursing and Health, 2,* 45-51.

Heater, B.S., Becker, A., & Olson, M. (1988). Nursing interventions and patient outcomes: A meta-analysis of studies. *Nursing Research, 37*(5), 303-307.

Horsley, J.A., & Crane, J. (1983). *Using research to improve nursing practice: A guide.* New York: Grune & Stratton.

Institute of Medicine. (1992). *Guidelines for clinical practice: from development to use.* Washington, D.C.: National Academy Press.

Stetler, C.B., Brunell, M., Giuliano, K.K., Morsi, D., Prince, L., & Newell-Stokes, V. (1998). Evidence-based practice and the role of nursing leadership. *JONA, 28*(7/8), 45-53.

Tanner, C.A. (May 1998). *Clinical judgement and evidence-based practice.* Paper presented at the Western Institute of Nursing, Communicating Nursing Research Conference and WIN Assembly, Phoenix, Ariz.

Thomson, M.A. (Jan. 1998). Closing the gap between nursing research and practice. *Evidence-Based Nursing 1*(1), 7-8.

52

The Carondelet Community-Based Nurse Case Management Program

Yesterday, Today, and Tomorrow

Gerri S. Lamb
Donna Zazworsky

CHAPTER OVERVIEW

For more than a decade, the Carondelet Nurse Case Management program has been a model for leadership and innovation in nursing practice. This nationally recognized program anticipated and evolved with major trends in managed care, disease management, and outcome-based performance evaluation. In this final chapter, two of Carondelet's well-known leaders chronicle and celebrate the history of case management at Carondelet and highlight its lessons for the future.

Carondelet's nurse case management program has a well-deserved reputation for innovation and commitment to excellence in professional nursing and patient care. Many of the case management programs that have been recognized recently as best practices contain features that have characterized Carondelet's model for over a decade (Boult, Kane, Pacala, & Wagner, 1999). Carondelet's model is best known for patient-centered care across the continuum. Within this model, at-risk patients and their families have direct access to highly skilled professional nurses who provide education and support and assist them to manage their health needs across multiple settings.

Over the course of approximately 15 years, Carondelet's case management program took shape and became a leading example of "the beyond-the-walls" model of care coordination for numerous at-risk populations. It evolved through and took advantage of significant changes in the Tucson marketplace. The rapid growth of managed care in the late 1980s set the stage for the first nursing health maintenance organization (HMO) and the development of one of four national Community Nursing Organizations (CNOs). Carondelet's case managers were among the first nurses to experiment with capitated financing

Acknowledgment: This chapter was written and the story updated with respect, humility, and love. The case managers of Carondelet are an extraordinary group of nurses. We believe that the story of Carondelet's nurse case managers belongs to each one of the nurses who contributed to the creation of a dynamic and ever-evolving professional practice model. This is our version of the story, what we have learned, and our vision and hope for the future.

for high-risk case management services. Ten years later, dramatic shifts in financing arrangements between health plans and providers established new priorities and directions for case managers.

The evolution of case management at Carondelet illuminates a fascinating interplay between vision and financial reality. It offers an extraordinary case study in the stages of development of new practice models from innovation to consolidation to a struggle for survival. The story is rich with numerous nurses who were and continue to be passionate about the potential for nurses to improve health care for vulnerable populations.

The purpose of this Chapter is to trace the history of case management at Carondelet and to share our interpretation of the implications of its evolution for the future of nurse case management practice.

THE STORY UNFOLDS

The story of Carondelet's case management program is best understood in the context of the history of professional nursing at Carondelet and the growth of what ultimately became a turbulent and unpredictable managed care environment. In the early years, prospective payment and managed care were the backdrop for the emergence of a new community-based case management model. In the later years, managed care moved to center stage and played a pivotal role in shaping case management practice and payment for it. The interplay between Carondelet's case management model and health care reimbursement and reform is shown in Figure 52-1.

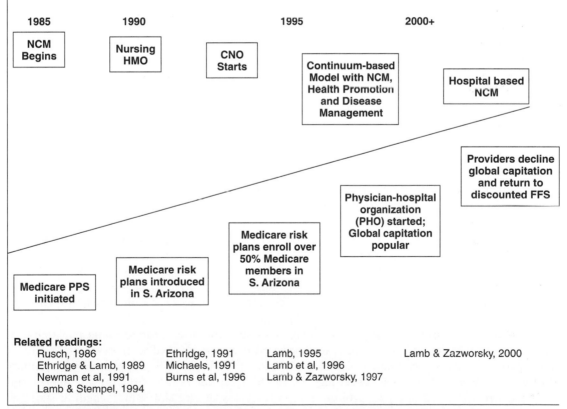

FIGURE **52-1**   Landmarks in Carondelet Nurse Case Management (NCM) and health care reimbursement and reform.

The foundation of the Carondelet model has been and remains professional nursing practice and the nurse-patient relationship (Hey, 1993). The model is firmly grounded in an understanding and respect for the patient's and family's right to identify their own health care needs and priorities. The nurse case manager's role is that of facilitator, advocate, and coach. One of Carondelet's most significant contributions to the evolution of nurse case management has been the exploration and description of the process of how a nurse case manager assists at-risk individuals to build self-care skills and negotiate the health care system. Carondelet nurse case managers have been in the forefront of developing systems of care that foreshadowed and ultimately transitioned into current models of population-based care and health and disease management.

The changing health care scene in Tucson, Arizona, offered an incredible opportunity to experiment with practice elements that subsequently became core to successful care coordination systems. In the course of 15 years, the case management program expanded to include automated risk assessment and chronic illness management. It was linked to health promotion and risk reduction services for less at-risk populations. Practice guidelines were integrated and outcomes measured. What began as a pilot program to empower hospital-based nurses to work with vulnerable patients across the care continuum evolved into a cutting-edge delivery system for healthy and at-risk populations.

THE EARLY YEARS

The story begins with the introduction of the new prospective payment system for Medicare and the vision of one nurse. Not long after diagnosis-related groups (DRGs) and prospective payment were initiated, policy people and health care administrators noted the decline in hospital length of stay accompanied by higher readmission rates, particularly for debilitating chronic illnesses like heart failure and obstructive pulmonary disease.

Phyllis Ethridge, who was Vice President for Patient Care Services at Carondelet, saw this scenario as an opportunity for innovation and change. Her initial plan was to prepare hospital-based nurses to transition home with patients requiring skilled nursing care. Selected nurses from each hospital unit were educated about home care practices and documentation. With the support and mentoring of home health nurses led by Susan Rusch, Carondelet's Home Health Director, these nurses began to work with patients from hospital to home (Rusch, 1986).

The patients and families loved having the same nurse during their hospital stay and their transition to home. The nurses who participated in this experiment reported vast new insights into the challenges patients and their families face in managing their health care needs after hospitalization. Unfortunately, the nurses did not grasp the nuances of home health documentation quickly enough to avoid significant numbers of Medicare denials for home health services. After several months of learning and refining, Ethridge and colleagues decided to build on the strengths of a professional nursing care delivery model for transitional care that they had discovered and, at the same time, distinguish this model from traditional home health care. Thus from the lessons of a brief experiment in hospital-based home health emerged the seeds of Carondelet's nurse case management program.

Armed with the knowledge that patients and nurses valued transitional care from hospital to home, Ethridge decided to try an experiment. Two unit-based nurses were asked to observe admission and readmission patterns on their units, to identify patients they thought would benefit from better continuity of care, and to work with them across settings. Salaries for these nurses came from the unit budget, and expenses were attributed to a pilot project to improve quality of care and reduce length of stay. The nurses were given little structure or guidelines—only the encouragement to use the nursing process and exercise their professional judgment. The two nurses became the core of a new nurse case management practice. In retrospect, it is interesting to note that the model emerged from a population-based practice focused on two high-risk patient groups.

By the beginning of 1989, the nurse case manager group had grown from 2 to 10 nurses, some of whom were unit-based specializing in selected populations, including patients with orthopedic, pulmonary, oncology, cardiac, and behavioral health conditions. Other case managers were generalists, including one nurse who focused on high-risk Native American patients. During these early years, there were few regulatory demands or payment constraints on case management practice. The nurses were free to explore how their relationships evolved with patients, the effectiveness of various nursing interventions, and the impact of their work within a broader health care delivery perspective.

At the same time that the nurse case management practice was evolving, core elements of professional nursing systems were being developed and debated locally and nationally. The nurse case managers of Carondelet designed new systems of care coordination in a broader nursing environment that had previously been recognized as a magnet hospital and embraced shared governance and exempt salary status for all nurses. Although the relationship between these has not been formally studied, it was clearly a fertile time for innovation and Carondelet nurses worked in an environment that resonated with professional development and pride.

As the first nurse case managers were encouraged to explore their practices with at-risk populations, efforts began to translate their experiences into outcome data and information. Two doctorally prepared nurses, Cathy Michaels and Gerri Lamb, were brought into the practice to assist with the evaluation. Initial discussions with the nurse case managers highlighted their passion for understanding their relationships with patients, the process of case management, as well as their insights into their impact on patient outcomes. Observations about the process of case management practice led to collaboration with Margaret Newman, a prominent nurse theorist, who discovered that Carondelet's nurse case management model embodied key concepts within her theory of health as expanding consciousness (Newman, Lamb, & Michaels, 1991). The nurse case managers' belief that "something different was going on" in their nursing care led to qualitative research from which the theory of nurse case manager as "insider-expert" emerged (Lamb & Stempel, 1994). This study stands as one of the few systematic qualitative explorations of the nurse case manager–patient relationship.

At the same time that the process of case management was being explored, members of the group practice made beginning attempts to demonstrate the link between case management interventions and patient outcomes. Initially, extensive descriptive data were compiled to look at common diagnoses of nurse case manager patients, visit frequencies, and visit patterns over time. Interviews with patients and nurses conducted as part of qualitative studies suggested several key outcomes for further evaluation, including quality of life, self-care abilities, symptom management, functional status, and service use outcomes of reduced hospitalization and emergency room visits.

Initial exploration of descriptive data led to important insights about potential differences in impact with acute and chronic conditions (Ethridge & Lamb, 1989). Many of the case managers pursued their hypotheses about their practice in their graduate work and subsequent theses (Chapman, 1990; Doerge, 1992; Huggins, 1996). An experimental study of the impact of case management on well-being, symptom management, personal power, satisfaction, and health service use for individuals with progressive multiple sclerosis reinforced the importance of the nurse-patient relationship in understanding the process-outcome connection (Lamb et al., 1993).

THE MANAGED CARE YEARS

Toward the end of the 1980s and into the beginning of the 1990s, managed care plans entered the local market and grew rapidly. The first Medicare risk plan in southern Arizona attracted thousands of members, and soon several other plans followed. Within a short time, payment shifted from discounted fee-for-service to capitation as plans and providers experimented with various risk-sharing arrangements. Capitated payment seemed to be an ideal way to drive the development of more integrated delivery systems and generate financial profit.

For nursing, participation in managed care and new capitated arrangements was an exciting invitation to shaping new delivery systems, particularly for at-risk populations. As the local market moved rapidly through the stage of managed care from low to high penetration and from limited to global capitation, interest grew in effective strategies for managing high-cost populations as well as in health promotion, disease prevention, and more integration across settings.

Seeing the opportunities and the fit for nurse case management in this new environment, Phyllis Ethridge went to the first Medicare risk plan on the scene and offered them case management services. She proposed that Carondelet would provide case management and home health care within the same capitated package for approximately the same monthly capitation the plan paid for home health care alone. This venture would accomplish several goals. Most important, the agreement would launch case management as a reimbursed service within managed care (Ethridge, 1991). Within this pilot, Carondelet would identify the costs of nurse case management for subsequent contracting efforts and gain experience delivering services in a new venue. It also provided an opportunity for the nurse case managers to better differentiate and integrate their care with home health services.

Entry into capitated contracting was an eye-opening, invigorating, and occasionally overwhelming experience for the nurse case managers. Virtually overnight, the nurse case managers became responsible for identifying and coordinating services for at-risk members of a large and growing Medicare risk plan (Michaels, 1991). Risk assessment systems had to be put in place. New referral systems to communicate with primary care physicians and home health and community providers were needed. Meanwhile, the clock was ticking and every admission and readmission began to be examined as a potentially preventable event.

Carondelet's plunge into managed care capitalized on and consolidated many of the strengths of the case management program. Insights about how to identify at-risk individuals were translated into screening tools used by the case managers and nursing staff. In the world of managed care, it was essential to find at-risk people early and offer case management assistance in monitoring, symptom management, and coordination.

Initially, the nurse case managers found that they were more effective and efficient in identifying risk than other members of the health care team. Waiting for others to find vulnerable patients often resulted in missed opportunities and readmissions. The nurse case managers began to explore differences between patient and professional perceptions of risk (Nichols, 1996). The demands for patient and data tracking systems became evident. Hand-tallied readmission rates were common and a source of significant frustration. Smooth hand-offs to home health nurses required extensive dialogue about referral criteria and scope of practice and service. Carondelet's Nursing HMO was off and running! The stories behind the scenes told as much about hard work, perseverance, and commitment to a vision as they did to the exhilaration of playing at the contract table.

Evaluation of the nursing HMO experience took many forms. There were the monthly data runs to evaluate admission and readmission rates. Managed care terms and indicators, such as bed days/1000 members, became very familiar. Judi Papenhausen worked extensively with the nurse case managers to measure and track their interventions (Papenhausen, 1996). In the most extensive quantitative analysis conducted to that point, Burns, Lamb, and Wholey (1996) compared hospitalization and service use in the nursing HMO patients and a control group. Amassing and cleaning the required demographic, clinical, and financial data for this study required months of tedious work getting separate and distinct information systems to talk to each other. After rigorous methodological review, these findings were published in the journal *Inquiry* and represent one of the first efforts to evaluate the impact of integrated nursing care delivery systems.

THE COMMUNITY NURSING ORGANIZATION AND BEYOND

After years of waiting for the CNO legislation passed in 1987 to be implemented, Carondelet applied for and was selected to participate in the national CNO Medicare demonstration in 1992. The goal of the CNO was to design, implement, and evaluate a nurse-managed model of community-based services for Medicare beneficiaries. Services included in the CNO were specified in the original legislation and included home health, outpatient therapies, durable medical equipment, and ambulance service. Case management was mentioned in the legislation as an optional service. Implemented as a randomized controlled experiment, the CNOs would be evaluated on the health status of their members as well as their functional status, satisfaction with health care services, service use, and Medicare costs.

At Carondelet the CNO was viewed as a wonderful vehicle to showcase and advance everything that had been learned about nurse case management within a fully capitated program. In addition, the CNO offered the opportunity to extend and link a primarily high-risk model with nursing delivery systems for low- and moderate-risk individuals. The CNO was required to enroll all eligible individuals, which included anyone who applied who had Medicare Part A and Part B and lived in the specified geographic areas. Members in the CNO range from older adults who are active and have few health problems to those who are extremely high risk with complex sets of acute and chronic conditions.

Carondelet's experience with case management formed the core of the CNO design. Carondelet and the other three CNO sites convinced the Health Care Financing Administration (HCFA), the sponsoring organization for the demonstration, that case management should be a mandatory rather than an optional feature of the CNO. HCFA used the experience of the CNO sites to establish initial rates for case management services.

The Carondelet CNO model incorporated and advanced case manager tools for risk assessment, documentation, and evaluation (Lamb, 1995). While Carondelet was the only site that differentiated case management practices for at-risk and low- or moderate-risk populations in the beginning of the demonstration, all four sites moved to some form of risk-adjusted practice model during the first few years.

The CNO currently is in its sixth year of operation after several extensions by HCFA and Congress. Nurse case managers in the CNO continue to provide their care and services to targeted high-risk populations. They work closely with the "nurse partners" for low- and moderate-risk members, assisting them to identify cues for changes in risk status and transition patients when their health care needs intensify. The impact of the nurse case managers is of particular importance in the CNO, because their care is targeted to the highest risk and potentially most expensive members of the CNO population.

CASE MANAGEMENT, DISEASE MANAGEMENT, AND INTEGRATED CARE DELIVERY

As the CNO was growing, the health care scene in southern Arizona rapidly progressed from a Stage II to a Stage IV highly penetrated managed care market with hospitals and physicians taking on greater financial risk under capitation. In the mid to late 1990s, attention turned, along with significant financial incentives, to integrated delivery systems and managing care. Innovations from case management and the CNO were exported for use in managed care contracts. More systematic processes for risk assessment and disease management were developed and implemented.

Soon after the shift to global capitation, Carondelet called on the case management and community programs to design and implement a network-wide program to manage high-volume and high-cost populations across the continuum. The initial pilot study focused on congestive heart failure, the diagnosis associated with the greatest number of hospital admissions in the Carondelet system. Designed by an interdisciplinary team consisting of nurse case managers, home health nurses, social workers, and physicians, the Heart Failure Project incorporated evidence-based guidelines for risk assessment and nurse case management interventions for symptom management, exercise, and nutrition (Lamb, Mahn, & Dahl, 1996). Results of the pilot showed significant improvement in health status, patient functional performance, and self-care performance, as well as a significant reduction in 30-day readmission rates.

The Heart Failure Project led the way to a network-wide, continuum-based model for disease management. Rather than waiting for high-risk patients to be admitted or readmitted to the hospital, standardized risk assessment tools used in the CNO were used with all managed care members with high-risk diagnoses. A systematic approach for finding, triaging, and intervening with at-risk patients was developed and implemented (Lamb & Zazworsky, 2000). Once identified, these patients were tracked over time to assure timely access to services that would enable them to manage their health care needs in the least acute and costly setting.

The shift to global capitation provided the long-awaited incentive to integrate services across the continuum, particularly for the high-risk members of managed care plans. Finally, the time was ripe for one systematic approach to risk assessment and the implementation of interdisciplinary, continuum-based practice guidelines, reaching from the primary care offices into the hospitals, the skilled facilities, home health services, and the home. Case management figured prominently in all of the disease management guidelines, in new efforts at integrating information system support, and in referral tools used throughout the network. Along with the rest of the network, the nurse case managers experimented with new strategies to improve care for their patients and increase the efficiency and effectiveness of the evolving systems of care.

THE WIND CHANGES

Unlike the smooth-staged progression of managed care outlined in the literature, the market in southern Arizona progressed through Stage IV penetration and global capitation and went into meltdown. Plans continued to reduce provider rates beyond what was considered sustainable. In a matter of months, hospitals and physicians began refusing capitated contracts and demanded to return to discounted fee-for-service payment. Financial incentives for prevention, risk assessment, disease management, and service integration declined on the provider side and shifted almost immediately back to the plans. Once again, the plans assumed the majority of risk for managing the health needs of their enrolled populations.

The combination of capitation and the effects of the new Balanced Budget Act regulations took a severe toll on many of the health care organizations in southern Arizona. Profit margins, which had been diminishing, now plummeted. Carondelet, along with other hospitals, home health agencies, and skilled facilities, took stock, prioritized its core business, and went into a cost-cutting strategy designed to align priorities and resource use with current incentives. Case management, a centerpiece of disease management and integrated delivery systems under global capitation, now was needed to shift attention back into managing hospital stays under reduced fee-for-service and prospective payment.

In anticipation of the dramatic and rapid shift in incentives, administrators of Carondelet's community and hospital-based case management programs moved quickly to redesign the case management system. The new model incorporated risk assessment and population-based approach with emphasis on management of the hospital stay. The model built in the opportunity for case managers to transition from hospital to the community for particularly vulnerable and expensive populations, including high-risk mothers and infants. The intent in designing this new model was to shift case management skill sets to the emergent need as well as to maintain a strong "memory trace" of community-based management when sanity and money were restored.

The community case managers who applied for the newly redesigned hospital-based case manager positions were viewed as extraordinary models for professional practice and systems expertise. Not surprisingly, the community nurse case managers also were seen as highly desirable by the health plans that now held most of the risk for effective population-based care. Several of the case managers chose to continue their community practice on the plan side rather than to return to hospital-based practice.

Today, community nurse case managers continue to practice in the CNO at Carondelet and as members of a predominantly hospital-oriented model of case management. Several have left Carondelet and are spreading their knowledge and experience in new nursing roles.

THE LEGACY OF CARONDELET: YESTERDAY, TODAY, AND TOMORROW

For the past 15 years, Carondelet's nurse case management program has epitomized what we now consider the hallmarks of successful health care programs: leadership, professionalism, vision, flexibility, and innovation. In many cases the nurses of Carondelet anticipated and led the changes and, in some, worked furiously to keep vision and dreams alive as health care plunged into the vast unknown.

It is important to highlight the features of Carondelet's nurse case management model that have stood fast for more than a decade, and still characterize the practice of Carondelet nurses who have remained at Carondelet and have now spread into the surrounding communities. These features are central to the vision of nurse case management as professional nursing practice.

Carondelet's model of nurse case management is first and foremost a model that demands, acknowledges, and celebrates nursing. While the nurse-patient relationship has evolved through face-to-face, group, and telephonic versions over the past 15 years, this relationship remains central to the work of case managers and is the core context in which quality and cost outcomes are achieved. Concepts of health as expanding consciousness and insider-expert are just as important today as when they were first explored at Carondelet. Interviews with patients and families today reveal the same themes that were heard 15 years ago. Patients of nurse case managers value their caring presence, their accessibility, their expert knowledge, and their commitment to making systems work better for highly vulnerable people.

Although the essence of the nurse-patient relationship has not changed significantly, competencies and skills required for nurse case manager practice have evolved substantially. Group and telephonic case management require a new model of interpersonal negotiation and collaboration. Maintaining a strong relationship over time and settings via the whole new range of communication technologies is challenging. Demands for more systematic risk assessment have required transitioning from experiential and paper-based tools to automated standardized instruments. Practical experience and expertise in case management have been critical in ensuring that these tools and other instruments used by case managers are relevant to their practice and will achieve the desired goals.

The Carondelet case managers anticipated the demand for outcome data. Over the course of 15 years, hundreds of reports, presentations, and publications attempted to capture the impact of community-based nursing practice on quality of care and cost outcomes. Even today, however, there has still not been sufficient advances in information technology support to bring together the requisite clinical and cost data in a timely way. While there are exciting and effective software available to support continuum-based case management, the majority of case managers practice in settings without them. Demonstrating the value of case management remains one of the most daunting and frustrating challenges. At Carondelet and for nurse case managers nationwide, the lack of "real-time" outcome data is the greatest threat to survival.

Carondelet's nurse case management program was among the first of the nursing programs to enter into risk contracts with managed care plans. Today, this is not as uncommon as it was 10 years ago. In several states, nursing programs hold Medicare, Medicaid, and commercial contracts. However, many of the same barriers to contracting continue to reduce opportunities to influence health care delivery, including financial payment systems that encourage fragmentation over integration, unaligned incentives across providers and settings, and contractors who understand finance much better than clinical practice.

Carondelet's story certainly would not be complete without a final emphasis on the close ties between nursing innovation and our national health care scene. What evolved at Carondelet was not coincidental. It was, in fact, a cataclysmic coming together of vision, opportunity, and a willingness to take risk. From Phyllis Ethridge's leap into managed care to the CNO to the crisis-precipitated redesign of Carondelet's care coordination system, at the center of it all is a fervent belief that nursing is integral to making our health care system better. Carondelet's story is a tribute to the drive to keep trying and the belief that our American health care system will be infinitely improved if nurses can get to the table and stay there.

References

Boult, C., Kane, R.L., Pacala, J.T., & Wagner, E. (1999). Innovative healthcare for chronically ill older persons: Results of a national survey. *The American Journal of Managed Care 5*(8), 1-11.

Burns, L.R., Lamb, G.S., & Wholey, D.R. (1996). Impact of integrated community nursing on hospital utilization and costs in a Medicare risk plan. *Inquiry 33*(1), 30-41.

Chapman, E. (1990). *Nurse case management and hospital length of stay*. Unpublished master's thesis, University of Arizona, Tucson, Ariz.

Doerge, J. (1992). *Cost effectiveness of nurse case management compared to an existing system of care*. Unpublished master's thesis, University of Arizona, Tucson, Ariz.

Ethridge, P. (1991). A nursing HMO: Carondelet St. Mary's experience. *Nursing Management 22*(7), 22-27.

Ethridge, P., & Lamb, G.S. (1989). Professional nursing case management improves quality, access and costs. *Nursing Management 20*(3), 30-35.

Hey, M. (1993). Nursing's renaissance: An innovative continuum of care takes nurses back to their roots. *Health Progress, 74*(8), 26-32.

Huggins, D.B. (1996). *Nurse case management: Impact on costs and outcomes*. Unpublished master's thesis. University of Arizona, Tucson, Ariz.

Lamb, G.S. (1995). Early lessons from a capitated community-based nursing model. *Nursing Administration Quarterly 19*, 18-26.

Lamb, G.S., Donaldson, N., & Kellogg, J. (1998). *Case management: A guide to strategic evaluation*. St. Louis: Mosby.

Lamb, G.S., Mahn, V., & Dahl, R. (1996). Using data to design systems of care for adults with chronic illness. *Managed Care Quarterly 4*(3), 46-53.

Lamb, G.S., & Stempel, J. (1994). Nurse case management from the client's view: Growing as insider-expert. *Nursing Outlook 42*(1), 7-14.

Lamb, G.S. & Zazworsky, D. (1997). The Carondelet experience. *Nursing Management 28*(3), 27-28.

Lamb, G.S., & Zazworsky, D. (2000). Improving outcomes fast. *Advances for Providers for Post-Acute Care 3*(1), 28-29.

Lamb, G.S., Zazworsky, D., Stempel, J., Martin, D., Gibson, B., Carlson, A., & Rapacz, K. (1993). Comprehensive case management for individuals with progressive multiple sclerosis: An experimental study. Report to the National Multiple Sclerosis Society.

Lancero, A. (1994). *Work satisfaction among nurse case managers*. Unpublished master's thesis. University of Arizona, Tucson, Ariz.

Michaels, C. (1991). A nursing HMO: 10 months with Carondelet St. Mary's hospital-based nurse case management. *Aspen's Advisor for Nurse Executives 6*(11), 1, 3-4.

Newman, M., Lamb, G.S., & Michaels, C. (1991). Nurse case management: The coming together of theory and practice. *Nursing & Health Care 12*(8), 404-408.

Nichols, C. (1996). Older adults who remain at risk: uncertainty in decision-making. Unpublished master's thesis. University of Arizona, Tucson, Ariz.

Papenhausen, J.L. (1996). Discovering and achieving client outcomes. In E. Cohen (Ed.), *Nurse case management in the 21st century* (pp. 257-268). St. Louis: Mosby.

Rusch, S. (1986). Continuity of care: From hospital unit into home. *Nursing Management 17*(12), 38-41.

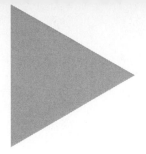

Index

A

ABC codes (Alternative Link), 448
Abused persons, 377
Access (Medicare), 205
Accountability
  changing procedures due to, 95
  in collaborative CM triad, 81
  in competing loyalties, 377-378
  in nursing case management, 16
  for own lifestyle, 377-378
  responsibility for, 363-364
  during startup, 95-96
Accreditation
  of case management program, 305
  commissions/associations for, 305-307, 309b
  concerns related to development of, 309b
  of disease management program, 40
  history of process for, 297
  process/benefits of, 307-308
Accreditation Association for Ambulatory Health Care (AAAHC), 309b
Accreditation Commission for Health Care, Inc. (ACHC), 309b
Acquired immunodeficiency syndrome (AIDS)
  community-based CM of, 184-185
  community-based nurse CM of, 136, 137
  computer networks to patients with, 380, 382
  demographics affecting management of, 184-185
  implementing CM in facility for, 337
  Medicaid challenges managing, 224
Activities of daily living (ADLs)
  dependency in, 181-182
  prospective payment system and, 191
  psychiatric CM model and, 106
Acute care-based nursing case management. *See also* Hospital-based.
  contemporary models for, 55-67
  vs. managing across continuum of care, 37

Acute care-based nursing case management—cont'd
  trend-setting models for, 28-31
Adherence, patient. *See* Compliance, patient.
Adkins, K., 4
Administration, hospital
  CM education for, 251-254
  using executive dashboards, 457
  marketing CM to, 242-244
  obtaining support of, 462
  presenting change in CM to, 95
  supporting standardized plans, 245
Administrative claims data, 45
Admission process
  to CM program, 22
  in emergency department CM, 173-175
  to enhance outcomes, 424, 425
  patient variances at time of, 344, 474
Advance directives
  advocacy for patients with, 372
  attending to patients needing, 430
  ethical dimensions of, 365
  prolonging dying vs. life and, 373
  responsibility for aiding, 364
Advanced Practice RN (APRN)
  in Carle Clinic model, 135
  in faculty CM practice, 162-163
  first generation of model using, 31
  in telehealth, 392
ADvantage Program of Oklahoma, 158-160
Advocacy agency model, 20
Advocacy role
  in case management, 23, 416
  competencies of, 375b
  in different decision-making models, 370-371
  as ethical competency, 364
  of nurse case manager, 290-291, 370-371
  promoting individualized care, 376
  supporting autonomy, 372, 375b
Africa, AIDS CM in, 185
Age factors. *See also* Elderly clients/population.
  affecting health care, 181-184
  length of stay and, 196-197